Complications in Orthopaedics: Spine Surgery

Complications in Orthopaedics: Spine Surgery

FIRST EDITION

Editors:

Vikas V. Patel MD, MA, BSME, FAAOS

Professor
Executive Vice Chair, Department of Orthopedic Surgery
Endowed Chair of Spine Innovation.
University of Colorado
Aurora
CO
United States

Christopher John Kleck, MD

Chief of Spine
Orthopedics
University of Colorado
Aurora
CO
United States

Associate Professor
Orthopedics
University of Colorado
Aurora
CO
United States

Spine Fellowship Program Director
Orthopedics
University of Colorado
Aurora
CO
United States

Series Editor:

Stephen R. Thompson, MD, MEd, FRCSC

Associate Professor of Sports Medicine,
Northern Light Eastern Maine Medical Center
University of Maine Bangor
Maine
United States

ELSEVIER

Elsevier
1600 John F. Kennedy Blvd.
Ste 1800
Philadelphia, PA 19103-2899

COMPLICATIONS IN ORTHOPAEDICS: SPINE SURGERY ISBN: 978-0-323-88066-4

Executive Content Strategist: Belinda Kuhn
Senior Content Development Specialist: Himanshi Chauhan
Publishing Services Manager: Deepthi Unni
Project Manager: Nandhini Thanga Alagu
Design Direction: Ryan Cook

Printed in the United States of America

Last digit is the print number: 9 8 7 6 5 4 3 2

To my wonderful family, especially Lisa, Sarita, and Shayan for all the love and support, for putting up with my humor, and for keeping me grounded.

Vikas V. Patel

To my amazing family, Melody, Ada, and Jed, your love and support have made this all possible and without you it comes to nothing.

C.J. Kleck

Contributors

Venu Akuthota, MD
Professor
SOM and Chair Dept. of Physical Medicine and Rehabilitation
University of Colorado, Boulder
Colorado
United States

Joseph L. Albano, DO, MBA
Orthopaedic and Spine Surgeons of NJ
Montclair
New Jersey
United States

Afshin Aminian, MD
Medical Director
Orthopedic Institute
CHOC Children's, Orange
California
United States

Neel Anand, MD, MBBS, MS, Mch.Orth(UK), FAAOS
Professor of Orthopaedics
Dpartment of Orthopaedics
Cedars Sinai Medical Center, Los Angeles
California
United States
Director
Spine Center
Cedars Sinai Medical Center, Los Angeles
California
United States

Kasra Araghi, BS
Research Fellow
Spine
Hospital for Special Surgery, New York
New York
United States

Ayush Arora, BSE
Medical Student
Department of Orthopaedic Surgery
University of California, San Francisco, San Francisco
California
United States

Alicia Asturias, BA, MD
Resident
Department of Orthopedic Surgery
University of California San Francisco, San Francisco
California
United States

Alla Balabanova, MD
Department of Orthopaedics
University of Colorado Medical School
Anschutz Medical Campus
Aurora, CO
United States

David Geoffrey Barnes, DO
Orthopedic Spine Surgeon
Spine Surgery
St. George Orthopedic Spine, St. George
Utah
United States

Mark Basilious, BS
Medical Student
Medical College
Weill Cornell, New York City
New York
United States

Sigurd H. Berven, MD
Chief of Spine Service
Orthopaedic Surgery
UC San Francisco, San Francisco
California
United States

Nitin Bhatia, MD
Professor and Chair
Orthopaedic Surgery
University of California, Irvine, Orange
California
United States

Shane Burch, MD
Associate Professor in Residence
Orthopedic Surgery
University of California, San Francisco
California
United States

Christopher Marden John Cain, MBBS, MD, FRACS, FAOrthA
Professor
Orthopedics
University of Colorado, Denver
Colorado
United States

Gaston Camino-Willhuber, MD
Attending Physician
Orthopaedic Department
Asuncion Klinika, Donostia-San Sebastian
Spain
Orthopaedic Spine Surgeon
Orthopaedic and Traumatology
Hospital Italiano de Buenos Aires
Argentina

Michael V. Carter, BS, BA
Research Assistant
Rothman Institute
Thomas Jefferson University, Philadelphia
Pennsylvania
United States

Justin P. Chan, MD
Physician
Orthopaedic Surgery
University of California, Irvine, Orange
United States

Jens Chapman, MD
Orthopaedic Spine Surgeon
Neurosurgery
Swedish Hospital, Seattle
Washington
United States

Andrew S. Chung, DO
Spine Surgeon
Orthopedics
Banner Health, Phoenix
Arizona
United States

Deanna Claus, MD
Physician
Department of Physical Medicine and Rehabilitation
University of Colorado Anschutz, Aurora
Colorado
United States

Alexander M. Crawford, MD, MPH
Resident
Harvard Combined Orthopaedic Residency Program
Harvard Medical School, Boston
Massachusetts
United States

Srikanth N. Divi, MD
Assistant Professor
Orthopaedic Surgery
Northwestern University Feinberg School of Medicine, Chicago
Illinois
United States

Robert K. Eastlack, MD
Division Head/Professor, Spine Surgery
Orthopaedic Surgery
Scripps Clinic, San Diego
California
United States

Meagan DelBaggio Fernandez, DO
Chief, Pediatric Orthopaedic Surgery
Orthopaedic Surgery
Geisinger, Danville
Pennsylvania
United States

Mitchell S. Fourman, MD, MPhil
Assistant Professor of Orthopaedic Surgery
Orthopaedic Surgery
Montefiore Einstein, Bronx
New York
United States

Yevgeniy Freyvert, MD
Assistant Professor
Neurological Surgery
Houston Methodist, Houston
Texas
United States

Sumeet Garg, MD
Associate Professor
Department of Orthopedics
University of Colorado, Aurora
Colorado
United States

Jacob L. Goldberg, MD
Physician
Neurosurgery
New York Presbyterian Hospital, New York
New York
United States

Munish C. Gupta, MD, MBA
MB Simon Distinguished Professor of Orthopaedics
Department of Orthopaedic Surgery
Washington University in St. Louis, St. Louis
Missouri
United States
Professor of Neurological Surgery

Roger Härtl, MD
Director of Neurosurgery Spine
Neurological Surgery
Weill Cornell Medicine, New York
New York
United States

Sohaib Hashmi, MD
Assistant Clinical Professor of Orthopaedic Surgery
Orthopaedic Surgery
University of California, Irvine, Orange
California
United States

Michael J. Heffernan, MD
Associate Professor
Orthopaedic Surgery
Children's Hospital Los Angeles, Los Angeles
California
United States

Ibrahim Hussain, MD
Assistant Professor
Neurological Surgery
Weill Cornell-New York Presbyterian Och Spine, New York
New York
United States

Kevin C. Jacob, BS
Research Coordinator
Orthopedics
Rush University Medical Center, Chicago
Illinois
United States

Diana Johnson, MD
Resident Physician
Physical Medicine and Rehabilitation
McGovern Medical School at The University of Texas Health Science Center at Houston, Houston
Texas
United States

Han Jo Kim, MD
Professor
Orthopaedic Surgery
Hospital for Special Surgery, New York
New York
United States

Stanley Kisinde, MB.ChB, PGD(DS,PPM), MMed
Dr
Clinical Research
Scoliosis and Spine Tumor Center, Texas Back Institute, Plano
Texas
United States

Eric O. Klineberg, MS, MD
Professor and Vice Chair
Orthopaedics
University of Texas, Houston, Houston
Texas
United States
Chief of Spine
Orthopaedics
University of Texas, Houston, Houston
Texas
United States

Jay I. Kumar, MD, MBA
Resident
Department of Neurosurgery and Brain Repair
University of South Florida, Tampa
Florida
United States

Mark J. Lambrechts, MD
Doctor
Orthopaedic Surgery
Rothman Orthopaedic Institute at Thomas Jefferson University, Philadelphia, PA
Pennsylvania
United States

Anh X. Le, MD, FAAOS
Alpine Orthopaedic and Spine Medical Group
Orthopaedic Surgery
St. Joseph's Medical Center, Stockton
California
United States
Assistant Clinical Professor
Orthopaedic Surgery
University of California, Davis, Sacramento
California
United States

Hai V. Le, MD, MPH
Assistant Professor
Orthopaedics
UC Davis, Sacramento
California
United States

Yu-Po Lee, MD
Clinical Professor
Orthopaedic Surgery
UC Irvine, Orange
California
United States

Jean-Christophe Leveque, MD
Section Head
Neurosurgery
Virginia Mason Franciscan Health, Seattle
Washington
United States

Isador H. Lieberman, MD
Director
Scoliosis and Spine tumor center
Texas Back Institute, Plano
Texas
United States

Elizabeth Lord, MD
Assistant Professor
Orthopaedic Surgery and Neurosurgery
University of California, Los Angeles, Los Angeles
California
United States

Francis C. Lovecchio, MD
Assistant Attending Orthopedic Surgeon
Spine Service
Hospital for Special Surgery, New York
New York
United States

Jessica Lu, MD
Resident Physician
PM&R
Stanford University, Palo Alto
California
United States

Keith W. Lyons, MD
Central Maine Healthcare Orthopedics, Aauburn
Maine
United States

Gabriel S. Makar, MD
Orthopaedic Surgery Resident
Orthopaedic Surgery
Geisinger Medical Center, Danville
Pennsylvania
United States

Michael H. McCarthy, MD, MPH
Spine Surgeon
Spine Surgery
Indiana Spine Group, Carmel
Indiana
United States
Assistant Professor
Orthopaedics
Indiana University School of Medicine, Indianapolis
Indiana
United States

Justin S. Merkow, MD
Assistant Professor
Anesthesiology
University of Colorado, Aurora
Colorado
United States
Marco Uribe
Anesthesiology
University of Colorado, Aurora
Colorado
United States

Robert Bruce Metter, MD
Assistant Professor of Medicine
Division of Hospital Medicine
University of Colorado School of Medicine, Aurora
Colorado
United States

Paul D. Minetos, MD, MBA
Resident
Orthopaedic Surgery
Indiana University School of Medicine, Indianapolis
Indiana
United States

John Ngo, DO
Resident Physician
Orthopaedic Surgery
Community Memorial Health, Ventura
California
United States

Jennifer Marie O'Donnell, MD
Resident Physician
Orthopaedic Surgery
University of California San Francisco, San Francisco
California
United States

Nathan Odom, MD
Assistant Professor
Physical Medicine and Rehabilitation
University of Colorado, Aurora
Colorado
United States

Kamil Okroj, MD
Orthopaedic Spine Surgery Fellow
Orthopaedic Surgery
Northwestern University (McGaw), Chicago
Illinois
United States

Rod J. Oskouian, MD
Chief of Spine
Swedish Hospital, Chicago
Illinois
United States

David Ou-Yang, MD
Assistant Professor
SOM, Dept. of Orthopedics
University of Colorado, Boulder
Colorado
United States

Alexander W. Parsons, MS
Research Intern
Orthopedics
Rush University, Chicago
Georgia
United States

Alpesh A. Patel, MD, MBA
Professor
Orthopaedic Surgery
Northwestern University Feinberg School of Medicine, Chicago
Illinois
United States
Professor
Neurosurgery
Northwestern University Feinberg School of Medicine, Chicago
Illinois
United States
Director
Northwestern Center for Spine Health, Chicago
Illinois
United States

Hemali Patel, MD
Associate Professor
Department of Medicine
University of Colorado, Aurora
Colorado
United States

Madhav R. Patel, MD
Department of Orthopaedic Surgery
Rush University Medical Center
Chicago, Illinois
United States

Shyam Ajit Patel, MD
Assistant Professor
Orthopaedic Surgery
NYU Langone, Mineola
New York
United States

Kemly Philip, MD, PhD, MBE
Assistant Professor
Physical Medicine and Rehabilitation
McGovern Medical School at UTHealth, Houston
Texas
United States

Danyal A. Quraishi, BS
Research Assistant
Department of Neurosurgery
Weill Cornell Brain and Spine Center, New York
New York
United States

Sheeraz A. Qureshi, MD MBA
Orthopaedic Surgeon
Orthopaedics
Hospital for Special Surgery, New York
United States

Brennan Roper, BS, MD
Fellow
Orthopedic Surgery
Children's Hospital Colorado, Aurora
Colorado
United States
Assistant Professor
Orthopedic Surgery
University of Texas - Houston, The Woodlands
Texas
United States

J. Manuel Sarmiento, MD
Spine Surgery Fellow
Spine and Scoliosis Service
Hospital for Special Surgery, New York
United States

Rick Sasso, MD
Professor
Chief of Spine Surgery
Department of Orthopaedic Surgery
Indiana University School of Medicine
Indiana
United States

Alexander M. Satin, MD, ABOS Certified
Spine Surgeon
Orthopaedic Surgery
Texas Back Institute, Plano
Texas
United States

Zachary T. Sharfman, MD
Ventura Orthopedics, Ventura
California
United States

Jesse Shen, MD, PhD, FRCSC
Orthopedic Surgeon
Surgery
Centre Hospitalier de l'Université de Montréal, Montréal
Quebec
Canada
Assistant professor
Surgery
Université de Montréal, Montréal
Quebec
Canada

Kern Singh, MD
Vice Chair, Clinical Affairs - Department of Orthopaedic Surgery
Professor and Director, Division of Spine Surgery
Rush University Medical Center, Chicago
Illinois
United States

Aaron W. Stevenson, MBBS, FRACS (Orth), BMedSci (Hons), FAOrthA
Head of Unit
Spinal Surgery
Royal Adelaide Hospital, Adelaide
South Australia
Australia

Lauren E. Stone, MD
Physician Surgeon
Neurological Surgery
University of Caifornia, San Diego, La Jolla
California
United States

Brendan Michael Striano, MD, MPH
Orthopaedic Resident
Orthopaedic Surgery
Harvard Combined Orthopaedic Residency Program, Boston
Massachusetts
United States

William Summers, MD
Fellow Physician
Physical Medicine and Rehabilitation
Vanderbilt Univsersity School of Medicine, Nashville
Tennessee
United States

Bobby K-B Tay, MD
Professor of Clinical Orthopedics
Department of Orthopedic Surgery
UCSF, San Francisco
California
United States
Vice Chair of Quality and Safety
Orthopedic Surgery
UCSF, San Francisco
California
United States

Tyler A. Tetreault, MD
Assistant Professor
Jackie and Gene Autry Orthopedic Center
Children's Hospital Los Angeles, Los Angeles
California
United States

Daniel G. Tobert, MD
Assistant Professor
Orthopaedic Surgery
Massachusetts General Hospital, Boston
Massachusetts
United States

Gregory R. Toci, MD
Resident
Orthopaedic Surgery
Rothman Orthopaedics at Thomas Jefferson University Hospital, Philadelphia
Pennsylvania
United States

Marco A. Uribe, IIIMD
Fellow Physician
Anesthesiology
University of Utah, Salt Lake City
Utah
United States

Alexander R. Vaccaro, MD, PhD, MBA
Professor
Department of Orthopaedic Surgery
Rothman Orthopaedic Institute, Philadelphia
Pennsylvania
United States

Wyatt D. Vander Voort, MD
Resident
Orthopaedic Surgery
University of California Davis Medical Center, Sacramento
California
United States

Alexander C. Wulff, DO
Resident Physician
Department of Family Medicine
Community Memorial Health System, Ventura
California
United States

Preface

"We look for medicine to be an orderly field of knowledge and procedure. But it is not. It is an imperfect science, an enterprise of constantly changing knowledge, uncertain information, fallible individuals, and at the same time lives on the line."

Atul Gawande

For better or worse, it is the path that we have chosen as physicians to touch the lives of people-individuals, who are our patients. In their care, we strive to take every possible precaution, yet complications are bound to be encountered. Some may be avoidable and many are not, but the more we can reflect on and study our complications, the more we can learn and apply towards better outcomes in our future patients. Learning from our mistakes is integral to advancing medicine. And, unfortunately, the complexity of spine surgery makes encountering complications that much more likely.

We are honored to have been asked to organize this book on complications with the hopes that these chapters can add to the body of knowledge in spine surgery and help our colleagues to avoid some of the complications we have encountered. We are even more honored to have such an esteemed group of authors willing to share with us lessons from their incredibly vast experience! The authors assembled in this book represent hundreds of years of collective spine experience whose filtered and organized knowledge provides invaluable insights into the advancement of spine patient care.

In addition, this book could not have been possible without Stephen Thompson whose concept has grown into a tremendous series of textbooks that truly make a difference in clinical practice. We also thank the team he has assembled together with Elsevier to make it possible!

Vikas V. Patel
Christopher J. Kleck

Contents

1 Introduction

Complications in spine surgery can be daunting. While the likelihood of a significant complication is typically a fraction of a percent, when your patient has one, it is devastating, for the patient and the surgeon. The task of compiling these is difficult but absolutely necessary, as the field of spine surgery continues to evolve. Many surgeries and technologies, such as Lueke wires and Harrington Rods evolving to pedicle screw fixation, led the way in advancing surgical techniques, and with this the complications changed. Yet, some issues (i.e., non-union, hardware failure, and adjacent level degeneration) continue in the discipline of spine surgery. While research is ongoing, and great progress has been made in reducing complications, many of the topics in the following chapters will continue.

Rapidly advancing techniques have produced both excellent and poor results and require more detailed scrutiny. The complications can vary by experience, and many publications can be found in the spine literature outlining the learning curves for these. While surgical techniques that are not discussed may exist, great efforts were made to include any and all current surgical treatments. This includes many of the new parameters that have been introduced in spine surgical planning.

To create the most effective manuscript on the topic, we organized topics by location and approach to the spine. This allows more specific discussions on global spine complications while providing discussion on issues specific to the anatomic area and the surgical approach. Although this creates some inherent duplication, it is important to ensure no topic is lost. Further, significant work has progressed in the preoperative evaluation and optimization of spine patients. This work is highlighted and is key in selecting the correct surgery, and even the correct patient for spine surgical care.

While complications are something all spine surgeons are attempting to avoid, and the conversation can be difficult, the editors hope this book will provide a guide for surgeons experienced and new in the field. As Louis Pasteur says, "in the field of observation, chance favors the prepared mind." Spine surgery is more than observation, but preparation and understanding give a surgeon the best chance at avoiding complications.

2 Optimization to Avoid Complications

DAVID OU-YANG AND ALLA BALABANOVA

CHAPTER OUTLINE

Introduction

Numerous risk factors have been correlated with increased complications in spinal surgery. Assessment and management of some of these risk factors fall outside the scope of typical spine surgery practice, i.e., cardiopulmonary, renal, hepatic, hematologic, immunologic, and endocrine comorbidities, and require thorough evaluation by anesthesia and respective medical specialists. Other risk factors are easily assessed with laboratory studies and tools common to spinal surgery practice, many of which can be modified preoperatively. As such, standard work protocols can potentially be employed for assessment and alteration of these modifiable risk factors. The following chapter discusses numerous modifiable risk factors that can be routinely assessed in a spine surgery practice, and suggests preoperative goals based on the current literature if available.

Preoperative Hemoglobin

Transfusion in spine surgery is associated with longer in-hospital stay and morbidity (OR 2.54) including infection (OR 4.59), thromboembolism (OR 2.03), and ischemic events (OR 14.53).[1,2] Thus, many advocate for more stringent criteria for perioperative transfusion and preoperative evaluation and management of anemia.

Nuttall et al. and Zheng et al. both found that lower preoperative hemoglobin was associated with need for perioperative transfusion, and Carabini et al, reported that preoperative hemoglobin in those undergoing three or greater levels of fusion was independently associated with need for major transfusion (≥4U pRBCs).[3–5] Lenoir et al. identified that preoperative hemoglobin less than 12 g/dL was an independent risk factor for perioperative transfusion with an odds ratio of 6.7, and in an American College of Surgeons National Surgical Quality Improvement Program (ACS-NSQIP) study Kim et al. reported that preoperative hemoglobin less than 12 g/dL for females and less than 13 g/dL for males resulted in increased transfusion rates.[6,7]

Corroborating the link between preoperative anemia, increased need for transfusion, and increased complication rate, Seicean et al. stratified patients based on severity of anemia using serum hematocrit levels (Severe <26%, Moderate 26% to 29%, Mild 30% to 37%, No >38%).[8,9] The authors reported a clear association between all levels of anemia and increase in both major and minor complications, length of stay, and 30-day mortality. Likewise, Veeravagu et al. performed a Veterans Affair NSQIP database evaluation and found that hematocrit less than 36% resulted in a 1.37-fold increase rate of wound infection.[10]

Ultimately, there is fair evidence that preoperative anemia is associated with increased need for perioperative transfusion, and, secondarily, increased rates of postoperative complications. Current literature supports preoperative targets for hemoglobin ≥12 g/dL in females, ≥13 in males, and hematocrit >36%. Preoperative screening with complete blood count should be included in all standard work protocols followed by evaluation and management of at-risk patients by medical specialists prior to surgery.

Bone Mineral Density

Bone mineral density (BMD) has long been associated with complications related to spinal surgery including pedicle screw loosening, implant subsidence, pseudarthrosis, and proximal junctional kyphosis (PJK) and failure. Dual x-ray absorptiometry (DEXA) is the gold standard diagnostic modality and can be used both for vertebral body fracture risk assessment and monitoring changes over time. Quantitative computed tomography (CT) appears to be similarly predictive of vertebral body fracture in postmenopausal women, but its predictive capabilities in men is less clear. The drawbacks of quantitative CT include increased cost and radiation exposure when compared to DEXA. A DEXA scan T score <–2.5, Hounsfield unit measurement <97.9, and serum vitamin D_3 level <20 ng/mL has been found to be associated with increased risk of adverse event in patients undergoing spinal instrumentation.[11] The Bone Health and Osteoporosis Foundation (BHOF) recommends DEXA scan evaluation in women 65 years and older, men 70 years and older, postmenopausal women under 65 with risk factors, men 50 to 69 years of age with risk factors, and in both men and women who sustain a fracture after age 50. Further recommendations can be found on the BHOF website (www.bonehealthandosteoporosis.org).

Multiple level III studies have demonstrated a correlation between preoperative BMD and pedicle screw loosening. Bredow et al. reported that 12.3% (45/365) of their thoracolumbar fusions demonstrated postoperative pedicle screw loosening with a mean bone density measuring 116 HU compared to 133 HU in those without loosening.[12] Both Kim et al. and Okuyama et al. demonstrated that lower BMD on DEXA was also correlated with pedicle screw loosening in lumbosacral interbody fusion patients.[13,14] Kim et al. found those with loosened screws demonstrated an average preoperative T score of –1.6 versus –0.8 in those without loosening. Okuyama et al. demonstrated a BMD of 0.72 g/cm^2 in those with loosening versus 0.922 g/cm^2 in those without loosening and noted those with pseudarthrosis demonstrated an average BMD of 0.674 g/cm^2 versus 0.934 g/cm^2 in those with fusion.

Similarly, correlations between lower BMD and both PJK have been confirmed by numerous authors including in a retrospective case review by Park et al. who reported that osteoporosis was a risk factor for proximal junctional failure (PJF) with a hazard ratio of 6.4675.[15] Likewise, in a meta-analysis by Liu et al., three studies were found that correlated low BMD with PJK with and odds ratio of 2.37.[16] Also, in a retrospective review of 364 adult deformity patients, Kim et al. demonstrated a significant increased risk of PJK in those with osteoporosis (T score < –2.5) versus those without.[17] Intuitively, low BMD has also been linked to interbody graft subsidence. In a retrospective evaluation of 80 lateral interbody fusion patients by Tempel et al., a mean T score of –1.65 was found in patients with subsidence versus –0.45 in those without subsidence.[18] Formby et al. confirmed this finding using preoperative CT scans and noted that preoperative osteoporosis (HU ≤ 112.4) was associated with subsidence (72.2% vs 45.7%) and iatrogenic fracture (16.7% vs 1.4%).[19] Finally, Puvansarajah et al. performed a multivariate analysis of patients with 5-year follow-up and noted that osteoporosis increased the risk of revision surgery (OR 1.98) with nearly 45% of patients undergoing revision surgery having osteoporosis.[20]

Current strategies to address preoperative osteoporosis include addressing secondary causes of osteoporosis, treatment with antiresorptive agents, and treatment with anabolic agents. The Congress of Neurological Surgeons task force provides a grade B recommendation that preoperative osteoporosis treatment with an anabolic agent can increase bone mineral density, induce earlier and more robust fusion, and may improve patient outcomes.[21–24] There is currently insufficient evidence for preoperative treatment with antiresorptive agents alone as it pertains to patient outcomes.[11] The ideal duration of treatment pre- and postoperatively has not been clearly delineated, but most of the literature is based on 3 to 6 months of treatment preoperatively and 12 months postoperatively.

Body Mass Index

While there are a few studies that fail to demonstrate association between BMI and complication rates in spinal surgery, there is a large body of literature that shows a consistent correlation with overall complication rates.[25–33]

Several large level II ACS-NSQIP and Medicare database studies have found that increased BMI is associated with surgical site infection (SSI) or wound complication in lumbar spine surgery.[20,29,34–37] Glassman et al. pooled three large spine surgery databases including the National Neurosurgery Quality and Outcomes Database, DaneSpine 1993, and the Japan Multicenter Spine Database and reported that increased BMI correlated with increased risk of SSI.[38] Non-database studies corroborate this finding, including The Spine Patient Outcomes Research Trial (SPORT) that reported that those with BMI ≥30 undergoing treatment for spondylolisthesis had higher postoperative infection rates than those with BMI <30 (5% vs 1%).[39] Additionally, multiple single center studies for lumbar spine surgery have also found increased BMI to be a risk factor for SSI including those by Ilyas et al., Koutsoumbelis et al., and Klemencsics et al.[40–42] Soroceanu et al. reported that BMI ≥30 in adult spinal deformity patients was associated with higher rates of major complications and wound infections, but BMI was not associated with minor complications, radiographic complications, or neurologic deficit.[27]

This association appears to apply to cervical spine surgery as well, as evidenced by numerous level II studies demonstrating association between increased BMI and SSI. Jalai et al. reviewed 3057 cervical spondylotic myelopathy patients and reported an overall infection rate of 1.15% with logistic regression analysis revealing a correlation between increased BMI and SSI.[43] Likewise, Pahys et al. reviewed posterior cervical spine fusion patients noting a 1.86% infection rate, higher in those with BMI >30 (OR 4.1).[44] This was corroborated by Sebastian et al. who reviewed 5441 posterior cervical patients and noted a 2.94% infection rate. Multivariate analysis noted BMI >35 was a risk factor for SSI.[45] Interestingly, in an ACS-NSQIP database study by Buerba et al., no association with increased BMI and SSI was found in anterior and posterior cervical fusion patients.[46]

The rates of complication also appear correlated with the severity of obesity. In an ASC-NSQIP database study by Marquez-Lara et al., an association was found between obesity and both superficial wound infection as well as PE. Beginning in the overweight category, as obesity class increased, the risk of deep vein thrombosis (DVT) increased accordingly. Finally, the risk of urinary tract infection (UTI), acute renal failure, and sepsis dramatically increased in class 3 obesity patients (BMI ≥40).[31]

The role that obesity plays in mechanical failure and PJK/PJF is less well understood. Literature for both complications is heterogeneous, with Smith et al. demonstrating that adult spinal deformity patients with rod fracture had an average BMI greater than those without fracture (30.6 vs 26.7) and Wang et al. identifying BMI >27 as a risk factor for rod fracture in 35 consecutive adult spinal deformity (ASD) patients.[47,48] In contrast Cho et al. evaluated 190 ASD patients with long construct instrumentation and found no correlation with BMI and implant failure.[49] Bridwell et al. evaluated 90 ASD patients reported that higher BMI was a significant risk factor for PJK.[50] This was corroborated by Park et al. in a study of 160 ASD patients where they reported a correlation between elevated BMI and PJK, but not PJF.[15] Curiously, Yagi et al., who evaluated 157 adult idiopathic scoliosis patients treated with long construct fusion, noted no difference in PJK rates based on BMI.[51]

Also controversial is the effect BMI has on reoperation and readmission rates. Multiple studies have indicated that elevated BMI is correlated with increased reoperation rates, including a subgroup analysis of the SPORT by McGuire et al. that reported reoperation rates in the obese group twice that of the nonobese group.[30,33,52] Several studies have, however, argued that such a correlation does not exist, including a study by Scheer et al. who reported an average BMI in those with no-reoperation of 27.3 versus 26.7 in the reoperation group.[53–55] Currently, there are limited studies evaluating the effect of BMI on readmission rates and the results are heterogeneous. Puvanesarajah et al. evaluated Medicare data for patients undergoing one- and two-level lumbar fusion and found a significantly higher rate of readmission in obese (30≤ BMI <40) versus nonobese patients (7.8% vs 4.9%) and in morbidly obese (BMI >40) versus matched nonobese patients (10.1% vs 5.2%).[20] Onyekwelu et al., in contrast, queried the Quality Outcomes Database and found no difference in 30-day readmission rates between obese and nonobese patients.[56] In studies dedicated to evaluating cervical spine surgery, no correlation has been found between BMI and reoperation.[57–59]

Ultimately, there is fair evidence to support a correlation between obesity and increased complications as well as increased risk with increasing severity of obesity. The effect of obesity on mechanical failure rates, PJK/PJF rates, and reoperation and readmission rates is less clear. Patients should be rigorously counseled about these complications and the potential effect obesity may have. Diet and exercise for healthy weight loss should always be recommended and facilitated by hospital sponsored programs when possible. Consultation with dieticians, nutritionists, metabolic disease specialists, and bariatric surgery can be considered in refractory cases, and in cases where prescription medication and bariatric surgery is deemed appropriate. Ideally, a BMI of <30 would be achieved in all surgical candidates, but patient pathology, severity of symptoms, patient function, and comorbidities also dictate the timing of surgery. In elective cases where BMI <30 is not feasible, the authors recommend a reasonable weight loss goal of 10% body weight prior to surgery.

Albumin/Prealbumin

Numerous studies have evaluated the association between serum nutrition markers and complications with spinal surgery. A variety of markers exists, but the most studied in spine surgery include albumin and prealbumin.

Schoenfeld et al. retrospectively evaluated preoperative albumin levels for 2150 patients from the NSQIP who had undergone spinal arthrodesis. Patients with albumin levels 3.5 g/dL or lower demonstrated increased all-cause complications rate 3 times greater than those with higher albumin levels. This finding was corroborated by several subsequent studies, including those by Adogwa et al.[60] and Fu et al.,[61] which both identified albumin levels less than 3.5 g/dL as an independent risk factor for any complication among those undergoing spinal fusion in general and anterior cervical discectomy and fusion (ACDF), respectively. Interestingly, Inose et al. evaluated 74 consecutive patients undergoing lumbar decompression and fusion and found that low preoperative serum albumin was an independent predictor of nonunion.[62]

Specifically, malnutrition appears to be associated with postoperative wound complication including infection. Schoenfeld et al.[63] reported increased risk of wound infection with albumin levels less than 3.5 g/dL with an odds ratio of 2.5. A subsequent NSQIP database study by Bohl et al. of 4310 patients confirmed that serum albumin less than 3.5 g/dL was an independent risk factor for wound dehiscence, UTI, and SSI.[64] Moreover, in a single center retrospective review of 83 postoperative wound infections by Tempel et al., 82 of the patients were found to have preoperative prealbumin levels less than 20 mg/dL.[65] Khanna et al. performed a review of the ACS-NSQIP database and identified 3000 patients undergoing revision spinal surgery. Eleven percent of these patients had preoperative hypoalbuminemia, which was significantly more common in those undergoing revision surgery for infection versus for other reasons (49.1% vs 8.5%, $P < 0.001$).[66]

Finally, both Adogwa et al. and Bohl et al. reported increased rates of unplanned 30 day readmission following spinal surgery with preoperative hypoalbuminemia.[64,67,68]

Adogwa specifically reports nearly a threefold increased rate of readmission (27% vs 9.5%) for those with serum albumin less than 3.5 g/dL. This was confirmed by Phan et al., who reported that hypoalbuminemia resulted in a 2.7-fold risk for unplanned readmission after lumbar fusion.[69] Unfortunately, malnourished patients also demonstrate increased rates of mortality with a reported odds ratio of 13.8 as reported by Schoenfeld et al.[63]

Malnutrition appears linked to all complications, wound complication, infection, readmission, extended length of stay, and mortality. Ultimately, the current body of literature supporting this claim consists primarily of level III and IV evidence. Regardless, the consistent correlations identified are worth noting as cursory evaluation for malnutrition with serum albumin and prealbumin measurements is straightforward. Based on current literature, albumin and prealbumin screening targets of greater than 3.5 g/dL and 20 mg/dL appear reasonable. However, given the multitude of nutrition assessment/screening tools as well as the myriad of biomarkers available for assessment (i.e., transferrin, C-reactive protein (CRP), cholesterol, lymphocyte count, α1-acid glycoprotein), consultation with diet/nutrition specialists and/or metabolic disease specialists is prudent when attempting to modify this risk factor prior to surgery.

Smoking

The biological effects of smoking on the spine include increased end plate porosity, decreased trabecular bone thickness, increased cortisol with decreased periosteal cell proliferation, interference with osteoprogenitor cell differentiation, estrogen imbalance, osteoblast death, interference with calcitonin, decreased oxygen supply, and decreased calcium absorption. The culmination of these processes is increased bone resorption and decreased bone formation. In the setting of fusion, smoking appears to exert most dramatic effects by inhibiting angiogenesis during the inflammatory and repair stage of bone healing and interference with signaling molecules involved with osteoprogenitor cell differentiation.

The evidence correlating smoking with complications in lumbar spine and adult spinal deformity surgery is heterogeneous. Tang et al. and Soroceanu et al. both identified significant correlation between smoking and postoperative complication in adult spinal deformity surgery, including medical complications.[70,71] Similarly, Martin et al. in a review of 35,477 patients undergoing lumbar spine surgery demonstrated an increased risk of superficial wound infection, overall wound complication, and 30-day morbidity in smokers compared to nonsmokers.[72] This was confirmed by Macki et al. who reviewed 209 instrumented lumbar fusions and found that tobacco use was the highest predictor of reoperation for SSI (OR 5.75).[73] McCunniff et al. reported that smoking was an independent risk factor for increased estimated blood loss (EBL) and perioperative transfusion in lumbar spine surgery.[74] In contrast, numerous studies by De la Garza et al., Seicean et al., and Cho et al. have failed to identify such correlations either in degenerative or adult spinel deformity surgery.[8,49,75]

Likewise, the literature correlating smoking with pseudarthrosis and mechanical failure of instrumentation in thoracolumbar fusion is heterogeneous. Kim et al. and Smith et al. identified no significant difference in pseudarthrosis and mechanical failure rates, respectively, when comparing smokers and nonsmokers undergoing adult spinal deformity surgery.[47,76] This was corroborated by Gerling et al. in a multicenter randomized control trial for lumbar spondylolisthesis.[77] While studies by Andersen et al., Glassman et al., Macki et al., Inoue et al., and Hofler et al. all demonstrated statistically significant increased rates of pseudarthrosis and mechanical failure among smokers undergoing thoracolumbar spinal fusion.[59,78–81] Macki et al. demonstrated this despite the use of recombinant bone morphogenic protein-2 (rhBMP-2).

The effect of smoking on fusion rates in the cervical spine is less clear. In one-level ACDF, several studies have demonstrated no significant difference in fusion rates between smokers and nonsmokers.[82,83] Likewise, Hilibrand et al. demonstrated no difference in fusion rates for those undergoing anterior corpectomy and Eubanks et al. demonstrated no difference in fusion rates with use of lateral mass instrumentation and iliac crest autograft.[84,85] In contrast, Hilibrand et al. did demonstrate significantly lower rates of fusion for multilevel ACDF in smokers. Hofler et al. also reviewed 107,420 cervical spinal fusion patients in the Healthcare Cost and Utilization Project State Inpatient Databases in NY, CA, FL, and WA, and found that smoking was significantly correlated with pseudarthrosis.[59]

The impact of smoking on reoperation rates and readmission rates in adult spinal deformity is somewhat limited and is heterogenous as well. Mok et al. and Puvanesarajah et al. both report that smoking was an independent risk factor for reoperation in adult spinal deformity with a risk ratio of 2.59 and odds ratio of 1.37, respectively (trended toward significance).[86,87] In contrast, Scheer et al. found no correlation between smoking and reoperation rates, and Manoharan et al. found no correlation between smoking and readmission rate in a NSQIP database evaluation of spinal deformity patients.[53,88] In the cervical spine, however, multiple retrospective studies have concluded that smoking was a risk factor for reoperation due to adjacent segment pathology after fusion.[89,90]

The heterogeneity within the literature suggests further investigation into the effects of nicotine alone, and other cigarette components is still necessary. Moreover, investigation into the effect of smoking on success rates for specific spine procedures, reoperation rates, and readmission rates is ongoing. However, given the clear molecular effects of smoking on bone healing biology, and the fair evidence suggesting association with pseudarthrosis, smoking cessation prior to fusion surgery remains a strong recommendation among most spine surgeons. The timing and duration of smoking cessation remains a matter of contention. As the first 3 to 4 weeks postoperatively are most critical for angiogenesis and most of the bone formation occurs over the first 6 months postoperatively, smoking cessation for 6 months after surgery would likely be beneficial. The effect of smoking cessation preoperatively on complications is less well understood. The authors of this text suggest cessation 4 to 6 weeks prior to surgery.

Mental Health Disorders

Various studies have evaluated the effect of mental health on postoperative outcomes in spine surgery. Multiple psychological assessment tools have been used. Hägg et al. performed a multicenter randomized controlled trial and reported that low neuroticism as measured by the Karolinksa Scale of Personality (KSP) was predictive of higher functional improvement in surgical patients. Interestingly, depression, as measured by the Zung Depression Scale (ZDS), was predictive of better outcomes in nonoperative treatment.[91] This has been contradicted by numerous studies using the ZDS to evaluate the correlation between depression and outcomes. For example, Chaichana et al. found those with preoperative depression and somatic anxiety were less likely to reach minimum clinically important difference (MCID) 12 months after single level lumbar discectomy.[92] This was corroborated by three sequential studies by Adogwa et al. in patients undergoing revision surgery for recurrent stenosis, adjacent segment disease, or pseudarthrosis. In these studies, the authors identified increasing ZDS scores as a predictor of poorer patient dissatisfaction and Oswestry Disability Index (ODI) scores.[93–95]

Further emphasizing the effect of mental health on spine surgery, multiple authors have linked preoperative Short Form 36 (SF-36) Mental Component Scores (MCS) with postoperative outcomes. Trief et al. found that in lumbar spinal fusion patients, those with lower MCS reported greater postoperative back pain, leg pain, and lower improvement at 12 months.[96] Carr et al. reported that low MCS was correlated with lower satisfaction and higher disability following ACDF.[97] Urban-Baeza et al. used the Beck Depression Inventory to show that postoperative spinal stenosis patients with depression at 1 year had worse outcomes compared to those without depression.[98]

Moreover, mental health disorder also appears to affect outcomes beyond subjective metrics. Menendez et al. evaluated 5000 patients from the National Hospital Discharge Survey and identified those with preoperative depression, anxiety, schizophrenia, and dementia. They reported higher rates of unusual discharge, in-hospital mortality, and increased incidences of adverse events in patients with a psychiatric disorder.[99] Likewise, Adogwa et al. found that depression was an independent risk factor for readmission.[67]

In summary, there is a fair amount of literature demonstrating the effect of mental health on spine surgery outcomes. Unfortunately, there are a myriad of psychological assessment tools currently being used to evaluate mental health and, as such, there is no consensus regarding preoperative optimization targets. Nonetheless, all the aforementioned studies suggest reduced improvement after spine surgery when preoperative mental health disorders are present regardless of which assessment tool is utilized. Moreover, the severity of mental health disorders appears inversely related to postoperative improvement and is potentially modifiable. Thus, the authors strongly recommend preoperative screening in spine clinic for depression, somatic anxiety, and dementia. Patients identified as at risk or with a history of mental health disorder should be under psychiatric evaluation and management prior to surgery.

Frailty

The modified Frailty Index (mFI) utilizes 11 components of the Canadian Study of Health and Aging Frailty Index (CSHA-FI). Numerous level III studies have evaluated the relationship between mFI and complications, readmission, and reoperation.[100]

Four level III studies querying the ACS-NSQIP identified an association between increasing mFI and overall complication rates within 30 days of surgery.[101–104] Leven et al. reported an association between higher mFI and increased complication, need for blood transfusion, venous thromboembolism (VTE), and mortality in spinal deformity surgeries.[104] This also appears to apply to shorter segment surgeries, as Flexman et al, evaluated 53,080 patients undergoing degenerative spine surgery and reported a higher odds ratio of major complication with increasing mFI (OR 1.15 for each increase of 0.1 in mFI).[101] This was also found in cervical spine fusion in a study by Shin et al. who found increased odds of life-threatening complications in ACDF or posterior cervical foraminotomy (PCF) with increasing mFI.[103] Ali et al. also noted increased rates of SSI, life-threatening complications, and mortality with increasing mFI.[102] Both Flexman and Leven also reported increased odds of reoperation with increased mFI, specifically for infection in the Flexman study.

Overall, there is fair evidence to support an association between frailty and development of complications in spinal surgery and need for reoperation. Given the nature of the studies available, all of which are database studies, specific correlations between comorbidities contributing to frailty and specific complications cannot be identified. At this juncture, mFI is best used as an instrument to counsel patients about their overall risk of complication, rather than as a target for optimization.

Vitamin D Deficiency

Vitamin D plays a critical role in bone metabolism, regulation of calcium and phosphorus, and bone remodeling. Thus, it has long been thought that vitamin D deficiency could have major impact on short- and long-term outcomes after spinal surgery. The current criteria for deficiency is defined as serum 25-hydroxyvitamin D levels <20 ng/mL while insufficiency is 20 to 30 ng/mL.

A recent systematic review and meta-analysis by Khalooeifard et al. included seven studies with 1188 patients in the evaluation of this issue.[105] They reported an aggregate vitamin deficiency incidence of 38.9% with insufficiency ranging from 57% to 73.6%. A variety of outcome metrics were reported, but only visual analog scale (VAS) and ODI were ubiquitous among the included studies. No correlation was found between preoperative vitamin D deficiency and postoperative VAS. The authors did, however, find that, in aggregate, those with vitamin D deficiency demonstrated worse ODI (4.82 points greater) than those without deficiency.

The association between vitamin D deficiency and pseudarthrosis has also been evaluated by numerous studies with conflicting results. Donnally et al. found no significant correlation between vitamin D levels and rates of pseudarthrosis after lumbar spinal fusion, while Ravindra et al. showed significantly higher pseudarthrosis rates (OR 3.449) and longer time to fusion (12 months vs 6 months) in vitamin D–deficient patients undergoing elective lumbar spinal fusion.[106,107] Xu et al. divided 44 patients with vitamin D deficiency undergoing transforaminal lumbar interbody fusion (TLIF) into a group receiving supplementation and a group receiving placebo. The fusion rates were significantly higher in the supplementation group (95.24% vs 65.22%, $P = 0.02$).[108]

Overall, the current body of literature suggests that vitamin D concentration may be associated with postoperative health-related quality of life (HRQOL) metrics and fusion rates. However, the data are conflicting, and the majority of studies have been limited by modest sample size, heterogeneity in study populations, confounding due labile serum vitamin D levels in individual patients, and dissimilarities in methodology. Moreover, few studies have evaluated the role of vitamin D supplementation in spinal surgery. Nonetheless, as evaluation for vitamin D deficiency is straightforward and the potential benefit of supplementation is great, the authors of this chapter recommend that surgeons strongly consider routine preoperative screening with serum 25-hydroxyvitamin D and supplementation for those with deficiency. This is particularly the case for those with risk factors for vitamin D deficiency such as BMI >40, male gender, age 40 to 60 years, and diagnosis of diabetes. Consensus has not been reached regarding target serum vitamin D levels, duration of supplementation, and frequency of screening. Of note, the Institute of Medicine Committee to Review Dietary Reference Intakes for Vitamin D and Calcium state that optimal bone mineral density is achieved with an average serum vitamin D of 50 ng/mL.

Hemoglobin A1c

The association between diabetes and postoperative complication has been reported in several studies, but the methodologies are heterogeneous. Cancienne et al. evaluated 3341 ACDF patients requiring reoperation and noted that HbA1c was an independent risk factor for reoperation. Preoperative serum glucose was not identified as a risk factor, but a HbA1c cutoff value of 7.5 mg/dL was 46% sensitive and 68% specific for reoperation.[109] Cancienne et al. also evaluated the effect of diabetes in lumbar decompression in 5194 patients where he identified a HbA1c >7.5 mg/dL as a risk factor for deep SSI (OR 2.9).[110] Likewise, in a retrospective review of 36 patients with diabetes by Hikata et al., diabetics demonstrated a higher rate of infection than nondiabetics, and preoperative HbA1c values were significantly higher in those with SSI than those without (7.6 mg/dL vs 6.9 mg/dL). Hikata reported that in those with "controlled diabetes" (HbA1c <7.0 mg/dL), no infections occurred, whereas 35.3% of those with HbA1c >7.0 mg/dL had infections.[111] In contrast, while both Caputo et al. and Koutsoumbelis et al. identified diabetes as a risk factor for SSI, they did not identify preoperative HbA1c as a risk factor.[42,112] In the case of the Caputo study, this was likely due to use of a higher HbA1c cutoff of 8%. Interestingly, both studies identified higher perioperative serum glucose levels as a predictor for SSI, with Caputo reporting that serum glucose levels >140 mg/dL doubled the risk of SSI. Finally, in a retrospective evaluation of 165 patients undergoing lumbar spine surgery, Takahashi et al. reported that those with a HbA1c >6.5% had higher rates of pseudarthrosis and were less likely to demonstrate improvement in preoperative leg pain and numbness.[113]

Overall, several level II and III studies provide fair evidence to support an association between diabetes and postoperative adverse events, particularly infection. Serum HbA1c and serum glucose levels appear to be the most common preoperative assessment tools, with preoperative HbA1c and perioperative serum glucose levels being associated with infection. While there is no consensus target for perioperative serum glucose, the Congress of Neurological Surgeons recommends preoperative HbA1c testing prior to surgery and counseling for increased complication risk for levels >7.5%.[114] Patients should be encouraged to work with their primary care providers to achieve this target prior to surgery, and to maintain appropriate diabetes control thereafter. Endocrinology referral should be considered in refractory cases.

Conclusion

While a myriad of other predictive factors likely exists, the current body of literature has elucidated numerous risk factors for perioperative morbidity, reoperation, and readmission that can be easily evaluated in a spine surgery practice. These include, but are not limited to, low preoperative hemoglobin, low BMD, elevated BMI, poor nutrition, tobacco use, mental health disorders, poor frailty, vitamin D deficiency, and elevated HbA1c. Unfortunately, the effect of "optimizing" these risk factors is largely unclear and a subject of future study. Nonetheless, it is our duty to attenuate risk to the extent we are capable.

References

1. Purvis TE, Goodwin CR, De la Garza-Ramos R, et al. Effect of liberal blood transfusion on clinical outcomes and cost in spine surgery patients. *Spine J.* 2017;17(9):1255–1263.
2. He YK, Li HZ, Lu HD. Is blood transfusion associated with an increased risk of infection among spine surgery patients?: Ameta-analysis. *Medicine.* 2019;98(28):e16287.
3. Carabini LM, Zeeni C, Moreland NC, et al. Development and validation of a generalizable model for predicting major transfusion during spine fusion surgery. *J Neurosurg Anesthesiol.* 2014;26(3):205–215.
4. Nuttall GA, Horlocker TT, Santrach PJ, Oliver Jr WC, Dekutoski MB, Bryant S. Predictors of blood transfusions in spinal instrumentation and fusion surgery. *Spine.* 2000;25(5):596–601.
5. Zheng F, Cammisa Jr FP, Sandhu HS, Girardi FP, Khan SN. Factors predicting hospital stay, operative time, blood loss, and transfusion in patients undergoing revision posterior lumbar spine decompression, fusion, and segmental instrumentation. *Spine.* 2002;27(8):818–824.
6. Lenoir B, Merckx P, Paugam-Burtz C, et al. Individual probability of allogeneic erythrocyte transfusion in elective spine surgery: the predictive model of transfusion in spine surgery. *Anesthesiology.* 2009;110(5):1050–1060.
7. Kim BD, Edelstein AI, Patel AA, Lovecchio F, Kim JYS. Preoperative anemia does not predict complications after single-level lumbar fusion: a propensity score-matched multicenter study. *Spine.* 2014;39(23):1981–1989.
8. Seicean A, Seicean S, Alan N. Effect of smoking on the perioperative outcomes of patients who undergo elective spine surgery. *Spine.* 2013;38(15):1294–1302.
9. Seicean A, Seicean S, Alan N, et al. Preoperative anemia and perioperative outcomes in patients who undergo elective spine surgery. *Spine.* 2013;38(15):1331–1341.
10. Veeravagu A, Patil CG, Lad SP, Boakye M. Risk factors for postoperative spinal wound infections after spinal decompression and fusion surgeries. *Spine.* 2009;34(17):1869–1872.
11. Dimar J, Bisson EF, Dhall S, et al. Congress of Neurological Surgeons systematic review and evidence-based guidelines for perioperative spine: Preoperative osteoporosis assessment. *Neurosurgery.* 2021;89(Suppl 1):S19–S25.
12. Bredow J, Boese CK, Werner CML, et al. Predictive validity of preoperative CT scnas and the risk of pedicle screw loosening in spinal surgery. *Arch Orthop Trauma Surg.* 2016;136(8):1063–1067.
13. Kim JB, Park SW, Lee YS, et al. The effects of spinopelvic parameters and paraspinal muscle degeneration on S1 screw loosening. *J Korean Neurosurg Soc.* 2015;58(4):357–362.
14. Okuyama K, Abe E, Suzuki T, Tamura Y, Chiba M, Sato K. Influence of bone mineral density on pedicle screw fixation: a study of pedicle screw fixation augmenting posterior lumbar interbody fusion in elderly patients. *Spine J.* 2001;1(6):402–407.
15. Park SJ, Lee CS, Chung SS, Lee JY, Kang SS, Park SH. Different risk factors of proximal junctional kyphosis and proximal junctional failure following long instrumented fusion to the sacrum for adult spinal deformity: survivorship analysis of 160 patients. *Neurosurgery.* 2017;80(2):279–286.
16. Liu FY, Wang T, Yang SD, Wang H, Yang DL, Ding WY. Incidence and risk facotrs for proximal junctional kyphosis: a meta-analysis. *Eur Spine J.* 2016;25(8):2376–2383.
17. Kim HJ, Bridwell KH, Lenke LG, et al. Proximal junctional kyphosis results in inferior SRS pain subscores in adult deformity patients. *Spine.* 2013;38(11):896–901.
18. Tempel ZJ, Gandhoke GS, Okonkwo DO, Kanter AS. Impaired bone mineral density as a predictor of graft subsidence following minimally invasive transpsoas lateral lumbar interbody fusion. *Eur Spine J.* 2015;24(Suppl 3):414–419.
19. Formby PM, Kang DG, Helgeson MD, Wagner SC. Clinical and radiographic outcomes of transforaminal lumbar interbody fusion in patients with osteoporosis. *Global Spine J.* 2016;6(7):660–664.
20. Puvanesarajah V, Werner BC, Cancienne JM, et al. Morbid obesity and lumbar fusion in patients older than 65 years: complications, readmissions, costs, and length of stay. *Spine.* 2017;42(2):122–127.
21. Ohtori S, Inoue G, Orita S, et al. Teriparatide accelerates lumbar posterolateral fusion in women with postmenopausal osteoporosis: prospective study. *Spine.* 2012;37(23):E1464–E1468.
22. Ohtori S, Inoue G, Orita S, et al. (2013). Comparison of teriparatide and bisphosphonate treatment to reduce pedicle screw loosening after lumbar spinal fusion surgery in postmenopausal women with osteoporosis from a bone quality perspective. *Spine (Phila Pa 1976).* 2013;38(8):E487–492.
23. Wang M, Meng X, Li Y, feng Y, Chang Z, Hai Y. Effects of anti-osteoporosis treatment in the elderly with anterior cervical discectomy and fusion. *Acta Orthop Traumatol Turc.* 2016;50(2):186–190.
24. Kim SM, Rhee W, Ha S, Lim JH, Jang IT. Influence of alendronate and endplate degeneration to single level posterior lumbar spinal interbody fusion. *Korean J Spine.* 2014;11(4):221–226.
25. Higgins DM, Mallory GW, Planchard RF, et al. (2016). Understanding the impact of obesity on short-term outcomes and in-hospital costs after instrumented spinal fusion. *Neurosurgery.* 2016;78(1):127–132.
26. Sing DC, Yue JK, Metz LN, et al. Obesity is an independent risk factor of early complications after revision spine surgery. *Spine.* 2016;41(10):E632–640.
27. Soroceanu A, Burton DC, Diebo BG, et al. Impact of obesity on complications, infection, and patient-reported outcomes in adult spinal deformity surgery. *J Neurosurg Spine.* 2015;23(5):656–664.
28. Basques BA, Fu MC, Buerba RA, Bohl DD, Golinvaux NS, Grauer JN. Using the ACS-NSQIP to identify factors affecting hospital length of stay after elective posterior lumbar fusion. *Spine.* 2014;39(6):497–502.
29. Buerba RA, Fu MC, Gruskay JA, Long 3rd WD, Grauer JN. Obese class III patients at significantly greater risk of multiple complications after lumbar surgery: an analysis of 10,387 patients in the ACS NSQIP database. *Spine J.* 2014;14(9):2008–2018.
30. Jiang J, Teng Y, Fan Z, Khan S, Xia Y. Does obesity affect the surgical outcome and complication rates of spinal surgery? A meta-analysis. *Clin Orthop Relat Res.* 2014;472(3):968–975.
31. Marquez-Lara A, Nandyala SV, Sankaranarayanan S, Noureldin M, Singh K. Body mass index as a predictor of complications and mortality after lumbar spine surgery. *Spine.* 2014;39(10):798–804.
32. McClendon Jr J, Smith TR, Thompson SE, et al. The impact of body mass index on hospital stay and complications after spinal fusion. *Neurosurgery.* 2014;74(1):42–50. discussion 50.
33. McGuire KJ, Khaleel MA, Rihn JA, Lurie JD, Zhao W, Weinstein JN. The effect of high obesity on outcomes of treatment for lumbar spinal conditions: subgroup analysis of the spine patient outcomes research trial. *Spine.* 2014;39(23):1975–1980.

34. Jain D, Berven SH, Carter J, Zhang AL, Deviren V. Bariatric surgery before elective posterior lumbar fusion is associated with reduced medical complications and infection. *Spine J.* 2018;18(9):1526–1532.
35. Lieber B, Han B, Strom RG, et al. Preoperative predictors of spinal infection within the National Surgical Quality Inpatient Database. *World Neurosurg.* 2016;89:517–524.
36. Ranson WA, Cheung ZB, Di Capua J, et al. Risk factors for perioperative complications in morbidly obese patients undergoing elective posterior lumbar fusion. *Global Spine J.* 2018;8(8):795–802.
37. Kurtz SM, Lau E, Ong KL, et al. Infection risk for primary and revision instrumented lumbar spine fusion in the Medicare population. *J Neurosurg Spine.* 2012;17(4):342–347.
38. Glassman S, Carreon LY, Andersen M, et al. Predictors of hospital readmission and surgical site infection in the United States, Denmark, and Japan: Is risk stratification a universal language? *Spine.* 2017;42(17):1311–1315.
39. Rihn JA, Radcliff K, Hilibrand AS, et al. Does obesity affect outcomes of treatment for lumbar stenosis and degenerative spondylolisthesis? Analysis of the Spine Patient Outcomes Research Trial (SPORT). *Spine.* 2012;37(23):1933–1946.
40. Ilyas H, Golubovsky JL, Chen JC, Winkelman RD, Mroz TE, Steinmetz MP. Risk factors for 90-day reoperation and readmission after lumbar surgery for lumbar spinal stenosis. *J Neurosurg Spine.* 2019;31(1):20–26.
41. Klemencsics I, Lazary A, Szoverfi Z, Bozsodi A, Eltes P, Varga PP. Risk factors for surgical site infection in elective routine degenerative lumbar surgeries. *Spine J.* 2016;16(11):1377–1383.
42. Koutsoumbelis S, Hughes AP, Girardi FP, et al. Risk factors for postoperative infection following posterior lumbar instrumented arthrodesis. *J Bone Joint Surg Am.* 2011;93(17):1627–1633.
43. Jalai CM, Worley N, Poorman GW, Cruz DL, Vira S, Passias PG. Surgical site infections following operative management of cervical spondylotic myelopathy: prevalence, predictors of occurence, and influence on peri-operative outcomes. *Spine J.* 2016;25(6):1891–1896.
44. Pahys JM, Pahya JR, Cho SK, et al. Methods to decrease postoperative infections following posterior cervical spine surgery. *J Bone Joint Surg Am.* 2013;95(6):549–554.
45. Sebastian A, Huddleston 3rd P, Kakar S, Habermann E, Wagie A, Nassr A. Risk factors for surgical site infection after posterior cervical spine surgery: an analysis of 5,441 patients from the ACS NSQIP 2005–2012. *Spine J.* 2016;16(4):504–509.
46. Buerba RA, Fu MC, Grauer JN. Anterior and posterior cervical fusion in patients with high body mass index are not associated with greater complications. *Spine J.* 2014;14(8):1643–1653.
47. Smith JS, Shaffrey E, Klineberg E, et al. Prospective multicenter assessment of risk factors for rod fracture following surgery for adult spinal deformity. *J Neurosurg Spine.* 2014;21(6):994–1003.
48. Wang H, Guo J, Wang S, et al. Instrumentation failure after posterior vertebral column resection in adult spinal deformity. *Spine.* 2017;42(7):471–478.
49. Cho W, Mason JR, Smith JS, et al. Failure of lumbopelvic fixaiton after long construct fusions in patientws with adult spinal deformity: clinical and radiographic risk factors: clinical article. *J Neurosurg Spine.* 2013;19(4):445–453.
50. Bridwell KH, Lenke LG, Cho SK, et al. Proximal junctional kyphosis in primary adult deformity surgery: evaluation of 20 degrees as a critical angle. *Neurosurgery.* 2013;72(6):899–906.
51. Yagi M, Akilah KB, Boachie-Adjei O. Incidence, risk factors and classification of proximal junctional kyphosis: surgical outcomes review of adult idiopathic scoliosis. *Spine.* 2011;36(1):E60–68.
52. Bridwell KH, Lenke LG, Cho SK, et al. Proximal junctional kyphosis in primary adult deformity surgery: evaluation of 20 degrees as a critical angle. *Neurosurgery.* 2013;72(6):899–906.
53. Scheer JK, Tang JA, Smith JS, et al. Reoperation rates and impact on outcome in a large, prospective, multicenter, adult spinal deformity database: clincal article. *J Neurosurg Spine.* 2013;19(4):464–470.
54. Owens 2nd RK, Djurasovic M, Onyekwelu I, Bratcher KR, McGraw KE, Carreon LY. Outcomes and revision rates in normal, overweight, and obese patients 5 years after lumbar fusion. *Spine J.* 2016;16(10):1178–1183.
55. Passias PG, Soroceanu A, Yang S, et al. Predictors of revision surgical procedure excluding wound complications in adult spinal deformity and impact on patient-reported outcomes and satisfaction: a two-year follow-up. *J Bone Joint Surg Am.* 2016;98(7):536–543.
56. Onyekwelu I, Glassman SD, Asher AL, Shaffrey CI, Mummaneni PV, Carreon LY. Impact of obesity oncomplications and outcomes: a comparison of fusion and nonfusion lumbar spine surgery. *J Neurosurg Spine.* 2017;26(2):158–162.
57. Bovonratwet P, Fu MC, Tyagi V, et al. Incidence, risk factors, and clinical implications of postoperative hematoma requiring reoperation following anterior cervical discectomy and fusion. *Spine.* 2019;44(8):543–549.
58. Narain AS, Hijii FY, Haws BE, et al. Impact of body mass index on surgical outcomes, narcotics consumption, and hospital costs following anterior cervical discectomy and fusion. *J Neurosurg Spine.* 2018;28(2):160–166.
59. Hofler RC, Swong K, Martin B, Wemhoff M, Jones GA. Risk of pseudoarthrosis after spinal fusion: analysis from the healthcare cost and utilization project. *World Neurosurg.* 2018:e194–e202.
60. Adogwa O, Martin JR, Huang K, et al. Preoperative serum albumin level as a predictor of posoperative complication after spine fusion. *Spine.* 2014;39(18):1513–1519.
61. Fu MC, Buerba RA, Grauer JN. Preoperative nutritional status as an adjunct predictor of major postooperative complications following anterior cervical discectomy and fusion. *Clin Spine Surg.* 2016;29(4):167–172.
62. Inose H, Yamada T, Mulati M, et al. Bone turnover markers as a new predicting factor for nonunion after spinal fusion surgery. *Spine.* 2018;43(1):E29–E34.
63. Schoenfeld AJ, Carey PA, Cleveland 3rd AW, Bader JO, Bono CM. Patient facots, comorbidities, and surgical characteristics that increase mortality and complication risk after spinal arthrodesis: a prognostic study based on 5,887 patients. *Spine J.* 2013;13(10):1171–1179.
64. Bohl DD, Shen MR, Mayo BC, et al. Malnutrition predicts infectious and wound complications following posterior lumbar spinal fusion. *Spine.* 2016;41(21):1693–1699.
65. Tempel Z, Grandhi R, Maserati M, et al. Prealbumin as a serum biomarker of impaired perioperative nutritional status and risk for surgicl site infection after spine surgery. *J Neurol Surg A Cent Eur Neurosurg.* 2015;76(2):139–143.
66. Khanna K, Yi PH, Sing DC, Geiger E, Metz LN. Hypoalbuminemia is associated with septic revisions after primary surgery and postoperative infection after revision surgery. *Spine.* 2018;43(6):454–460.
67. Adogwa O, Elsamadicy AA, Mehta AI, et al. Association between baseline affective disorders and 30-day readmission

rates in patients undergoing elective spine surgery. *World Neurosurg*. 2016;94:432–436.
68. Adogwa O, Elsamadicy AA, Mehta AI, et al. Preoperative nutritional status is an independent predictor of 30-day hospital readmission after elective spine surgery. *Spine*. 2016;41(17):1400–1404.
69. Phan K, Ranson W, White SJW, et al. Thirty-day perioperative complications, prolonged length of stay, and readmission following elective posterior lumbar fusion associated with poor nutritional status. *Global Spine J*. 2019;9(4):417–423.
70. Tang H, Zhu J, Ji F, Wang S, Xie Y, Fei H. Risk factors for postoperative complication after spinal fusion and instrumentation in degenerative lumbar scoliosis patients. *J. Orthop Surg Res*. 2014;9(1):15.
71. Soroceanu A, Burton DC, Oren JH, et al. Medical complications after adult spinal deformity surgyer: incidence, risk factors, and clinical impact. *Spine*. 2016;41(22):1718–1723.
72. Martin CT, Gao Y, Duchman KR, Pugely AJ. The impact of current smoking and smoking cessation on short-term morbidity risk after lumbar spine surgery. *Spine*. 2016;41(7):577–584.
73. Macki M, Uzosike A, Kerezoudis P, Bydon A, Bydon M, Gokaslan ZL. Duration of indwelling drain following instrumented posterolateral fusion of the lumbar spine does not predict surgical site infection requiring reoperation. *J Clin Neurosci*. 2017;40:44–48.
74. McCunniff PT, Young ES, Ahmadinia K, Ahn UM, Ahn NU. Smoking is associated with increased blood loss and transfusion use after lumbar spinal surgery. *Clin Orthop Relat Res*. 2016;474(4):1019–1025.
75. De la Garza Ramos R, Goodwin CR, Qadi M, et al. Impact of smoking on 30-day morbidity and mortality in adult spinal deformity surgery. *Spine*. 2017;42(7):465–470.
76. Kim YJ, Bridwell KH, Lenke LG, Rinella AS, Edwards 2nd C. Pseudarthrosis in primary fusions for adult indiopathic scoliosis: incidence, risk factors, and outcome analysis. *Spine*. 2005;30(4):468–474.
77. Gerling MC, Leven D, Passias PG, et al. Risk factors for reoperation in patients treated surgically for degenerative spondylolisthesis: a subanalysis of the 8-year data from the SPORT trial. *Spine*. 2017;42(20):1559–1569.
78. Andersen T, Christensen FB, Laursen M, Høy K, Hansen ES, Bünger C. Smoking as a predictor of negative outcome in lumbar spinal fusion. *Spine*. 2001;26(23):2623–2628.
79. Glassman SD, Anagnost SC, Parker A, Burke D, Johnson JR, Dimar JR. The effect of cigarette smoking and smoking cessation on spinal fusion. *Spine*. 2000;25(20):2608–2615.
80. Macki M, Syeda S, Rajjoub KR, et al. The effect of smoking status on successful arthrodesis after lumbar instrumentation supplemented with rhBMP-2. *World Neurosurg*. 2017;97:459–464.
81. Inoue S, Khashan M, Fujimori T, Berven SH. Analysis of mechanical failure associated with reoperation in spinal fusion to the sacrum in adult spinal deformity. *J Orthop Sci*. 2015;20(4):609–616.
82. Samartzis D, Shen FH, Goldberg EJ, An HS. Is autograft the gold standard in achiving radiographic fusion in one-level anterior cervical discectomy and fusion with rigid anterior plate fixation? *Spine*. 2005;30(15):1756–1761.
83. Luszczyk M, Smith JS, Fischgrund JS, et al. Does smoking have an impact on fusion rate in single-level anterior cervical discectomy and fusion with allograft and rigid plate fixation? *J Neurosurg Spine*. 2013;19(5):527–531.
84. Hilibrand AS, Fye MA, Emery SE, Palumbo MA, Bohlman HH. Impact of smoking on the outcome of anterior cervical arthrodesis with interbody or strut-grafting. *J Bone Joint Surg Am*. 2001;83(5):668–673.
85. Eubanks JD, Thorpe SW, Cheruvu VK, Braly BA, Kang JD. DOes smoking influence fusion rates in posterior cervical arthrodesis with lateral mass instrumentation? *Clin Orthop Relat Res*. 2011;469(3):696–701.
86. Mok JM, Cloyd JM, Bradford DS, et al. Reoperation after primary fusion for adult spinal deformity: rate, reason, and timing. *Spine (Phila Pa1976)*. 2009;34(8):832–839.
87. Puvanesarajah V, Shen FH, Cancienne WM, et al. Risk factors for reision surgery following primary adult spinal deformity surgery in patients 65 years and older. *J Neurosurg Spine*. 2016;25(4):486–493.
88. Manoharan SR, Baker DK, Pasara SM, Ponce B, Deinlein D, Theiss SM. Thirty-day readmissions following adult spinal deformity surgery: an analysis of the National Surgical Quality Improvement Program (NSQIP) database. *Spine J*. 2016;16(7):862–866.
89. Lee JC, Lee SH, Peters C, Riew KD. Adjacent segment pathology requiring reoperation after anterior cervical arthrodesis: the influence of smoking, sex, and number of operated levels. *Spine*. 2015;40(10):E571–E577.
90. Lee JC, Lee SH, Peters C, Riew KD. Risk-factor analysis of adjacent-segment pathology requiring surgery following anterior, posterior, fusion, and nonfusion cervical spine operations: survivorship analysis of 1358 patients. *J Bone Joint Surg Am*. 2014;96(21):1761–1767.
91. Hägg O, Fritzell P, Ekselius L, Nordwall A. Swedish Lumbar Spine Study. Predictors of outcome in fusion surgery for chronic low back pain. A report from the Swedish Lumbar Spine Study. *Eur Spine J*. 2003;12(1):22–33.
92. Chaichana KL, Mukherjee D, Adogwa O, Cheng JS, McGirt MJ. Correlation of preoperative depression and somatic perception scales with postoperative disability and quality of life after lumbar discectomy. *J Neurosurg Spine*. 2011;14(2):261–267.
93. Adogwa O, Parker SL, Shau DN, et al. Preoperative Zung Depression Scale predicts outcome after revision lumbar surgery for adjacent segment disease, recurrent stenosis, and pseudarthrosis. *Spine J*. 2012;12(3):179–185.
94. Adogwa O, Parker SL, Shau DN, et al. Preoperative Zung depression scale predicts patient satisfaction independent of the extent of improvement after revision lumbar surgery. *Spine J*. 2013;13(5):501–506.
95. Adogwa O, Verla T, Thompson P, et al. Affective disorders influence clinical outcomes after revision lumbar surgery in elderly patients with symptomatic adjacent-segment disease, recurrent stenosis, or pseudarthrosis. *J Neurosurg Spine*. 2014;21(2):153–159.
96. Trief PM, Ploutz-Snyder R, Fredrickson BE. Emotional health predicts pain and function after fusion: a prospective multicenter study. *Spine*. 2006;31(7):823–830.
97. Carr FA, Healy KM, Villavicencio AT, et al. Effect on clinical outcomes of patient pain expectancies and preoperative Mental Component Summary scores from the 36-Item Short Form Health Survey following anterior cervical discectomy and fusion. *J Neurosurg Spine*. 2011;15(5):486–490.
98. Urban-Baeza A, Zárate-Kalfópulos B, Romero-Vargas S, Obil-Chavarría C, Brenes-Rojas L, Reyes-Sánchez A. Influence of depression symptoms on patient expectations and

clinical outcomes in the surgical management of spinal stenosis. *J Neurosurg Spine.* 2015;22(1):75–79.

99. Menendez ME, Neuhaus V, Bot AGJ, Ring D, Cha TD. Psychiatric disorders and major spine surgery: epidemiology and perioperative outcomes. *Spine (Phila Pa 1976).* 2014:E111–122.
100. Saxton A, Velanovich V. Preoperative frailty and quality of life as predictors of postoperative complications. *Ann Surg.* 2011;253(6):1223–1229.
101. Flexman AM, Charest-Morin R, Stobart L, Street J, Ryerson CJ. Frailty and postoperative outcomes in patients undergoing surgery for degenerativespine disease. *Spine J.* 2016;16(11):1315–1323.
102. Ali R, Schwalb JM, Nerenz DR, Antione HJ, Rubinfeld I. Use of the modified frailty index to predict 30-day morbidity and mortality from spine surgery. *J Neurosurg Spine.* 2016;25(4):537–541.
103. Shin JI, Kothari P, Phan K, et al. Frailty index as a predictor of adverse postoperative outcomes in patients undergoing cervical spinal fusion. *Spine.* 2017;42(5):304–310.
104. Leven DM, Lee NJ, Kothari P, et al. Frailty index is a significant predictor of complications and mortality after surgery for adult spinal deformity. *Spine.* 2016;41(23):E1394–1401.
105. Khalooeifard R, Rahmani J, Tavanaei R, et al. The effect of vitamin D deficiency on outcomes of patients undergoing elective spinal fusion surgery: A systematic review and meta-analysis. *Int J Spine Surg.* 2022;16(1):53–60.
106. Donnally 3rd CJ, Sheu JI, Bondar KJ, et al. Is there a correlation between preoperative or postoperative vitamin D levels with pseudarthrosis, hardware failure, and revisions after lumbar spine fusion. *World Neurosurg.* 2019;130:e431–e437.
107. Ravindra VM, Godzik J, Dailey AT, et al. Vitamin D levels and 1-year fusion outcomes in elective spine surgery. *Spine.* 2015;40(19):1536–1541.
108. Xu Y, Zhou M, Liu H, et al. Effect of 1, 25-dihydroxyvitamin D3 on posterior transforaminal lumbar interbody fusion in patients with osteoporosis and lumbar disc degenerative disease. *Zhongguo Xiu Fu Chong Jian Wai Ke Za Zhi.* 2014;28(8):969–972.
109. Cancienne JM, Werner BC, Chen DQ, Hassanzadeh H, Shimer AL. Perioperative hemoglobin A1c as a predictor of deep infection following single-level lumbar decompression in patients with diabetes. *Spine J.* 2017;17(8):110–1105.
110. Cancienne JM, Werner BC, Hassanzadeh H, Singla A, Shen FH, Shimer AL. The association of perioperative glycemic control with deep postoperative infection after anterior cervical discectomy and fusion in patients with diabetes. *World Neurosurg.* 2017;102:13–17.
111. Hikata T, Iwanami A, Hosogane N, et al. High preoperative hemoglobin A1c is a risk factor for surgical site infection after posterior thoracic and lumbar spinal instrumentation surgery. *J Orthop Sci.* 2014;19(2):223–228.
112. Caputo AM, Dobbertien RP, Ferranti JM, Brown CR, Michael KW, Richardson WJ. Risk factors for infection after orthopaedic spine surgery at a high-volume institution. *J Surg Orthop Adv.* 2013;22(4):295–298.
113. Takahashi S, Suzuki A, Toyoda H, et al. Characteristics of diabetes associated with poor improvements in clinical outcomes after lumbar spine surgery. *Spine.* 2013;38(6):516–522.
114. Harrop JS, Mohamed B, Bisson EF, et al. Congress of Neurological Surgeons systematic review and evidence-based guidelines for perioperative spine: Preoperative surgical risk assessment. *Neurosurgery.* 2021;89(Suppl 1):S9–S18.

3

Managing Medical Complications

ROBERT BRUCE METTER AND HEMALI PATEL

CHAPTER OUTLINE

Cardiovascular Complications

Myocardial Infarction

Myocardial infarction (MI) is a known complication of spinal surgeries, with one study of elective spinal fusions identifying an incidence of 0.36% during the initial hospitalization.[1] Typical symptoms include substernal chest pain, shoulder/arm pain, shortness of breath, diaphoresis, nausea, or vomiting. However, the presentation may be subtle, especially in patients with preexisting diabetes or neurologic disease. Often, tachycardia may be the only initial clue. The assessment should be prompt with an electrocardiogram (EKG) and troponin assay.[2,3] An elevated troponin with or without dynamic EKG changes, in the presence of clinical signs and symptoms, warrants internal medicine or cardiology consultation. The treatment of acute ST elevation myocardial (MI) (STEMI) or non-ST elevation MI type 1 (NSTEMI) includes antiplatelet agents (aspirin and GP IIa/IIIb inhibitors), anticoagulation (typically with heparin products), beta blockade, and the use of a statin. Risks of each need to be weighed with the postoperative bleeding risk. Emergent percutaneous revascularization is required for STEMI. Current United States guidelines do not recommend routine preoperative troponin testing as a baseline, or routine postoperative troponin testing in the absence of symptoms.[4] One additional consideration is a type 2 NSTEMI, defined as an MI resulting from mismatched myocardial oxygen supply and demand that is not related to unstable coronary artery disease. This can be seen with large blood losses during surgery or postoperative hypoxia among other conditions. Unlike NSTEMI type 1, this is managed by correcting the underlying condition.

Venous Thromboembolism

Deep venous thrombosis (DVT) and pulmonary embolism (PE) are the two most common forms of venous thromboembolism (VTE) after surgery. PE has been noted to occur as frequently as 1.4% of patients after spinal operations.[5] Symptoms of DVT include distal edema of the affected extremity, with or without pain. Symptoms of PE include dyspnea, chest pain (often pleuritic), and occasionally cough or hemoptysis or unexplained hypoxia. Diagnosis of extremity DVT is most commonly established via Doppler ultrasound, while diagnosis of PE is made with contrasted chest NT computer tomography (CT) or, less commonly, ventilation-perfusion lung scan. Once diagnosed, treatment should immediately be initiated with intravenous unfractionated heparin (UFH), low-molecular-weight heparin (LMWH), or direct oral anticoagulant (DOAC).[6] In patients with high risk for intraoperative blood loss, the physician may opt to start with UFH. The advantage is that it typically comes in drip form, which can quickly be stopped in the event that bleeding occurs. Anticoagulation with DOACs is now preferred over LMWH or vitamin K antagonists.[7] Duration is typically 3 to 6 months for a provoked VTE associated with surgery.

Hypotension

Hypotension after surgery has a wide differential, which includes sepsis, acute blood loss, PE, medications, cardiomyopathy, adrenal insufficiency, and other etiologies. Hypotension can be defined as mean arterial pressure less than 65 or evidence of end-organ hypoperfusion. Initial stabilization may include administration of urgent intravenous isotonic fluids (normal saline or lactated Ringer's), and vasopressor therapy if fluids do not have the desired effect. Evidence of end-organ hypoperfusion can include elevated lactate, decreased urine output, cool extremities, sluggish capillary refill on physical exam, or altered mentation. Workup should begin with a careful review of recent history, comorbidities, current and prior medications, vitals, exam, and lab work. Any localizing infectious symptoms or fever should prompt infectious evaluation. If concern for bleeding, a head to toe examination and hemoglobin level should be performed, although stable hemoglobin does not exclude acute bleeding. Medications such as opiates, muscle relaxants, and antihypertensives are common iatrogenic culprits. Adrenal insufficiency, often in the setting of chronic steroid use, is managed with stress dose steroids.

Infectious Complications

Postoperative Fever

Postoperative fever is common; a recent study noted incidence as high as 12.1% after lumbar spinal surgery.[8] Fever can be a normal physiologic response to cytokine release after surgery, especially if occurring in the first 24 hours after surgery.[9,10] Postoperative fever differential diagnoses can be generated based on timing of the fever: immediate postoperative (hours after surgery), early postoperative (through postoperative day [POD]#3), late postoperative (POD#4-30), or delayed (after 30 days); see Table 3.1 below.[11] Factors that increase likelihood of a secondary cause being present include multiple days febrile and fever occurring after POD#3.[12] Workup of postoperative fever should be symptom directed rather than automatic; blood cultures are often low-yield in the absence of prolonged high fever or other symptoms of bacteremia. Similarly, chest x-ray and urinalysis are low-yield in the absence of localizing infectious symptoms.[12] Of note, atelectasis is no longer considered a typical cause of postoperative fever.[13,14]

TABLE 3.1 Common Etiologies of Postoperative Fever as Stratified by Time of Onset from Surgery

Timing of Fever	Potential Etiologies
Immediate postoperative (hours)	Cytokines (normal inflammatory response) Preexisting infection Malignant hyperthermia Transfusion related
Early postoperative (<POD#3)	Cytokines (normal inflammatory response) Urinary tract infection Pneumonia Medications
Late postoperative (POD#3-#30)	Surgical site infection Urinary tract infection Venous thromboembolism (DVT or PE) Catheter-related bloodstream infection Medications
Delayed postoperative (>POD#30)	Surgical site infection Venous thromboembolism

UTI and CAUTI

Urinary tract infection (UTI) is the most common hospital-acquired infection and was found to be responsible for postoperative fever in up to a third of patients in one study.[9] Most commonly it presents 3 to 5 days after surgery. The daily risk of bacteriuria is 3% to 7% per day in patients with indwelling urinary catheters.[15] UTI is a clinical diagnosis requiring symptoms and urinalysis (UA) findings. Typical symptoms include: dysuria, urinary frequency, flank pain, fever, and/or suprapubic pain. Dysuria will not be manifest in patients with indwelling transurethral catheters (such as Foley) which makes diagnosis more difficult. UA shows pyuria (elevated white blood cell count), positive leukocyte esterase, and sometimes positive nitrite. UA and urine culture should always be obtained prior to antibiotics. They should be obtained via a clean catch urine sample or straight catheterization if necessary; drawing from indwelling transurethral catheters results in frequent contamination. Indwelling catheters should be removed prior to obtaining the UA. Blood cultures are not typically necessary unless the patient is septic or has high fever. Treatment of uncomplicated UTI is typically 3 days of appropriate antibiotics; refer to the institution's antibiogram or antimicrobial guidelines for appropriate medication selection. Complicated UTI involves one or more of the following: fever >37.7°C (threshold varies), features of systemic illness (such as chills, rigors, or malaise), flank pain, costovertebral angle tenderness, or pelvic or perineal pain in men.[15] Catheter-associated urinary tract infections or complicated UTIs (pyelonephritis) require 7 or more days of treatment and exchange of the urinary catheter. For unresolving UTI, consider repeat urine cultures to rule out resistant organism, or imaging with renal ultrasound or CT scan to evaluate for a perinephric abscess.

Pneumonia

Pneumonia is a common postoperative complication and has an incidence of 0.45% to 14%.[16] It is defined as either community acquired (CAP; occurring <48 hours after admission), hospital acquired (HAP; occurring >48 hours after admission), or ventilator associated (VAP; developing after endotracheal intubation). Pneumonia occurs when pathogens colonize the upper airway and are aspirated into the lower respiratory tract, usually in the setting of impaired host defenses. Risk factors for postoperative pneumonia include poor baseline lung function due to chronic disease such as chronic obstructive pulmonary disease (COPD), older age, and concurrent medical comorbidities such as diabetes.[16] Symptoms typically include cough (usually productive), fever, and dyspnea. Patients are typically hypoxic and may be septic. A chest x-ray usually reveals focal or diffuse consolidation, infiltrate, or ground-glass opacities. Sputum and blood cultures are recommended to guide antimicrobial therapy. In the absence of an identified pathogen, antimicrobial therapy is empiric and should be based on an institutional antibiogram considering regional epidemiology and resistance patterns in typical pathogens.[17] Patients with CAP are typically treated for at least 5 days, whereas HAP and VAP are typically treated for a minimum of 7 days.

Surgical Site Infection

Surgical site infections (SSIs) occur in about 2% to 2.5% of spinal surgeries.[18] The average time to presentation is about 17 days postoperatively and thus most patients have been discharged before they occur.[19] SSIs can present with increased drainage from surgical site (often purulent), surrounding erythema of the skin, pain, and sometimes fever. Treatment typically entails washout and debridement of the surgical bed, and operative cultures should always be sent. If the patient is stable, empiric antimicrobial therapy can be withheld until operative cultures are sent to maximize microbial yield. However, if the patient is septic or otherwise decompensated, antibiotics should be started immediately. Empiric therapy typically includes agents with activity against staphylococcus species including methicillin-resistant Staphylococcus aureus (MRSA) and other skin flora. Infectious disease specialist consultation is recommended. Once culture results are available, antibiotic therapy can be tailored to susceptibilities and treatment usually involves several weeks of intravenous antibiotics.

GI Complications

Constipation, Ileus, and Bowel Obstruction

Constipation, ileus, and bowel obstruction often occur on a continuum in postsurgical patients. Lumbar spinal surgery is associated with increased risk of ileus as compared to cervical or thoracic spinal surgery.[20] The type of procedure also impacts the risk of ileus; anterior approach places the patient at increased risk compared with posterior approaches. Postoperative patients should be assessed daily regarding bowel movements, passing of flatus, nausea, or emesis. Prevention is key with standing postoperative bowel regimens. Any patient on postoperative opioid therapy should have standing laxatives ordered. If constipation has developed, current laxatives may be increased in frequency or additional laxatives may be added. It is often effective to use a combination of different modality laxatives such as an osmotic agent like polyethylene glycol and a motility agent like senna. In more severe cases, suppositories and enemas may be required to remove distal stool blockages.

In contrast to physiologic postoperative ileus, which can last up to 3 days after surgery, prolonged postoperative ileus is defined as gut dysmotility extending to day 4 postoperatively or beyond.[21] Typical features include absence of bowel movements and hypoactive bowel sounds, with or without nausea or emesis. Bowel obstruction also results in absence of stool and flatus, but additionally patients may have tympanitic bowel sounds on exam, and imaging (typically CT with oral contrast) reveals a discrete point of obstruction. Treatment of prolonged postoperative ileus and small bowel obstruction is multimodal including bowel rest, intravenous hydration, reduction of all opiates and anticholinergic medications, and aggressive mobilization. Daily electrolytes, including potassium, magnesium, calcium, and phosphorus, should be monitored and replenished as necessary to optimize bowel muscle motility.[22,23] Nasogastric tube decompression is indicated in overt bowel obstruction, and in ileus as well if the patient has significant nausea, emesis, or abdominal distention. General surgical and/or gastroenterology consultation may be required if the ileus or obstruction fails to improve after several days.

Pulmonary Complications

Hypoxia and Respiratory Failure

Postoperative hypoxia has a broad differential including pneumonia, pulmonary embolism, pneumothorax, atelectasis, or pulmonary edema. Initial evaluation of the hypoxic patient should differentiate impending respiratory failure from stable hypoxia. High oxygen requirements (above 6 liters per minute), accessory muscle use, increased work of breathing, speaking in short sentences, or cyanosis should all prompt consideration for transfer to higher level of care such as stepdown or intensive care. Arterial blood gas and a chest x-ray should be obtained promptly in any decompensating respiratory patient.

Atelectasis

Atelectasis is a common cause of postoperative hypoxia. Patients who lie in bed in typical Fowler's position are prone to developing bibasilar atelectasis. Splinting due to pain, especially in spinal surgery patients, decreases vital capacity and promotes atelectasis. All postoperative spine surgery patients should have an incentive spirometer placed within reach at all times and be instructed in its use. Incentive spirometry should be performed at least five to six times per hour to help reduce atelectasis by opening lung alveoli. Contrary to outdated teachings, atelectasis is not a cause of postoperative fever.[13,24]

Pulmonary Embolism

Pulmonary embolus (PE) occurs when deep venous thrombosis (DVT) embolizes to the lungs. Typical symptoms include pleuritic chest pain, dyspnea, and occasionally hemoptysis. Findings on exam include tachycardia and hypoxia. A chest x-ray will often be clear and this finding in conjunction with significant hypoxia should raise concern for a PE. While patients in the ambulatory setting are often evaluated first with D-dimer, this test is largely unhelpful in postoperative patients as it will be elevated due to postoperative inflammation. A contrasted CT of the chest is the gold standard for diagnosis of PE; if contrast is contraindicated, a ventilation-perfusion scan can be obtained instead.[25] Troponin, brain-natriuretic peptide, and echocardiogram are used to risk-stratify PEs. Treatment entails systemic anticoagulation with either heparin (unfractionated or low-molecular weight), Coumadin, or direct oral anticoagulants.[7] If the risk of postoperative bleeding is high, heparin may be preferred initially because of its short half-life and easy reversibility. Once stable, the patient may be transitioned to an oral agent. A bilateral lower extremity venous ultrasound should be obtained to evaluate for DVT and a transthoracic echocardiogram may be indicated based on imaging, lab, and ECG findings.

Neurologic Complications

Postoperative Pain

Postoperative pain is an expected and omnipresent complication of any surgical procedure. Main principles of perioperative pain management include utilizing nonnarcotic analgesics whenever possible, consideration of patient-controlled analgesia, and avoiding prolonged opioid pain medication usage.[26] Nonnarcotic analgesia should be utilized in all patients and includes acetaminophen, NSAIDs, neuropathic pain medications, topical analgesics, and nerve blocks when able. Scheduled acetaminophen, in doses up to 4 grams daily (and up to 2 grams daily in liver disease), should be a baseline in any postoperative pain regimen. NSAIDs such as oral ibuprofen or naproxen, or intravenous ketorolac, are effective either scheduled or as needed, provided the (small) bleeding risk is acceptable to the surgeon. NSAIDs should be used with caution in patients with acute kidney injury or chronic kidney disease, history of peptic ulcer disease, or those already on blood thinners. Neuropathic pain medications such as gabapentin or pregabalin can be effective adjuncts and decrease the amount of opioids needed. Adjunctive medications such as duloxetine or tricyclic antidepressants such as amitriptyline are other slower-onset neuropathic agents.[27] Nerve blocks can be considered if pain is localized.

Delirium

Risk factors for postoperative delirium include elderly age, multiple comorbidities, opioid and anticholinergic medications, duration of surgery, type of anesthesia, intensive care unit level of care, and underlying cognitive impairment among others.[28] Delirium can develop at any time during the hospitalization and contributes to longer length of stay and morbidity.[29,30] Diagnosis of delirium is clinical, and tools such as the Confusion Assessment Method (CAM) are useful. Workup should include a thorough physical exam, assessment of indwelling devices and tethers, medication review (both as-needed and scheduled) with attention to opioids, anticholinergics, benzodiazepines, and other Beers criteria medications.[31] Polypharmacy is frequently a cause of postoperative delirium, and offending medications should be discontinued. The possible presence of an infection should be assessed. Metabolic etiologies such as thyroid pathologies, hyperglycemia, and hepatic encephalopathy should be investigated. Hypercarbia can be assessed with a blood gas analysis. Full neurologic exam should be performed to exclude stroke. If the infectious, toxic/metabolic, and neurologic workup is unrevealing, a diagnosis of hospital-acquired delirium can be made. Treatment consists of supportive care and includes the removal of offending medications; removal of nonnecessary lines, catheters, and telemetry; frequent reorientation and early mobilization; maximizing day/night cycle cues; correcting any metabolic or electrolyte disturbances if present; and treating any infection if present. Resolution of delirium may take up to 24 to 48 hours to occur.

Genitourinary Complications

Urinary Retention

Acute urinary retention is diagnosed often in postoperative patients when the postvoid residual (PVR) volume in the bladder is greater than 350 to 400 milliliters. Patients should be straight catheterized to avoid urinary stasis, which can lead to urinary tract infection, bladder distention, delirium, and even rarely bladder rupture. Efforts should be made to preferentially utilize intermittent straight catheterization over the placement of indwelling transurethral catheters when possible, as indwelling catheters pose higher risk of catheter-associated UTI (CAUTI). In patients with urinary retention, PVR should be monitored frequently, at least every 6 to 8 hours. If patients require frequent intermittent catheterization, transurethral catheter placement may be necessary for a time. Common etiologies of postoperative urinary retention include: opioid pain medications, anticholinergic medications, constipation, immobility. Risk factors include preexisting prostatic hyperplasia and chronic urinary retention.

Acute Kidney Injury

Acute kidney injury (AKI) is defined when any of the following three criteria are met: a 50% increase in creatinine over 7 days, an increase in serum creatinine by >0.3 mg/dL in 48 hours, or oliguria.[32] Etiologies can be classified into prerenal, intrinsic, or postrenal. Prerenal etiologies include those that result in poor perfusion of the kidneys, including intra- or perioperative hypotension, decompensated heart or liver failure, severe dehydration, or sepsis.[33] Intrinsic causes include acute interstitial nephritis, acute tubular necrosis, and are often medication related. Postrenal causes include obstructive etiologies such as urinary blockage due to renal stones, or benign prostatic hyperplasia (BPH). Standard initial workup for AKI includes a complete urinalysis, urine electrolytes and creatinine, postvoid residual, and often a renal ultrasound. If a prerenal etiology such as hypotension or dehydration is suspected, intravenous fluids are the mainstay of treatment.[34] Early medical consultation and/or renal consultation is advised due to the myriad of potential etiologies for AKI.

Endocrine Complications

Adrenal Insufficiency

Patients with chronic adrenal insufficiency should receive stress dose steroids starting the day of surgery, based on the intensity of the procedure. For smaller procedures, doubling the outpatient chronic steroid dose may be sufficient. For more complex procedures, intravenous hydrocortisone can be used, starting immediately preoperatively at 50–100 mg every 8 hours, and continuing for 24 to 48 hours postop followed by a taper over 1 to 2 days back to the home replacement dose. Patients should be closely monitored perioperatively for signs of adrenal crisis including hypotension, nausea and emesis, abdominal pain, severe weakness, or encephalopathy. Adrenal crisis and/or insufficiency should be considered on the differential for any perioperative patient with unexplained hypotension, especially those previously receiving significant (≥20 mg/day) doses of steroids for longer than a month or chronic opiate use. A timed 8:00 a.m. cortisol level can be used as initial screening test for those suspected of having adrenal insufficiency, and if low, the diagnosis should be confirmed by an adrenocorticotropic hormone (ACTH) stimulation test. Internal medicine consultation should be considered in patients needing stress dose steroids, or who are suspected of having new or chronic adrenal insufficiency.

Hyperglycemia and Diabetic Ketoacidosis/Hyperosmolar Hyperglycemic State

For patients with diabetes, postoperative inflammation can often lead to hyperglycemia and difficult glucose control. Outpatient oral antihyperglycemic medications are typically held on admission prior to surgery, and patients are managed on insulin therapy while admitted due to inconsistent dietary intake. Inpatient glycemic goals are generally <180. Severe hyperglycemia can result in osmotic diuresis, increase risk of infection, and impaired wound healing. Tighter glycemic goals are not associated with improved outcomes and may result in medical complications such as syncope or cardiovascular events.[35] Patients on long-acting insulin should have it continued during admission; dosage reduction can be considered in those anticipated to have poor oral intake. In rare cases, surgery or another stimulus such as infection may precipitate diabetic ketoacidosis (DKA) or hyperosmolar hyperglycemic state (HHS). DKA occurs predominantly in type 1 diabetics and is characterized by hyperglycemia (typically in the hundreds), anion gap metabolic acidosis, and elevated urine and serum ketones, and is the result of inadequate insulin production leading to ketogenesis. HHS, in contrast, occurs predominantly in type 2 diabetics and is characterized by even more severe hyperglycemia (typically in high hundreds to thousands), lack of anion gap acidosis, severe dehydration and encephalopathy. The presence of either of these syndromes should prompt emergent internal medicine consultation, initiation of intravenous insulin infusion, and transfer to a critical care location.

Hematologic Complications

Bleeding

In the setting of postsurgical bleeding, the patient should be screened for coagulopathies with prothrombin time (PT) and activated partial thromboplastin time (aPTT). The platelet count should be checked as well. The medication administration record should be checked for the presence of anticoagulants, aspirin, NSAIDs, supplements, or other medications that can increase bleeding risk.

Thrombocytopenia

Isolated thrombocytopenia can be a sign of inadequate production, consumption, or sequestration of platelets. An acute drop postoperatively from a normal baseline is most commonly due to platelet consumption associated with postoperative hemostasis, but can also be caused by destructive conditions such as heparin-induced thrombocytopenia (HIT), disseminated intravascular coagulopathy (DIC) or idiopathic thrombocytopenic purpura (ITP), among others. Persistently dropping platelet counts greater than 2 to 3 days after surgery, or severe thrombocytopenia (<20) should prompt further workup. Workup should include peripheral smear to assess for platelet clumping (pseudothrombocytopenia) as well as PT and partial thromboplastin time (PTT), assessment of medications that can cause thrombocytopenia, and potentially a HIT assay if pretest probability is moderate-high as measured by the 4T score. Concurrent coagulopathy and/or evidence of schistocytes and microangiopathic hemolytic anemia on the peripheral blood smear should raise suspicion for DIC.

References

1. Arena PJ, Mo J, Liu Q, et al. The incidence of acute myocardial infarction after elective spinal fusions or joint replacement surgery in the United States: a large-scale retrospective observational cohort study in 322,585 patients. *Patient Saf Surg.* 2021;15:30.
2. O'Gara PT, Kushner FG, Ascheim DD, et al. 2013 ACCF/AHA guideline for the management of ST-elevation myocardial infarction: a report of the American College of Cardiology Foundation/American Heart Association Task Force on Practice Guidelines. *J Am Coll Cardiol.* 2013;61:e78–e140.
3. Amsterdam EA, Wenger NK, Brindis RG, et al. 2014 AHA/ACC guideline for the management of patients with Non–ST-elevation acute coronary syndromes: A report of the American College of Cardiology/American Heart Association Task Force on practice guidelines. *Circulation.* 2014;130:e344–e426.
4. Fleisher LA, Fleischmann KE, Auerbach AD, et al. 2014 ACC/AHA guideline on perioperative cardiovascular evaluation and management of patients undergoing noncardiac surgery: Executive summary: A report of the American College of Cardiology/American Heart Association Task Force on practice guidelines. *Circulation.* 2014;130:2215–2245.
5. Lee MJ, Konodi MA, Cizik AM, et al. Risk factors for medical complication after spine surgery: a multivariate Analysis of 1,591 patients. *Spine J.* 2021;12(3):197–206.
6. Kearon C, Akl EA, Comerota AJ, et al. Antithrombotic therapy for VTE disease: Antithrombotic Therapy and Prevention of Thrombosis, 9th ed: American College of Chest Physicians Evidence-Based Clinical Practice Guideline. *Chest.* 2012;141(2 Suppl):e419S–e496S.
7. Stevens SM, Woller SC, Kreuziger LB, et al. Antithrombotic therapy for VTE disease: Second update of the CHEST Guideline and Expert Panel Report. *Chest.* 2021;160(6):e545–e608.
8. Mayo BC, Haws BE, Bohl DD, et al. Postoperative fever evaluation following lumbar fusion procedures. *Neurospine.* 2018; 15(2):154–162.
9. Garibaldi RA, Brodine S, Matsumiya S, et al. Evidence for the non-infectious etiology of early postoperative fever. *Infect Control.* 1985;6:273–277.
10. Andres BM, Taub DD, Gurkan I, et al. Postoperative fever after total knee arthroplasty: the role of cytokines. *Clin Orthop Relat Res.* 2003;415:221–231.
11. Narayan M, Medinilla SP. Fever in the postoperative patient. *Emerg Med Clin North Am.* 2013;31:1045–1058.
12. Ward DT, Hansen EN, Takemoto SK, et al. Cost and effectiveness of postoperative fever diagnostic evaluation in total joint arthroplasty patients. *J Arthroplasty.* 2010;25((6) Suppl):43–48.
13. Crompton JG, Crompton PD, Matzinger M. Does atelectasis cause fever after surgery? Putting a damper on dogma. *JAMA Surg.* 2019;154(5):375–376.
14. Engoren M. Lack of association between atelectasis and fever. *Chest.* 1995;107:81–84.
15. Hooton TM, Bradley SF, Cardenas DD, et al. Diagnosis, prevention and treatment of catheter-associated urinary tract infection in adults: 2009 International Clinical Practice Guidelines from the Infectious Diseases Society of America. *Clin Infect Dis.* 2010;50:625–663.
16. Chughtai M, Gwam CU, Mohamed N, et al. The epidemiology and risk factors for postoperative pneumonia. *J Clin Med Res.* 2017;9(6):466–475.
17. Kalil AC, Metersky ML, Klompas M, et al. Management of adults with hospital-acquired and ventilator-associated pneumonia: 2016 Clinical Practice Guidelines by the Infectious Diseases Society of America and the American Thoracic Society. *Clin Inf Dis.* 2016;63(5):e61–e111.
18. Swan MC, Hoes KS, Aoun SG, et al. Postoperative complications of spine surgery. *Best Pract Res Clin Anaesthesiol.* 2016;30: 103–120.
19. Bohl DD, Webb ML, Lukasiewicz AM, et al. Timing of complications after spinal fusion surgery. *Spine.* 2015;40(19):1527e35.
20. Fineberg SJ, Nandyala SV, Kurd MF, et al. Incidence and risk factors for postoperative ileus following anterior, posterior, and circumferential lumbar fusion. *Spine J.* 2014;14(8):1680e5.
21. Vather R, Trivedi S, Bissett I. Defining postoperative ileus: Results of a systematic review and global survey. *J Gastrointest Surg.* 2013;17:962–972.
22. Luckey A, Livingston E, Tache Y. Mechanisms and treatment of postoperative ileus. *Arch Surg.* 2003;138:206–214.
23. Mattei P, Rombeau JL. Review of the pathophysiology and management of postoperative ileus. *World J Surg.* 2006;30:1382–1391.
24. Mavros MN, Velmahos GC, Falagas ME, et al. Atelectasis as a cause of postoperative fever: where is the clinical evidence? *Chest.* 2011;140(2):418–424.
25. Konstantinides SV, Meyer G, Becattini C, et al. 2019 ESC Guidelines for the diagnosis and management of acute pulmonary embolism developed in collaboration with the European Respiratory Society (ERS). *Eur Heart J.* 2020;41:543–603.
26. Chou R, Gordon DB, de Leon-Casasola OA, et al. Management of postoperative pain: A clinical practice guideline from the American Pain Society, the American Society of Regional Anesthesia and Pain Medicine, and the American Society of Anesthesiologists' Commitee on Regional Anesthesia, Executive Commitee, and Administrative Council. *J Pain.* 2016;17(2):131–157.
27. Dale R, Chen T, Ballantyne J. Planning for perioperative pain management. *Hosp Med Clin.* 2016;5:303–318.
28. Bilotta F, Lauretta MP, Borozdina A, et al. Postoperative delirium: risk factors, diagnosis and perioperative care. *Minerva Anestesiol.* 2013;79(9):1066–1076.
29. Kirfel A, Menzenbach J, Guttenthaler V, et al. Postoperative delirium after cardiac surgery of elderly patients as an independent risk factor for prolonged length of stay in intensive care unit and in hospital. *Aging Clin Exp Res.* 2021;33:3047–3056.
30. Dziegielewski C, Skead C, Canturk T, et al. Delirium and associated length of stay and costs in critically ill patients. *Crit Care Res Pract.* 2021;2021:1–8.
31. Fick DM, Semla TP, Steinman M, et al. American Geriatrics Society 2019 Updated AGS Beers Criteria for potentially inappropriate medication use in older adults. *J Am Geriatr Soc.* 2019; 67(4):674–694.
32. Kellum JA, Lameire N, KDIGO AKI. Diagnosis, evaluation, and management of acute kidney injury: a KDIGO summary (Part 1) Guideline Work Group. *Crit Care.* 2013;17:204.
33. Calvert S, Shaw A. Perioperative acute kidney injury. *Perioper Med.* 2012;1:6.
34. Prowle JR, Forni LG, Bell M, et al. Postoperative acute kidney injury in adult non-cardiac surgery: joint consensus report of the Acute Disease Quality Initiative and PeriOperatie Quality Initiative. *Nat Rev Nephrol.* 2021;17:605–618.
35. Finfer S, Chittock DR, Su SY, et al. Intensive versus conventional glucose control in critically ill patients. *N Engl J Med.* 2009;360(13):1283–1297.

4 Avoiding Complications in Pain Management Before and After Spine Surgery

MARCO A. URIBE AND JUSTIN S. MERKOW

CHAPTER OUTLINE

Introduction

Pain management in spine surgery patients can be uniquely challenging. These patients have complex pain patterns, often suffer from an extensive history of chronic pain, and may have considerable disability. For these reasons, they are vulnerable to pain complications in the perioperative realm. In this chapter we will explore complications related to pain and how to prevent them. We will divide this chapter into preoperative and postoperative considerations and will not cover intraoperative management or complications.

First, it is important to define opioid tolerance (OT) and opioid-induced hyperalgesia (OIH), as spine patients are often on or have previously been on chronic opioids. Mitigating these phenomena will be an underlying thread throughout the chapter. Opioid tolerance is defined as a physiologic adaptation in response to opioid exposure that results in lessening of the drug effects over time. Opioid-induced hyperalgesia, on the other hand, is defined as an increased sensitivity to painful stimuli secondary to opioid use. These conditions can be easily confused but have their own characteristics and mechanisms that are outlined in Table 4.1. The physiological changes resulting from chronic opioid use puts patients at an increased risk of perioperative pain complications. The primary treatment for both OT and OIH is weaning or discontinuing opioids.

Preoperative

The preoperative period is critical, not only in limiting preoperative issues, but also preventing postoperative complications. One of the key aspects of pain management prior to spine surgery is early identification of patients suffering from significant pain. A proactive interdisciplinary approach is essential in these patients. Current guidelines on the management of perioperative pain recommend a thorough preoperative evaluation including pain history, physical examination, review of current medications, and an assessment for psychiatric and substance abuse disorders. Evidence tells us that there is a strong correlation between presurgical mental health status and the postoperative resolution of pain and improved function.[1] Online prescription drug monitoring program databases should also be reviewed.

Multimodal Pain Therapy

Multimodal pain relief is a critical aspect of the perioperative management of spine patients. Decades ago, Kehlet and Dahl established the benefits of not relying on a single class of medication to treat pain and initiated the movement to "multimodal" or "balanced analgesia."[2] A multimodal

TABLE 4.1 **Opioid tolerance vs. opioid-induced hyperalgesia.**

	Opiod Tolerance (OT)	Opioid-Induced Hyperalgesia (OIH)
Definition	Diminishing effect over time secondary to exposure	Increasing sensitivity to pain stimuli secondary to exposure
Mechanism	Desensitization of receptors	Activation of pronociceptive circuits
	Internalized opioid receptors, changes in signaling proteins and receptor phosphorylation	Potentiated NMDA receptors, increased levels of CCK, spinal dynorphin, and neuroinflammatory mediators
Similarities	Develop secondary to a period of opioid exposure	
	Clinically obvious decreased analgesic effect of opioids	
Clinical Signs	Pain is limited to the original site of injury	Spreading of pain location and pattern
	Progressive diminishing response to opioids that can only be overcome with escalating the dose or frequency	Paradoxically increased pain with increased opioid dose and duration
		Allodynia-increased response to nonpainful stimuli

approach combines medications from different drug classes that work together, synergistically to alleviate pain while minimizing side effects from any single drug class.[3] The goal of using a multimodal regimen is to limit uncontrolled preoperative pain and also help with intraoperative and postoperative pain control. Further studies are required to elucidate an effective preoperative multimodal pain regimen specific for spine surgery.[4] However, a balanced preoperative multimodal pain regimen should focus on each of the different classifications of pain (nociceptive, neuropathic, inflammatory, and dysfunctional). Basic regimens commonly include therapies like acetaminophen, nonsteroidal anti-inflammatory drugs (NSAIDs), and various neuropathic pain medications.

Acetaminophen

Acetaminophen is a mainstay of multimodal pain therapy and a frequently used option for spine patients preoperatively. It is effective at treating nociceptive pain and a single preoperative dose of acetaminophen has shown to reduce postoperative pain, opioid use, and nausea.[4,5] While available in oral and parenteral formulations, recent studies have found no difference between the two when dosed preoperatively in postoperative opioid consumption.[6] The first dose is often administered preoperatively and is typically scheduled for patients with 1 gram every 6 hours with caution to not exceed 4 g/day. With chronic use some recommend not exceeding 3 g/day.

NSAIDs

NSAIDs have also been reviewed in-depth for perioperative pain management, and their side effects are a frequent topic of controversy. In a large retrospective study of total joint patients, Memtsoudis et al. found that NSAIDs resulted in the greatest decrease in postoperative complications when compared to other common multimodal analgesics.[7] The primary mechanism of action of NSAIDs is inhibition of COX enzymes and prostaglandin synthesis to inhibit inflammatory pathways. This collectively leads to decreased inflammatory and nociceptive signaling.

There are a number of different types of NSAIDs, but more broadly there are nonselective NSAIDs and COX-2-specific inhibitors. Nonselective NSAIDs carry a risk of GI ulcer formation and platelet dysfunction and most are relatively contraindicated in the setting of renal insufficiency, GI bleeding, reduced cardiac output, and uncontrolled hypertension. The COX-2 inhibitor class of NSAIDs are very useful for patients who have a history of GI ulcers or bleeding as they do not carry as high a risk in causing such issues. Table 4.2 summarizes some of the NSAIDs frequently used for a multimodal analgesia, and their suggested dosing. Data regarding stopping NSAIDs prior to surgery and when to re-start are limited and up to the discretion of the surgeon.

Neuropathic Agents

Spine patients being evaluated for surgery are frequently suffering from neuropathic pain resulting from spinal stenosis, nerve compression, or pain sensitization. Neuropathic medications like gabapentin and pregabalin are commonly prescribed and may be efficacious if titrated to therapeutic levels prior to surgery. In the past, providers have given a single dose of gabapentin preoperatively, as there has been some evidence it may improve postoperative pain.[8–10] Recently this has come into question with a newer study by Ohnuma et al. showing that exposure to gabapentin at any dose on the day of total hip or knee replacement was associated with minimal effects on perioperative opioid consumption, and more alarmingly with a dose-dependent increased odds of pulmonary complications.[11] We therefore caution providers regarding the use of one-time preoperative gabapentin dosing, and rather recommend having patients on a steady dose for a longer duration prior to surgery.

TABLE 4.2 Suggested preoperative and postoperative multimodal analgesic doses.

Class	Drug	Route	Suggested Dosing	Comments
Analgesic	Acetaminophen	PO/IV	*If >50 kg*: Preoperative: 1000 mg Postoperative: 1000 mg q6h	Maximum recommended daily dose is 4 g
NSAID (nonselective COX inhibitor)	Ibuprofen	PO	Preoperative: 600 to 800 mg Postoperative: 600 mg q6h	Use with caution in patients with GI ulcers, kidney disease, or coagulopathy
	Ketorolac	PO/IV/IM	Preoperative: 15 to 30 mg Postoperative: 15 to 30 mg q6h	
COX-2 selective inhibitor	Celecoxib (COX-2)	PO	Preoperative: 400 mg Postoperative: 200 mg q12h	Increases risk of MI, avoid in congestive heart failure
	Meloxicam (COX-2)	PO	Preoperative: 15 mg Postoperative: 7.5 to 15 mg q24h	
Gabapentinoid	Gabapentin	PO	Preoperative: 600 to 1200 mg Postoperative: 300 to 1200 mg q8h (must slowly uptitrate)	Can cause sedation, especially in elderly
	Pregabalin	PO	Preoperative: 150 mg Postoperative: 75 mg q12h	

Regional Anesthesia

The use of various preoperative regional anesthetic techniques have been described for spine surgery. Epidural catheters have been placed before and during spine surgery and showed great efficacy in managing perioperative pain, but each demonstrated unique challenges and complications. Because spine surgery incurs the risk of damage to the dura mater, there is a dangerous risk of intrathecal administration of local anesthetic through epidural catheters should this happen. For this reason, a regional anesthetic technique that is performed away from the neuraxial space is necessary for the spine surgery population.

A relatively new ultrasound-guided block that shows similar analgesic efficacy to epidural techniques is the erector spinae plane (ESP) block.[12] Recent studies have shown that ESP blocks reduced postoperative opioid requirements and improved patient satisfaction when compared to traditional analgesia in lumbar spine surgery.[13] The technique is procedurally simple, and with the use of an ultrasound it is relatively safe from injury to the spinal cord or pleura. It also does not cause the sympathectomy that is incurred with epidural or paravertebral blocks, thus imparting greater hemodynamic stability. Additionally, the block can be performed with the placement of an indwelling catheter that can offer continuous administration of local anesthetic for prolonged analgesic coverage. Some institutions have begun to offer this regional intervention prior to select spine surgeries, and it is worth considering with your acute pain service.

Chronic Opioid Use and Weaning

One of the most critical aspects of the preoperative management of spine surgery patients is addressing chronic opioid use if it exists. A multimodal medication approach as discussed above is one key strategy to accomplish this. Weaning patients' chronic opioids is difficult but often critical, especially if on high doses. This is designed to limit OT and OIH. It has been shown in multiple studies that limiting and/or weaning opioids in orthopedic and spine patients improves postoperative outcomes. A systematic review of preoperative opioid use and clinical outcomes in spine surgery found that preoperative opioid consumption was overwhelmingly associated with negative surgical and functional outcomes.[14,15] A retrospective review of patients on chronic opioid therapy before cervical spine fusion found that these patients were at increased risk for wound complications, emergency department (ED) visits, postoperative interventional pain treatment, repeat cervical fusions, and long-term opioid use.[16] While no clinical trials are published to date, it may be advisable to encourage weaning prior to surgery particularly for patients taking more than 90 morphine milligram equivalents daily.[17] Weaning does take time and considerable effort, but surgery can be a significant motivator to decrease or wean off these medications.

Another perioperative challenge and source of complications is with chronic pain or addiction patients undergoing treatment with medications such as Suboxone, methadone, and naltrexone. These medications can be extremely effective and even lifesaving, although they certainly pose a perioperative challenge. We will go through each medication and the recommended preoperative approach to patients taking them here.

Methadone

Methadone is a synthetic opioid agonist that works to eliminate withdrawal symptoms, relieve drug cravings, and treat chronic pain by acting on the same opioid receptors in the brain that are activated by other opioid pain medications or heroin. Although activating the same receptors, it does so in a slower and more controlled manner so that when given to an opioid-dependent patient, treatment does not produce any feelings of euphoria. An effective daily dose of methadone for addiction can vary from 60 to 120 mg/d, but higher doses are not uncommon. The optimal daily dose for a patient should successfully suppress withdrawal symptoms, eliminate cravings, and have minimal side effects. Methadone dosing for chronic pain is considerably smaller and administered multiple times per day as the analgesic effect is shorter lasting than the effect on drug craving.

Preoperatively and on day of surgery, the patient's daily outpatient methadone dose should be continued after confirmation of the dosage with the outpatient treatment program or prescriber. It is important to note that the patient's daily dose will undoubtedly be insufficient to provide acute pain relief in the postoperative setting and additional medications and strategies will be required to manage their acute pain. These patients will likely have significant opioid tolerance. In the preoperative setting, clinicians should consider early implementation of multimodal pain strategies and inpatient acute pain and/or addiction medicine consults as clinically indicated. Early education and communication of expectations with the patient, methadone prescriber, and support persons are critical. There should be a low threshold to have these patients evaluated in a preoperative anesthesia clinic.

Suboxone

Suboxone is a mixture of buprenorphine and naloxone and is also used to treat opiate addiction as well as chronic pain. Buprenorphine is a partial agonist at the mu receptor and an antagonist at the kappa receptor. It has a high affinity to its receptor targets. If given during withdrawal (while the mu receptors are unoccupied), buprenorphine will relieve withdrawal symptoms by its opioid agonist effect. If taken during a euphoric state (while mu receptors are occupied with a full agonist such as heroin), buprenorphine's high affinity will uncouple and replace the full agonist causing a decrease in the full agonist effect. This produces a precipitated withdrawal. The other component of Suboxone, naloxone, is an opioid antagonist that antagonizes opioid effects by competing for the same receptor sites and essentially reversing the effects of opioids. Naloxone is added in combination with the buprenorphine to decrease the likelihood of diversion and misuse. This is because when the product is taken as prescribed as sublingual tablets, buprenorphine's partial agonism dominates the naloxone effect. However, if the sublingual tablets are crushed and injected (misused), the naloxone reversal effect dominates and can bring on opioid withdrawal.

Treatment with Suboxone is usually started with 2 to 4 mg and can be increased to 8 to 12 mg over the subsequent 24 hours. Like methadone, it is often dosed once daily for addiction while multiple times per day for chronic pain. The effective dose of buprenorphine is typically around 8 to 24 mg/day. At therapeutic levels, buprenorphine occupies mu receptors and prevents other full agonists from binding if used concurrently, thus blocking the euphoric effect of the full agonists. A dose of 16 mg of buprenorphine blocks over 80% of mu receptors. There is an alarming potential for uncontrolled postoperative pain in patients continued on high buprenorphine doses because of its receptor binding affinity, long half-life, and partial agonism that can block or limit the analgesic effects of traditional opioids.[18] For this reason, the critical question for clinicians is whether Suboxone should be altered preoperatively to achieve effective analgesia.

Several options exist when formulating a plan for perioperative management of patients on Suboxone. This includes continuing Suboxone therapy, decreasing the dose, or holding Suboxone therapy for a defined period with or without bridging to alternative opioids. There is no current evidence that one strategy provides superior postoperative pain control for spine surgery specifically, but interruption of Suboxone may result in harm including failure to return to baseline Suboxone doses, continuation of non-Suboxone opioids, or relapse of opioid use disorder. Additionally, stopping Suboxone or buprenorphine therapy will cause a significant opioid debt that will need to be filled with another opioid, risking overdosing or underdosing. This is problematic in the postoperative period and potentially increases the risk of complications as well as prolonging hospital length of stay. A systematic review and meta-analysis found that the risk of mortality is considerably higher after discontinuing buprenorphine treatment.[19] Given the mounting evidence of favorable outcomes from patients continuing Suboxone and receiving adjunct opioid therapy perioperatively, we do not recommend discontinuing Suboxone in the preoperative period.[20]

By continuing Suboxone preoperatively, patients are maintained on stable doses of Suboxone throughout the perioperative period without fluctuations in the serum levels of the drug and without an increased logistical burden on the patients or providers. Patient's acute pain can be treated with multimodal analgesia and high-dose short-acting opioids can be used to overcome buprenorphine's strong mu receptor affinity. For patients on high-dose Suboxone, some institutions recommend tapering the dose preoperatively to 12 to 16 mg/day 2 to 3 days prior to surgery to provide more mu receptor availability.[21] This approach has not been formally studied although receptor binding studies in buprenorphine-treated heroin-addicted volunteers confirmed a dose–response curve of reduced but conserved receptors available for additional analgesia, even at high sublingual doses of buprenorphine.[22] Which opioids to use for additional analgesia has also not been formally studied, but using agents with high mu receptor affinity like sufentanil, fentanyl, or hydromorphone should be considered.

Naltrexone

Naltrexone is an opioid antagonist and competitively binds to opioid mu receptors, thus blocking the effect of endogenous and exogenous opioids. Naltrexone is available as both an oral formulation and as a monthly intramuscular injectable. After naltrexone is started, an increase in the density of opioid receptors develops and therefore an increase in the patient's sensitivity to the effects of opioids if naltrexone is discontinued. Current recommendations are for those on oral formulation to undergo a 72-hour washout period after the last dose and before the date of surgery. Patients on the intramuscular monthly injectable formulation should be scheduled for surgery at least 4 weeks after the last injection of the extended-release naltrexone. If surgery were to be performed while the patient is on injectable naltrexone, higher doses of opioids will likely be required to overcome the opioid blockade caused by naltrexone. However, if naltrexone is no longer occupying those receptors, opioids can elicit an exaggerated response due to the receptor upregulation and result in increased sensitivity. Given these possibilities of an altered response to opioids, a preoperative consult with a preoperative anesthesia clinic, pain or addiction specialist can be very informative.

Psychological Issues

Finally, addressing psychological comorbidities preoperatively is essential. This should be done early on as adequate management of psychiatric comorbidities takes time. Patients should be assessed and those at risk for chronic post-surgical pain—with uncontrolled depression, anxiety, pain catastrophizing, or other mental health issues—should be referred to the appropriate providers. This may include discussion with the patients primary care physician (PCP) or referral to a psychologist or psychiatrist. Systematic reviews of psychiatric risk factors for chronic post-surgical pain have demonstrated a positive predictive value of presurgical depression and chronic stress on risk of persistent pain following surgery.[23] Theunissen et al. found that patients with pre-surgical anxiety and pain catastrophizing are approximately twice as likely to go on to develop chronic postoperative pain.[24]

There are many psychology-focused therapies that can be helpful for these patients. Modalities such as biofeedback, relaxation techniques, cognitive behavioral therapy, and mindfulness have been shown to play an important role in pain management.[25] Preoperative education, relaxation, guided imagery, and clinical hypnosis have also been shown to improve postsurgical outcomes, reduce postoperative pain, opioid consumption, and length of stay.[26]

Postoperative

While pain is common and expected after surgery due to the inherent tissue damage with surgical procedures, it can be inadequately controlled in some patients despite excellent management. This is particularly true for spine surgery, as it is often associated with especially high levels of pain in the acute postoperative period compared to other surgeries. In a review of 179 surgical procedures, lumbar fusion (1 to 2 levels), lumbar fusion (greater than or equal to 3 levels), and complex spine reconstruction surgeries comprised three of the top six procedures ranked for highest pain scores on postoperative day one.[27] It has also been well proven that poorly controlled pain can cause reduced mobility that can in turn lead to postoperative complications like deep vein thrombosis, pulmonary embolus, and pneumonia. Quality and effective pain control in the postoperative period has been shown to be associated with improved surgical outcomes, reduced hospital stays, and decreased development of new chronic pain conditions.[28] Therefore, it is critical to be prepared for pain control in the postoperative period following spine surgery. Although the preoperative recommendations outlined previously are critical to optimize outcomes, there are important considerations in the postoperative period.

While there is good evidence that supports many of the common agents utilized in multimodal pain therapy regimens, there is a lack of evidence regarding optimal postoperative protocols or pathways to manage pain after spine surgery. Multimodal pain therapy arrangements that concurrently target pain pathways at different sites using distinctive mechanisms are linked with superior pain relief and less opioid consumption.[28] Opioid analgesics are often first-line agents in postoperative pain management, but overuse can lead to a list of adverse effects including: somnolence, confusion, urinary retention, ileus, respiratory depression, addiction, and even death. The goal of a multimodal regimen in the postoperative setting is to avoid these complications by limiting opioid requirements. Additionally, a multidisciplinary effort may be helpful to find an agreement regarding perioperative treatment protocols at the institutional level. Surgeons, anesthesiologists, pain management physicians, pharmacists, nurses, and physical therapists should optimally come together to organize a spine surgery specific approach.

Regardless of the institution's perioperative protocol for pain control, some basic concepts should always be reviewed in the postoperative setting. When the patient is able to tolerate PO medications, be sure to restart their baseline preoperative medications and then supplement additional multimodal therapies as well as short-acting opioids for acute breakthrough pain. As discussed previously, continue Suboxone or methadone in the postoperative setting. It may be advised to divide patient's methadone dose frequency into twice a day or three times a day dosing for better pain control. High-dose naltrexone, however, should be held until the patient is no longer requiring opioids. For patients on Suboxone, methadone, or naltrexone, it would be prudent for the primary surgical service to coordinate care at discharge with the prescribing provider.

At times, even with excellent pre- and postoperative management strategies, patients still experience uncontrolled pain in the postoperative setting. Rather than escalating the doses of acute acting opioids to dangerous levels, providers should first seek advice from their institution's acute pain, addiction medicine, or other pain consulting services. These provider teams can often offer alternative interventional techniques or pharmacologic strategies like ketamine or lidocaine infusions for severe situations. The mechanism of these medications is beyond the scope of this chapter, but it is important to consider that these therapies may require the patient to be escalated to higher levels of care for closer monitoring.

Conclusion

Spine surgery patients pose a unique challenge in terms of optimizing pain control and mitigating perioperative pain-related complications. The importance of early preoperative planning for at-risk patients cannot be understated. Postoperative strategies including use of a multimodal medication approach is also critical. Ultimately, when faced with challenging pain, we suggest eliciting the help of inpatient acute pain, addiction medicine if relevant, and coordinating with the patient's outpatient medical team.

References

1. Jaiswal P, Railton P, Khong H, Smith C, Powell J. Impact of preoperative mental health status on functional outcome 1 year after total hip arthroplasty. *Can J Surg.* 2019;6(5):300–304.
2. Kehlet H, Dahl JB. The value of "multimodal" or "balanced analgesia" in postoperative pain treatment. *Anesth Analg.* 1993;77(5):1048–1056.
3. Wenzel JT, Schwenk ES, Baratta JL, Viscusi ER. Managing opioid-tolerant patients in the perioperative surgical home. *Anesthesiol Clin.* 2016;34(2):287–301.
4. Maheshwari K, Avitsian R, Sessler DI, et al. Multimodal analgesic regimen for spine surgery. *Anesthesiology.* 2020;132(5):992–1002.
5. Apfel CC, Turan A, Souza K, Pergolizzi J, Hornuss C. Intravenous acetaminophen reduces postoperative nausea and vomiting: A systematic review and meta-analysis. *Pain.* 2013;154(5):677–689.
6. Cain KE, Iniesta MD, Fellman BM, et al. Effect of preoperative intravenous vs oral acetaminophen on postoperative opioid consumption in an enhanced recovery after surgery (ERAS) program in patients undergoing open gynecologic oncology surgery. *Gynecol Oncol.* 2021;160(2):464–468.
7. Memtsoudis SG, Poeran J, Zubizarreta N, et al. Association of multimodal pain management strategies with perioperative outcomes and resource utilization. *Anesthesiology.* 2018;128(5):891–902.
8. Verret M, Lauzier F, Zarychanski R, et al. Perioperative use of gabapentinoids for the management of postoperative acute pain. *Anesthesiology.* 2020;133(2):265–279.
9. Han C, Kuang MJ, Ma JX, Ma XL. The efficacy of preoperative gabapentin in spinal surgery: A meta-analysis of randomized controlled trials. *Pain Physician.* 2017;20(7):649–661.
10. Hurley R, Cohen S, Williams K, Rowlingson A, Wu C. The analgesic effects of perioperative gabapentin on postoperative pain: A meta-analysis. *Reg Anesth Pain Med.* 2006;31(3):237–247.
11. Ohnuma T, Raghunathan K, Moore S, et al. Dose-dependent association of gabapentinoids with pulmonary complications after total hip and knee arthroplasties. *J Bone Joint Surg Am.* 2020;102(3):221–229.
12. Forero M, Adhikary SD, Lopez H, Tsui C, Chin KJ. The erector spinae plane block: A novel analgesic technique in thoracic neuropathic pain. *Reg Anesth Pain Med.* 2016;41(5):621–627.
13. Singh S, Choudhary NK, Lalin D, Verma VK. Bilateral ultrasound-guided erector spinae plane block for postoperative analgesia in lumbar spine surgery: A randomized control trial. *J Neurosurg Anesthesiol.* 2020;32(4):330–334.
14. Yerneni K, Nichols N, Abecassis ZA, Karras CL, Tan LA. Preoperative opioid use and clinical outcomes in spine surgery: A systematic review. *Neurosurgery.* 2020;86(6):E490–E507.
15. Lee D, Armaghani S, Archer KR, et al. Preoperative opioid use as a predictor of adverse postoperative self-reported outcomes in patients undergoing spine surgery. *J Bone Joint Surg Am.* 2014;96(11):e89.
16. Kalakoti P, Volkmar AJ, Bedard NA, Eisenberg JM, Hendrickson NR, Pugely AJ. Preoperative chronic opioid therapy negatively impacts long-term outcomes following cervical fusion surgery. *Spine.* 2019;44(18):1279–1286.
17. Dowell D, Haegerich TM, Chou R. CDC Guideline for prescribing opioids for chronic pain—United States, 2016. *JAMA.* 2016;315(15):1624.
18. Anderson TA, Quaye ANA, Ward EN, Wilens TE, Hilliard PE, Brummett CM. To stop or not, that is the question. *Anesthesiology.* 2017;126(6):1180–1186.
19. Sordo L, Barrio G, Bravo MJ, et al. Mortality risk during and after opioid substitution treatment: systematic review and meta-analysis of cohort studies. *BMJ.* 2017;357:j1550. https://doi.org/10.1136/bmj.j1550.
20. Kohan L, Potru S, Barreveld AM, et al. Buprenorphine management in the perioperative period: educational review and recommendations from a multisociety expert panel. *Reg Anesth Pain Med.* 2021;46(10):840–859.
21. Lembke A, Ottestad E, Schmiesing C. Patients maintained on buprenorphine for opioid use disorder should continue buprenorphine through the perioperative period. *Pain Med.* 2019;20(3):425–428.
22. Greenwald MK, Johanson CE, Moody DE, et al. Effects of buprenorphine maintenance dose on μ-opioid receptor availability, plasma concentrations, and antagonist blockade in heroin-dependent volunteers. *Neuropsychopharmacology.* 2003;28(11):2000–2009.
23. Hinrichs-Rocker A, Schulz K, Järvinen I, Lefering R, Simanski C, Neugebauer EAM. Psychosocial predictors and correlates for chronic post-surgical pain (CPSP) - A systematic review. *Eur J Pain.* 2009;13(7):719–730.
24. Theunissen M, Peters ML, Bruce J, Gramke HF, Marcus MA. Preoperative anxiety and catastrophizing: A systematic review and meta-analysis of the association with chronic postsurgical pain. *Clin J Pain.* 2012;28(9):819–841.

25. Dunn LK, Durieux ME, Fernández LG, et al. Influence of catastrophizing, anxiety, and depression on in-hospital opioid consumption, pain, and quality of recovery after adult spine surgery. *J Neurosurg Spine*. 2018;28(1):119–126.
26. Weinrib AZ, Azam MA, Birnie KA, Burns LC, Clarke H, Katz J. The psychology of chronic post-surgical pain: new frontiers in risk factor identification, prevention and management. *Br J Pain*. 2017;11(4):169–177.
27. Gerbershagen HJ, Aduckathil S, van Wijck AJM, Peelen LM, Kalkman CJ, Meissner W. Pain intensity on the first day after surgery. *Anesthesiology*. 2013;118(4):934–944.
28. Devin CJ, McGirt MJ. Best evidence in multimodal pain management in spine surgery and means of assessing postoperative pain and functional outcomes. *J Clin Neurosci*. 2015;22(6): 930–938.

5

Avoiding Complications in Outpatient Spine Surgery

J. MANUEL SARMIENTO, KASRA ARAGHI, MITCHELL S. FOURMAN, KEITH W. LYONS, FRANCIS C. LOVECCHIO, AND SHEERAZ A. QURESHI

CHAPTER OUTLINE

Introduction

Minimally invasive spine surgery techniques have ushered in an era where procedures that have traditionally been performed in the hospital are now transitioning to the outpatient setting. Outpatient procedures have decreased postoperative length of stay (LOS) and healthcare costs, as well as improved overall patient satisfaction.[1,2] There is a growing body of evidence that supports the safety and efficacy of outpatient cervical and lumbar surgery.[3–6] However, as the prevalence of spine surgery increases and more procedures transition to the outpatient setting, it is increasingly important to understand and mitigate spine surgery complications, especially in light of the emphasis placed on cost-effective health care.[7,8] There is no universal agreement on a classification system for complications after spinal surgery, and there is wide variability in the recording and reporting of spine surgery complications in the literature. Perioperative spine surgery complications can significantly impact surgical outcomes, patient quality of life, and healthcare costs. This chapter discusses managing and avoiding perioperative complications in outpatient spine surgery. Specifically, we aim to focus on complications relating to outpatient spine surgeries performed at standalone ambulatory surgery centers (ASCs) that are not connected to a hospital. This is an interesting group of patients because they require more thoughtful consideration about proper patient selection, surgical indications, and preoperative risk stratification than their counterparts who undergo surgery in the inpatient setting.

Complication Risk Factors

Understanding and optimizing modifiable risk factors is crucial to improving surgical outcomes after spine surgery. Known risk factors for postoperative complications include advanced age, smoking, obesity, chronic preoperative opioid use, and medical comorbidities such as cardiac, renal, and pulmonary disease.[9] Obesity has also been shown to adversely affect patient outcomes after spine surgery, and increased BMI has been significantly associated with postoperative complications in several studies.[9,10] One study reported a 2.2-fold increased risk of surgical site infection in obese patients, and a 3.5-fold increased risk of surgical site infection in diabetics who underwent spinal surgery.[10] The American Society of Anesthesiologists (ASA) Physical Status Classification System is used to rate patient medical complexity and assess the control of their medical comorbidities in preparation for surgery (Fig. 5.1).[11] Increasing ASA grade has been shown to be a significant risk factor for major complications and increased healthcare costs after spine surgery.[12]

Intraoperative factors need to be considered to prevent complications from occurring. Appropriate patient positioning in the operating room is necessary to access the surgical corridor, achieve a desired spinal alignment, and prevent

Class	Definition	Examples
1	Normal health	Healthy, nonsmoking, no or minimal alcohol use
2	Mild systemic disease	Mild diseases only without substantive functional limitations. Examples include (but not limited to): current smoker, social alcohol drinker, pregnancy, 30 < BMI < 40, well-controlled DM/HTN, mild lung disease
3	Severe systemic disease	Substantive functional limitations. One or more moderate to severe diseases. Examples include (but not limited to): poorly controlled DM or HTN, COPD, morbid obesity (BMI ≥ 40), active hepatitis, alcohol dependence or abuse, implanted pacemaker, moderate reduction in ejection fraction, ESRD undergoing regularly scheduled dialysis, premature infant PCA< 60 weeks, history (> 3 months) of MI, CVA, TIA or CAD/stents
4	Severe systemic disease that is a constant threat to life	Examples include (but not limited to): recent (< 3 months) MI, CVA, TIA or CAD/stents, ongoing cardiac ischaemia or severe valve dysfunction, severe reduction in ejection fraction, sepsis, DIC, ARD or ESRD not undergoing regularly scheduled dialysis
5	Moribund: survival not expected without surgery	Examples include (but not limited to): ruptured abdominal/thoracic aneurysm, massive trauma, intracranial bleed with mass effect, ischaemic bowel in the face of significant cardiac pathology or multiple organ/system dysfunction
6	Brain-dead organ donor	

ARD, acute respiratory distress; BMI, body mass index; CAD, coronary artery disease; COPD, chronic obstructive pulmonary disease; CVA, cerebrovascular accident; DIC, disseminated intravascular coagulation; DM, diabetes mellitus; ESRD, end-stage renal disease; HTN, hypertension; MI, myocardial infarction; PCA, postconceptual age; TIA, transient cerebral ischaemic attack.

• **Fig. 5.1** The ASA classification of physical status, as revised in 2014. The addition of "E" denotes emergency surgery, defined as threat to survival or body part if delayed. With permission from Mayhew D, Mendonca V, Murthy BVS. A review of ASA physical status - historical perspectives and modern developments. Anaesthesia. Mar 2019;74(3):373–379. https://doi:10.1111/anae.14569.

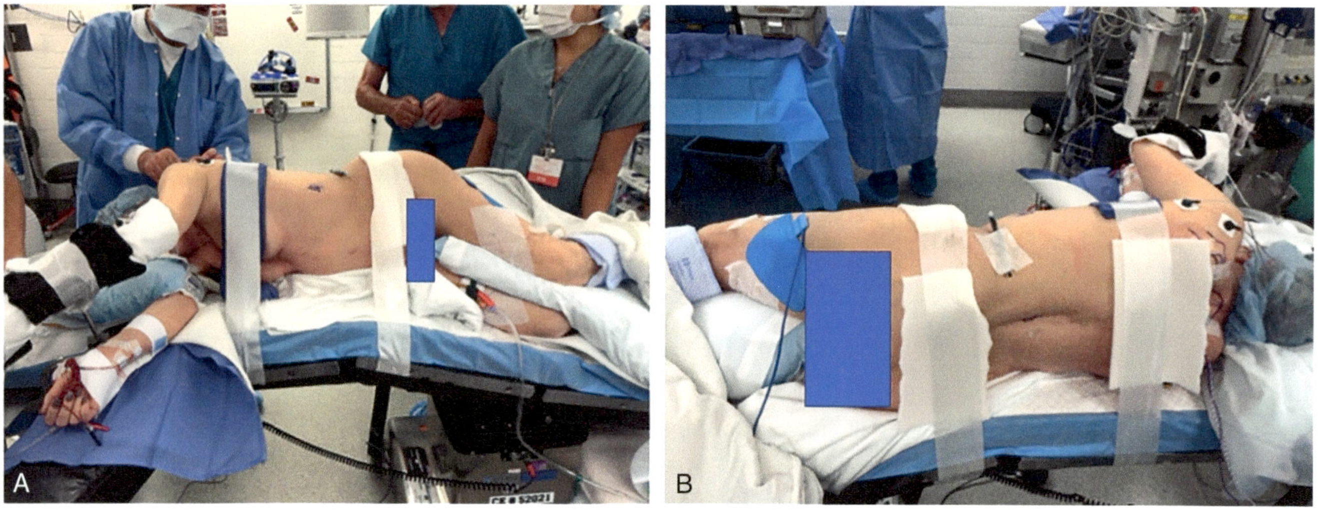

• **Fig. 5.2** Anterior view (A) and posterior view (B) of a right-sided lateral decubitus position for a left-sided lateral lumbar interbody fusion (LLIF). Note the axillary gel roll used to pad the right axilla.

peripheral nerve compression and skin breakdown. A bolster beneath the neck and the interscapular region during anterior cervical procedures enhances cervical extension. A gel roll should be placed under the axilla when utilizing the lateral decubitus position to avoid compression of the brachial plexus (Fig. 5.2). The lateral aspects of the knee and upper leg should be padded to prevent peroneal nerve compression. The inside of the elbow should be padded to prevent compression of the ulnar nerve. Patients who are undergoing a posterior thoracolumbar fusion are ideally positioned on a Jackson table with their hips extended to accentuate their lumbar lordosis and permit fusion of the spine in a favorable sagittal alignment. Patients who are undergoing a lumbar decompression may be placed on a Wilson frame in order to open their spinal canal and facilitate a safe laminotomy or laminectomy. Patients in the prone position should have their abdomen hanging free. Patients in the prone position with abdominal compression can have venal caval pressures greater than 300 mm H_2O (normal 0 to 40 mm H_2O).[13] Increased venal caval pressures not only increase bleeding during surgery due to congestion of the vertebral veins, but also can impair spinal cord perfusion. Positioning the shoulders at no more than 90 degrees of abduction with the arms palms down and the head in a neutral position is recommended to avoid brachial plexus injury in the prone position.[14,15] Risks factors that are associated with increased postoperative complications include increased surgical invasiveness (e.g., combined anterior-posterior approach), three-column osteotomy, increased blood loss, an increased number of operative levels, and increased surgical time.[16]

Cervical Spine Complications

Anterior Cervical Approaches

Airway Complications and Management

Preoperative evaluation of the patient for cervical spine surgery focuses on functional capacity, neurological assessment, and upper airway examination. A thorough preoperative evaluation is most important in patients undergoing anterior cervical spine surgery, such as an anterior cervical discectomy and fusion or artificial disc replacement. The upper airway is evaluated in the nontrauma patient by flexing and extending the neck without symptoms while awake. Extension at the craniocervical junction is needed for full mouth opening. A small mouth opening should therefore alert the anesthesiologists of the possibility of a difficult intubation. Respiratory compromise upon extubation or in the early recovery period occurs in less than 1% of cases (range 0.57% to 0.60%).[17,18] However, the incidence of respiratory compromise and unplanned reintubation after multilevel anterior cervical procedures can be as high as 6%.[19] Independent predictors of respiratory compromise include age ≥65, a 3-level or greater anterior decompression and fusion (ACDF), exposure of more rostral levels, preoperative myelopathy, operating room (OR) duration >3 hours, and ASA classification III/IV.[17,18,20] The most common complications after anterior cervical surgery are adjacent segment disease (8.1%), dysphagia (5.3%), C5 palsy (3%), and graft or hardware failure (2.1%).[21] Respiratory-related issues (i.e., pneumonia, tracheostomy complication, and respiratory failure) are the most common medical reasons for readmission following anterior cervical spine surgery.[18,22]

Dysphagia and Recurrent Laryngeal Nerve Palsy

Dysphagia is the second most common complication following anterior cervical surgery, and is associated with increased LOS postoperatively and is a predictor for patient readmission.[23] The use of bone morphogenic protein (BMP) was associated with increased rates of postoperative dysphagia in four retrospective studies and one prospective study.[24–28] A retrospective study of 1015 patients undergoing ACDF showed an increased risk of dysphagia in 3-level versus 1- or 2-level ACDF.[29] The use of local intraoperative steroids has been shown to reduce dysphagia at 90 days in patients undergoing an ACDF of 3 or more levels, but not in patients undergoing an ACDF of 1 or 2 levels.[30] Recurrent laryngeal nerve palsy is an uncommon ACDF-related complication with a reported incidence of 1.3%.[21] It is clinically expressed as postoperative hoarseness, dysphonia, or vocal cord paralysis.[29] Known risk factors for recurrent laryngeal nerve palsy include previous neck surgery, enlarged thyroid gland, and any preexisting hoarseness.[29] There is no convincing evidence that the use of BMP or performing a multilevel ACDF versus corpectomy affect the rate of recurrent laryngeal nerve palsy. There are mixed results about the association of recurrent laryngeal nerve palsy with the number of operative levels.[21] There is no convincing evidence that supports a higher rate of recurrent laryngeal nerve palsy after either a left- or right-sided approach.[31] Careful neck dissection and longus coli retraction minimizes the risk of this injury.

Postoperative Anterior Cervical Hematoma

Postoperative cervical hematoma is a rare complication after anterior cervical spine surgery, with a pooled incidence ranging from 0.4% to 1.0%.[21,32] While uncommon, postoperative hematoma is a feared complication because of the potential for devastating neurological and respiratory sequelae. Postoperative hematomas may cause mass effect on the spinal cord that leads to myelopathy and spinal cord injury. However, the most dangerous complication of a postoperative hematoma is compromise of the trachea and airway, which requires emergent intubation and/or emergent evacuation of the hematoma.[20] Due to the risk of airway compromise, evacuation of a symptomatic postoperative hematoma often needs to be performed expeditiously, even if this means cutting open the surgical wound in the post anesthesia care unit setting if the patient has already left the operating room. Hematoma evacuation is the most common reason for reoperation after anterior cervical spine surgery for patients with respiratory compromise.[18] While large postoperative hematomas may cause tracheal deviation on radiographs, postoperative hematoma is a clinical diagnosis that does not require imaging studies for confirmation as long as clinical suspicion is high. Risk factors for the development of postoperative hematoma requiring reoperation were multilevel procedures (most notably ≥3 levels), preoperative international normalized ratio >1.2, BMI ≤24, and ASA classification ≥3.[32]

Posterior Cervical Approaches

Posterior Cervical Epidural Hematoma

Postoperative epidural hematoma is one of the most concerning complications after posterior cervical spine surgery. This complication is rare, with a reported incidence of less than 1%.[33] However, because the cervical spine is such high-risk territory for potentially devastating spinal cord injury and severe neurological morbidity, high clinical suspicion and prompt identification are crucial for diagnosing a symptomatic postoperative epidural hematoma. Immediate surgical evacuation with a laminectomy, identifying the source of the bleeding (i.e., epidural vessel bleeding, osseous bleeding, or diffuse muscle bleeding), and stopping it is necessary.[34] Generalized diffuse bleeding in the surgical cavity generally represents a systemic coagulopathy and should prompt a hematologic workup and expedient transfusion. Preoperative risk factors for epidural hematoma formation are age >60 years, >5 operative levels, preoperative coagulopathy, preoperative nonsteroidal antiinflammatory agent use, prior posterior neck surgery, and increased international normalized ratio values.[35,36] Preoperative risk factor optimization and maintaining meticulous intraoperative hemostasis and perioperative blood pressure control can minimize the risk of a postoperative epidural hematoma.[37]

Lumbar Spine Complications

Anterior Approaches to the Lumbar Spine

Ileus

The most common gastrointestinal problem after spine surgery is ileus, which is the inability of the bowel to contract normally and move waste out of the body. Clinical findings and symptoms of ileus include nausea, vomiting, abdominal distention, and abdominal cramping/discomfort. A localized ileus will show one or two persistently dilated loops of small bowel on conventional upright radiographs, whereas generalized ileus will have gas within and dilation of the entire small and large bowel. Since ileus has no mechanical obstruction, there should be gas within the rectum and sigmoid colon. Common causes of ileus include general anesthesia, prolonged use of narcotics, immobility after surgery, and significant manipulation of intestinal contents during anterior surgical procedures. The rate of postoperative ileus after anterior lumbar approaches has been found to be more than two times than that of posterior lumbar approaches.[38] Prolonged ileus occurs after 3% to 5% of anterior lumbar interbody fusions (ALIFs).[39,40] The incidence and duration of postoperative ileus can potentially be diminished by optimizing oral medication regimens and nutrition, and using nonnarcotic pain control strategies.[41] Patients may be started on ice chips after spinal fusion after bowel patency is confirmed on abdominal examination based on the presence of bowel sounds. If this is well-tolerated then the patient may progress to a clear liquid diet followed by a regular diet. In the setting of postoperative ileus, diet restriction and intravenous fluids are the initial treatment. Nasogastric suction and antiemetic agents are provided for symptomatic relief as needed. In severe cases of ileus with acute massive dilation of the cecum and the ascending and transverse colon—a condition known as Ogilvie syndrome—treatment involves decompressing the colon with a rectal tube and sometimes colonoscopy for refractory cases.

Vascular Injury

The most dangerous injuries during anterior approaches to the lumbar spine are vascular injuries, which are estimated to occur in 6% to 12% of cases.[39,40,42] A vascular injury should be suspected in the postoperative patient when the lower extremity ipsilateral to the side of the exposure becomes cold, with severe associated pain and decreased distal pulses. An emergent arteriogram and vascular surgery consultation are indicated in such cases. The most common injuries are venous and most commonly occur during exposure of L4-5. Risk factors for vascular injuries are exposure of both L4-5 and L5-S1 spinal levels, spondylolisthesis, previous radiation exposure, and transitional anatomy.[43] In general, small venous lacerations less than 5 mm long can be treated with pressure and hemostatic agents. Larger tears and arterial injuries require a more involved repair using sutures and/or vascular clips (Fig. 5.3).[44,45] The vessels at highest risk of injury are the iliac veins, the iliolumbar vein, and the

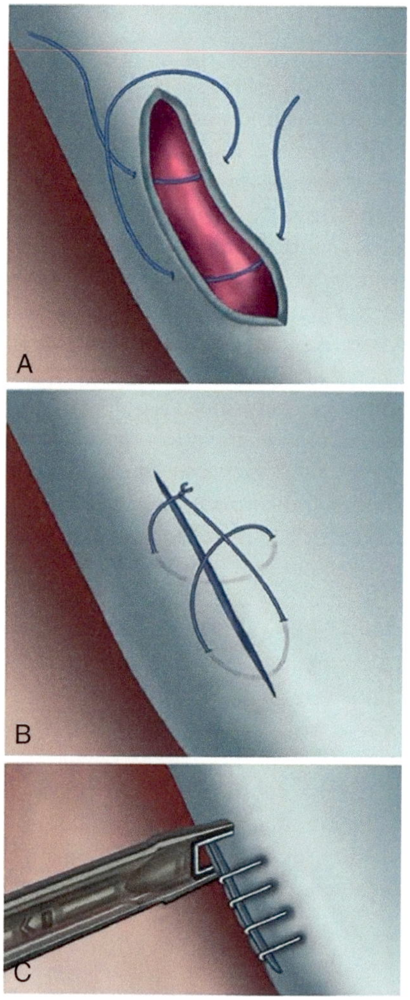

• **Fig. 5.3** Lateral repair of a iliac vein with 5-0 prolene suture placed in figure-of-eight fashion (A, B) and vascular clips placed in "railroad tract" fashion (C). With permission from Fantini GA, Pawar AY. Access related complications during anterior exposure of the lumbar spine. *World J Orthop*. Jan 18 2013;4(1):19–23. https://doi:10.5312/wjo.v4.i1.19.

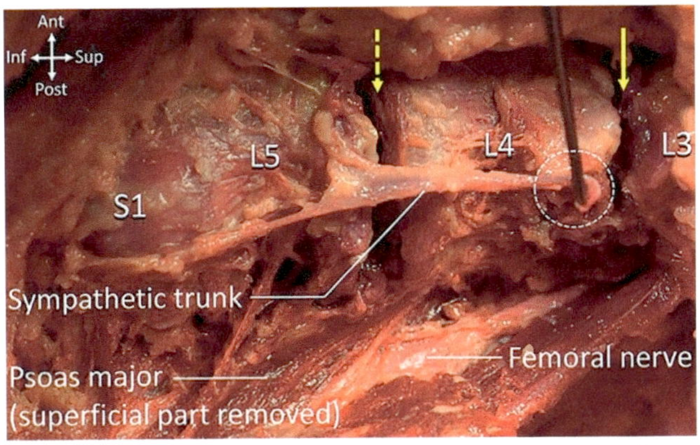

• **Fig. 5.4** Cadaveric specimen following direct lateral transpsoas approach for total discectomy of the L3-4 (arrow) and L4-5 (dashed arrow) intervertebral discs. The lumbar sympathetic trunk was completely transected at the L3 level. From Iwanaga J, Zeoli T, Scullen T, Maulucci C, Tubbs RS. Cadaveric Evidence of Complete Transection of the Lumbar Sympathetic Trunk After Extreme Lateral Transpsoas Approach to the Lumbar Spine: A Word of Caution. *Cureus*. Apr 07 2021;13(4):e14346. https://doi:10.7759/cureus.14346.

left iliac artery. If an iliac vessel is injured and needs to be repaired primarily, direct pressure should be immediately applied and then proximal and distal control of the injured vessel needs to be achieved before an actual repair can be performed.[40,42] Arterial injuries that cannot be repaired primarily may require an interposition graft. The assistance of a skilled exposure surgeon is crucial to avoiding and managing the vascular complications associated with anterior spinal exposures.[46] A spine surgeon and a vascular surgeon working in combination has resulted in low rates of total blood loss for both single-level and multilevel procedures.[40] In the rare instance of an intraoperative vascular injury where primary repair is unsuccessful, the patient should be stabilized and emergency protocols need to be in place for prompt transfer to a specialized medical center for continued management at a higher level of care.

Sympathetic Nerve Injury

The sympathetic chain is located on the lateral border of the vertebral bodies and is at risk for injury during an anterior surgical approach (Fig. 5.4).[47] Studies from standalone ALIFs report sympathetic dysfunction rates ranging from 6% to 10%.[39,40] A sympathectomy effect occurs by virtue of arterial vasodilation, permitting increased blood flow to the leg ipsilateral to the side of the sympathetic chain injury. This leads to a painless temperature increase and occasional swelling of the affected lower extremity. Anterior spine surgery at the L5-S1 level puts the superior hypogastric plexus at risk for injury. This sympathetic plexus traverses the anterior aspect of the L5-S1 disc, distal aorta, and the left common iliac vein, lying just beneath the peritoneum (Fig. 5.5).[48,49] Injury may occur when dividing the peritoneum, with traction on the plexus and surrounding vessels, and with accidental ligation.[50] The superior hypogastric plexus is ultimately responsible for controlling bladder neck closure during ejaculation. Thus, injury to this important nerve leads to failure of closure of the bladder neck during ejaculation, causing ejaculate to travel in a retrograde direction into the bladder that can sometimes result in sterility. Reported rates of retrograde ejaculation during standalone ALIFs range from 1.8% to 3.3%.[39,40]

Lateral Approaches to the Lumbar Spine

A popular method of interbody fixation is lateral lumbar interbody fusion (LLIF), which utilizes a minimally invasive retroperitoneal, transpsoas corridor to access the intervertebral disk space and avoids disruption of the posterior spinal musculature and posterior tension band. The psoas major muscle is the key muscle that is dissected during the LLIF approach, and functions as a hip flexor, abductor, and lateral rotator. Within the psoas major lies the lumbar plexus that receives nerve input from the T12 to L5 spinal nerves. Lumbar plexus nerves are commonly encountered specifically within the posterior psoas at the level of L4-5. Electromyography guidance is used to avoid these intervening nerves and safely access the intervertebral disk space.[51] An important lumbar plexus nerve at risk at the L4-5 level is the femoral nerve, which is formed by the L2, L3, and L4 spinal nerves and travels to the thigh to innervate the quadriceps. A study by Grimm et al. reports a single surgeon's first 108 patients who underwent an extreme lateral interbody fusion (XLIF; NuVasive Inc., San Diego, CA) of ≥1 level to highlight the learning curve and complication profile of the procedure.[52] Twenty-five complications (23%) were reported, of which 4 (3.7%) were major that required revision surgery or were functionally limiting, and 21 (19.4%) were minor that did not impair long-term function or required revision surgery. Out of 21 patients who sustained minor complications, 19 complained of some degree of antero-lateral thigh numbness and/or pain or hip flexor weakness on the ipsilateral side of the surgical approach. These symptoms resolved 3 to 6 months postoperatively. The L4-5 level was instrumented alone or included in multilevel cases in 18 (94%) out of these 19 patients. The largest series of LLIF complications was published by Rodgers et al. who reported an overall perioperative complication rate of 6.2% (up to 6 weeks postoperative) in 600 patients treated with a lateral approach to fusion for degenerative spinal conditions.[53] Three patients developed postoperative quadriceps weakness and one developed anterior tibialis weakness for a total neurological complication rate of 0.7%. Each patient's weakness resolved within 3 months. In both aforementioned studies by Grimm et al. and Rodgers et al., none of the patients experienced an infection, visceral, vascular, or dural injury.

There is increasing evidence that shows that a LLIF may be safely performed in the outpatient setting, but careful patient selection and a high degree of surgical expertise to prevent complications is necessary.[54] A comparative analysis study by Chin et al. showed no difference in complications

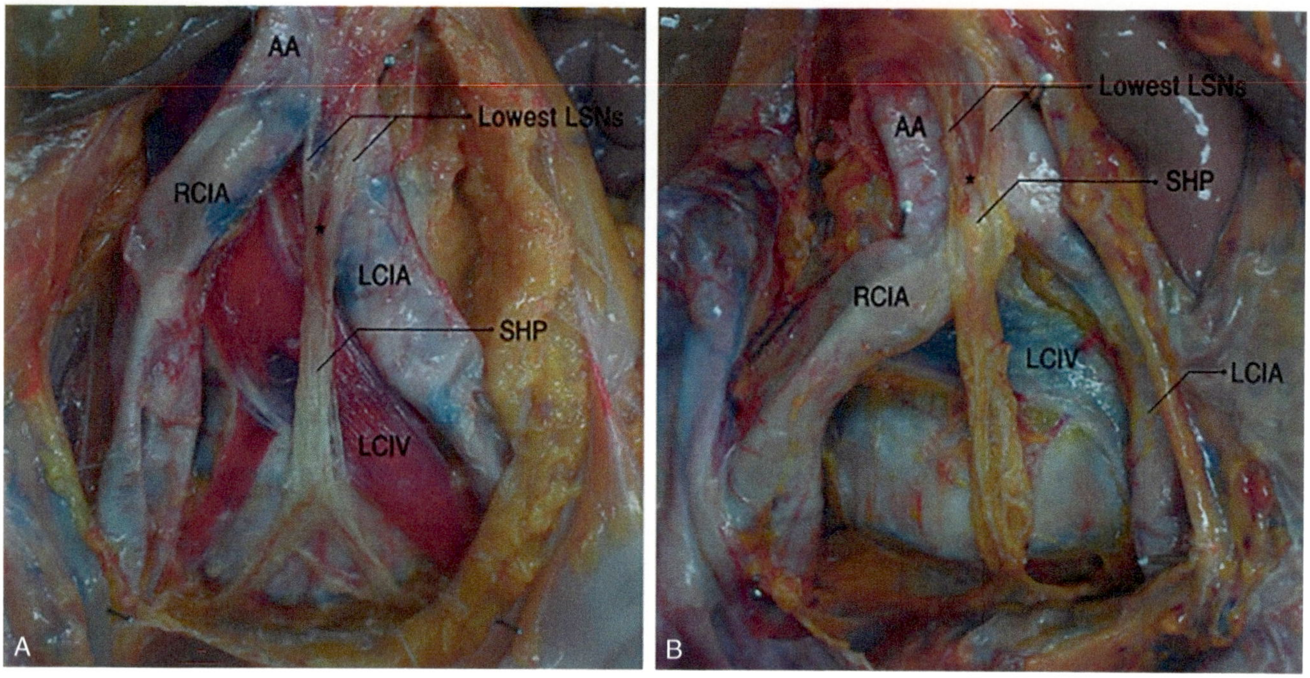

• **Fig. 5.5** Ventral view of the superior hypogastric plexus (SHP). (A) The SHP is formed by the bilateral lowest lumbar splanchnic nerves (LSNs) below the aortic bifurcation. The SHP is located anterior to the left common iliac artery (LCIA), the left common iliac vein, and the fifth lumbar vertebral body. (B) The SHP is formed above the aortic bifurcation. The SHP is located anterior to the right common iliac artery (RCIA), the left common iliac vein, and the fifth lumbar vertebral body. The asterisk (*) indicates the origin of the SHP. Between the bilateral LSNs, multiple fibers from the abdominal aortic plexus were observed; AA, abdominal aorta; LCIV, left common iliac vein. Image used with permission from Kim H, Nam YS, Lee UY, Kim IB, Kim YS. Anatomy of the superior hypogastric plexus and its application in nerve-sparing paraaortic lymphadenectomy. *Folia Morphol (Warsz)*. 2021;80(1): 70–75. https://doi.org/10.5603/FM.a2020.0037.

between 30 patients who underwent single-level LLIF with supplemental posterior fixation performed in the outpatient setting and 40 patients who had LLIF performed in the inpatient setting.[1] The most common complaint was dermatome numbness (20% and 7% in the hospital and ASC groups, respectively), and the level affected most commonly in each group was L4-5. To diminish the chances of neuropraxia, especially at the L4-5 level, retractor time should be minimized as much as possible. Dilator and retractor placement should be placed at or anterior to the midline at L4-5 to avoid the femoral nerve. The outrigger arm can be loosened so that the retractor may slide posteriorly and bring the femoral nerve with it and out of the surgical field behind the retractor blade.[52] A 2022 study by Silverstein et al. demonstrates that monitoring femoral nerve evoked potentials, particularly saphenous nerve somatosensory evoked potentials, can reliably alert the surgeon to hyperacute femoral nerve conduction failure and enable prompt surgical countermeasures in order to avoid femoral nerve injury.[55] The ideal patient for an outpatient LLIF would be relatively young, require a one-level fusion without significant spinal deformity, have minimal comorbidities, and possess retroperitoneal anatomy that lends itself to the lateral approach.[54]

Posterior Approaches to the Lumbar Spine

Postoperative Lumbar Epidural Hematoma

Postoperative epidural hematomas are rare but dreaded complications after lumbar spine surgery (Fig. 5.6).[56] The incidence of a postoperative symptomatic hematoma ranges from 0.2% to 0.67%.[33] Most spine surgery procedures provoke a small and clinically insignificant epidural hematoma. However, it is important to maintain a high clinical suspicion of epidural hematoma in patients who complain of new postoperative numbness, lower extremity weakness, pain, and/or urinary incontinence. Risk factors for a symptomatic epidural hematoma include multilevel spinal procedures, preoperative coagulopathy, preoperative nonsteroidal antiinflammatory agent use, large intraoperative blood loss (>1 liter), advanced age, and increased international normalized ratio values.[35] Symptomatic postoperative epidural hematomas are a true surgical emergency because, depending on the spinal level of the hematoma, epidural compression against the dura may lead to postoperative conus medullaris syndrome or cauda equina syndrome. Rapid diagnosis and emergent surgical treatment of the postoperative symptomatic epidural hematoma has been shown

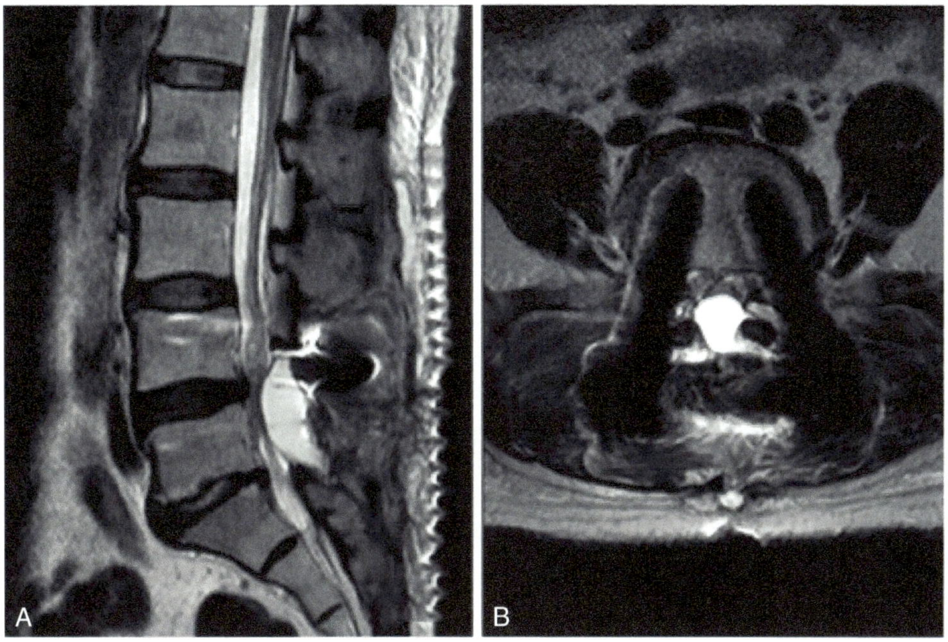

• **Fig. 5.6** Sagittal T2-weighted magnetic resonance imaging (MRI) with an epidural hematoma at L5 level (A). Axial T2-weighted MRI showing the epidural hematoma compressing the thecal sac and the nerve root (B). With permission from Shin HK, Jeong HJ, Kim E, Park JH, Park SJ, Cho Y. Should We Check the Routine Postoperative MRI for Hematoma in Spinal Decompression Surgery? *Clin Orthop Surg*. Jun 2017;9(2):184–189. https://doi.org/10.4055/cios.2017.9.2.184.

to maximize neurological recovery.[34] The ability of a postoperative subfascial drain to prevent epidural hematoma is controversial, and does not replace appropriate preoperative optimization and meticulous intraoperative hemostasis.

Cerebrospinal Fluid Leak

Incidental dural tears and durotomies can lead to cerebrospinal fluid (CSF) leaks. The reported incidence of intraoperative durotomies during spine surgery range from 1% to 17%.[57] Adverse consequences of untreated or ongoing CSF leaks after spinal surgery are increased risk of postoperative meningitis, pain and radicular symptoms from nerve roots herniating out from the dural sac, and wound dehiscence/infection if CSF traverses the fascial closure and leaks from the wound. An ongoing postoperative CSF leak is suspected if patients complain of new-onset positional headaches (headaches that worsen with standing upright and improve or resolve completely in the recumbent position). MRI of the spine can confirm the diagnosis and typically reveal a large epidural fluid collection at the surgical site.[58] The definitive treatment for a dural leak is primary repair, and the majority of dural tears are amendable to this strategy and heal spontaneously. An intraoperative Valsalva maneuver held at 40 mmHg for 5 seconds should be used to test the integrity of the closure. If the defect is large or the dura is too shredded to reapproximate with sutures alone, then a muscle or fascial patch may be sewn to normal dura and over the dural defect for direct closure. If the dural defect is too large to accommodate a patch graft or if it is located in a difficult to reach location, such as the lateral and/or ventral aspects of the thecal sac, then a synthetic dural graft is used in onlay fashion followed by fibrin sealant for closure.[59] Cerebrospinal fluid diversion in the form of lumbar drainage promotes dural healing and may be utilized for large dural defects or persistent CSF leaks for 3 to 5 days postoperatively. Laying the patient flat for 48 to 72 hours postoperatively may also promote dural healing in the lumbar spine by reducing intrathecal pressure. In the largest reported series of dural tears secondary to a lumbar spine operation, watertight primary repair with the use of dural silk suture followed by an average of approximately 3 days of bedrest resulted in resolution of the cerebrospinal fluid leak in 86 out of 88 patients (97.7%).[60]

Conclusion

While spine surgery will always carry inherent risks of complications, the rates and severity of these complications vary widely depending on the location of the spinal procedure, the surgical approach, preoperative patient risk factors, and the surgeons' technical expertise. Spine surgeons who are operating in the ambulatory setting and away from the safety net provided by hospitals should have extensive surgical experience, a thoughtful preoperative surgical plan, and a thorough understanding of the patients' preoperative imaging. The current literature has repeatedly shown favorable safety profiles and postoperative outcomes in outpatient spine procedures. Appropriate patient selection, cardiopulmonary risk stratification, and preoperative optimization are some of the most important factors in ensuring patient safety and minimizing complications in spine surgeries performed in the outpatient setting.

References

1. Chin KR, Pencle FJ, Coombs AV, et al. Lateral lumbar interbody fusion in ambulatory surgery centers: Patient selection and outcome measures compared with an inhospital cohort. *Spine (Phila Pa 1976)*. 2016;41(8):686–692.
2. Chin KR, Coombs AV, Seale JA. Feasibility and patient-reported outcomes after outpatient single-level instrumented posterior lumbar interbody fusion in a surgery center: preliminary results in 16 patients. *Spine (Phila Pa 1976)*. 2015;40(1):E36–42.
3. Chin KR, Pencle FJR, Seale JA, Pencle FK. Clinical outcomes of outpatient cervical total disc replacement compared with outpatient anterior cervical discectomy and fusion. *Spine (Phila Pa 1976)*. 2017;42(10):E567–E574.
4. Vaishnav A, Hill P, McAnany S, et al. Comparison of multilevel anterior cervical discectomy and fusion performed in an inpatient versus outpatient setting. *Global Spine J*. 2019;9(8):834–842.
5. Vaishnav AS, McAnany SJ. Future endeavors in ambulatory spine surgery. *J Spine Surg*. 2019;5(Suppl 2):S139–S146.
6. Sivaganesan A, Hirsch B, Phillips FM, McGirt MJ. Spine surgery in the ambulatory surgery center setting: Value-based advancement or safety liability? *Neurosurgery*. 2018;83(2):159–165.
7. Schuermans VNE, Smeets AYJM, Boselie AFM, et al. Cost-effectiveness of anterior surgical decompression surgery for cervical degenerative disk disease: a systematic review of economic evaluations. *Eur Spine J*. 2022;31(5):1206–1218.
8. Ghogawala Z, Whitmore RG, Watters WC, et al. Guideline update for the performance of fusion procedures for degenerative disease of the lumbar spine. Part 3: assessment of economic outcome. *J Neurosurg Spine*. 2014;21(1):14–22.
9. Schoenfeld AJ, Ochoa LM, Bader JO, Belmont PJ. Risk factors for immediate postoperative complications and mortality following spine surgery: a study of 3475 patients from the National Surgical Quality Improvement Program. *J Bone Joint Surg Am*. 2011; 93(17):1577–1582.
10. Olsen MA, Nepple JJ, Riew KD, et al. Risk factors for surgical site infection following orthopaedic spinal operations. *J Bone Joint Surg Am*. 2008;90(1):62–69.
11. Mayhew D, Mendonca V, Murthy BVS. A review of ASA physical status - historical perspectives and modern developments. *Anaesthesia*. 2019;74(3):373–379. https://doi.org/10.1111/anae.14569.
12. Whitmore RG, Stephen JH, Vernick C, et al. ASA grade and Charlson Comorbidity Index of spinal surgery patients: correlation with complications and societal costs. *Spine J*. 2014;14(1):31–38.
13. PEARCE DJ. The role of posture in laminectomy. *Proc R Soc Med*. 1957;50(2):109–112.
14. Cunha PD, Barbosa TP, Correia G, et al. The ideal patient positioning in spine surgery: a preventive strategy. *EFORT Open Rev*. 2023;8(2):63–72.
15. Lee MJ, Konodi MA, Cizik AM, Bransford RJ, Bellabarba C, Chapman JR. Risk factors for medical complication after spine surgery: a multivariate analysis of 1,591 patients. *Spine J*. 2012;12(3):197–206.
16. Blamoutier A, Guigui P, Charosky S, Roussouly P, Chopin D. (GES) GdÉdlS. Surgery of lumbar and thoracolumbar scolioses in adults over 50. Morbidity and survival in a multicenter retrospective cohort of 180 patients with a mean follow-up of 4.5 years. *Orthop Traumatol Surg Res*. 2012;98(5):528–535.
17. Lim S, Kesavabhotla K, Cybulski GR, Dahdaleh NS, Smith ZA. Predictors for airway complications following single- and multilevel anterior cervical discectomy and fusion. *Spine (Phila Pa 1976)*. 2017;42(6):379–384.
18. Boddapati V, Lee NJ, Mathew J, et al. Respiratory compromise after anterior cervical spine surgery: Incidence, subsequent complications, and independent predictors. *Global Spine J*. 2022; 12(8):1647–1654.
19. Swann MC, Hoes KS, Aoun SG, McDonagh DL. Postoperative complications of spine surgery. *Best Pract Res Clin Anaesthesiol*. 2016;30(1):103–120.
20. Sagi HC, Beutler W, Carroll E, Connolly PJ. Airway complications associated with surgery on the anterior cervical spine. *Spine (Phila Pa 1976)*. 2002;27(9):949–953.
21. Yee TJ, Swong K, Park P. Complications of anterior cervical spine surgery: a systematic review of the literature. *J Spine Surg*. 2020;6(1):302–322.
22. Schafer E, Bazydlo M, Schultz L, et al. Rates and risk factors associated with 90-day readmission following cervical spine fusion surgery: analysis of the Michigan Spine Surgery Improvement Collaborative (MSSIC) registry. *Spine J*. 2020;20(5):708–716.
23. Shields LB, Raque GH, Glassman SD, et al. Adverse effects associated with high-dose recombinant human bone morphogenetic protein-2 use in anterior cervical spine fusion. *Spine (Phila Pa 1976)*. 2006;31(5):542–547.
24. Vaidya R, Carp J, Sethi A, Bartol S, Craig J, Les CM. Complications of anterior cervical discectomy and fusion using recombinant human bone morphogenetic protein-2. *Eur Spine J*. 2007;16(8):1257–1265.
25. Cahill KS, Chi JH, Day A, Claus EB. Prevalence, complications, and hospital charges associated with use of bone-morphogenetic proteins in spinal fusion procedures. *JAMA*. 2009;302(1):58–66.
26. Fineberg SJ, Ahmadinia K, Oglesby M, Patel AA, Singh K. Hospital outcomes and complications of anterior and posterior cervical fusion with bone morphogenetic protein. *Spine (Phila Pa 1976)*. 2013;38(15):1304–1309.
27. Cole T, Veeravagu A, Jiang B, Ratliff JK. Usage of recombinant human bone morphogenetic protein in cervical spine procedures: analysis of the MarketScan longitudinal database. *J Bone Joint Surg Am*. 2014;96(17):1409–1416.
28. Burkus JK, Dryer RF, Arnold PM, Foley KT. Clinical and radiographic outcomes in patients undergoing single-level anterior cervical arthrodesis: A prospective trial comparing allograft to a reduced dose of rhBMP-2. *Clin Spine Surg*. 2017; 30(9):E1321–E1332.
29. Fountas KN, Kapsalaki EZ, Nikolakakos LG, et al. Anterior cervical discectomy and fusion associated complications. *Spine (Phila Pa 1976)*. 2007;32(21):2310–2317.
30. Cancienne JM, Werner BC, Loeb AE, et al. The effect of local intraoperative steroid administration on the rate of postoperative dysphagia following ACDF: A study of 245,754 patients. *Spine (Phila Pa 1976)*. 2016;41(13):1084–1088.
31. Beutler WJ, Sweeney CA, Connolly PJ. Recurrent laryngeal nerve injury with anterior cervical spine surgery risk with laterality of surgical approach. *Spine (Phila Pa 1976)*. 2001;26(12): 1337–1342.
32. Bovonratwet P, Fu MC, Tyagi V, et al. Incidence, risk factors, and clinical implications of postoperative hematoma requiring reoperation following anterior cervical discectomy and fusion. *Spine (Phila Pa 1976)*. 2019;44(8):543–549.
33. Aono H, Ohwada T, Hosono N, et al. Incidence of postoperative symptomatic epidural hematoma in spinal decompression surgery. *J Neurosurg Spine*. 2011;15(2):202–205.

34. Lawton MT, Porter RW, Heiserman JE, Jacobowitz R, Sonntag VK, Dickman CA. Surgical management of spinal epidural hematoma: relationship between surgical timing and neurological outcome. *J Neurosurg.* 1995;83(1):1–7.
35. Awad JN, Kebaish KM, Donigan J, Cohen DB, Kostuik JP. Analysis of the risk factors for the development of post-operative spinal epidural haematoma. *J Bone Joint Surg Br.* 2005;87(9): 1248–1252.
36. Halvorsen CM, Lied B, Harr ME, et al. Surgical mortality and complications leading to reoperation in 318 consecutive posterior decompressions for cervical spondylotic myelopathy. *Acta Neurol Scand.* 2011;123(5):358–365.
37. Tomii M, Mizuno J, Kazama K, Matsushima T, Watanabe K. Delayed postoperative spinal epidural hematoma after cervical laminoplasty. *NMC Case Rep J.* 2018;5(1):35–38.
38. Qureshi R, Puvanesarajah V, Jain A, Shimer AL, Shen FH, Hassanzadeh H. A comparison of anterior and posterior lumbar interbody fusions: Complications, readmissions, discharge dispositions, and costs. *Spine (Phila Pa 1976).* 2017;42(24): 1865–1870.
39. Rajaraman V, Vingan R, Roth P, Heary RF, Conklin L, Jacobs GB. Visceral and vascular complications resulting from anterior lumbar interbody fusion. *J Neurosurg.* 1999;91(1 Suppl):60–64.
40. Mobbs RJ, Phan K, Daly D, Rao PJ, Lennox A. Approach-related complications of anterior lumbar interbody fusion: Results of a combined spine and vascular surgical team. *Global Spine J.* 2016;6(2):147–154.
41. Than KD, Wang AC, Rahman SU, et al. Complication avoidance and management in anterior lumbar interbody fusion. *Neurosurg Focus.* 2011;31(4):E6.
42. Hamdan AD, Malek JY, Schermerhorn ML, Aulivola B, Blattman SB, Pomposelli FB. Vascular injury during anterior exposure of the spine. *J Vasc Surg.* 2008;48(3):650–654.
43. Nourian AA, Cunningham CM, Bagheri A, Bruffey JD, Eastlack RK. Effect of anatomic variability and level of approach on perioperative vascular complications with anterior lumbar interbody fusion. *Spine (Phila Pa 1976).* 2016;41(2):E73–77.
44. Xu DS, Walker CT, Godzik J, Turner JD, Smith W, Uribe JS. Minimally invasive anterior, lateral, and oblique lumbar interbody fusion: a literature review. *Ann Transl Med.* 2018;6(6):104.
45. Fantini GA, Pawar AY. Access related complications during anterior exposure of the lumbar spine. *World J Orthop.* 2013; 4(1):19–23. https://doi.org/10.5312/wjo.v4.i1.19.
46. Anderson DG, Sayadipour A, Shelby K, Albert TJ, Vaccaro AR, Weinstein MS. Anterior interbody arthrodesis with percutaneous posterior pedicle fixation for degenerative conditions of the lumbar spine. *Eur Spine J.* 2011;20(8):1323–1330.
47. Iwanaga J, Zeoli T, Scullen T, Maulucci C, Tubbs RS. Cadaveric evidence of complete transection of the lumbar sympathetic trunk after extreme lateral transpsoas approach to the lumbar spine: A word of caution. *Cureus.* 2021;13(4):e14346. https://doi.org/10.7759/cureus.14346.
48. Bateman DK, Millhouse PW, Shahi N, et al. Anterior lumbar spine surgery: a systematic review and meta-analysis of associated complications. *Spine J.* 2015;15(5):1118–1132.
49. Kim H, Nam YS, Lee UY, Kim IB, Kim YS. Anatomy of the superior hypogastric plexus and its application in nerve-sparing paraaortic lymphadenectomy. *Folia Morphol (Warsz).* 2021;80(1):70–75. https://doi.org/10.5603/FM.a2020.0037.
50. Czerwein JK, Thakur N, Migliori SJ, Lucas P, Palumbo M. Complications of anterior lumbar surgery. *J Am Acad Orthop Surg.* 2011;19(5):251–258.
51. Alluri RK, Vaishnav AS, Sivaganesan A, Ricci L, Sheha E, Qureshi SA. Multimodality intraoperative neuromonitoring in lateral lumbar interbody fusion: A review of alerts in 628 patients. *Global Spine J.* 2023;13(2):466–471.
52. Grimm BD, Leas DP, Poletti SC, Johnson DR. Postoperative complications within the first year after extreme lateral interbody fusion: Experience of the first 108 patients. *Clin Spine Surg.* 2016; 29(3):E151–156.
53. Rodgers WB, Gerber EJ, Patterson J. Intraoperative and early postoperative complications in extreme lateral interbody fusion: an analysis of 600 cases. *Spine (Phila Pa 1976).* 2011; 36(1):26–32.
54. Basques BA, Ferguson J, Kunze KN, Phillips FM. Lumbar spinal fusion in the outpatient setting: an update on management, surgical approaches and planning. *J Spine Surg.* 2019;5(Suppl 2):S174–S180.
55. Silverstein JW, Block J, Smith ML, et al. Femoral nerve neuromonitoring for lateral lumbar interbody fusion surgery. *Spine J.* 2022;22(2):296–304.
56. Shin HK, Jeong HJ, Kim E, Park JH, Park SJ, Cho Y. Should we check the routine postoperative MRI for hematoma in spinal decompression surgery? *Clin Orthop Surg.* 2017;9(2): 184–189. https://doi.org/10.4055/cios.2017.9.2.184.
57. Kamenova M, Leu S, Mariani L, Schaeren S, Soleman J. Management of incidental dural tear during lumbar spine surgery. To suture or not to suture? *World Neurosurg.* 2016;87: 455–462.
58. You SH, Son KR, Lee NJ, Suh JK. Remote cerebral and cerebellar hemorrhage after massive cerebrospinal fluid leakage. *J Korean Neurosurg Soc.* 2012;51(4):240–243.
59. Takenaka S, Makino T, Sakai Y, et al. Prognostic impact of intra- and postoperative management of dural tear on postoperative complications in primary degenerative lumbar diseases. *Bone Joint J. 101-B.* 2019;9:1115–1121.
60. Wang JC, Bohlman HH, Riew KD. Dural tears secondary to operations on the lumbar spine. Management and results after a two-year-minimum follow-up of eighty-eight patients. *J Bone Joint Surg Am.* Dec 1998;80(12):1728–1732.

6

Managing Spinal Cord Injuries

DEANNA CLAUS, WILLIAM SUMMERS, JESSICA LU, AND NATHAN ODOM

CHAPTER OUTLINE

Introduction

Spinal cord injuries (SCI) are a known indication for, and a known complication of, orthopedic spine surgery. SCI is defined by damage to the spinal cord, which can result in sensory and motor abnormalities, neurogenic bowel, neurogenic bladder, autonomic dysfunction, and other conditions that require attention from medical specialists.

Neuroanatomy Overview

When considering how a surgical complication could result in a SCI, a basic appreciation of neuroanatomy is helpful. The central nervous system is made up of the brain and spinal cord, which communicates with the rest of the body through the peripheral nervous system. The spinal cord does not traverse the entire vertebral column in adults, and typically terminates at the L1 vertebral level, though this can vary from T12 to L3.[1] The end of the spinal cord is named the **conus medullaris**. The collection of lumbar and sacral nerve roots caudal to the distal tip of the spinal cord is called the **cauda equina.**[2] Of note, while damage to the cauda equina affects peripheral nerves, these injuries can be managed with similar principles used for other types of SCI.

The spinal cord contains grey matter, primarily neuron cell bodies, and white matter composed of myelinated axons. Fig. 6.1 demonstrates important white matter tracts that help explain common deficits noted in SCI. The **corticospinal tract** is responsible for voluntary motor signals. The **dorsal column-medial lemniscus pathway** (running through the fasciculus cuneatus and fasciculus gracilis, or dorsal columns) carries vibration, proprioceptive input, and two point discrimination information. Pain and temperature sensation is contained in the **spinothalamic tract.**[2] Damage to these tracts, and others, can lead to impaired function below the level of injury.

Fig. 6.2 illustrates the vascular supply of the spinal cord. The anterior two-thirds of the spinal cord is supplied by the anterior spinal artery. Damage to this artery, including an acute infarct, leads to **anterior cord syndrome.** This presents with loss of motor function, pain, and temperature sensation below the lesion, due to damage to the corticospinal and spinothalamic tracts. The patient retains light touch and proprioception, as the dorsal columns remain intact.[2] The paired posterior spinal arteries provide blood to the posterior portion of the spinal cord. **Posterior cord syndrome** presents with lack of vibration and proprioception, with retained motor function.[2] The **artery of Adamkiewicz** is well known to surgeons, as it provides blood supply to the caudal two-thirds of the spinal cord and can cause significant spinal cord ischemia if damaged. It is typically found on the left side, originating between the levels of T8 and L1, though significant variation exists within the population.[3]

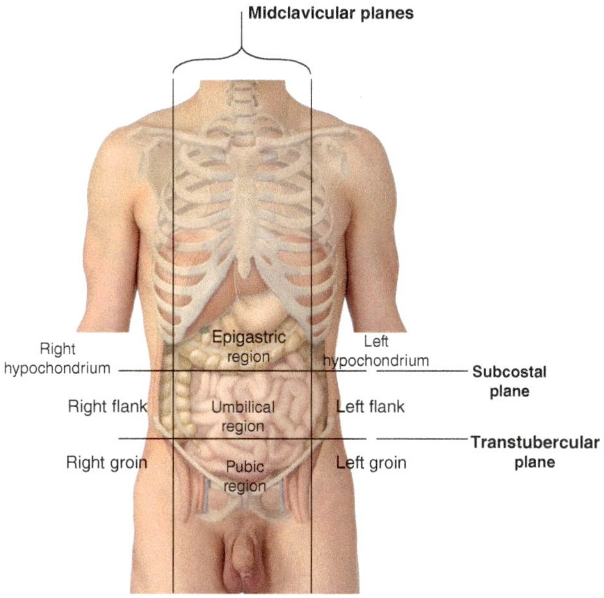

• **Fig. 6.1** Spinal cord cross-section with labeled white matter tracts. Cross-sectional anatomy of the spinal cord demonstrates the white matter tracts that run throughout the spinal cord. These tracts carry important information, such as voluntary motor signals (the corticospinal tract), light touch and proprioception (dorsal column medial lemniscus), as well as pain and temperature (spinothalamic tract). (From Sebesteny T, Deller T. *Fotoatlas Neuroanatomie*, 1. A. Munich: Elsevier GmbH, Urban & Fischer; 2007.)

SCI Overview

Spinal cord injuries have a vast array of injury subtypes and etiologies. To appropriately manage SCI and its complications, an understanding of SCI classification and general SCI syndromes is necessary.

SCI Classification

A thorough exam should be performed after any new SCI to determine the level and completeness of the patient's injury. This standardized exam by the International Standards for Neurological Classification of SCI (ISNCSCI) will produce an ASIA (American Spinal Injury Association) Impairment Scale grade.[4] These grades are referred to as **ASIA Impairment Scale (AIS)** A, B, C, D, and E. The nuances of this exam are beyond the scope of this chapter. Briefly, it includes a motor, sensory, and rectal exam. The grades range from AIS A, which refers to a complete injury (see "Complete and Incomplete" section), to AIS E, which refers to a patient with history of SCI but now has a normal exam.[4] This grade allows for classification and prognostication about the patient's injury (see "Navigating Prognosis, Function, and Uncertainty" section).

Acute and Chronic

Patients can acquire an SCI abruptly from an acute injury, such as a stroke during surgery or fractured vertebrae from a car accident. Alternatively, patients can develop a SCI slowly over time. A common example is cervical stenosis that leads to cervical myelopathy. Both types of injuries to the spinal cord can lead to similar presentations and need to be managed with special attention to the complications of SCI mentioned in this chapter.

Paraplegia and Tetraplegia

A SCI can result in damage that leads to involvement of two limbs (**paraplegia**) or all four limbs (**tetraplegia**, sometimes called quadriplegia). Due to the level of their injury, patients with tetraplegia may have more significant instability of their cardiovascular, pulmonary, autonomic, and thermoregulatory systems compared to those with paraplegia.[5,6]

Complete and Incomplete

Injuries can be classified as a complete injury where no signal can cross the injured level of the spinal cord, or an incomplete injury where some information is able to pass. Preserved sensation in the lowest sacral dermatomes, voluntary anal contraction, or deep anal pressure sensation, indicates the presence of an incomplete SCI.

Upper Motor Neuron Signs and Lower Motor Neuron Signs

SCI can lead to upper motor neuron (UMN) or lower motor neuron (LMN) injury depending on the location of the lesion. UMN refers to presynaptic primary neurons contained in spinal cord tracts. UMN injuries develop hyperreflexia, muscle spasticity, and can lead to a spastic bladder and anal sphincter.[7–9] Conversely, LMN refers to postsynaptic neurons, such as alpha motor neurons in the ventral horn of the grey matter of the spinal cord. On exam, LMN injuries can present with hyporeflexia, flaccid paralysis, as well as decreased tone of the bladder and anal sphincter.[8,9] Due to these differences in presentation, differentiating between UMN and LMN damage has important management and prognostic implications.

Management

Acute Management

Early identification of a SCI, either through a neurologic exam or imaging, is essential for many reasons.

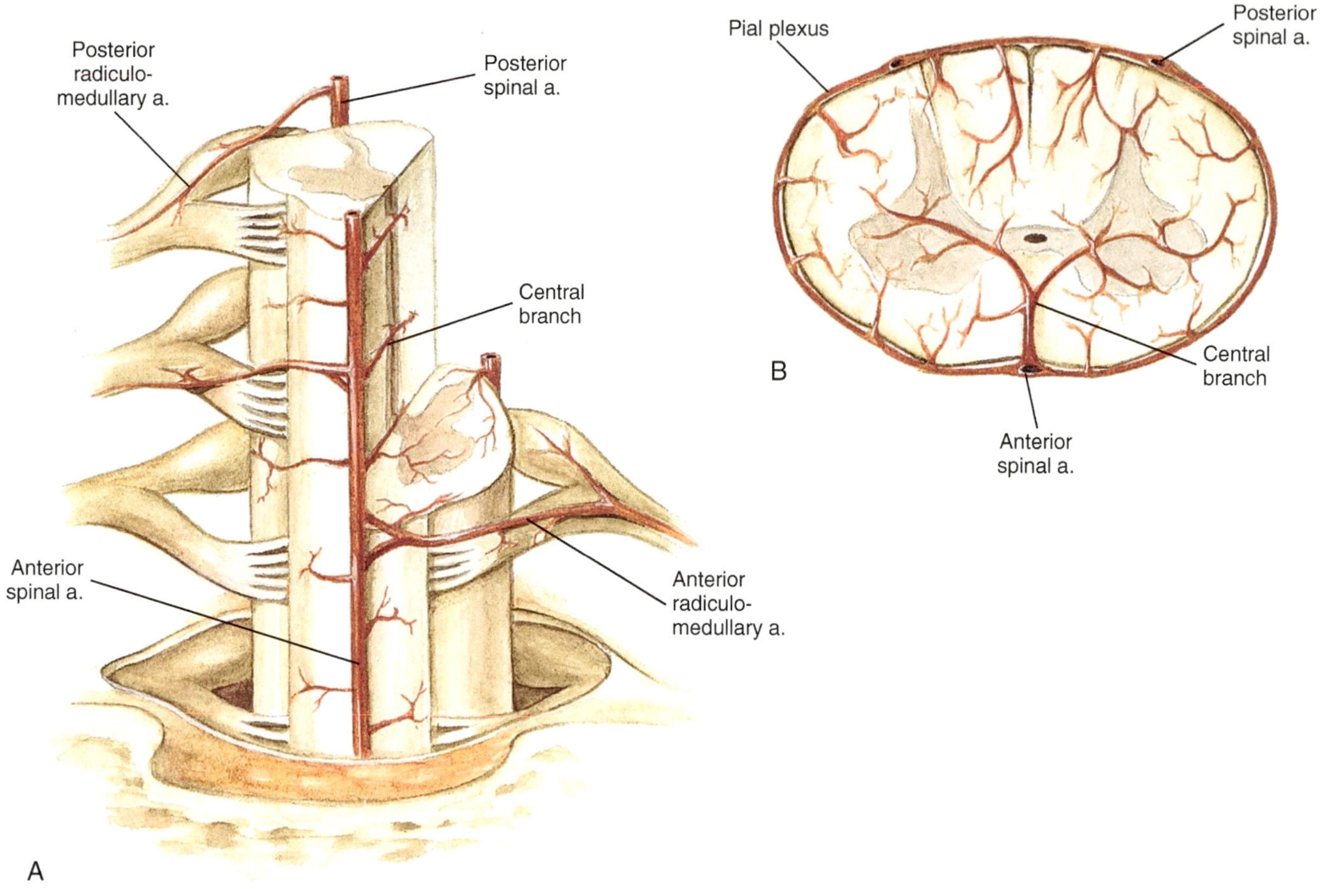

• **Fig. 6.2** Longitudinal (A) and cross-sectional (B) view of the vascular supply of the spinal cord. The anterior spinal artery provides blood flow to the anterior two-thirds of the spinal cord and the paired posterior spinal arteries provide blood flow to the posterior spinal cord. Reproduced with permission from Darby SA. Chapter 3: General anatomy of the spinal cord. In: Cramer GD, Darby SA, eds. *Clinical Anatomy of the Spine, Spinal Cord, and ANS*. 3rd ed. Mosby; 2014: 65–97.

One critical consideration is that patients with a new SCI may require intensive care unit (ICU) level care. Depending on the level and completeness of the injury, the patient may become hemodynamically unstable or require respiratory support. If an SCI is suspected, frequent monitoring of vital signs is important. From a cardiovascular standpoint, bradycardia and hypotension can result from dysregulation of the autonomic nervous system (**neurogenic shock**).[5,6] It may be so profound that vasopressor medications and intensive monitoring are required. From a pulmonary perspective, respiratory muscle weakness and autonomic dysregulation can lead to inadequate ventilation and decreased ability to clear secretions.[10] Both cervical and thoracic injuries demonstrate varied degrees of respiratory impairment. The risk of respiratory failure is directly associated with injury level. High cervical injuries are the most likely to require endotracheal intubation.[10] Involvement of pulmonology, respiratory therapy, and speech therapy may be necessary.

Medical interventions to mitigate or reverse damage to the spinal cord are an active area of research. For example, the use of steroids, specifically methylprednisolone, has been investigated extensively. Data supporting their use initially seemed encouraging, but more recent, larger studies have not found any significant neurologic difference in those patients treated with steroids compared to those treated without.[11–13] Furthermore, a high incidence of adverse effects, such as gastrointestinal bleeding, pneumonia, and hyperglycemia have been noted.[12,13] Current recommendations either recommend against or recommend careful consideration prior to administration of methylprednisolone.[12,13]

Surgical techniques after acute damage to the spinal cord are discussed outside of this chapter.

The rest of this chapter will focus on how to approach many of the expected complications after an SCI.

Neurogenic Bowel

SCI often causes bowel dysfunction, termed **neurogenic bowel**. SCI can result in two general patterns of neurogenic bowel depending on the location and extent of the damage.[9,14] Injuries above T12 typically lead to UMN lesions, termed a **reflexic bowel**, as the defecation reflexes connecting the spinal cord and bowel are intact. Waste moves through the digestive tract, utilizing the preserved gastric and colonic reflexes, but it is challenging to pass stool due to increased muscle tone of the anal sphincter. Lumbar or sacral spinal cord injuries can produce a LMN lesion, leading to loss of reflex coordination (**areflexic bowel**) and a flaccid anal sphincter.[9] Both types can lead to incontinence and constipation.

The mainstay of neurogenic bowel management is promoting predictable bowel movements. Bowel programs are necessary from the onset of the SCI to facilitate regular bowel movements and prevent fecal incontinence or impaction.[9] Oral bowel medications including stool softeners and peristaltic stimulants can be used to establish a regular bowel pattern. Sufficient water intake, exercise, and a regular diet with adequate fiber content is recommended to promote digestive health and regular bowel movements.[14,15] Additionally, when they are able, patients should be seated on a toilet or padded commode chair, which allows gravity to assist with evacuation.

For those with a reflexic bowel, the bowel program can take advantage of the body's natural defecation reflexes. Eating or drinking 30 minutes before the program is recommended, as it promotes peristalsis via the **gastrocolic reflex**. Digital stimulation, or manually stimulating the rectum with slow and gentle rotation of the finger, utilizes the **rectocolic reflex** to propel stool down the rectum and induce relaxation of the internal anal sphincter.[14] A reflexic bowel program often includes inserting a rectal suppository and performing digital stimulation, which can be repeated until stool evacuation is complete.[9,16]

Areflexic bowels do not respond to suppositories or digital stimulation, due to lack of intact reflex arcs. Often, stool must be removed manually.[9] Patients can promote evacuation using maneuvers like abdominal massage, deep breathing, Valsalva maneuvers, or leaning forward.[16] Stool bulking agents can be useful in specific situations, as a firmer stool consistency can facilitate manual evacuation and prevent leaking through the anal sphincter.[9]

Neurogenic Bladder

Similar to the bowel, the bladder is also affected by autonomic dysregulation from SCI. Appropriate acute management of a **neurogenic bladder** is pivotal in SCI to prevent long-term consequences.

Both UMN and LMN lesions cause difficulty urinating and incontinence. UMN physiology results in overactive, disinhibited voiding reflexes and bladder spasms.[8] In addition, the detrusor muscle of the bladder and the urethral sphincter can act in an uncoordinated fashion, leading to inadequate emptying and high bladder pressures.[8,17] LMN physiology results in a flaccid detrusor, unable to fully empty, which can lead to high bladder volumes and overflow incontinence.[8] Urodynamic studies may be helpful in distinguishing these different pathologies. When patients chronically retain urine, it can lead to complications such as vesicoureteral reflux, hydroureter, hydronephrosis, and renal failure.[8,17,18]

When SCI is suspected, an indwelling Foley catheter should be inserted and maintained while the patient is stabilized. Practically, the Foley catheter is sometimes left in place until the patient is having regular bowel movements. Once the Foley catheter is removed, frequently monitoring bladder volumes to ensure the patient is not retaining urine is very important. Patients may require a variety of techniques to achieve continence, ranging from timed toileting programs to surgical techniques.[8] Clean intermittent catheterization (CIC) is frequently used as a management strategy and is often the treatment of choice. Patients are taught to perform CIC every 4 to 6 hours, depending on fluid intake, voiding volumes, and incontinence.[18] CIC is thought to decrease the risk for urinary tract infections (UTIs) compared to indwelling Foley catheters.[19,20] See Box 6.1 for further information about UTIs in SCI.

Adequate bowel and bladder management are crucial first steps in promoting a patient's independence. Neurogenic bowel and bladder can have a significant impact on all aspects of a person's life, including health, self-esteem, participation in activities, and quality of life.[18,21,22] Ultimately, the goal of the bowel and bladder program is to determine the best strategies to create a predictable bowel movement and complete, regular voiding with minimal incontinence.

Skin and Pressure Injury

Monitoring a patient's skin is essential after an SCI, as there is significant morbidity and mortality from pressure injuries.

• BOX 6.1

Urinary tract infections (UTIs) are a major cause of morbidity and mortality in patients with SCI. However, asymptomatic bacteriuria is common in SCI and should not be treated. Treatment is recommended when the patient has clinical signs of systemic infection, which may present differently if the patient has altered abdominal or pelvic sensation. These signs and symptoms may include cloudy urine with increased odor, incontinence, autonomic dysreflexia, lethargy, and worsened spasticity.[8]

Pressure-sensitive areas of skin with absent or altered sensation are at high risk for breakdown causing ulcers, wounds, and infections such as osteomyelitis. Severe enough pressure injuries may require excision of the ulcer and necrotic tissue, as well as resurfacing the area with a musculocutaneous flap.[23] Treatment for pressure-induced ulcers are costly and can lead to their own complications. For example, the prolonged bedrest required for surgical healing after a musculocutaneous flap procedure can induce further debility. Prevention of these types of wounds is crucial. In the hospital, patients need to be repositioned in bed at least every 2 hours, have pressure-reducing support surfaces positioned beneath them, and undergo frequent, thorough skin checks.[23] Seating systems should be properly fitted and well padded. As time goes on, patients and caregivers must learn how to appropriately weight shift themselves throughout the day and perform daily skin checks to evaluate for areas of breakdown.[23] These routines require vigilance and should become a lifelong commitment.

Blood Pressure Regulation

Blood pressure abnormalities, including **orthostatic hypotension** (OH) and **autonomic dysreflexia** (AD), are common in patients with SCI. These are especially seen in patients with lesions at or above the level of T6 in the spinal cord.

OH often accompanies SCI. In a patient without an SCI, the transition to an upright position causes an initial decrease in blood pressure that is sensed by aortic and carotid baroreceptors, which leads to a compensatory sympathetic signal to vasoconstrict peripheral blood vessels. However, in SCI, the injury can interrupt that compensatory response, resulting in hypotension.[24] Symptoms include nausea, lightheadedness, and syncope. Initial management includes supine or even Trendelenburg positioning, lower extremity and abdominal compression, and, in certain cases, fluid resuscitation. If the orthostasis persists despite conservative management, titration of medications, such as midodrine or fludrocortisone, with the assistance of specialists and pharmacists can be helpful.

AD is a life-threatening complication of SCI due to uncontrolled sympathetic activity. A noxious stimulus below the level of the spinal cord lesion creates a sympathetic response. This leads to regional vasoconstriction and hypertension.[25] The high blood pressure is sensed by aortic and carotid baroreceptors, but it is unable to suppress the response because of the injury to the spinal cord. This sympathetic surge builds without any negative feedback, due to interruption of the descending central sympathetic control from the brain.[25] The patients often experience headache, sweating, and flushing above the level of SCI, alongside a variety of other symptoms including blurred vision, piloerection, stuffy nose, and anxiety.[25] Some patients also experience reflex bradycardia, though this is not always present.[25] Management of AD includes immediately sitting the patient upright and loosening any tight clothing.[26] This is followed by identifying and treating the noxious stimuli causing AD. The noxious stimulus is most often related to the bladder, bowel, or skin, but can be related to any number of conditions.[26] For example, a clogged Foley catheter, an infection, constipation, a wound, or constrictive clothing are all common causes of AD. The hypertension should resolve once the stimulus is removed or treated.[25,26] If blood pressure remains significantly elevated after these steps and a source of AD is not identified, medications to lower BP should be initiated. Nitrates and other short-acting antihypertensives are often used as first-line agents.[26] Frequent blood pressure monitoring after administration is required to assess the response. If all the above measures are unsuccessful, ICU monitoring and intravenous antihypertensives may be required. Untreated AD can lead to hypertensive encephalopathy, stroke, cardiac arrest, seizure, or death.[25,26]

Venous Thromboembolism

Venous thromboembolism (VTE) is a common complication following SCI, due to acute onset of venous stasis from immobility, often in the setting of accompanying endothelial injury or orthopedic trauma.[27] SCI also leads to a transient hypercoagulable state.[27] Proposed mechanisms for this change include alterations in the circadian rhythm of hemostasis and fibrinolysis,[28] impaired fibrinolytic activity,[29] and increased platelet affinity for collagen and elevated Factor VIII activity.[30] VTE is a significant cause of morbidity and mortality for SCI patients.[27] Pulmonary emboli are a frequent cause of death in the first year after SCI.[31]

Low-molecular-weight heparin (LMWH) is recommended within 72 hours of SCI to minimize the occurrence of VTE and is preferred over unfractionated heparin.[27] In the surgical setting, if possible, LMWH should be held on the morning of surgery and resumed within 24 hours following surgery.[32] The optimal duration of therapy remains under investigation. Thromboprophylaxis is recommended for at least 8 weeks after initial injury, though this should be considered on an individualized patient basis.[27]

Other Important Chronic Considerations

- **Temperature regulation** can be impaired in patients with SCI, especially with cervical and high thoracic injuries.[5]
- **Pain** frequently accompanies SCI. Studies indicate that approximately half of patients have neuropathic pain after SCI and should be treated.[33]
- **Spasticity**, or an increase in muscle tone due to lack of inhibition from the cerebral cortex, is often a chronic complication of SCI.[7,34] Patients may require systemic medication, targeted injections, or other interventions if the spasticity impacts the patient's daily life.[34]

- **Emotional adjustment** after SCI can be challenging. Common psychosocial complications include depression, suicide, drug addiction, and divorce.[35,36] Depression has a higher prevalence in patients after SCI, compared to the general population.[15,37] This has devastating consequences, as suicide is a leading cause of death in SCI patients younger than 55 years old.[15] Due to the high prevalence, regular screening for depression and suicidality is critical. Recommended treatment includes counseling for patients and families, pharmacologic intervention, and peer support groups.[37]

Rehabilitation

Generally, managing SCI is complex and requires a multidisciplinary team. Physical medicine and rehabilitation (PM&R) physicians, physical therapists, occupational therapists, and speech therapists are essential to help patients return to the life they led prior to the injury. Recognition of injury should prompt consultation of these specialties as early as possible. Patients need to learn skills to physically navigate their environment and perform their activities of daily living after their injury.[15] In addition, a key aspect of the rehabilitation process is education about SCI, because the patient and their caregivers will be responsible for managing many of the medical conditions associated with SCI after discharge.[15] Rehabilitation serves to empower the patient and their caregivers to move forward in their life after SCI.

Navigating Prognosis, Function, and Uncertainty

SCI is a chronic, lifelong condition. Patients with spinal cord injuries often face significant changes in their life and will have questions about what to expect moving forward. One challenge of caring for patients with SCI is navigating the uncertainty of the future.

Spinal cord injury recovery is measured on a scale of months. The most rapid rate of recovery is observed within the first 3 months after a traumatic spinal cord injury.[38] The majority of recovery occurs within the first 6 to 9 months.[38] A plateau in motor recovery often occurs around 12 to 18 months.[38]

Naturally, patients and loved ones will have questions about their ultimate prognosis. For example, they may wonder if the patient will regain the ability to ambulate or live independently. PM&R physicians can assist with discussing functional and neurologic prognostication. Generally, less recovery is expected from more complete spinal cord injuries, which is the most important determinant of long-term prognosis.[39] In addition, the more cranial the lesion, the more likely the patient may require assistance in the future. Patients with incomplete paraplegia are more likely to ambulate compared to incomplete tetraplegia.[40] The age of the patient is also a significant predictive factor, as patients greater than 50 years old have a decreased likelihood of recovering walking ability 1 year postinjury, compared to patients less than 50 years old.[41,42] Spasticity, balance, proprioception, trunk control, and cognition also play a role in whether the patient ambulates in the future.[40] The team should help prepare the patient to return to life as independently as possible with their current deficits, knowing they may improve with time and therapy.

Conclusion

Surgeons and other providers should understand general complications and management principles when working with a patient with SCI. SCI is complex and affects almost all organ systems, and serious complications can result from SCI if cared for improperly. Patients benefit from a multidisciplinary approach, including rehabilitation professionals, as they navigate a life that may look very different after their injury.

References

1. Saifuddin A, Burnett SJ, White J. The variation of position of the conus medullaris in an adult population. A magnetic resonance imaging study. *Spine (Phila Pa 1976)*. 1998;23(13):1452–1456. https://doi.org/10.1097/00007632-199807010-00005.
2. Bican O, Minagar A, Pruitt AA. The spinal cord: a review of functional neuroanatomy. *Neurol Clin*. 2013;31(1):1–18. https://doi.org/10.1016/j.ncl.2012.09.009.
3. Taterra D, Skinningsrud B, Pękala PA, et al. Artery of Adamkiewicz: a meta-analysis of anatomical characteristics. *Neuroradiology*. 2019;61(8):869–880. https://doi.org/10.1007/s00234-019-02207-y.
4. American Spinal Injury Association. International Standards for Neurological Classification of SCI (ISNCSCI) Worksheet. American Spinal Injury Association. https://asia-spinalinjury.org/international-standards-neurological-classification-sci-isncsci-worksheet/.
5. Hagen EM. Acute complications of spinal cord injuries. *World J Orthop*. 2015;6(1):17. https://doi.org/10.5312/wjo.v6.i1.17.
6. Ruiz IA, Squair JW, Phillips AA, et al. Incidence and natural progression of neurogenic shock after traumatic spinal cord injury. *J Neurotrauma*. 2018;35(3):461–466. https://doi.org/10.1089/neu.2016.4947.
7. Segal M. Muscle overactivity in the upper motor neuron syndrome: Pathophysiology. *Phys Med Rehabil Clin N Am*. 2018;29(3):427–436. https://doi.org/10.1016/j.pmr.2018.04.005.
8. Consortium for Spinal Cord Medicine Bladder management for adults with spinal cord injury: a clinical practice guideline for health-care providers. *J Spinal Cord Med*. 2006;29(5):527–573.
9. Johns J, Krogh K, Rodriguez GM, et al. Management of neurogenic bowel dysfunction in adults after spinal cord injury suggested citation: Jeffery Johns, Klaus Krogh, Gianna M. Rodriguez, Janice Eng, Emily Haller, Malorie Heinen, Rafferty Laredo, Walter Longo, Wilda Montero-Colon, Mark Korsten. Management of neurogenic bowel dysfunction in adults after spinal cord injury: Clinical practice guideline for healthcare providers. *J Spinal Cord Med*. 2021;44(3):442–510. [published

correction appears in *J Spinal Cord Med.* 2021;44(4):684]. https://doi.org/10.1080/10790268.2021.1883385.
10. Berlowitz DJ, Wadsworth B, Ross J. Respiratory problems and management in people with spinal cord injury. *Breathe (Sheff).* 2016;12(4):328–340. https://doi.org/10.1183/20734735.012616.
11. Canseco JA, Karamian BA, Bowles DR, et al. Updated review: The steroid controversy for management of spinal cord injury. *World Neurosurg.* 2021;150:1–8. https://doi.org/10.1016/j.wneu.2021.02.116.
12. Liu Z, Yang Y, He L, et al. High-dose methylprednisolone for acute traumatic spinal cord injury: A meta-analysis. *Neurology.* 2019;93(9):e841–e850. https://doi.org/10.1212/WNL.0000000000007998.
13. Sultan I, Lamba N, Liew A, et al. The safety and efficacy of steroid treatment for acute spinal cord injury: A Systematic Review and meta-analysis. *Heliyon.* 2020;6(2):e03414. https://doi.org/10.1016/j.heliyon.2020.e03414.
14. Lynch AC, Antony A, Dobbs BR, Frizelle FA. Bowel dysfunction following spinal cord injury. *Spinal Cord.* 2001;39(4):193–203. https://doi.org/10.1038/sj.sc.3101119.
15. Kirshblum SC, Priebe MM, Ho CH, Scelza WM, Chiodo AE, Wuermser LA. Spinal cord injury medicine. 3. Rehabilitation phase after acute spinal cord injury. *Arch Phys Med Rehabil.* 2007;88(3 Suppl 1):S62–S70. https://doi.org/10.1016/j.apmr.2006.12.003.
16. Krassioukov A, Eng JJ, Claxton G, Sakakibara BM, Shum S. Neurogenic bowel management after spinal cord injury: a systematic review of the evidence. *Spinal Cord.* 2010;48(10):718–733. https://doi.org/10.1038/sc.2010.14.
17. Hamid R, Averbeck MA, Chiang H, Garcia A, Al Mousa RT, Oh SJ, Patel A, Plata M, Del Popolo G. Epidemiology and pathophysiology of neurogenic bladder after spinal cord injury. *World J Urol.* 2018;36(10):1517–1527. https://doi.org/10.1007/s00345-018-2301-z.
18. Taweel WA, Seyam R. Neurogenic bladder in spinal cord injury patients. *Res Rep Urol.* 2015;7:85–99. https://doi.org/10.2147/RRU.S29644.
19. Esclarín De Ruz A, García Leoni E, Herruzo Cabrera R. Epidemiology and risk factors for urinary tract infection in patients with spinal cord injury. *J Urol.* 2000;164(4):1285–1289. https://doi.org/10.1016/S0022-5347(05)67157-1.
20. National Institute On Disability And Rehabilitation Research Prevention and management of urinary tract infections among people with SCI: Consensus statement. *NeuroRehabilitation.* 1994;4(4):222–236. https://doi.org/10.3233/NRE-1994-4405.
21. Glickman S, Kamm MA. Bowel dysfunction in spinal-cord-injury patients. *Lancet.* 1996;347(9016):1651–1653. https://doi.org/10.1016/s0140-6736(96)91487-7.
22. Liu CW, Attar KH, Gall A, Shah J, Craggs M. The relationship between bladder management and health-related quality of life in patients with spinal cord injury in the UK. *Spinal Cord.* 2010;48(4):319–324. https://doi.org/10.1038/sc.2009.132.
23. Consortium for Spinal Cord Medicine Clinical Practice Guidelines Pressure ulcer prevention and treatment following spinal cord injury: A clinical practice guideline for health-care professionals. *J Spinal Cord Med.* 2001;24(sup1):S40–S101. https://doi.org/10.1080/10790268.2001.11753592.
24. Claydon VE, Steeves JD, Krassioukov A. Orthostatic hypotension following spinal cord injury: understanding clinical pathophysiology. *Spinal Cord.* 2006;44(6):341–351. https://doi.org/10.1038/sj.sc.3101855.
25. Eldahan KC, Rabchevsky AG. Autonomic dysreflexia after spinal cord injury: Systemic pathophysiology and methods of management. *Auton Neurosci.* 2018;209:59–70. https://doi.org/10.1016/j.autneu.2017.05.002.
26. Krassioukov A, Linsenmeyer TA, Beck LA, et al. Evaluation and management of autonomic dysreflexia and other autonomic dysfunctions: Preventing the highs and lows: Management of blood pressure, sweating, and temperature dysfunction. *Top Spinal Cord Inj Rehabil.* 2021;27(2):225–290. https://doi.org/10.46292/sci2702-225.
27. Prevention of venous thromboembolism in individuals with spinal cord injury: Clinical practice guidelines for health care providers, 3rd ed.: Consortium for Spinal Cord Medicine. *Top Spinal Cord Inj Rehabil.* 2016;22(3):209–240. https://doi.org/10.1310/sci2203-209.
28. Iversen PO, Groot PDE, Hjeltnes N, Andersen TO, Mowinckel MC, Sandset PM. Impaired circadian variations of haemostatic and fibrinolytic parameters in tetraplegia: Haemostatic and fibrinolytic oscillations in tetraplegia. *Br J Haematol.* 2002;119(4):1011–1016. https://doi.org/10.1046/j.1365-2141.2002.03953.x.
29. Winther K, Gleerup G, Snorrason K, Biering-Sørensen F. Platelet function and fibrinolytic activity in cervical spinal cord injured patients. *Thromb Res.* 1992;65(3):469–474. https://doi.org/10.1016/0049-3848(92)90178-D.
30. Green D, Rossi EC, Yao JST, Flinn WR, Spies SM. Deep vein thrombosis in spinal cord injury: effect of prophylaxis with calf compression, aspirin,and dipyridamole. *Spinal Cord.* 1982;20(4):227–234. https://doi.org/10.1038/sc.1982.41.
31. National Spinal Cord Injury Statistical Center. 2021 Annual Statistical Report for the Spinal Cord Injury Model Systems – Complete Public Version. University of Alabama at Birmingham: Birmingham, Alabama.
32. Christie S, Thibault-Halman G, Casha S. Acute pharmacological DVT prophylaxis after spinal cord injury. *J Neurotrauma.* 2011;28(8):1509–1514. https://doi.org/10.1089/neu.2009.1155-A.
33. Burke D, Fullen BM, Stokes D, Lennon O. Neuropathic pain prevalence following spinal cord injury: A systematic review and meta-analysis. *Eur J Pain.* 2017;21(1):29–44. https://doi.org/10.1002/ejp.905.
34. Adams M, Hicks A. Spasticity after spinal cord injury. *Spinal Cord.* 2005;43:577–586. https://doi.org/10.1038/sj.sc.3101757.
35. Hagen EM, Lie SA, Rekand T, Gilhus NE, Gronning M. Mortality after traumatic spinal cord injury: 50 years of follow-up. *J Neurol Neurosurg Psychiatry.* 2010;81(4):368–373. https://doi.org/10.1136/jnnp.2009.178798.
36. North NT. The psychological effects of spinal cord injury: a review. *Spinal Cord.* 1999;37(10):671–679. https://doi.org/10.1038/sj.sc.3100913.
37. Consortium for Spinal Cord Medicine. *Depression Following Spinal Cord Injury: A Clinical Practice Guideline for Primary Care Physicians.* Washington, DC: Paralyzed Veterans of America; 1998.
38. Kirshblum S, Snider B, Eren F, Guest J. Characterizing natural recovery after traumatic spinal cord injury. *J Neurotrauma.* 2021;38(9):1267–1284. https://doi.org/10.1089/neu.2020.7473.

39. Kirshblum SC, O'Connor KC. Levels of spinal cord injury and predictors of neurologic recovery. *Phys Med Rehabil Clin N Am.* 2000;11(1):1-vii.
40. Chay W, Kirshblum S. Predicting outcomes after spinal cord injury. *Phys Med Rehabil Clin N Am.* 2020;31(3):331–343. https://doi.org/10.1016/j.pmr.2020.03.003.
41. Oleson CV, Marino RJ, Leiby BE, Ditunno JF. Influence of age alone, and age combined with pinprick, on recovery of walking function in motor complete, sensory incomplete spinal cord injury. *Arch Phys Med Rehabil.* 2016;97(10):1635–1641. https://doi.org/10.1016/j.apmr.2016.01.024.
42. Penrod LE, Hegde SK, Ditunno Jr. JF. Age effect on prognosis for functional recovery in acute, traumatic central cord syndrome. *Arch Phys Med Rehabil.* 1990;71(12):963–968.

7 Managing Nerve Root Injuries

DIANA JOHNSON, KEMLY PHILIP, AND VENU AKUTHOTA

CHAPTER OUTLINE

Introduction

Radiculopathy, or radicular syndrome, refers to the broad collection of symptoms secondary to injury of the spinal nerve root, whether by mechanical compression or inflammation.[1] Lumbosacral radiculopathy is common and, in fact, accounts for up to 32.4% of the 577 million cases worldwide of lower back pain.[1] Similarly, neck pain is considered the fourth leading cause of disability worldwide after low back pain, of which the annual incidence of cervical radiculopathy is 1.79 per 1000 person-years.[2,3] Patients will often present with radiating pain, paresthesias, or numbness along a dermatome or myotomal weakness in the distribution of the involved nerve root.[1,4] Radicular pain may be used to describe symptoms in a dermatomal pattern without neurologic weakness or sensory deficit. Of note, the term radiculopathy implies neurologic deficit.[1]

Mechanical etiologies of nerve root injury include bony overgrowth of the spinal vertebrae, herniated or degenerative disc disease, spinal stenosis, spondylolisthesis, and facet synovial cysts.[5] Other causes include trauma, mass, inflammation, infection (e.g., shingles), metabolic, or vascular lesions that involve the nerve root.[5]

Nerve Root Injuries: Clinical Evaluation

A comprehensive history should include identifying any red flag symptoms that suggest malignancy, infection, fracture, or other threat to neurologic function such as acute cauda equina syndrome. To this end, other considerations that may warrant expedited diagnostic imaging include whether a patient is younger than 20 or older than 50 years of age, presence of constitutional symptoms including fevers or night sweats, bowel, bladder, or sexual dysfunction, saddle anesthesia, or history of trauma, cancer, immunosuppression, or IV drug use.[6] Evaluating for autoimmune or genetic disease such as rheumatoid arthritis or Down syndrome should raise suspicion for other causes of nonnerve root or radicular neck pain such as atlantoaxial instability.[2] Similarly, clinical history should assess the quality of pain, neuropathic versus nociceptive, and any exacerbating or alleviating factors that support a diagnosis of nerve root injury.

Physical evaluation for diagnosing radiculopathy includes a complete neurologic and focused musculoskeletal exam to evaluate for myotomal weakness or dermatomal changes in sensation, assessment of upper motor neuron signs and gait disturbances.[6] Provocative maneuvers to reproduce radicular symptoms due to nerve root injury include neural tension maneuvers (e.g., the Spurling maneuver or Straight Leg Raise test). The Spurling maneuver, shoulder abduction relief test, and neck distraction tests have moderate sensitivity but high specificity greater than 85% in distinguishing cervical radiculopathy from other mechanical causes of neck or arm pain.[2] Neural tension maneuvers can be nuanced further to evaluate different nerve roots. For example, the femoral stretch test evaluates nerve root irritation of the L2, L3, or L4 nerve roots.[1]

Nerve Root Injuries: Diagnosis

The diagnosis of nerve root injury or radiculopathy can be made largely on clinical history and physical exam as discussed above. Further diagnostic evaluation with advanced imaging is not recommended for patients with radicular pain lasting less than 4 to 6 weeks.[6] Additionally, as many as 27% up to 80% of asymptomatic patients may have imaging findings of disc herniation on magnetic resonance imaging (MRI), emphasizing the need to correlate with history and physical exam.[1] If symptoms do not resolve with conservative management, then further diagnostic imaging should be considered.

Plain radiographs are easily accessible and may reveal skeletal bony abnormalities including fractures, transitional vertebrae, disc space narrowing, spondylosis, or segmental instability; however, soft tissue assessment is limited.[7] Magnetic resonance imaging is considered the gold standard for diagnosis given its superior resolution of the spinal cord, canal, neural foramen, nerve roots, and discs. Limitations of MRI, however, include cost, claustrophobia, presence of metal, and is contraindicated in patients with pacemakers or aneurysmal metal clips; for this reason, computed tomography (CT) or CT myelogram may serve as an alternative with improved evaluation of the cortical bone.[7] Electrodiagnostic studies have high sensitivity for radiculopathy ranging from 50% to 80% although they do not reveal the cause of nerve root injury like the cross-sectional imaging modalities above.[2,4] Additional diagnostic workup including cell blood count or evaluation of inflammatory markers may be ordered if suspicion exists for infectious, inflammatory, or neoplastic cause of nerve root injury.[6]

Nonoperative Management

Most cases of radiculopathy are often self-limited.[3,4] However, guidelines suggest that initial treatment for nerve root injuries should include conservative management with a combination of patient education, oral anti-inflammatory medications, focused physical therapy, therapeutic exercise, and/or psychological programs, or targeted injections before considering invasive operative treatment.[4,6,8,9] A recent prospective observational cohort showed that patients with motor deficits due to lumbosacral radiculopathy can still regain strength and function at 12 months regardless of intervention with surgery or a comprehensive pain management and rehabilitation program.[10] The following section discusses features to consider in a comprehensive treatment program

Physical Therapy

A comprehensive rehabilitation program to manage spine-related musculoskeletal pain and dysfunction consists of acute, recovery, and maintenance phases.[11] The acute phase incorporates education on how to protect the injured tissue and proper body mechanics to avoid further injury.[11] Relative rest and gentle return to activity are encouraged. Immobilization is avoided as it results in decreased muscle strength, endurance, and flexibility. Therapeutic exercise aimed at improving muscle strength, flexibility, and aerobic capacity is incorporated early alongside modalities and medications for symptom control in this phase.[11]

The recovery phase aims to optimize range of motion, strength, and balance with minimal pain.[11] For spine-related conditions, stabilization exercises are often used to emphasize the synergistic activation of the trunk and paraspinal musculature in the mid-range position.[12] Developing muscular support of the trunk and spine reduces stress on the intervertebral disk and other static stabilizers of the spine, thereby decreasing the recurrence of low back pain from spondylolysis and spondylolisthesis.[11,13] Mechanical diagnosis and treatment (MDT) or McKenzie therapy is often an extension-biased program that aims to centralize peripheral symptoms to the spine.[12] Patients are divided into subgroups based upon the historical and mechanical properties of their pain.[14] Most patients centralize their pain with extension exercises, but others respond to side bending or flexion exercises.[11] In the short term, McKenzie therapy has been shown to be more effective than comparison treatments such as nonsteroidal anti-inflammatory medications, general mobility exercises, strength training with therapist guidance, and spinal mobilization.[14] Assessment of long-term efficacy is limited by the lack of randomized controlled trials comparing McKenzie therapy to placebo or no treatment.[14]

Finally, the maintenance phase of the comprehensive rehabilitation program involves return to work and other activities to promote continued fitness and education regarding ergonomics, posture training, and reinforcing awareness of biomechanics during activities of daily living to prevent reinjury.[11]

Modalities

Therapists might employ modalities to exchange energy between tissues including the delivery of heat, cold, light waves, sound waves, or electricity to alter the transmission or perception of the pain message, thereby achieving a therapeutic response.[11,15] Modalities are best used in the acute period after injury as an adjunct to an active treatment program.[12]

Superficial heat causes cutaneous vasodilation and increased blood flow to local tissues and has been shown to decrease pain and alleviate muscle spasms.[11,15] Cryotherapy, or therapeutic use of cold, achieves local analgesia via vasoconstriction, decreasing the delivery of inflammatory vasodilators to the injured area and desensitizing local nociceptors.[15]

Ultrasound diathermy generates vibrations that heat high protein–concentrated tissues such as muscle, ligament, tendon, nerve, and bones.[15] Ultrasound diathermy is capable of heating deeper structures than superficial heat modalities (5 cm vs 0.5 cm from surface, respectively), but does not alleviate pain or muscle spasms as effectively as superficial heating.[11,15] Most studies failed to demonstrate a statistically significant benefit of the use of ultrasound diathermy in an array of musculoskeletal conditions, limiting its incorporation into the therapeutic plan of care.[11,15]

Transcutaneous electrical nerve stimulation (TENS) stimulates cutaneous nerve fibers using surface electrodes emitting a mild electrical current to directly affect pain signal transmission.[11] Frequency and intensity can be adjusted to optimize patient tolerance and modulate various types of pain.[11]

Traction and manipulation are thought to provide symptomatic relief from radicular pain by relieving compression on nerve roots.[16] Cervical traction is easier to apply than lumbar traction as less weight needs to be countered. Manual manipulation can be trialed by a therapist or chiropractor; however, if the patient has failed to improve after three to four treatments, manipulation should be discontinued and the patient should be reassessed.[11]

Acupuncture attenuates pain through activation of bioactive chemicals through peripheral, spinal, and supraspinal mechanisms.[17] Clinical studies on the efficacy of acupuncture support its temporary benefits for ailments such as neck pain, tension headache, migraines, and pain from osteoarthritis of the knee and low back.[17] Like other modalities, acupuncture may serve as an adjunct to multimodal pain management to reduce pharmacologic analgesic doses and thus reduce risk of adverse side effects.[17]

Oral Medications

The goal of oral medications is to provide adequate analgesia, targeting central and peripheral pain pathways, to ultimately increase patient participation in the comprehensive rehabilitation program. Pain medications often do not eliminate pain entirely; therefore, careful counseling and establishing patient expectations is crucial in the prescription of both opioid and nonopioid analgesics.[18]

Nonopioid analgesics frequently encountered in the treatment of spine-related musculoskeletal complaints include acetaminophen, nonsteroidal anti-inflammatory drugs (NSAIDs), corticosteroids, muscle relaxants, anticonvulsants, antidepressants, and antispasmodics.[11] Acetaminophen is a safe and cost-effective analgesic, especially in the elderly where it is considered first-line therapy for pain given its low risk side effect profile and limited drug–drug interactions.[19] Its use in the treatment of nerve root injury or irritation is limited due to its weak anti-inflammatory effects and it has not been shown to be effective in the treatment of cervical or lumbar radiculopathy.[12,19]

NSAIDs attenuate pain and inflammation in a dose-dependent fashion and are best utilized in the acute period following injury.[19] The dose to achieve analgesic effects is substantially lower than the dose to reduce inflammation.[18] Care should be taken when titrating this class of medications to mitigate adverse side effects such as cardiovascular events, gastrointestinal bleeding, and acute kidney injury.[18] In fact, prolonged NSAID use is generally not indicated for most musculoskeletal complaints and should be avoided.[18]

Oral corticosteroids with high glucocorticoid effects are potent anti-inflammatories and can be used to relieve acute pain in conditions with an inflammatory component, such as acute cervical or lumbar radiculopathy.[20] The use of oral corticosteroids beyond the acute period is not recommended and practitioners should exercise caution when prescribing oral steroids to immunosuppressed or diabetic patients to avoid adverse side effects.[18]

Muscle spasm is a frequent complaint in patients afflicted with cervical or lumbar radiculopathy.[18] A review by Chou et al. examining the comparative efficacy and safety of skeletal muscle relaxants concluded there was fair evidence that antispasmodic medications such as cyclobenzaprine, carisoprodol, tizanidine, and methocarbamol were effective in treating acute neck or low back pain.[21] Cyclobenzaprine in particular has consistently been found to be effective in most clinical trials.[18] Antispasmodics can cause QT prolongation and significant anticholinergic side effects and should be used cautiously in the elderly or in those with cardiac arrhythmias or conduction disturbances.[18]

Gabapentin and pregabalin exert their analgesic effects by binding to a subunit of voltage-gated calcium channels and are frequently used in the treatment of pain associated with diabetic peripheral polyneuropathy and postherpetic neuralgia.[22] A prospective study of 1304 subjects with cervical and lumbar radiculopathy found that pregabalin monotherapy resulted in significant pain reduction and resource consumption.[23] Associated side effects with these medications include dizziness, fatigue, sleepiness, and difficulty with mentation.[22]

Selective serotonin reuptake inhibitors (SSRIs) and serotonin–norepinephrine reuptake inhibitors (SNRIs) are antidepressants with applications in the treatment of neuropathic pain. SSRIs do not have primary analgesic properties but are useful in treating the affective component of pain.[24] SNRIs differ from SSRIs because they inhibit both serotonin and norepinephrine reuptake, the latter of which has been shown to improve analgesia.[24] Duloxetine and venlafaxine are the most well-studied medications in this group. Duloxetine is usually selected owing to its more favorable side effect profile although common side effects include nausea, constipation, dry mouth, sleeping difficulties, and dizziness.[24]

Tricyclic antidepressants (TCAs) are an older class of medications that treat neuropathic pain via nonselective inhibition of norepinephrine and serotonin reuptake.[24] TCAs are widely available, inexpensive, and well-studied in the treatment of neuropathic pain. Their use is primarily limited by their extensive anticholinergic side effect profile.[24]

The decision to incorporate opioids into the patient's oral pain regimen should account for the cause, acuity, functional status, and expected clinical course of the patient's pain.[22] Opioids have not been shown to be effective in the treatment of nerve root–related symptoms and neuropathic pain, even when combined with other neuropathic pain medications.[24] Consideration may be given to relieve severe, acute pain as a bridge to return to activity and initiation of therapy. When using opioids for the treatment of acute pain, clinicians should prescribe the lowest effective dose of immediate-release opioids and should prescribe no greater quantity than needed for the expected duration of severe pain.[25] Clinicians should consider incorporating alternative treatments, such as nonopioid medications, physical therapy, and interventional pain procedures, which may reduce the opioid dose necessary to achieve adequate analgesia.[22]

Intervention With Injections

If patients do not respond to the above interventions, then image-guided injection can be considered as a next step. These injections often consist of a combination of corticosteroid and anesthetic that is targeted into the epidural space utilizing fluoroscopic and/or CT guidance. Targeted intervention towards the area of nerve root injury can provide not only therapeutic relief but also serve a diagnostic purpose in patients that may have multiple pain generators. It is believed that epidural steroid injections (ESIs) function by decreasing inflammation, nociceptive somatic input, synthesis of pain-modulating neuropeptides, and inhibit C-fiber activity in the dorsal root ganglion.[3]

There is Level 1 evidence to support lumbar transforaminal ESIs in symptomatic patients with lumbar radiculopathy due to disc herniation with the goal of improving pain and function in the short term, although the data are mixed regarding efficacy in the long term.[4] On the other hand, cervical transforaminal ESI has only been shown to provide 60% relief and only 25% of patients referred for surgical management may experience short-term relief.[26] In fact, there are some data that suggest the addition of steroid to anesthetic did not provide any additional pain relief at the 3-month mark.[4]

Different fluoroscopic approaches can be utilized to enter the epidural space; however, there is little evidence to suggest whether interlaminar, transforaminal, or caudal alters the effectiveness of ESIs nor whether there exists an optimal steroid type, dosing, or frequency of injections.[4] Given proximity of the cervical nerve root to the vertebral artery, some practitioners consider the interlaminar cervical ESI approach to be safer to avoid inadvertent vascular uptake that could cause cerebral infarction. Other factors to consider with ESI include assessing coagulopathy or anticoagulation therapy, ongoing bodily or local skin infection that may increase the risk of bleeding or infection related to the procedure. Steroid injections can have systemic effects including suppression of the hypothalamus-pituitary-adrenal axis, osteoporosis, or hyperglycemia so should be used cautiously in patients who may have premorbid conditions predisposing them to these adverse effects.[26]

Surgical management of nerve root injury in the long term can more quickly resolve radicular pain; however, it does not come without increased risks and costs. A single-center study of 100 patients with lumbar radiculopathy showed that at least 46% of patients avoided the need for surgery due to intervention with interlaminar ESI.[27] A more recent, multicenter, randomized control trial of transforaminal ESI in comparison to microdiscectomy amongst patients with a 12-month history of radicular pain due to disc herniation led to decreased pain and disability with an unsurprisingly, improved cost-effectiveness ratio per quality-adjusted year of life.[28] Ultimately, clinicians should seriously evaluate the effectiveness of injections as a step in conservative treatment, especially among patients without progressive or serious neurologic deficit.

Operative Management

Predictors of response to conservative treatment after nerve root injury include negative crossed straight leg raise, absence of leg pain with spinal extension, lack of stenosis on imaging, favorable response to ESIs, return of neurologic function within 12 weeks, along with motivated and fit patients with no workers compensation claims or psychological illness.[29] However, patients who do not respond to conservative management or minimally invasive intervention may ultimately benefit from surgical treatment.

Surgical Intervention

Operative management for patients with radiculopathy due to nerve root injury include percutaneous disc decompression, disc replacement, or decompression with discectomy or laminectomy. Surgery may be indicated for patients with persistent and disabling pain after at least 6 to 12 weeks of conservative management, progression of neurologic deficits, or in the presence of red flags suggesting acute cauda equina syndrome or worsening myelopathy.[30]

Given that spinal nerve roots are at risk for direct injury during operations involving the insertion of pedicle screws or in patients with canal and/or foraminal narrowing, intraoperative electromyography (EMG) serves to monitor nerve root and peripheral nerve.[31] Free-run EMG or triggered EMG is commonly used for neurophysiologic monitoring. In free-run EMG, nerve root irritation from surgical trauma leads to spontaneous discharges and muscle activation.[31] The utility of free-run EMG may be impaired in the setting of chronic irritation at the site of measurement or if neuromuscular blocking agents are used.[31] Triggered EMG is primarily used during the creation of pedicle screw tracks during major corrective spine surgery. A ballpoint stimulating electrode is inserted into the screw track and can identify a breech in the medial or lateral wall of the track prior to screw insertion, allowing for correction of the screw trajectory.[31]

The Spine Patients Outcomes Research Trial (SPORT) was a randomized clinical trial that examined the outcomes of surgical and nonoperative treatment for lumbar intervertebral disk herniation, spinal stenosis, or degenerative spondylolisthesis.[32] Both surgical and nonoperative groups substantially improved and the trial was not able to establish superiority or equivalence of either treatment due to significant bidirectional crossover between groups.[32] A subsequent as-treated analysis of both groups at 4 years demonstrated surgery was superior to nonoperative treatment in relieving symptoms and improving function.[33] It should be noted that the nonoperative group improved significantly over the same time period as well.[33]

Tendon Transfer for Nerve Injuries

Tendon transfer after nerve root injury is intended to restore function to nonfunctioning neuromuscular units through the transfer of force from functional neuromuscular units to nonfunctional units.[34] When considering tendon transfer to enhance function, there are many factors to consider. The functional loss associated with harvesting a donor tendon should be less than the expected functional gain expected after transfer. Furthermore, consideration should be paid to the strength of the donor tendon, as strength can be expected to decrease by one grade after transfer.[34] One should consider the force vector through which the donor tendon will act and whether this vector is aligned with the recipient site. The recipient site should be a stable and flexible soft tissue bed with minimal scar tissue to allow the donor tendon to move easily in its recipient site.[34] Finally, unlike nerve transfers, tendon transfers can be performed many years after injury, making this an attractive option in the reconstructive algorithm.

Postoperative Orthotic Management

Bracing serves to immobilize and unload forces on the spine.[35] Spinal orthoses offer proprioceptive feedback to encourage the patient to move more slowly than he or she might move in an unbraced state.[35] This can be accomplished with both a soft or rigid orthosis.[35] Bracing is routinely used after surgery for a number of spinal pathologies including cervical and lumbar degenerative disease, vertebral fractures, and scoliosis.[36] However, current evidence suggests postoperative bracing in patients with degenerative cervical myelopathy, radiculopathy, or lumbar degenerative disease does not improve pain, fusion rate, or the incidence of complications.[36] Therefore, the use of spinal orthoses in these situations should be primarily as a psychological reminder to avoid sudden movements that might reinjure healing tissue.[35]

Psychological Considerations

The stress associated with chronic pain can unveil premorbid, semidormant personality characteristics that affect mood, thought patterns, and coping abilities that can influence tolerance to treatment, adverse side effects, or compliance with rehabilitation.[37] Clinicians should approach a patient's pain experience from the biopsychosocial perspective, which is multidimensional and influenced by the interaction of biological factors, psychological comorbidities, social support, and environmental circumstances.[37]

Dorow et al. found that persistent pain after surgery may be associated with psychological factors and pain that existed premorbidly, including anxiety, depression, or somatization.[38] To mitigate pain chronification, numerous authors suggest psychological screenings to identify at-risk individuals and expansion of preventative approaches and psychological interventions, alongside routine surgical treatment.[38]

Conclusions

Low back pain is the 15th cause of disability worldwide with a yearly incidence of 245.9 million cases.[39] The annual prevalence of neck pain is as high as 52%.[2] Nerve root injuries causing radicular pain or radiculopathy account for a fair portion of pain in these patients. Robust clinical trials are needed to investigate impact of ESI or surgery; however, there is sufficient evidence to support the value and utilization of a multidisciplinary and comprehensive pain program to yield functional gains and improve the quality of life of the millions impacted due to this burden of disease.

References

1. Malik K, Benzon HT. Chapter 21: Low back pain. In: Hurley R, ed. *Essentials of Pain Medicine*. 4th ed. Elsevier; 2017.
2. Cohen S. Epidemiology, diagnosis, and treatment of neck pain. *Mayo Clin Proc*. 2015;90(2):284–299.
3. Iyer S, Kim HJ. Cervical radiculopathy. *Curr Rev Musculoskeletal Medicine*. 2016;9:272–280.
4. Kreiner D, Hwang S, Easa J, et al. An evidence-based clinical guideline for the diagnosis and treatment of lumbar disc herniation with radiculopathy. *Spine J*. 2014;14(1):180–191.
5. Tarulli AW, Raynor EM. Lumbosacral radiculopathy. *Neurol Clin*. 2007;25(2):387–405.
6. Bigos S, Braen G. Acute low back problems in adults: Clinical practice guidelines, quick reference guide. Number 14. Ed. US Department of Health and Human Services, Public Health Service, Agency for Healthcare Policy and Research (AHCPR). 1994.
7. Lateef H, Patel D. What is the role of imaging in acute low back pain? *Curr Rev Musculoskelet Med*. 2009;2(2):69–73.
8. Wong JJ, Cote P, Sutton DA, et al. Clinical practice guidelines for the noninvasive management of low back pain: A systematic review by the Ontario Protocol for Traffic Injury Management Collaboration. *Eur J Pain*. 2017;21:201–216.
9. Kjaer P, Kongsted A, Hartvigsen J, et al. National clinical guidelines for non-surgical treatment of patients with recent onset neck pain or cervical radiculopathy. *Eur Spine J*. 2017;26:2242–2257.
10. Akuthota V, Marshall B, Boimbo S, et al. Clinical course of motor deficits from lumbosacral radiculopathy due to disc herniation. *PMR*. 2019;11(8):807–814.
11. Scholten P, Stanos SP, Rivers WE, Prather H, Press J. *Physical medicine and rehabilitation approaches to pain management. Essentials of Pain Medicine*. Elsevier; 2018:531–538.e1.
12. Malanga GA, Nadler SF. Nonoperative treatment of low back pain. *Mayo Clin Proc*. 1999;74(11):1135–1148.
13. O'Sullivan PB, Phyty GDM, Twomey LT, Allison GT. Evaluation of specific stabilizing exercise in the treatment of chronic low back pain with radiologic diagnosis of spondylolysis or spondylolisthesis. *Spine*. 1997;22(24):2959–2967.

14. Busanich BM, Verscheure SD. Does McKenzie therapy improve outcomes for back pain? *J Athl Train*. 2006;41(1):117–119.
15. Fishman S, Ballantyne J, Rathmell JP, Bonica JJ, eds. *Bonica's Management of Pain*. 4th ed. Lippincott, Williams & Wilkins; 2010.
16. Bernard K, Portugal SE. Cervical radiculopathy. In: Kahn SB, Xu RY, eds. *Musculoskeletal Sports and Spine Disorders: A Comprehensive Guide*. Springer International Publishing; 2017: 353–355.
17. Hsu ES, Wu I, Lai B. *Acupuncture. Essentials of Pain Medicine*. Elsevier; 2018:545–550.e1.
18. Berger JM, Zaghi S. Nonopioid analgesics in pain management. In: Vadivelu N, Urman RD, Hines RL, eds. *Essentials of Pain Management*. Springer; 2011:117–150.
19. Williams BS. Nonopioid analgesics *Essentials of Pain Medicine*. 457-468. Elsevier; 2018.e2.
20. Tolba R. Radiculopathy. In: Pope JE, Deer TR, eds. *Treatment of Chronic Pain Conditions: A Comprehensive Handbook*. Springer; 2017:253–255.
21. Chou R, Peterson K, Helfand M. Comparative efficacy and safety of skeletal muscle relaxants for spasticity and musculoskeletal conditions: a systematic review. *J Pain Symptom Manage*. 2004;28(2):140–175.
22. Maher DP, Shah BJ, Vorobeychik Y. Opioid and non-opioid therapy. In: Mao J, ed. *Spine Pain Care: A Comprehensive Clinical Guide*. Springer International Publishing; 2020:231–257.
23. Saldaña MT, Navarro A, Pérez C, Masramón X, Rejas J. A cost-consequences analysis of the effect of pregabalin in the treatment of painful radiculopathy under medical practice conditions in primary care settings. *Pain Practice*. 2010;10(1):31–41.
24. Visco CJ, Cheng DS, Kennedy DJ. Pharmaceutical therapy for radiculopathy. *PMR*. 2011;22(1):127–137.
25. Sheth S, Holtsman M, Mahajan G. Major opioids in pain management. *Essentials of Pain Medicine*. Elsevier; 2018:373–384.e2.
26. Shim E, Lee J, Lee E, et al. Fluoroscopically guided epidural injections of the cervical and lumbar spine. *Radiographics*. 2017; 37:537–561.
27. Buttermann GR. Treatment of lumbar disc herniation: epidural steroid injection compared with discectomy. A prospective, randomized study. *J Bone Joint Surg Am*. 2004;86:670–679.
28. Wilby MJ, Best A, Wood E, et al. Surgical microdiscectomy versus transforaminal epidural steroid injection in patients with sciatica secondary to herniated lumbar disc (NERVES): a phase 3, multicentre open-label, randomised controlled trial and economic evaluation. *Lancet Rheumatol*. 2021;3:e347–e356.
29. Van Tulder MW, Malmivaara A, Esmail R, et al. Exercise therapy for low back pain. *Cochrane Database Syst Rev*. 2000;2: CD000335.
30. Carette S, Fehlings MG. Cervical radiculopathy. *N Engl J Med*. 2005;353(4):392–399.
31. Rabai F, Sessions R, Seubert CN. Neurophysiological monitoring and spinal cord integrity. *Best Pract Res Clin Anaesthesiol*. 2016;30(1):53–68.
32. Weinstein JN, Tosteson TD, Lurie JD, et al. Surgical vs nonoperative treatment for lumbar disk herniation: the spine patient outcomes research trial (Sport): a randomized trial. *JAMA*. 2006; 296(20):2441.
33. Weinstein JN, Lurie JD, Tosteson TD, et al. Surgical versus non-operative treatment for lumbar disc herniation: four-year results for the spine patient outcomes research trial (Sport). *Spine*. 2008;33(25):2789–2800.
34. Aziz KT, Shores JT, Ingari J. Restoring function: Tendon and nerve transfers. In: *The Mangled Extremity: Evaluation and Management*. Cham: Springer International Publishing; 2021: 153–173.
35. Agabegi SS, Asghar FA, Herkowitz HN. Spinal orthoses. *J Am Acad Orthop Surg*. 2010;18(11):657–667.
36. Zhu MP, Tetreault LA, Sorefan-Mangou F, Garwood P, Wilson JR. Efficacy, safety, and economics of bracing after spine surgery: a systematic review of the literature. *Spine J*. 2018; 18(9):1513–1525.
37. Leo RJ, Quinton WJ, Ebert MH. Psychological and psychosocial evaluation of the chronic pain patient. In: Vadivelu N, Urman RD, Hines RL, eds. *Essentials of Pain Management*. Springer; 2011:203–235.
38. Dorow M, Löbner M, Stein J, et al. Risk factors for postoperative pain intensity in patients undergoing lumbar disc surgery: a systematic review. *PLoS ONE*. 2017;12(1):e0170303.
39. Mattiuzzi C, Lippi G, Bovo C. Current epidemiology of low back pain. *J Hosp Manag Health Policy*. 2020;4:15.

8

Prevention, Diagnosis, and Management of Postoperative Spine Infections

BRENDAN MICHAEL STRIANO, ALEXANDER M. CRAWFORD, AND DANIEL G. TOBERT

CHAPTER OUTLINE

Introduction

Infection is a dreaded, and relatively frequent, complication following spine surgery. In a large, pooled meta-analysis of greater than 22,000 spine operations, postoperative surgical site infection (SSI) varied from 0.2% to 16.1% with a pooled estimate of 3.1%.[1] Despite the available data on SSI and many effective interventions to reduce SSI rate, infection continues to be a troubling problem. Recent data on 1-year postoperative outcomes following SSI demonstrated no significant difference from uninfected patients.[2,3] However, SSI is a significant financial burden and represents a considerable functional setback at the individual level.[4]

Infection mitigation techniques are unlikely to eradicate SSI completely. However, an understanding of preoperative risk factors, perioperative reduction strategies, and treatment options for SSIs is important to minimize infection rates and impact. The purpose of this chapter is to provide a working framework in each perioperative period to reduce risk and manage postoperative infections after spine surgery.

Preoperative Considerations

Effective mitigation of postoperative spine infection risk begins with preoperative assessment. Many risk factors for postoperative spine infections have been identified. Some, but not all, of these factors are modifiable and therefore are viable targets for optimization. Nonetheless, it is important to incorporate all preoperative risk factors, modifiable and nonmodifiable, into shared decision making prior to undergoing surgical intervention.

Age

The association between age and postoperative spine infection has been studied several times. Though there are inconsistent cutoffs used to categorize age,[5] advanced age does consistently seem to confer increased infection risk.[6–9] Though age is nonmodifiable, knowledge of increased infection risk with increased age can help surgeons understand the global risk profile and scale risk reduction strategies accordingly.

Body Habitus

Body mass index (BMI) has similarly been studied in detail. In a 2013 meta-analysis, increased BMI was not only identified as a risk factor for infection but was also found to have a dose-dependent effect with each additional 5 kg/m^2 increase in BMI conferring additional risk.[10] Further, distribution of weight (i.e., subcutaneous tissue thickness at incision site) has been associated with increased rates of SSI in the cervical spine.[11] Though such factors are modifiable, preoperative weight loss can be difficult to achieve. Even with the help of dedicated outpatient weight loss programs, patients still struggle to meaningfully lose weight.[12–14] Therefore, it is suggested to utilize preoperative BMI in the calculus regarding perioperative risk, but a strict cutoff value is not recommended.

Diabetes Mellitus

Many studies have evaluated the risk associated with DMII. In a systematic review, Schuster et al. found that DMII had a significant association with SSI in five of the seven studies.[6] Importantly, the point estimate for the odds ratios for these associations was markedly elevated, ranging from 3.5 to ∞. In a 2016 meta-analysis, pooled data from 13,476 patients similarly identified DMII as a robust risk factor for infection (RR 2.2; 95% CI 1.38-3.60; $P = 0.001$).[15] A retrospective review of 4778 patients reported worse overall postoperative outcomes with hemoglobin A1c (HbA1c) greater than 8%.[16] In a systematic review published by the Congress of Neurologic Surgeons, patients with HbA1c greater than 7.5% had higher infection rate.[17] In light of the evidence, involving the patient's endocrinologist or primary care provider in HbA1c optimization and deferring elective spine surgery until it is below 8% is recommended.

Nicotine

Tobacco smoking has demonstrated a mixed association with spine SSIs in the literature. Fei et al., in a meta-analysis of multiple SSI risk factors, found no association between smoking and infection risk (RR 1.81; 95% CI 0.70–4.69).[15] In contrast, meta-analysis of 67,000 patients dedicated to interrogating smoking and SSI identified a significant, though minor, association (OR 1.26; 95% CI 1.05–1.51).[18] Regarding smoking risk mitigation, it is commonly suggested that all patients have ceased smoking prior to the surgical date, particularly in cases where fusion is sought. In instances where there is doubt regarding abstinence from tobacco, nicotine, and cotinine levels from the urine can be used to verify abstinence.[19] The extended plasma half-life of cotinine, a nicotine metabolite, allows identification of tobacco smoking in the past 7 to 10 days.

Nutrition

Nutritional status has been consistently demonstrated to be associated with infectious outcomes following elective spine surgery. In a case-control study design, as well as a retrospective cohort study, Salvetti et al. identified prealbumin levels less than 20 mg/dL as significantly associated with postoperative infection.[20,21] The infection in malnourished patients was nearly three times that of patients with normal prealbumin levels.

Nares MRSA Colonization

There has been growing interest with utilization of preoperative methicillin-resistant *Staphylococcus aureus* (MRSA) swab of the nares to help risk stratify for SSI. Much of this interest stems from the arthroplasty literature, but few studies have investigated spine surgery specifically. In a review of all orthopaedic patients, positive MRSA nasal swab was associated with increased infection risk.[22] However, in a dedicated group of elective spine surgery patients, it was recently demonstrated that no association between MRSA swab result and infection exists.[23,24] It is not clear if MRSA decolonization with topical antibiotics decreases the risk of SSI in spine surgery. As research on this topic continues, it is hypothesized that MRSA colonization acts as an indication of host immunologic dysfunction rather than directly causative.

Renal Disease

End-stage renal disease (ESRD) has been noted to confer significant risk of SSI. In a national review, dialysis-dependent patients were noted to have a deep infection rate of 6.40% compared to only 0.71% in the nondialysis-dependent group.[25] In large part, this risk factor cannot be modified, but understanding its impact can lead to more comprehensive shared decision making, motivation to optimize other risk factors, and scaling other risk reduction strategies.

Surgical Approach

Surgical approach represents a spectrum of risk for SSI development. Anterior surgical approaches have lower infection rates than do posterior approaches in both the cervical and lumbar spine.[6,9,26,27] The surgical goal may preclude the ability to take advantage of this difference in risk profiles. However, if a surgical goal is reasonably achievable with either approach, it can be worth lower SSI risk with surgical approach if there are overwhelming host risk factors. This assumes that surgeon comfort and experience for either option is present.

In summary, there are many preoperative factors that must be considered when trying to minimize infection risk. Some risk factors are modifiable and warrant focused attention and optimization prior to surgery, but others are simply important to acknowledge in order to conduct appropriate shared decision making and to dose intraoperative and postoperative risk mitigation strategies. As an example, a malnourished, diabetic, obese smoker on dialysis warrants different consideration than a healthy, active individual with no medical comorbidities. Several authors have made preliminary attempts to quantify these risks,[28,29] but no definitive algorithm has yet been developed, externally validated, and widely put into use. In the next section, perioperative risk factors will be addressed, as well as strategies to reduce infection risk.

Perioperative Management

The perioperative phase is critical not only for its continued opportunity to identify risk factors, but it also allows for intervention to reduce SSI risk.

Perioperatively, infection risk reduction begins with topical surgical site cleansing. This process begins with an at-home chlorhexidine gluconate (CHG) bath for all patients without an explicit allergy. This practice falls in line with spine surgery specific data wherein patients who utilized a 4% CHG bath at home had a reduced rate of infection.[30] Nonetheless, it is also important to note that the 2015 Cochrane review assessing the role for preop CHG bath was not able to identify efficacy of this practice, but this review grouped all surgical procedures together and was not specific to spine surgery.[31] Within the operating room, a randomized controlled trial demonstrated that neither ChloraPrep nor DuraPrep was clearly superior regarding skin preparation.[32]

About routine perioperative antibiotics, institutional protocols emphasizes administration of antibiotics within 1 hour of skin incision, which has been shown to significantly reduce SSI compared to antibiotics >60 minutes before incision.[33] The antibiotic of choice in spine surgery is cefazolin, except for the rare case of a distinct allergy or other contraindication.[34] In the event of a documented allergy preventing the use of a cephalosporin antibiotic, most institutional protocols utilize clindamycin or vancomycin. Antibiotic prophylaxis is routinely extended for 24 hours postoperatively. Some surgeons have advocated for extension of antibiotics until the removal of any postoperative drain, but this has not been proven in the literature with evidence lacking.

Intraoperatively, the surgeon must be cognizant of multiple factors that can increase SSI risk. Blood loss is a major contributor because it is a compounding risk factor. First, patients receiving allogeneic blood transfusions have been found to have increased risk of infection compared to patients not requiring blood transfusion.[6,35] This finding was confirmed in a population of arthroplasty patients and confirmed within a spine-specific cohort.[36,37] Additionally, increased bleeding is often associated with larger surgeries and longer operative times, which have both been found to increase SSI risk in spine surgery or other surgical disciplines.[6,38]

There are several interventions that can be undertaken to mitigate both these intraoperative and preoperative risks. Intraoperative irrigation presents an opportunity to reduce infection risk. Both the identity of the irrigation and the volume of irrigate have been studied. Cheng et al. found that dilute betadine irrigation (0.35% betadine) resulted in fewer postoperative deep infections compared to saline irrigation (2.9% reduction; $P = 0.0146$).[39] Further, Watanabe and colleagues found that patients who went on to develop SSI had been irrigated with significantly lower volumes than patients without infection.[40] The noninfected group had been treated with more than 2000 cc of irrigation per hour. In this manner, copious irrigation can, to some degree, be scaled to match patients' risk profile. Further research has been dedicated to the use of vancomycin powder directly into the wound at the completion of the operation. Use of vancomycin powder has been shown to significantly reduce SSI without reported serious or pervasive side effects.[41] There are multiple reported techniques for the placement of vancomycin including sub or suprafascial placement. Likely both is the most successful employment strategy.

Wound closure also has effect on SSI and a layered fashion closure beginning with tight approximation of the fascia is key. A complete and robust fascial closure is paramount in reducing SSI risk. In the event of a particularly high-risk wound such as for patients with metastatic disease who are expected to undergo postoperative radiation, an additional closure of the subfascial muscular layer is typically performed. Additionally, a nonabsorbable skin suture, such as interrupted nylon stitches, can be used to provide a measure of control over skin tension based on the progress of epithelialization. The use of plastic surgeons for wound closure has been published with positive results as well.[42]

In addition to a layered closure, a subfascial drain can be used based on the appearance of the wound at the conclusion of the surgery. Minimally invasive or same-day procedures do not typically receive a drain. A subfascial drain serves both to prevent compressive epidural hematoma as well as to reduce pressure on the wound and facilitate healing. Drain use has been studied and, despite concern that it represents a communication between the outside world and the surgical wound, has not been found to be associated with postoperative infection.[43] To mitigate this theoretical risk, however, drains are dressed with an occlusive, sterile dressing and removed when output has diminished sufficiently (usually less than 30 cc/8-hour shift). In high-risk wounds, subfascial (and occasionally suprafascial) drains are often left for a prolonged duration and can even be maintained until outpatient follow-up. Based on the Healthcare Infection Control Practices Advisory Committee guidelines, postdischarge PO antibiotic prophylaxis is not used unless recommended by an infectious disease specialist.[44] While wound dressing has not been significantly studied, a simple, occlusive, dry sterile dressing is typical. However, in situations when multiple risk factors have been identified, a negative pressure wound dressing may be utilized. Dyck et al. studied the use of negative pressure wound therapy (NPWT) in spine surgery patients at increased risk of infection and discovered a 50% reduction in infections.[45]

Diagnosis and Management of Postoperative Infection

Critical to the management of postoperative infection is early, prompt identification. The Centers for Disease Control definition of surgical site infection is the most widely cited definition. The core components for this definition are occurrence of the infection within 90 days of the index procedure and meeting clinical criteria for infection. Infections can be defined as superficial or deep surgical site infection, based on the depth of involvement of the infection.[46]

It is important to have a mental schema when considering postoperative spine incisions. An algorithm for the consideration of postoperative wounds is presented in Fig. 8.1. First are well-appearing wounds without issue. This is the ideal scenario and warrants just routine follow-up (Fig. 8.1A). On the other end of the spectrum are patients who present with leukocytosis, fever, purulent drainage, and an obvious dehiscence (Fig. 8.1C). These patients warrant surgical irrigation and debridement (I&D) and will be addressed specifically later in this chapter. The third group of patients are those with a somewhat troubling wound, but not so obviously problematic as to warrant surgical I&D (Fig. 8.1B). Patients in this intermediary category can either go on to successful wound healing or develop frank dehiscence and infection. Multiple treatment options have been proposed and are utilized to attempt to salvage a wound of

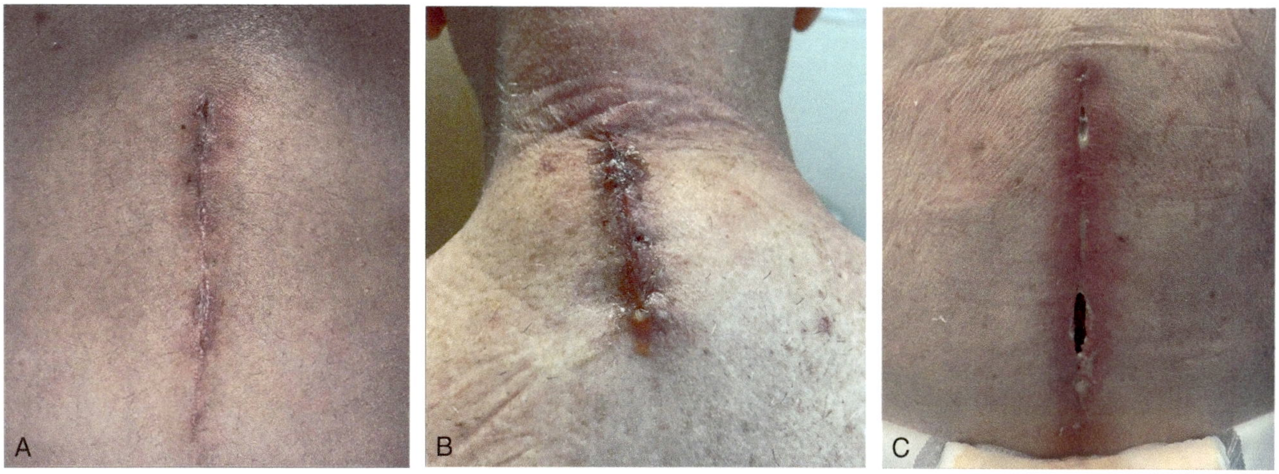

• **Fig. 8.1** Examples of different postoperative wound healing. (A) Well-healed incision. (B) Posterior cervical incision 2 weeks postop with mild but persistent inferior pole drainage. (C) Posterior thoracolumbar incision with multiple sites of dehiscence at 1 month postoperatively.

this type, though discrete data on this topic are minimal. Oral antibiotics and the addition of incisional negative pressure wound therapy (e.g., Prevena, 3M, St. Paul, MN) can be utilized to aid in the healing of these wounds. It may be preferred to resterilize the incision prior to application of the wound vac. Regarding antibiotics, it is important to cover skin flora, which can be achieved with cephalexin or, for ease of dosing schedule, cefadroxil. For patients at risk for MRSA (e.g., those with positive preoperative nares swab, baseline immunocompromise, discrete risk factors, etc.), coverage with trimethoprim-sulfamethoxazole (TMP-SMX), doxycycline, or clindamycin can be pursued. Lastly, it is important to maximize offloading of the incision, which can be accomplished with increased physical activity, or for infirmed patients, increased repositioning.

Work-Up

Diagnostic work-up of a potential postoperative spine infection involves a detailed history, physical exam, lab work, and diagnostic imaging. Patients with postoperative infection will often present with one or several of the following complaints: excessive pain at the incision site, a history of persistent drainage that may be foul smelling or frankly purulent, and/or fever.[47,48] Physical examination should assess for the presence of peri-incisional erythema, dehisced areas of the incision, native drainage, an expressible fluid collection, and/or new/evolving neurologic deficits.

Basic blood work including complete blood count with differential, erythrocyte sedimentation rate (ESR) and C-reactive protein (CRP) can also help to identify infection. These lab values must be interpreted within the context of each patient's recovery, as one would still expect elevated inflammatory markers early in the recovery process. In their investigation into how these values change after spine surgery, Mok and colleagues discovered that CRP values formally peaked in 78% of their patients, with a mean value 165.8 mg/L (SD 69) on postoperative day 2.68 (SD 0.81).[49] ESR values only demonstrated a formal peak in 47% of patients, with a mean value of 10.9 (SD 12.9) on POD 4.20 (SD 1.94).[49] In this study, the authors concluded that CRP is superior to ESR in the early detection of postoperative infections. They additionally found that a second peak in CRP or a failure of CRP to decline with the expected kinetics showed a sensitivity of 82% for postoperative infection.

In the setting of wound drainage, the treating physician must consider the possibility of cerebrospinal fluid leakage as the etiology of persistent drainage. Patients should be questioned about the presence of headache and special note made regarding any positional nature of the headache. In instances of uncertainty, peri-incisional fluid can be analyzed for beta-2 transferrin, which can confirm the diagnosis of CSF leak.[50]

For suspected deep infection, magnetic resonance imaging (MRI) with and without gadolinium can prove helpful.[48,51] The sensitivity, specificity, and accuracy of such imaging in the detection of a postoperative spine infection has been reported as 96%, 94%, and 92%, respectively.[52] Findings consistent with infection can include but are not limited to a postoperative fluid collection with rim enhancement, rim-enhancing epidural collections, endplate erosion, loss of disc height, progressive marrow edema, and bony destruction[48,51] (Figs. 8.2 and 8.3). However, it should be noted that postoperative fluid collections are common following any spine surgery. In a prospective cohort, Yeo and colleagues performed an immediate postoperative MRI on 121 patients and discovered a fluid collection in 73.8% of single-level laminectomies and 88.5% of two-level laminectomies.[53] For this reason, it is important to keep the entire clinical gestalt in mind.

Surgery

Once an SSI has been diagnosed, prompt surgical irrigation and debridement is paramount. Specific anatomy associated with the infection site and how much of the bony and/or

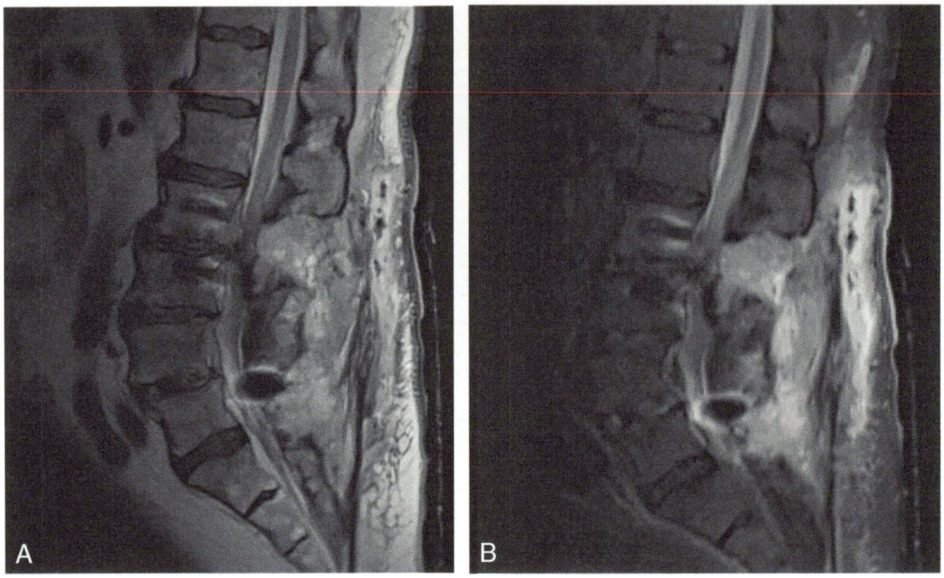

• **Fig. 8.2** Parasagittal T2 (A) and STIR (B) weighted images of postoperative abscess following lumbar decompression and instrumented fusion with communicating subfascial and suprafascial components.

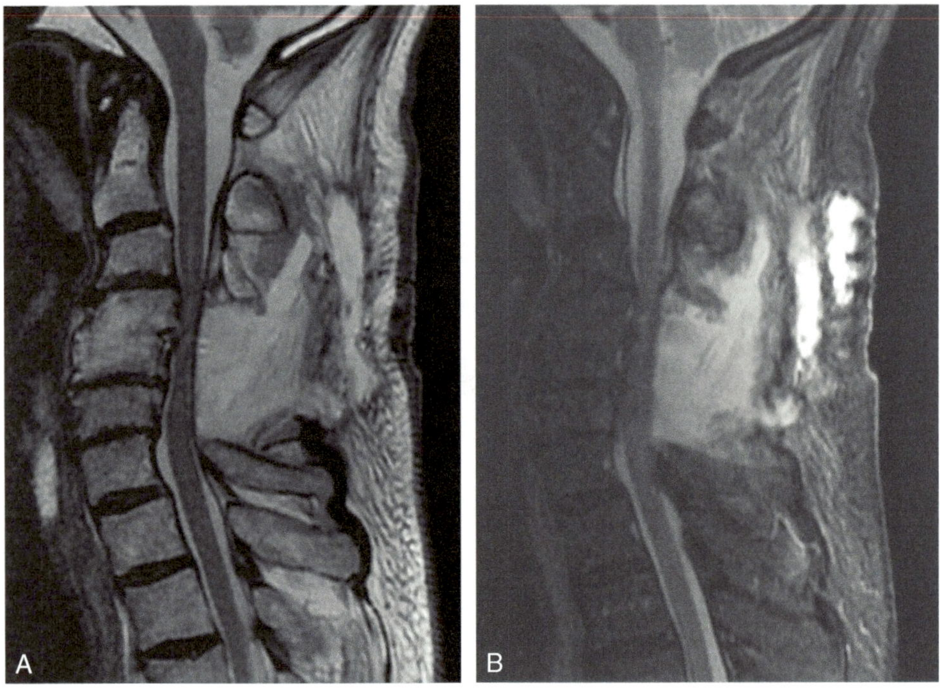

• **Fig. 8.3** Parasagittal T2 (A) and STIR (B) weighted images of postoperative abscess following cervical decompression and instrumented fusion with communicating subfascial and suprafascial components and cord compression.

discogenic spine are involved will dictate specific surgical considerations. For example, an infection that manifests as diffuse purulence shortly after a lumbar laminectomy may necessitate only reopening the incision and performing a thorough irrigation and debridement. However, a more latent infection involving the postoperative cervical spine that has gone on to epidural abscess and spondylodiscitis with diffuse vertebral body erosion that threatens mechanical stability may benefit from a multilevel corpectomy. The specific surgeries performed for postoperative spine infections may be innumerable based on these considerations, but their principles are the same: debride all potential sites of infection, copious irrigation of the wound, and stabilize the spine if necessary (Fig. 8.4).

Despite early concerns about the use of implants in the setting of spine infections, subsequent research has demonstrated its safety.[54–61] In the setting of infection, however, some

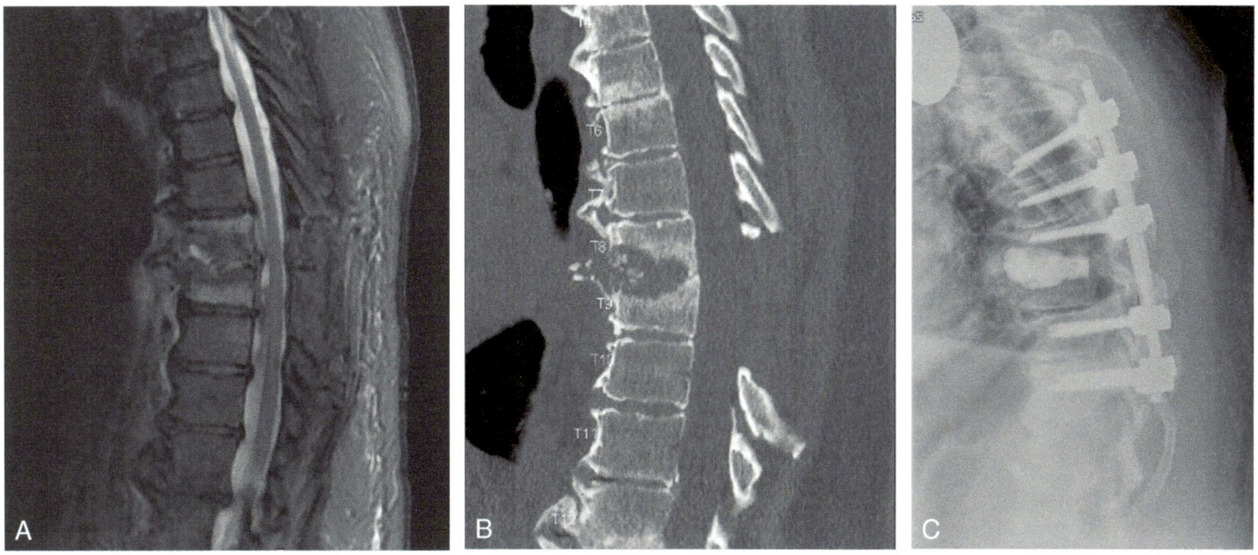

• **Fig. 8.4** MRI and CT sagittal images of an adult female who underwent thoracic laminectomy for spinal cord stimulator and developed MRSA SSI treated with one-stage I&D at an outside hospital. Despite 3 months of IV antibiotics, she developed osteomyelitis/discitis (A) with intractable pain, resultant bony erosion, and biomechanical instability (B). She underwent instrumented fusion to provide biomechanical stability and antibiotic-impregnated PMMA to fill bone loss and elute local antibiotics (C). *I&D,* Irrigation and debridement; *MRSA*,methicillin-resistant Staphylococcus aureus; *PMMA*, polymethyl methacrylate; *SSI*, surgical site infection.

authors do advocate for the use of titanium instead of stainless steel due to increased porosity and a potentially improved risk profile with regard to glycocalyx formation.[58] Nonetheless, further research is needed to definitively show superiority of one type of implant versus another in this setting.

The efficacy of single versus multiple debridements in the setting of spine SSI has also been a topic of research. In a retrospective single-center review of patients undergoing surgical debridement, Dipaola et al. report MRSA microbiology and bacteremia as independent predictors of multiple debridements.[62] If these predictors are known in advance, it may be useful to plan staged debridements before definitive closure. This is best discussed with the patient, including the possibility of multiple debridements, and the decision based on intraoperative appearance and postoperative clinical course.

Antibiotics

In the setting of a postoperative spine infection, it is often prudent to involve the infectious disease consultants for a multidisciplinary approach. It may also be recommended to hold empiric intravenous antibiotics (except in the setting of hemodynamic instability) until the wound bed has been cultured in the operating room. This practice includes holding immediate preoperative antibiotics and is intended to maximize yield for culture-driven antibiosis. Although it would likely benefit from further research, this practice has been proven effective in periprosthetic joint infections upon systematic review.[63]

Following sampling, an extended course of culture-guided antibiotics (at least 6 weeks) is recommended by infectious disease colleagues, consistent with previously published standards.[48,64] Although these antibiotics are usually intravenous, certain antibiotics with good oral bioavailability (e.g., linezolid) may represent a situationally viable alternative depending on local bacterial sensitivity profiles.[65] Additionally, rifampin may be indicated as an adjunct in the setting of a Staphylococcal infection with underlying hardware.[66,67]

Bacteria

The microbial etiology of postoperative spinal infections is key to understanding not only the best empiric antibiotic therapies, but also potential preventive measures, and even potential explanations of the source of infection. *Staphylococcus* species are very common, with *S. aureus* being most common; in some studies it is reported as the etiology in up to 50% of cases.[68–70] Coagulase negative staphylococci, such as *Staphylococcus epidermidis*, are commonly found associated with implant-related infection. Likely routes of staphylococcal inoculation include intraoperative contamination as well as wound contamination.[71] With regard to wound contamination from local skin, *Cutibacterium acnes* (formerly known as *Propionobacterium acnes*) is becoming an increasingly appreciated source of postoperative spinal infection.[72] This diagnosis is particularly challenging because *C. acnes* is an anaerobic, low virulence organism that is difficult to grow in culture and requires extended periods of incubation. The difficulty with culturing *C. acnes* may explain previously cited high rates of "culture-negative" infection.[69] Gram-negative postoperative infections represent a separate entity and often are the result of either hematogenous seeding or contamination from the anogenital region in the case of lumbosacral incisions[68,70,72]). Common causative organisms include *Escherichia coli*, *Pseudomonas aeruginosa*,

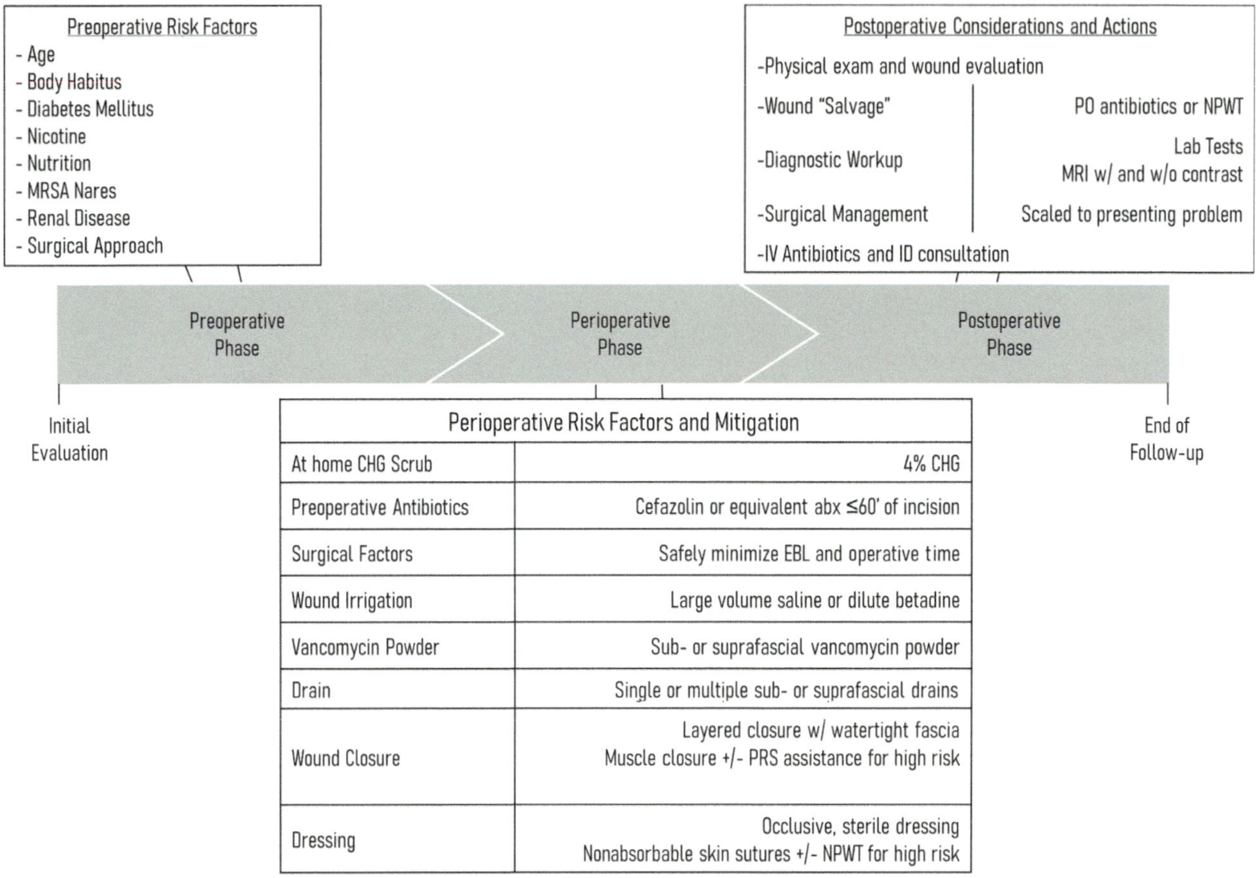

• **Fig. 8.5** Schematic representation of schema to conceptualize SSI risk management. *Abx*, Antibiotics; *CHG*, chlorhexidine gluconate; *NPWT*, negative pressure wound therapy; *PRS*, plastic and reconstructive surgery.

Enterobacter cloacae, and several *Proteus* species.[73] The final consideration is polymicrobial infections. Data on polymicrobial infections vary with studies citing 13% to 35% of infections isolating multiple organisms.[74,75] These challenging infections have also been noted to be associated with a three times increased odds of relapse.[75]

Conclusions

Surgical site infection is a dreaded complication following spinal surgery that continues to haunt spine surgeons and patients alike. To best prevent, identify, and manage infections, spine surgeons must have a working model to think about postoperative infection, focusing on risk factors, ways to risk mitigate, infection detection, and appropriate treatment (Fig. 8.5). With this model in mind, surgeons cannot only have a working concept of postoperative infection risk, but also can employ infection reduction strategies to minimize likelihood of infection.

References

1. Zhou J, Wang R, Huo X, et al. Incidence of surgical site infection after spine surgery: a systematic review and meta-analysis. *Spine.* 2020;45(3):208–216.
2. Urquhart JC, Gurr KR, Siddiqi F, et al. The impact of surgical site infection on patient outcomes after open posterior instrumented thoracolumbar surgery for degenerative disorders. *J Bone Joint Surg Am.* 2021;103(22):2105–2114.
3. Karamian BA, Mao J, Toci GR, et al. Clinical outcomes at one-year follow-up for patients with surgical site infection after spinal fusion. *Spine (Phila Pa 1976).* 2022;47(15):1055–1061.
4. Blumberg TJ, Woelber E, Bellabarba C, et al. Predictors of increased cost and length of stay in the treatment of postoperative spine surgical site infection. *Spine J.* 2018;18(2):300–306.
5. Fang A, Hu SS, Endres N, et al. Risk factors for infection after spinal surgery. *Spine (Phila Pa 1976).* 2005;30(12):1460–1465.
6. Schuster JM, Rechtine G, Norvell DC, et al. The influence of perioperative risk factors and therapeutic interventions on infection rates after spine surgery: a systematic review. *Spine (Phila Pa 1976).* 2010;35(9 Suppl):S125–37.
7. Apisarnthanarak A, Jones M, Waterman BM, et al. Risk factors for spinal surgical-site infections in a community hospital: a case-control study. *Infect Control Hosp Epidemiol.* 2003;24(1):31–36.
8. Kanafani ZA, Dakdouki GK, El-Dbouni O, et al. Surgical site infections following spinal surgery at a tertiary care center in Lebanon: incidence, microbiology, and risk factors. *Scand J Infect Dis.* 2006;38(8):589–592.
9. Maragakis LL, Cosgrove SE, Martinez EA, et al. Intraoperative fraction of inspired oxygen is a modifiable risk factor for surgical site infection after spinal surgery. *Anesthesiology.* 2009;110(3):556–562.

10. Abdallah DY, Jadaan MM, McCabe JP. Body mass index and risk of surgical site infection following spine surgery: a meta-analysis. *Eur Spine J.* 2013;22(12):2800–2809.
11. Donnally CJ, Henstenburg JM, Pezzulo JD, et al. Increased surgical site subcutaneous fat thickness is associated with infection after posterior cervical fusion. *Surg Infect (Larchmt).* 2022; 23(4):364–371.
12. Unick JL, Beavers D, Bond DS, et al. The long-term effectiveness of a lifestyle intervention in severely obese individuals. *Am J Med.* 2013;126(3):236–242. 242.e1-2.
13. Hofsø D, Nordstrand N, Johnson LK, et al. Obesity-related cardiovascular risk factors after weight loss: a clinical trial comparing gastric bypass surgery and intensive lifestyle intervention. *Eur J Endocrinol.* 2010;163(5):735–745.
14. Aadland E, Robertson L. Physical activity is associated with weight loss and increased cardiorespiratory fitness in severely obese men and women undergoing lifestyle treatment. *J Obes.* 2012;2012:810594.
15. Fei Q, Li J, Lin J, et al. Risk factors for surgical site infection after spinal surgery: A meta-analysis. *World Neurosurg.* 2016; 95:507–515.
16. Lim S, Yeh HH, Macki M, et al. Preoperative HbA1c > 8% is associated with poor outcomes in lumbar spine surgery: A Michigan Spine Surgery Improvement Collaborative study. *Neurosurgery.* 2021;89(5):819–826.
17. Harrop JS, Mohamed B, Bisson EF, et al. Congress of Neurological Surgeons systematic review and evidence-based guidelines for perioperative spine: Preoperative surgical risk assessment. *Neurosurgery.* 2021;89(Suppl 1):s9–s18.
18. Kong L, Liu Z, Meng F, et al. Smoking and risk of surgical site infection after spinal surgery: A systematic review and meta-analysis. *Surg Infect (Larchmt).* 2017;18(2):206–214.
19. Benowitz NL. Cotinine as a biomarker of environmental tobacco smoke exposure. *Epidemiol Rev.* 1996;18(2):188–204.
20. Salvetti DJ, Tempel ZJ, Gandhoke GS, et al. Preoperative prealbumin level as a risk factor for surgical site infection following elective spine surgery. *Surg Neurol Int.* 2015;6(Suppl 19):S500–3.
21. Salvetti DJ, Tempel ZJ, Goldschmidt E, et al. Low preoperative serum prealbumin levels and the postoperative surgical site infection risk in elective spine surgery: a consecutive series. *J Neurosurg Spine.* 2018;29(5):549–552.
22. Yano K, Minoda Y, Sakawa A, et al. Positive nasal culture of methicillin-resistant Staphylococcus aureus (MRSA) is a risk factor for surgical site infection in orthopedics. *Acta Orthop.* 2009;80(4):486–490.
23. Xiong GX, Greene NE, Hershman SH, et al. Nasal screening for methicillin-resistant Staphylococcus aureus does not reduce surgical site infection after primary lumbar fusion. *Spine J.* 2022;22(1):113–125.
24. Xiong GX, Greene NE, Hershman SH, et al. Does nasal screening for methicillin-resistant Staphylococcus aureus (MRSA) prevent deep surgical site infections for elective cervical spinal fusion? *Clin Spine Surg.* 2023;36(1):E51–E58.
25. Ottesen TD, McLynn RP, Zogg CK, et al. Dialysis is an independent risk factor for perioperative adverse events, readmission, reoperation, and mortality for patients undergoing elective spine surgery. *Spine J.* 2018;18(11):2033–2042.
26. Olsen MA, Mayfield J, Lauryssen C, et al. Risk factors for surgical site infection in spinal surgery. *J Neurosurg.* 2003;98(2):149–155.
27. Olsen MA, Nepple JJ, Riew KD, et al. Risk factors for surgical site infection following orthopaedic spinal operations. *J Bone Joint Surg Am.* 2008;90(1):62–69.
28. Hopkins BS, Mazmudar A, Driscoll C, et al. Using artificial intelligence (AI) to predict postoperative surgical site infection: A retrospective cohort of 4046 posterior spinal fusions. *Clin Neurol Neurosurg.* 2020;192:105718.
29. Veeravagu A, Li A, Swinney C, et al. Predicting complication risk in spine surgery: a prospective analysis of a novel risk assessment tool. *J Neurosurg Spine.* 2017;27(1):81–91.
30. Chan AK, Ammanuel SG, Chan AY, et al. Chlorhexidine showers are associated with a reduction in surgical site infection following spine surgery: an analysis of 4266 consecutive surgeries. *Neurosurgery.* 2019;85(6):817–826.
31. Webster J, Osborne S. Preoperative bathing or showering with skin antiseptics to prevent surgical site infection. *Cochrane Database Syst Rev.* 2015;2015(2):CD004985.
32. Savage JW, Weatherford BM, Sugrue PA, et al. Efficacy of surgical preparation solutions in lumbar spine surgery. *J Bone Joint Surg Am.* 2012;94(6):490–494.
33. Hawn MT, Richman JS, Vick CC, et al. Timing of surgical antibiotic prophylaxis and the risk of surgical site infection. *JAMA Surg.* 2013;148(7):649–657.
34. Sousa-Pinto B, Blumenthal KG, Courtney L, et al. Assessment of the frequency of dual allergy to penicillins and cefazolin: A systematic review and meta-analysis. *JAMA Surg.* 2021; 156(4):e210021.
35. Hill GE, Frawley WH, Griffith KE, et al. Allogeneic blood transfusion increases the risk of postoperative bacterial infection: a meta-analysis. *J Trauma.* 2003;54(5):908–914.
36. Kim JL, Park JH, Han SB, et al. Allogeneic blood transfusion is a significant risk factor for surgical-site infection following total hip and knee arthroplasty: A meta-analysis. *J Arthroplasty.* 2017;32(1):320–325.
37. Kato S, Chikuda H, Ohya J, et al. Risk of infectious complications associated with blood transfusion in elective spinal surgery—a propensity score matched analysis. *Spine J.* 2016;16(1):55–60.
38. Wang Q, Goswami K, Shohat N, et al. Longer operative time results in a higher rate of subsequent periprosthetic joint infection in patients undergoing primary joint arthroplasty. *J Arthroplasty.* 2019;34(5):947–953.
39. Cheng M-T, Chang M-C, Wang S-T, et al. Efficacy of dilute betadine solution irrigation in the prevention of postoperative infection of spinal surgery. *Spine.* 2005;30(15):1689–1693.
40. Watanabe M, Sakai D, Matsuyama D, et al. Risk factors for surgical site infection following spine surgery: efficacy of intraoperative saline irrigation. *J Neurosurg Spine.* 2010;12(5):540–546.
41. Xiong L, Pan Q, Jin G, et al. Topical intrawound application of vancomycin powder in addition to intravenous administration of antibiotics: a meta-analysis on the deep infection after spinal surgeries. *Orthop Traumatol Surg Res.* 2014;100(7):785–789.
42. Xu H, Rozanski C, Taub PJ. The value of plastic surgery spinal closures: A review of 782 spine cases. *Ann Plast Surg.* 2019; 83(2):201–205.
43. Aleem IS, Tan LA, Nassr A, et al. Surgical site infection prevention following spine surgery. *Global Spine J.* 2020;10 (1 Suppl):92s–98s.
44. Berríos-Torres SI, Umscheid CA, Bratzler DW, et al. Centers for Disease Control and Prevention guideline for the prevention of surgical site infection, 2017. *JAMA Surg.* 2017;152(8):784–791.

45. Dyck BA, Bailey CS, Steyn C, et al. Use of incisional vacuum-assisted closure in the prevention of postoperative infection in high-risk patients who underwent spine surgery: a proof-of-concept study. *J Neurosurg Spine.* 2019;31(3):430–439.
46. Centers for Disease Control. *National Healthcare Safety Network (NHSN) Patient Safety Component Manual.* 2022:125–163. (cdc.gov).
47. Weinstein MA, McCabe JP, Cammisa FP. Postoperative spinal wound infection: a review of 2,391 consecutive index procedures. *J Spinal Disord.* 2000;13(5):422–426.
48. Meredith DS, Kepler CK, Huang RC, et al. Postoperative infections of the lumbar spine: presentation and management. *Int Orthop.* 2012;36(2):439–444.
49. Mok JM, Pekmezci M, Piper SL, et al. Use of C-reactive protein after spinal surgery: comparison with erythrocyte sedimentation rate as predictor of early postoperative infectious complications. *Spine (Phila Pa 1976).* 2008;33(4):415–421.
50. Skedros DG, Cass SP, Hirsch BE, et al. Beta-2 transferrin assay in clinical management of cerebral spinal fluid and perilymphatic fluid leaks. *J Otolaryngol.* 1993;22(5):341–344.
51. Ortiz AO, Levitt A, Shah LM, et al. ACR Appropriateness Criteria® suspected spine infection. *J Am Coll Radiol.* 2021; 18(11s):S488–s501.
52. Arbelaez A, Restrepo F, Castillo M. Spinal infections: clinical and imaging features. *Top Magn Reson Imaging.* 2014;23(5):303–314.
53. Yeo JB, Lee E, Lee JW, et al. Immediate postoperative MRI findings after lumbar decompression surgery: Correlation of imaging features with clinical outcome. *J Clin Neurosci.* 2021; 89:365–374.
54. Bluman EM, Palumbo MA, Lucas PR. Spinal epidural abscess in adults. *J Am Acad Orthop Surg.* 2004;12(3):155–163.
55. Duarte RM, Vaccaro AR. Spinal infection: state of the art and management algorithm. *Eur Spine J.* 2013;22(12):2787–2799.
56. Cornett CA, Vincent SA, Crow J, et al. Bacterial spine infections in adults: Evaluation and management. *J Am Acad Orthop Surg.* 2016;24(1):11–18.
57. Sharfman ZT, Gelfand Y, Shah P, et al. Spinal epidural abscess: A review of presentation, management, and medicolegal implications. *Asian Spine J.* 2020;14(5):742–759.
58. Hsieh PC, Wienecke RJ, O'Shaughnessy BA, et al. Surgical strategies for vertebral osteomyelitis and epidural abscess. *Neurosurg Focus.* 2004;17(6):E4.
59. Abramovitz JN, Batson RA, Yablon JS. Vertebral osteomyelitis. The surgical management of neurologic complications. *Spine (Phila Pa 1976).* 1986;11(5):418–420.
60. Redfern RM, Miles J, Banks AJ, et al. Stabilisation of the infected spine. *J Neurol Neurosurg Psychiatry.* 1988;51(6):803–807.
61. Atesok K, Vaccaro A, Stippler M, et al. Fate of hardware in spinal infections. *Surg Infect (Larchmt).* 2020;21(5):404–410.
62. Dipaola CP, Saravanja DD, Boriani L, et al. Postoperative infection treatment score for the spine (PITSS): construction and validation of a predictive model to define need for single versus multiple irrigation and debridement for spinal surgical site infection. *Spine J.* 2012;12(3):218–230.
63. Wouthuyzen-Bakker M, Benito N, Soriano A. The effect of preoperative antimicrobial prophylaxis on intraoperative culture results in patients with a suspected or confirmed prosthetic joint infection: a systematic review. *J Clin Microbiol.* 2017; 55(9):2765–2774.
64. Sasso RC, Garrido BJ. Postoperative spinal wound infections. *J Am Acad Orthop Surg.* 2008;16(6):330–337.
65. Theil C, Schmidt-Braekling T, Gosheger G, et al. Clinical use of linezolid in periprosthetic joint infections - a systematic review. *J Bone Jt Infect.* 2020;6(1):7–16.
66. Cho OH, Bae IG, Moon SM, et al. Therapeutic outcome of spinal implant infections caused by Staphylococcus aureus: A retrospective observational study. *Medicine (Baltimore).* 2018; 97(40):e12629.
67. Zimmerli W, Widmer AF, Blatter M, et al. Role of rifampin for treatment of orthopedic implant-related staphylococcal infections: a randomized controlled trial. Foreign-Body Infection (FBI) Study Group. *JAMA.* 1998;279(19):1537–1541.
68. Chahoud J, Kanafani Z, Kanj SS. Surgical site infections following spine surgery: eliminating the controversies in the diagnosis. *Front Med (Lausanne).* 2014;1:7.
69. McClelland S 3rd, Takemoto RC, Lonner BS, et al. Analysis of postoperative thoracolumbar spine infections in a prospective randomized controlled trial using the Centers for Disease Control surgical site infection criteria. *Int J Spine Surg.* 2016;10:14.
70. Striano BM, Refakis CA, Anari JB, et al. Site-specific surgical site infection rates for rib-based distraction. *J Pediatr Orthop.* 2019;39(9):e698–e702.
71. Chahoud J, Kanafani Z, Kanj SS. Surgical site infections following spine surgery: eliminating the controversies in the diagnosis. *Front Med (Lausanne).* 2014;1:7.
72. McDermott H, Bolger C, Humphreys H. Postprocedural discitis of the vertebral spine: challenges in diagnosis, treatment and prevention. *J Hosp Infect.* 2012;82(3):152–157. 2012.
73. Nasto LA, Colangelo D, Rossi B, et al. Post-operative spondylodiscitis. *Eur Rev Med Pharmacol Sci.* 2012;16(Suppl 2): 50–57.
74. Maruo K, Berven SH. Outcome and treatment of postoperative spine surgical site infections: predictors of treatment success and failure. *J Orthop Sci.* 2014;19(3):398–404.
75. Wille H, Dauchy FA, Desclaux A, et al. Efficacy of debridement, antibiotic therapy and implant retention within three months during postoperative instrumented spine infections. *Infect Dis (Lond).* 2017;49(4):261–267.

9

When to Operate on the Cervical Spine?

ALICIA ASTURIAS, ANH X. LE AND BOBBY TAY

CHAPTER OUTLINE

Introduction

The first seven vertebrae in the spine work in concert to protect the spinal cord and exiting nerve roots while providing multiplanar range of motion of the head and neck. As with any vital structure, the delicate balance of protection and function lays the foundation for pathology. Akin to other orthopaedic structures, the cervical spine is susceptible to degenerative, traumatic, and oncologic pathologies with interventions ranging from the nonoperative to the operative. Unlike the appendicular skeleton in which the operative benefits of function preservation largely outweigh the risks of functional limitation—in the spine, and in particular the cervical spine—operating even in the most mundane of pathologies comes with considerable functional and mortality risk. Keeping these risks and benefits in mind, the purpose of this chapter is to provide a framework for operative indications within the cervical spine. We will start by briefly summarizing an approach to the standard operative indications for the cervical spine. Subsequently, we will discuss nuanced circumstances in which cervical spine pathology, symptom chronicity, and patient factors combine to cloud the standard algorithm for operative intervention and provide a summation of the literature to guide decision making. The hope is that after reading this chapter, there will be a better understanding of the complexity of operative decision making for unique cervical spine scenarios and a framework for guiding operative management.

Standard Indications

Despite the operative and perioperative risks involved, standard indications for operating in the cervical spine do not differ substantially from other orthopaedic pathologies. The goals of preserving function via the restoration of length, alignment, and rotation can be similarly applied to the cervical spine regarding preserving neurologic function through stabilization and decompression. Further, it is important to delineate urgent or emergent operative interventions in the cervical spine from standard elective interventions. Lastly, as with all surgical interventions, the decision to operate is one that is made jointly with your patient, and this cannot be overstated as the risk of iatrogenic and perioperative complications can be paramount.

Neurologic function is quantified clinically as balance, coordination, gait, protective sensation, and strength. In regard to patient experience, clinical neurologic function translates into an applied ability to perform activities of daily living. Anecdotally, it's a patient's ability to eat, to maintain their basic hygienic needs, and to ambulate that correlate to their physical and mental well-being. When determining operative indications in the cervical spine, it is important to assess these neurologic metrics through both objective and subjective means.

Operative assessment in the cervical spine begins with a thorough history and physical to better understand the cause, duration, progression, and functional limitations of a patient's current condition. While pain is not considered a metric of objective neurologic function, subjectively it can greatly impair a patient's ability to perform activities of daily living and must also be evaluated for duration, severity, and progression. Similarly, duration can be useful to determine the likelihood of neurologic restoration after operative intervention. Acute neurologic dysfunction often warrants acute operative interventions with an increased likelihood of return to function.[1–3] Conversely, chronic neurologic dysfunction may be due to significant compressive or unstable neurologic damage and may be less likely to be restored.[4] It is also important to consider the overall health status and prognostic factors for individual patients when considering operative interventions in the cervical spine. This applies to all organ systems including cardiac, pulmonary, and hematologic systems, but also orthopaedic health correlates such as bone density, endocrine disorders, or aberrant anatomy. Finally, it is important to consider the psychosocial and environmental factors that may impact a patient's likelihood of complications, nonunion, and postoperative compliance. This includes age, smoking status, housing status, nutrition, mental status, and social support. While the impact of age and smoking on perioperative cervical spine complications has been well documented, literature focusing on the impact of mental illness, social support, and socioeconomic status is in its infancy. Perhaps future iterations of this chapter will have online calculators to help risk stratify cervical spine patients holistically, but for now, we continue to rely on clinical judgment and joint decision making.

With these preoperative considerations in mind, the following can be used as a framework for operative considerations in the cervical spine (see Table 9.1).

TABLE 9.1 Standard Surgical Indications for the Cervical Spine.

- Acute neurologic functional loss (severe pain or motor deficit)
- Progressive motor deficits
- Failed conservative management
- Instability

Controversial Considerations for Operative Intervention

Generally, the above indications for operative intervention can outweigh the risks of surgery in a healthy population. With advances in navigation, implant augmentation, and designated spinal and trauma services, cervical spine surgery is well tolerated.[4–9] However, there are instances in which patient factors add complexity to the risk–benefit analysis of surgery and thus a topic of reflection and guidance within this chapter.

In addition to the general indications for some of the most common pathologies in the cervical spine, this chapter will discuss the timing of operative intervention in acute spinal cord injury, as well as the rare scenario of multiple cervical spinal fractures. We will also discuss applications in the geriatric population in regard to odontoid fractures and cervical stenosis. Lastly, we discuss the operative considerations of oncologic pathologies and how patient's risk–benefit analysis leans on quality of life and overall prognosis to guide operative interventions for neurologic symptoms.

Traumatic Cervical Spine

Introduction

Cervical spinal injuries represent 20% of all spinal cord injuries and can lead to catastrophic sequelae of neurologic dysfunctions ranging from paresthesia to tetraplegia.[1–3,10–12] Although the incidence of spinal cord injury (SCI) is relatively low compared to chronic widespread illnesses, the cost to patients and our medical system is disproportionately high. In the United States alone, the cost of SCI-related hospitalization estimations per patient ranges widely from \$290 to \$620,590, and the overall cost to the healthcare system is estimated at 1.7 billion dollars.[13,14] Unsurprisingly, cervical spinal injuries comprise the largest acute and long-term care costs within this total.[13] Thus, for both patients and our healthcare system, appropriate and timely interventions for cervical spine injuries is of the utmost importance.

Evaluating the Cervical Trauma Patient

- Basic and advanced trauma life support considerations
- Assessing the level and pattern of skeletal injury
- Assessing the neurologic injury
- Assessing for distal spinal injuries and extremity injuries

Basic and advanced trauma life support is highly protocolized and is not the focus of this chapter; however, it is important to know that within such protocols is the assumption of cervical spine injury for each patient. It is also important to recognize that 80% of upper cervical spine injuries have a second injury within the cervical spine.[12] Therefore, it is up to the orthopaedic or neurosurgeon to determine the extent of the assumed injury as well as those distally, as this guides management. Assessing the level and pattern of injury is done with combinatory imaging modalities such as cervical spine radiographs and noncontrast CT scans of the head/neck and the consideration of more advanced imaging with MRI.

The surgeon's goal with categorizing the pattern of injury is to assess for instability of the cervical spine. Instability can be defined as "the loss of the ability of the spine under physiological loads to maintain its pattern of displacement so that there is no initial or additional neurological deficit, no major deformity and no incapacitating pain." Instability can cause active cord compression or represent injuries that have a substantial risk for displacement and later cord compression.

Considerations regarding instability and displacement differ in the upper and subaxial cervical spine largely due to the anatomic differences between these two regions. We know from imaging and cadaveric studies that the diameter of the C1-C2 canal levels is 15 to 29 mm while the subaxial cervical spine canal width is 14 to 23 mm.[12,15,16] Therefore, given the additional epidural space, fractures within the upper cervical levels rarely lead to primary mechanical neurological deficits. However, there remains consequences of chronic intermittent myelopathic compression after C1-C2 injuries for which operative interventions are necessary but may be dependent on patient considerations for which there are controversies to discuss later in this chapter. General surgical indications are summarized below (see Table 9.2).

TABLE 9.2 General surgical indications in the cervical trauma patient.

Neurologic Considerations

- Presenting neurologic deficits, motor or sensory
- Progressive neurological deterioration
- Failure of closed reduction

Imaging Considerations

Upper Cervical Spine (C1-C2)

- Assess instability via the integrity of the transverse ligament
- Atlano-Dens Interval (ADI): >3 mm suggestive of injury to transverse ligament
- Lateral Mass Displacement: >7 mm suggestive of injury to transverse ligament
- Type II odontoid fractures in a healthy population

Subaxial Cervical Spine (C3-C7)

- Assess instability via the integrity of the posterior ligamentous complex (PLC)
- >11 degrees of kyphosis
- >5 mm posterior displacement
- Bilateral facet dislocation of more than 25%
- Compression fractures with kyphosis of 30 degrees or height loss of more than 50%

A combination of physical examination, patient stability, and imaging findings can help guide operative management in the cervical spine.[11] While these principles are generally accepted, the timing of such interventions have prompted considerable controversy within the field of orthopaedics and will be discussed below.

A. Cervical Spinal Cord Injury

As mentioned previously, the economic and social burden for patients and our medical system is immense, affecting mostly young patients who will endure the sequelae of their injury for the duration of their lifetime. The prognosis of neurologic recovery in traumatic spinal cord injuries remains low, and thus defining the risk and benefits of operative intervention is imperative to minimize further complications and promote optimal outcome.

SCI is thought to have both primary and secondary insults. The primary insult can be complete (all motor/sensory function below the lesion) or incomplete (some remaining sensory or motor) and involves rapid spinal cord compression in the setting of fracture dislocation or burst injury. What follows is a secondary insult that involves ischemia, hemorrhage, electrolyte disturbances, and lipid peroxidation that places the remaining spinal cord tissue at risk of further neurologic injury. While the primary injury is irreversible, secondary injury may benefit from surgical intervention and is a topic of considerable debate.[5–9,17]

Timeline of Controversy

Historically, cervical spine injuries were treated nonoperatively, prescribing to the notion that stabilization and reduction can be achieved through nonoperative postural and bedrest techniques.[10,11,18] Adhering to this dogma, Frankel et al.[18] in 1969 demonstrated in his historic nonoperative cohort of 612 patients that through nonoperative stabilization techniques, a subset of cervical spine patients improved functional levels by discharge. Specifically, 11/123 complete cervical spinal cord patients had return of functional motor status and 16/21 patients with motor useless functional status had improvement to useful or recovered functional status with nonoperative means alone. Continued research demonstrated some recovery of function for ~11% nonoperative patients (except for in the case of locked bilateral facet dislocations) but also demonstrated neurologic deterioration in 10% to 24% in nonoperative treatment groups.[19,20] Thus, while some patients recover, many patients do not. Additionally, there is a subset of patients who deteriorate, and that prompted further research in animal modeling alongside the modernization of surgical implants, techniques, and critical care for SCI.

Animal studies in the late 1990s and early 2000s suggested the duration of compressive injury was inversely proportional to the return of function.[10,11,17] Specifically, the longer a cord was artificially compressed, the less likely it was to recover. Further, animals in these compressive groups that underwent an urgent decompressive intervention had better functional outcomes than those animals for which intervention was delayed.[21,22] This prompted a distinct shift in the dogma regarding acute surgery in spinal cord injury. While many operative interventions previously recommended stabilization alone as early laminectomies suggested worse outcomes, clinical applications trended toward stabilization and decompression, some institutional recommendations as early as <6 hour.[12] However, cumulative prospective and retrospective data on patient applications had mixed results. While expedited operative interventions had few documented complications as compared to delayed interventions, the impact on neurologic outcomes were not as linear as suggested by animal models. Two primary systematic reviews have compiled data over the last two decades to suggest that there is prospective evidence to recommend <24 hour decompression and stabilization for SCI than compared to interventions at >24 hour, specifically in regards to improvements in ASIA motor scoring at 6 months.[20–22] Further, there is insufficient evidence to suggest differences in intensive care unit (ICU) stay, complications, or hospital stay duration between early and delayed interventions. A recent retrospective analysis also suggested for a rare subset of patients who have clinical findings of SCI but are without radiographic evidence, also known spinal cord injury without radiographic abnormality (SCIWORA), optimal time to intervention for stabilization and decompression for improvement in ASIA grades was delayed. Specifically, intervention 3 to 7 days after injury can significantly improve the short-term and long-term follow-up effects in this subgroup.[23]

Discussion

There is a role for operative decompression and stabilization in cervical spine trauma. There is type II evidence to suggest that operating within the first 24 hours impacts functional outcome.[4–9] While it is prudent to have randomized clinical trials to guide clinical recommendations, the complexity and heterogeneous nature of cervical spine trauma and overall patient hemodynamic stability makes randomization difficult. Prior studies have been significantly confounded, and thus we must continue to rely on clinical judgment and available data to guide interventions. Adding to the complexity, there is budding evidence to suggest that the size of the intramedullary lesion may be more predictive of recovery than operative timing.[24] A recent prospective study of 32 cervical spine patients by Aarabi et al. compared the efficacy of Ultra-Early (<12 hour), Early (12–24 hour), and Late (>24–138.5 hour) interventions alongside preoperative and postoperative intramedullary lesion length on MRI (IMLL). Their multivariate regression model suggested that preoperative IMLL and postoperative IMLL confirmation of decompression were correlated to return of function, not the timing of surgery. However, outside of the research setting, there are patient and systemic factors that interfere with the attainment of timely imaging studies. Further, postoperative imaging can be costly and potentially confounded by metal artifact. Thus, room remains for continued research on the operative recommendations in the acute cervical spine injury patient; however, some key points can be emphasized and are summarized below.

A Summary: Operative Considerations in Acute Spinal Cord Injury SCI

- There remains insufficient evidence to provide standard recommendations regarding the optimal timing and role of acute decompression in SCI
- There are limitations in the current data given the heterogeneity of stability in trauma patients, spinal injury patterns, subjectivity of initial functional assessments, and lack of control groups
- Level II Evidence to suggest some functional improvements after stabilization and decompression within <24 hour of SCI, pending hemodynamic stability of the patient
- Level II Evidence to suggest <24 hour results appear to have increased reliability in the incomplete spinal cord and Acute Traumatic Central Cord Syndrome (ATCCS) groups
- Level II Evidence to support urgent closed reduction of bilateral locked facets in an SCI patient with neurologic deterioration; in the experienced, these interventions are safe
- Insufficient evidence to support that early <24 hour intervention impacts ICU stay, length of hospital stay, or late medical complications
- More research is warranted for rare subcohort of spinal cord injury without radiographic abnormality (SCIWORA) group, single center Level III retrospective analysis suggests stabilization and decompression in 3 to 7 days

B. Geriatric Odontoid Fractures

Geriatric odontoid fractures represent a particularly complex clinical scenario for the surgeon and is the topic of debate. The surgeon must balance medical comorbidities in an aging, osteoporotic population with anatomic considerations of healing vascular watershed areas at the odontoid waist. Upper cervical spine trauma in the elderly patient is reported at 69% as compared to 36% in a younger population, with half representing odontoid fractures.[25] Thus, low energy odontoid fractures in the elderly population are becoming increasingly common and mortality rates of 18% to 45 % after 1 year and 44% to 51% after 2 years for type II odontoid fractures have been reported.[1–3,26,27] Further, there are complications related to both operative and non-operative treatment strategies—the former with possible implant failures, iatrogenic vascular injury, and infection and the latter compromising union and stability as well as aspiration risks.

Classification

The most used classification system was described by Anderson/D'Alonzo in 1974.[2] It defines odontoid fractures by their location, with type 2 associated with the highest pseudoarthrosis rate with a fracture line extending at the poorly vascularized odontoid waist. Given the high rate of pseudoarthrosis or nonunion, in 1993 Eysel and Roosen developed a subclassification of the type 2 variants based on the obliquity of the fracture line to help guide operative techniques. A subsequent, widely adopted modification was developed by Grauer in 2005.[27,28] The AO Spine division recently developed the Upper Cervical Spine Injury Classification System that has been applied in the research setting but has not yet been adopted clinically.

Additionally, to these classifications, nearly 50% of patients over 70 years of age with a type 2 odontoid fracture have an additional atlas fracture.[27,29] Unusual in the younger population, this concomitant injury is likely the result of underlying arthritis of the C1-C2 joint causing a varied distribution of force across the stiffened upper cervical segment. The majority are stable atlas fractures with 56% Gehweiler 1 and 22% Gehweiler 2. Some fractures do not fit the classic patterns and are known as atypical C2 body fractures and have unique coronal or sagittal fracture lines as described by Benzel. There is little summative research to stratify unique treatment strategies for atypical fractures or concomitant atlas fractures, but in general follow classic pattern considerations that will be discussed below.

Management Considerations

There are three main types of treatment options: rigid cervical collar immobilization (CC), halo vest (HV), and surgical intervention. The goal of treatment interventions for odontoid fractures focuses on stability and mortality.

For displaced fractures of the odontoid with neurologic compromise, surgical intervention is recommended. Controversy largely stems from the treatment of nondisplaced type II odontoid fractures that are typically asymptomatic. Not surprisingly, there are differences in union rates between the treatment strategies. Harrop et al. performed a meta-analysis focusing on type II and type III fractures of the odontoid process and found rates of nonunion for CC and HV 70% versus 78%, respectively. Surgical intervention had lower nonunion rates from 0% to 65.5%.[28] However, it is not clear if union rate in nondisplaced Type II odontoid fractures correlates to neurologic compromise. Delcourt et al.'s 2015 meta-analysis suggests neurologic sequelae from nonunion is rare.[25] Hart et al. followed five elderly patients >80 years of age for 55.2 months with an odontoid nonunion and none of them developed secondary myelopathy or displacement >1 mm.[28] Kalsi-Ryan et al. treated a cohort of 30 patients with CC fractures and although nonunion was 77%, there was no evidence of secondary displacement or neurological deterioration for any patient at 21 months.[30] Additionally, Koech et al. reported a case series of 42 patients, and although their union rate was 50% with CC, there was 90% dynamic x-rays in 90% (CC) or 100% (HV) of the patients.[31] Therefore, for patients who present with nondisplaced type 2 dens fracture, a stable fibrous union is adequate and can be achieved by nonoperative means.[27,29,31]

Regarding mortality and medical complications, halo-vest has the greatest compilation risk for both the apparatus and medical morbidity.[28,32–35] The apparatus complications include pin site infections, screw loosening, medical complications, and others. The most common complication is pin site infections, occuring in 14.6% to 59.5% of patients.[27,29,32] Screw loosening, halo dislocations, and decubitus ulceration are also not uncommon, representing 12% to 60%, 3% to 13%, and 0% to 11%, respectively. Medical complications can be severe. In studies where specific analysis of nonconservative treatment measures were available, the mortality rate after CC varied from 0.0% to 35.0%, compared to HV mortality rate, which varied from 0.0% to 42.1%. Generally, a rigid cervical collar is well tolerated by patients; however, the summative complications from the halo vest apparatus and mortality are significant.[28,33,36,37]

Similarly, Schoenfeld et al. found a 1-year mortality rate of 36% after isolated odontoid fractures and nonoperative treatment, whereas this rate dropped to 21% after surgical treatment.[38] Josten et al. in their cohort of 83 patients reported an overall surgical mortality rate of 16%, subgroup analysis showing that patients <85 years old had postoperative mortality of 15% whereas those >85 had mortality of 36%.[27] Additional studies have noted similar results with >85 postoperative group having higher mortality, but comparable to nonoperative interventions. Surgical revision rates in the Schoenfeld group were comparable in all age groups.[38]

Overall, summative data are lacking in definitive data for the operative and nonoperative management for geriatric odontoid fractures. Generally, rigid cervical collars are low risk, affordable interventions that are appropriate for a large majority of odontoid fractures. More data are needed for individual age groups, preoperative function, and comorbidities to better stratify the optimal patient for surgical intervention, but some data suggest that for the older but not elderly population, surgical intervention is both safe and effective for definitive management of odontoid fractures.

A Summary: Operative Considerations for Geriatric Odontoid Fractures

- Mortality rate is high regardless of intervention and may represent overall health deterioration akin to that of a hip fracture
- Displaced odontoid fractures with neurologic compromise are operative fractures and require reduction and fixation
- Fractures type 1, type 3, and nondisplaced fractures type 2 according to Anderson/D'Alonzo can be treated conservatively with rigid cervical collar; however, close follow-up for symptomatic radiographic displacement is necessary
- Surgical intervention for type 2 odontoid fracture affords higher union rates, but more data are needed to determine if the nonunion rates impact mortality. Some data suggest this may be the case for patients <85
- Halo vest should not be used in the treatment of odontoid fractures in the absence of significant contraindications to operative fixation for displaced, neurologically compromised patients

Cervical Polytrauma—Multiple Cervical Spinal Fractures

The final cervical trauma topic in the chapter is the cervical polytrauma patient, specifically patients who have multiple fractures within the cervical spine. This is a rare subtype of cervical trauma and covers axial and subaxial contiguous and noncontiguous patterns.[39] Due to the rarity of this occurrence, data are limited largely to case reviews that have relied on both operative and nonoperative interventions.[40–46]

Gliezes et al. report on the largest single center cohort of combined cervical spine fractures. Their review demonstrated 31 of 116 cervical trauma patients that had 2 or 3 cervical spine fractures. 61.2% of the combined fractures involved C1 and C2, whereas the remaining 38.8% involved combined axial and subaxial injuries.[45] Out of 31 patients who had combined lesions, 13 received surgical treatment (41.9%) compared to single cervical vertebral injuries of 21.7%. Surgical interventions were single staged and included a modified Gallie arthrodesis in seven cases, posterior C1-C2 screw fixation in two, C2 pedicle screw fixation in three, and posterior plate fixation of the low contact stress (LCS) in five.[45] A peripheral injury was present in 10 cases, and severe head trauma in 6 (19.4%). Two patients were Frankel A, 1 C, and 27 E. One patient could not be examined due to severe head trauma. No complications occurred in these cases and all patients healed within 3 months.[45]

Letts et al. report on a case of a 14-year-old male who sustained fractures of every cervical vertebrae after a snowmobile accident. Per their report, the multiple cervical spine fractures included fracture to the anterior arch of the first cervical vertebra, Type 2 odontoid fracture with anterior displacement, and a combination of lateral and bilateral fractures of vertebrae.[3–7,41] There was no canal impingement at any level and the boy was neurologically intact. He was treated with a halo vest urgently that was kept in place for 10 weeks with a transition to Minerva spinal bracing thereafter. He developed a scapular ulcer at week 3 that was debrided, and anterior 2 mm displacement of his odontoid was noted 3 weeks after injury but was asymptomatic and stable on flexion/extension views obtained at 3 months. His overall health status was complex, requiring two below-knee amputations (BKAs), multiple finger amputations, and sequelae of a large pulmonary embolism on injury day 5, but was ultimately discharged on hospital day 146 with some ambulatory function with BKA arthroses.

Vargas-Mena et al. report on a case of a 46-year-old male involved in a motor vehicle accident who sustained spine and spinal cord injuries consisting of ASIA C C2-C6 fractures.[42] The operative team proceeded with surgery. It was decided to do the procedure in two stages with posterior and anterior instrumentation, a C4-6 anterior cervical discectomy and fusion (ACDF), posterior to anterior odontoid lag screw, and C2-C6 posterior fusion. At 19-month follow-up he had ASIA D neurologic function and had returned to work with some left-sided arm deficit.[41]

A Summary: Operative Considerations in Combined Cervical Spine Fractures

There are insufficient data to offer standard operative guidelines in the combined cervical spinal fracture group. There is evidence to suggest that a majority of patients present with remarkably preserved function, despite the apparent severity of their injury. The mechanisms of this are not known, but one theory suggests that displaced, contiguous fracture patterns widen the spinal canal to limit compressive insults such as those seen with single level injuries. The pediatric case series reported skeletally mature epiphyseal plates, and could be considered adult; however, the success of nonoperative treatment in a halo vest with remarkably few side effects could be explained by the known resilience of this age group than superiority of nonoperative treatment.[41,43]

- Combined injuries of the cervical spine are poorly documented in the literature
- There is insufficient evidence to suggest specific operative treatment strategies in combined injuries; however, there have been few reported complications by applying the standard indications of restoring stability and alignment of the spine surgically in this population in the acute setting

Degenerative Cervical Spine

A. Degenerative Cervical Stenosis

Cadaveric studies note the incidence of cervical stenosis is 4.9% of the adult population, 6.8% of the population 50 years of age or older, and 9% of the population 70 years of age or older.[15,16] Although not all patients become symptomatic, those who do contribute to make it one of the most common causes of spinal cord dysfunctions. The symptoms of cervical stenosis are myelopathic in nature, but can be concurrent with radicular symptoms in the setting of degenerative disease. Myelopathic symptoms include clumsiness of the hands, difficulty walking, impaired balance and coordination, and sensory complaints of numbness or tingling in the hands and feet. Radicular symptoms can be both pain and paresthesia. As with most pathologies, there was a historical emphasis on nonoperative management of cervical stenosis.[4,47–50] However, with the main symptom caused by anatomic cord compression, nonoperative interventions do not halt the progression of disease and can lead to well-documented worsening outcomes compared to operative management.[5–9] Where the controversy lies is in the timing of operative intervention, the complexities of concomitant radicular symptoms, and asymptomatic incidental cord compression.

Classification

There are three classifications for cervical myelopathy. They include the Nurick Classification, the Ranawat Classification, and the Japanese Orthopaedic Association Classification (JOA). The Nurick classification is the least comprehensive, but in addition to myelopathic symptoms, looks to classify radicular pathology, work status, and gait. While important in assessing functional limitations and goals of treatment, it is difficult to apply to the elderly population who may have confounding reasons for poor ambulation or alternative reasons for unemployment. The Ranawat Classification attempts clinical objectivity with formal strength assessment. Lastly, the JOA classification is the most comprehensive and has the highest reliability; however, due to its length it can be cumbersome.[51] Assessment for severity and lifestyle limitations are thus combinatory between subjective and objective measures, including the above classifications.

Historical Indications

It is known that the natural history of cervical stenosis with myelopathy includes prolonged periods of stasis, followed by intermittent exacerbations, thought to have been caused by minor trauma.[4] Despite these prolonged periods of stasis, neurologic decline in conservatively managed patients occurs in 20% to 62% of patients at 3- to 6-year follow-up.[5–9,30,47,52–54] Fehlings et al.'s retrospective analysis similarly found that 37% of patients managed nonoperatively and were converted to operative management within 6.5 years. So, while the progression can be slow, many patients continue to decline and are at risk for acute decompensation in the setting of trauma. Thus, there is a role for expedited operative intervention.

In 1993 Law et al. summarized the literature to provide the following recommendations; their team understood the pitfalls of nonoperative management, offering a timeline for progression.[55] An AO Global Spine Consensus suggests a similar emphasis on operative management, focusing on symptoms progression and counseling, as opposed to a definitive timeline. Both indication guidelines are summarized below (see Table 9.3).

TABLE 9.3 Historical operative indications in cervical myelopathy.

- Progression of symptoms
- Duration of symptoms greater than 6 months
- Compression ratio (cord sagittal diameter/transverse diameter) 0.4 or less, or transverse area of the cord less than 40 mm^2

2017 AO Global Spine Consensus

- Based on the mJOA score, mild myelopathy is defined as >15, moderate as 12 to 14, and severe as >11
- Severe DCM: Surgical intervention (Grade: Strong Recommendation; Moderate Evidence)
- Moderate DCM: Surgical intervention for patients with moderate DCM (Grade: Strong Recommendation; Moderate Evidence)
- Mild DCM: Offer surgical intervention or a supervised trial of structured rehabilitation for patients with mild DCM. Should there be subsequent neurological deterioration or should symptoms fail to improve, operative intervention is recommended (Grade: Weak Recommendation; Very Low to Low Evidence)
- Asymptomatic radiographic cord compression: Consensus does not offer surgery for nonmyelopathic patients with evidence of cervical cord compression without signs or symptoms of radiculopathy. We suggest that these patients be counseled as to potential risks of progression, educated about relevant signs and symptoms of myelopathy, and followed clinically. (Grade: Weak Recommendation; No Evidence Identified, based on expert opinion)
- Cord compression +/– EMG confirmed radiculopathy without myelopathy: Offer either surgical intervention or nonoperative treatment consisting of close serial follow-up or a supervised trial of structured rehabilitation. In the event of myelopathic development, the patient should be managed according to the recommendations above. (Grade: Weak Recommendation; Low Evidence)

Controversy

The AO Global Spine Consensus provides a necessary framework for operative considerations in cervical stenosis. It also emphasizes gaps in the current literature regarding operative considerations for asymptomatic cord compression and cervical stenosis in the geriatric trauma population.

Asymptomatic cord compression, when considering the optimal timing of operative intervention, is important to consider the timeline of disease progression for patient counseling. These authors similarly cannot provide well-evidenced recommendations for prophylactic treatment in these groups, but it is important to discuss disease progression and understand which patients may be at particular risk for progression that may warrant future intervention. Wilson et al. found that approximately 8% of asymptomatic patients at 1-year follow-up develop myelopathic symptoms and 23% at a median of 44-month follow-up.[54] Further, their analysis suggested that certain patient characteristics could be predictive of the development of cervical myelopathy and found the strongest correlation to the prolonged motor-evoked potentials (MEPs) and symptomatic radiculopathy.[54]

Additionally, how do these recommendations apply to the geriatric cervical trauma patient? Specifically geriatric patients who fall under the SCIWORA trauma subgroup, but have underlying stenosis?[53,56] Unfortunately, at this time there is limited direct analysis of this subgroup. However, we can appreciate the complexity of acute operative considerations for stable or asymptomatic myelopathy in the setting of trauma. Recalling that 62% of patients develop myelopathic symptoms within 3 to 6 years, the progression of cervical myelopathy in the elderly population is of particular concern when considering the mortality rate of hip fractures and odontoid fractures already discussed in this chapter.

In 2015 Nakashima et al. reported that there was no difference in patient reported outcomes after decompression in patients >75 years old compared to patients <75, suggesting that even within this age group there can be meaningful functional gains.[56,57] Madhavan et al. performed a meta-analysis on 1169 patients >75 years old and found that the only significant difference between operative decompression outcomes in the elderly and nonelderly patients was the incidence of delirium.[58] Specifically, patients >74 who underwent decompression were 15.9 times more likely to develop delirium than their younger counterparts.[59] Thus, there is summative research to suggest decompression in this age group is not only safe but can offer functional improvements. How this translates into operating in the acute setting for elderly patients without evidence of traumatic acute on chronic cord compression has not been established yet.

Summary

- The AO Global Spine Recommendations are a useful tool for operative indications in cervical stenosis
- For asymptomatic patients or minimally symptomatic patients, a proportion of patients begin to feel symptomatic as early as 1 year
- There is weak evidence to support that cervical decompression in the elderly population is comparative to decompression in the <75 year old population
- More analysis is needed in the asymptomatic or stable geriatric cervical stenosis trauma patient and the value of operative decompression in the acute setting

Oncology

Within this last section, we discuss the nuances of when to operate in the oncologic cervical spine. This includes both the prognostic considerations unique to spinal tumors, but also the timing of intervention in the case of cord compression and the timing of radiation (if indicated). Although not the focus of this chapter, prior to surgical intervention it is important to characterize and stage the lesion, the histopathology of the lesion, and its extent. Specifically, with the appropriate systemic laboratory work-up, advanced imaging, and biopsy if the primary tumor is unknown. Further, it is important to distinguish if the patient's symptoms are caused by the tumor itself or if their symptoms are secondary sequelae of compression or instability. This can guide not only the timing of intervention but also the type of intervention.

Classification

As with all operative decisions, it is important to classify the pathology. The first decision point is determining if the lesion is primary or metastatic as well as their location as intramedullary, extradural, or intramedullary/extradural. Some of the most common spinal-associated tumors are listed below; this is by no means a comprehensive list and focuses on adult pathologies versus pediatric[59] (see Table 9.4).

Subsequently comes classifying the extent of the disease, cord compression, the prognosis of the patient, and finally the stability of the spine. Scoring systems have been developed to help the surgeon with these considerations. While not specific to just the cervical spine, these include the Tomita, Weinstein-Boriani-Biagini (WBB), Tokuhashi, and Spinal Instability Neoplasm Scoring (SINS) systems.

The Tomita scoring system focuses on classifying the anatomic location of the tumor. The WBB staging system

TABLE 9.4 Spinal tumors

Intramedullary - Within the spinal cord (5% of spinal tumors)
- Astrocytoma
- Ependymoma
- Intramedullary lipoma

Extramedullary - Outside the spinal cord/dura (55% of spinal tumors)
- Metastatic lesions (most common lung, breast, prostate) ~95% of extramedullary)
- Lipoma
- Sarcoma
- Chordoma

Intradural - Extramedullary (40% of spinal tumors)
- Meningiomas
- Schwannoma
- Neurofibroma

similarly takes into consideration anatomy but focuses on intradural or extradural extent to guide a specific lesional dependent tumor resection. The Tokuhashi Scoring System focuses on patient prognosis to guide palliative versus excisional management by considering the severity of spinal cord palsy, primary tumor pathology, and organ involvement. Within this scoring system, palliative options are considered for patients with a predicted survival of <6 months, while those with lesions isolated to one vertebrae with predicted survival >6 months are amenable to excisional procedures such as primary corpectomy. But, beyond the prognosis of the patient, stability of the spine can also be a unique indicator of operative intervention. Specifically, the SINS can help better classify the impact the lesion has on spinal stability as a cause for debilitating mechanical pain or risk of future spinal cord injury.[60] There are six classifying variables that include location, mechanical pain, lytic vs blastic qualities, alignment, vertebral collapse, and posterolateral alignment. A score of 6 is indicative of a stable lesion, 7–12 a possibly unstable lesion, and a score of 13–18 representing an unstable lesion requiring operative stabilization.

Controversy—Evolution of the Timing of Surgical Intervention

The utility of the above classifications is of paramount importance when guiding treatment of primary and metastatic lesions in the outpatient setting; however, what about patients who present emergently with metastatic cord compression (MSCC)?

It has been estimated that 5% to 14% of patients with cancer experience metastatic cord compression within the course of their disease.[61,62] In the past, primary treatments focused on palliative care with either radiation or laminectomy alone. These did not have a significant impact on functional outcomes for patients.[63,64] However, as treatments have advanced, the necessity for prompt recognition and intervention to preserve quality of life for these patients has become the focus of treatment algorithms. Delayed intervention has been associated with significant urologic and bowel dysfunction that, outside of the pathology of their specific lesion, can add to patient mortality and decrease quality of life.[65]

In 2008, The National Institute of Care and Excellence (NICE) emphasized the importance of prompt diagnosis and treatment after a Scottish audit showed a delay in referral of 3 months from the onset of back pain or nerve root pain, finding ultimately that nearly 50% of patients with metastatic cord compression were unable to walk at the time of diagnosis. Of these, 67% recovered no additional function within 1 month. The full recommendations can be found here, https://www.nice.org.uk/guidance/cg75. However, main takeaways include prompt referral and access to MRI within 24 hours of symptom onset.

Beyond diagnosis, Quraishi et al. retrospectively reviewed 153 cases of MSCC and found that the cohort of patients who underwent operative intervention within 48 hours had significantly greater improvement in Frankel functional scores than those who underwent intervention >48 hours. There was no difference with operative stay, complications, and overall patient survival.[65] It is important to note that the severity of symptoms at presentation is also predictive of outcome. In a small cohort of 35 patients, Furstenberg et al. found that patients who presented with bowel and bladder sphincter symptoms were more likely to have a poor functional outcome than those who did not.[66] Finally, like traumatic injuries of the cervical spine, the duration of compression was also predictive of outcome. Chaichana et al. found that patients who presented with symptoms <48 hours were more likely to recover.[67]

With these recommendations in place, surgical intervention in the metastatic spinal patient has become more common, but functional outcomes go beyond the neurologic. Bourassa-Moreau found that preoperative factors such as sarcopenia or cancer cachexia, as measured by L3 Total Psoas Area/Vertebral body Area (L3-TPA/VB) technique on computed tomography (CT), is a significant predictor of adverse outcomes after spinal surgery for metastatic lesions as well as 3-month survival, independent of tumor histology.[68]

Thus, although we have progressed in our treatment of various cancers as well as the perioperative care of medically complex patients, preoperative assessment remains paramount when considering the risks of operative intervention. However, if medically safe, early intervention for cord compression within <48 hours can result in preservation or improvement in function for patients with cervical spine metastatic pathology.

Controversy—Radiation and Surgery in the Cervical Spine

In a landmark paper in 2006, Falicov et al. demonstrated the positive impact of surgical intervention on quality of life for patients with spinal metastasis.[69] While stabilization and decompression procedures become more commonplace in the spinal oncologic setting, so too becomes the role of integrating radiation therapy with operative intervention.[70,71] We know from other fields that operative wound complications arise after radiation.[72,73] Further factors contributing to wound healing issues in this population include sarcopenia, immunocompromise, and malnourishment. However, the literature is distinctly lacking for randomized or even retrospective guidance on the optimal timing of radiation treatment and spinal surgery for metastasis despite the seemingly gold standard of care for spinal metastasis.

A meta-analysis by Itshayek el al. noted from 46 reports that operative timing ranged from 5 to 21 days after radiation and, based on their review, suggested surgical intervention should be delayed from radiation by at least 1 week.[74] A recent *2020 Journal of Spine Surgery* article regarding expert opinion surveyed spine surgeons and radiation oncologists on their practice and the timing of surgical intervention. Spine surgeons recommended at least 16 days, on average, after radiation therapy until surgical intervention. Radiation oncologists, conversely, suggested 21 days. Although a significant difference, both parties agreed anecdotally and within their personal practice to avoid surgical intervention for >2 weeks after radiation.[15,16]

While it would seem appropriate to wait for operative intervention after radiation in the context of wound complications, the optimal timing has yet to be established in an evidence-based fashion. We patiently await guidance from the literature on this topic on future iterations of this chapter.

Conclusion

In this chapter we discussed a generic framework for operating in the cervical spine that included acute neurologic functional loss (severe pain or motor deficit), progressive motor deficits, failed conservative management, and instability. As with most orthopaedic pathologies, our review of the literature demonstrated expedited interventions had improved outcome measures compared to delayed interventions, most notably in acute spinal cord injury and in acute metastatic cord compression. Further, we discussed the nuances of operating in the traumatized cervical spine and the considerations for multiple, contiguous cervical spinal fractures. We also discussed the increasingly common situation of the geriatric odontoid fracture in which surgical intervention is safe and has a higher union rate compared to nonoperative measures, although it may not significantly change clinical outcome. We also discussed the timing of surgery for cervical stenosis, emphasizing the likely progression of disease within 1 to 3 years and the positive impact of surgical decompression and stabilization. Lastly, we discussed the combination of surgery and radiation therapy for spinal metastasis and the distinct need for further randomized trials to guide evidence based management for this increasingly common scenario. Overall, while operating in the cervical spine comes with unique risks, an exploration of these topics continues to show benefits of operative intervention for many populations and pathologies as we look to the future for even more clarity within these groups.

References

1. Anderson KK, Tetreault L, Shamji MF, Singh A, Vukas RR, Harrop JS, Fehlings MG, Vaccaro AR, Hilibrand AS, Arnold PM. Optimal timing of surgical decompression for acute traumatic central cord syndrome: A systematic review of the literature. *Neurosurgery*. 2015;77(Suppl 4):S15–S32.
2. Anderson LD, D'Alonzo RT. Fractures of the odontoid process of the axis. *J Bone Joint Surg Am*. 1974;56:1663–1674.
3. Anderson PA, Matz PG, Groff MW, et al. Laminectomy and fusion for the treatment of cervical degenerative myelopathy. *J Neurosurg Spine*. 2009;11:150–156.
4. Rothman RH, Simeone FA, Herkowitz HN.*Rothman-Simeone and Herkowitz's the Spine*. 7th ed. Elsevier; 2018.
5. Fehlings MG, Wilson JR, Yoon ST, Rhee JM, Shanji MF, Lawrence BD. Symptomatic progression of cervical myelopathy and the role of nonsurgical management: a consensus statement. *Spine*. 2013;38:S19–S20.
6. Fehlings MG, Sekhon L. Cellular, ionic and biomolecular mechanisms of the injury process. In: Benzel E, Tator CH, eds.*Contemporary Management of Spinal Cord Injury: From Impact to Rehabilitation*. American Association of Neurological Surgeons; 2000.
7. Fehlings MG, Tetreault LA, Riew KD, Middleton JW, Wang JC. A clinical practice guideline for the management of degenerative cervical myelopathy: Introduction, rationale, and scope. *Global Spine J*. 2017;7(3 Suppl):21S–27S.
8. Fehlings MG, Vaccaro A, Wilson JR, et al. Early versus delayed decompression for traumatic cervical spinal cord injury: results of the Surgical Timing in Acute Spinal Cord Injury Study (STASCIS). *PLoS One*. 2012;7(2):e32037.
9. Fehlings MG, Perrin RG. The timing of surgical intervention in the treatment of spinal cord injury: A systematic review of recent clinical evidence. *Spine*. 2006;31(11):S28–S35.
10. Bedbrook GM, Sedgley GI. The management of spinal injuries--past and present. *Int Rehabil Med*. 1980;2(2):45–61.
11. Bedbrook GM. Spinal injuries with tetraplegia and paraplegia. *J Bone Joint Surg Br*. 1979;61-B(3):267–284.
12. O'Dowd JK. Basic principles of management for cervical spine trauma. *Eur Spine J*. 2010;19(Suppl 1(Suppl 1)):S18–S22.
13. Malekzadeh H, Golpayegani M, Ghodsi Z, et al. Direct cost of illness for spinal cord injury: A systematic review. *Global Spine J*. 2022;12(6):1267–1281.
14. Hall OT, McGrath RP, Peterson MD, et al. The burden of traumatic spinal cord injury in the United States: disability-adjusted life years. *Arch Phys Med Rehabil*. 2019;100(1):95–100.
15. Lee MJ, Cassinelli EH, Riew KD. Prevalence of cervical spine stenosis: anatomic study in cadavers. *J Bone Joint Surg Am*. 2007;89:376–380.
16. Lee RS, Batke J, Weir L, Dea N, Fisher CG. Timing of surgery and radiotherapy in the management of metastatic spine disease: expert opinion. *J Spine Surg*. 2018;4(2):368–373.
17. Collins WF. A review and update of experiment and clinical studies of spinal cord injury. *Paraplegia*. 1983;21(4):204–219.
18. Frankel H, Hancock D, Hyslop G, et al. The value of postural reduction in the initial management of closed injuries of the spine with paraplegia and tetraplegia. *Spinal Cord*. 1969;7:179–192.
19. Bose B, Northrup BE, Osterholm JL, Cotler JM, DiTunno JF. Reanalysis of central cervical cord injury management. *Neurosurgery*. 1984;15:367–372.
20. Divi SN, Schroeder GD, Mangan JJ, et al. Management of acute traumatic central cord syndrome: A narrative review. *Global Spine J*. 2019;9(1 Suppl):89S–97S.
21. Fehlings MG, Perrin RG. The role and timing of early decompression for cervical spinal cord injury: update with a review of recent clinical evidence. *Injury*. 2005;36(Suppl 2):B13–B26.
22. La Rosa G, Conti A, Cardali S, et al. Does early decompression improve neurological outcome of spinal cord injured patients? Appraisal of the literature using a meta-analytical approach. *Spinal Cord*. 2004;42:503–512.
23. Qi C, Xia H, Miao D, Wang X, Li Z. The influence of timing of surgery in the outcome of spinal cord injury without radiographic abnormality (SCIWORA). *J Orthop Surg Res*. 2020;15(1):223.

24. Aarabi B, Akhtar-Danesh N, Chryssikos T, et al. Efficacy of ultra-early (< 12 h), early (12-24 h), and late (>24-138.5 h) surgery with magnetic resonance imaging-confirmed decompression in American Spinal Injury Association Impairment Scale Grades A, B, and C cervical spinal cord injury. *J Neurotrauma.* 2020;37(3):448–457.
25. Delcourt T, Begue T, Saintyves G, et al. Management of upper cervical spine fractures in elderly patients. Current trends and outcomes. *Injury.* 2015;46(Suppl. 1):S24–S27.
26. Osterhoff G, Schnake K, Scheyerer MJ, et al. Recommendations for diagnosis and treatment of odontoid fractures in geriatric patients. *Z Orthop Unfall.* 2020;158(6):647–656.
27. Josten C, Jarvers JS, Glasmacher S, et al. Anterior transarticular atlanto- axial screw fixation in combination with dens screw fixation for type II odontoid fractures with associated atlanto-odontoid osteoarthritis. *Eur Spine J.* 2016;25:2210–2217.
28. Harrop JS, Hart R, Anderson PA. Optimal treatment for odontoid fractures in the elderly. *Spine.* 2010;35:S219–227.
29. Josten C, Jarvers JS, Glasmacher S, et al. Odontoid fractures in combination with C1 fractures in the elderly treated by combined anterior odon- toid and transarticular C1/2 screw fixation. *Arch Orthop Trauma Surg.* 2018;138:1525–1531.
30. Kalsi-Ryan S, Karadimas SK, Fehlings MG. Cervical spondylotic myelopathy: the clinical phenomenon and the current pathobiology of an increasingly prevalent and devastating disorder. *Neuroscientist.* 2013;19:409–421.
31. Koech F, Ackland HM, Varma DK, Williamson OD, Malham GM. Nonoperative management of type II odontoid fractures in the elderly. *Spine (Phila Pa 1976).* 2008;33(26):2881–2886.
32. Chapman J, Smith JS, Kopjar B, Vaccaro AR, Arnold P, Shaffrey CI, Fehlings MG. The AOSpine North America geriatric odontoid fracture mortality study: a retrospective review of mortality outcomes for operative versus nonoperative treatment of 322 patients with long-term follow-up. *Spine (Phila Pa 1976).* 2013;38(13):1098–1104.
33. Tashjian RZ, Majercik S, Biffl WL, Palumbo MA, Cioffi WG. Halo-vest immobi- lization increases early morbidity and mortality in elderly odontoid fractures. *J Trauma.* 2006;60:199–203.
34. Daentzer D, Florkemeier T. Conservative treatment of upper cervical spine injuries with the halo vest: an appropriate option for all patients independent of their age? *J Neurosurg Spine.* 2009;10:543–550.
35. Horn EM, Theodore N, Feiz-Erfan I, Lekovic C, Dickman CA, Sonntag VK. Complications of halo fixation in the elderly. *J Neurosurg Spine.* 2006;5:46–49.
36. Majercik S, Tashjian RZ, Biffl WL, Harrington DT, Cioffi WG. Halo vest immobilization in the elderly: a death sentence? *J Trauma.* 2005;59:350–356.
37. Venkatesan M, Northover JR, Wild JB, et al. Survival analysis of elderly patients with a fracture of the odontoid peg. *Bone Joint J.* 2014;96-B(1):88–93.
38. Schoenfeld AJ, Bono CM, Reichmann WM, et al. Type II odontoid fractures of the cervical spine: do treatment type and medical comorbidities affect mortality in elderly patients? *Spine (Phila Pa 1976).* 2011;36(11):879–885.
39. Li F, Chen Q, Xu K. The treatment of concomitant odontoid fracture and lower cervical spine injuries. *Spine.* 2008;33(19):E693–698.
40. Phipatanakul W, Minster G. Fractures of the second through the fifth cervical vertebra with multilevel bilateral pedicle involvement: a case report. *J Bone Joint Surg Am.* 2003;85:1347–1350.
41. Letts M, Davidson D, Healey D. Simultaneous fracture of every cervical vertebra: a case study. *Spine (Phila Pa 1976).* 2002;27(20):E446–E450.
42. Vargas-Mena R, Dufoo-Olvera M, García-López OF, et al. Multiple cervical spine fractures. Case report. *Acta Ortop Mex.* 2014;28(5):315–318.
43. Tannoury T, Zmurko M, Tannoury CH, Anderson G, Chan D. Multiple unstable cervical fractures with cord compromise treated nonoperatively. A case report. *Spine.* 2006;28(11):E234–238.
44. Vaccaro AR, An HS, Lin S, et al. Noncontiguous injuries of the spine. *J Spinal Disord.* 1992;5:320–329.
45. Gleizes V, Jacquot FP, Signoret F, Feron JM. Combined injuries in the upper cervical spine: clinical and epidemiological data over a 14-year period. *Eur Spine J.* 2000;9(5):386–392.
46. Iencean SM. Double noncontiguous cervical spinal injuries. *Acta Neurochir (Wien).* 2002;144:695–701.
47. Gregorius FK, Estrin T, Crandall PH. Cervical spondylotic radiculopathy and myelopathy:along-termfollow-upstudy. *ArchNeurol.* 1976;33:618–625.
48. Emery SE. Cervical spondylotic myelopathy: diagnosis and treatment. *J Am Acad Orthop Surg.* 2001;9:376–388.
49. Riley 3rd LH, Skolasky RL, Albert TJ, et al. Dysphagia after anterior cervical decompression and fusion: prevalence and risk factors from a longitudinal cohort study. *Spine.* 2005;30:2564–2569.
50. Xu R, Bydon M, Macki M, et al. Adjacent segment disease after anterior cervical discectomy and fusion: clinical outcomes after first repeat surgery versus second repeat surgery. *Spine.* 2014;39:120–126.
51. Fukui M, et al. Japanese Orthopaedic Association Cervical Myelopathy Evaluation Questionnaire: part 3. Determination of reliability. *J Orthop Sci.* 2007;12:321–326.
52. Nurick S. The pathogenesis of the spinal cord disorder associated with cervical spondylosis. *Brain J Neurol.* 1972;95:87–100.
53. Boden SD, McCowin PR, Davis DO, Dina TS, Mark AS, Wiesel S. Abnormal magnetic-resonance scans of the cervical spine in asymptomatic subjects. A prospective investigation. *J Bone Joint Surg Am.* 1990;72:1178–1184.
54. Wilson JR, Barry S, Fischer DJ, et al. Frequency, timing, and predictors of neurological dysfunction in the nonmyelopathic patient with cervical spinal cord compression, canal stenosis, and/or ossification of the posterior longitudinal ligament. *Spine (Phila Pa 1976).* 2013;38(22 Suppl 1):S37–S54.
55. Law MD, Bernhardt M, White AA. Cervical spondylotic myelopathy: a review of surgical indications and decision making. *Yale J Biol Med.* 1993;66:165–177.
56. Nakashima H, Yukawa Y, Suda K, Yamagata M, Ueta T, Kato F. Abnormal findings on magnetic resonance images of the cervical spines in 1,211 asymptomatic subjects. *Spine (Phila Pa 1976).* 2015;40:392–398.
57. Nakashima H, Tetreault LA, Nagoshi N, Nouri A, Kopjar B, Arnold PM, et al. Does age affect surgical outcomes in patients with degenerative cervical myelopathy? Results from the prospective multicenter AOSpine International study on 479 patients. *J Neurol Neurosurg Psychiatry.* 2016;87(7):734–740.
58. Madhavan K, Chieng LO, Foong H, Wang MY. Surgical outcomes of elderly patients with cervical spondylotic myelopathy: a meta-analysis of studies reporting on 2868 patients. *Neurosurg Focus.* 2016;40(6):E13.
59. JO Jasmin, Schiff D.*Chapter 26 - Metastatic disease and the nervous system. In: Aminoff's Neurology and General Medicine.* 5th Edition. Academic Press; 2014:539–562.

60. Fox S, Spiess M, Hnenny L, Fourney DR. Spinal Instability Neoplastic Score (SINS): Reliability among spine fellows and resident physicians in orthopedic surgery and neurosurgery. *Global Spine J.* 2017;7(8):744–748.
61. Byrne TN. Spinal cord compression from epidural metastases. *N Engl J Med.* 1992;327(9):614–619.
62. Nelson KA, Walsh D, Abdullah O, et al. Common complications of advanced cancer. *Semin Oncol.* 2000;27(1):34–44.
63. Bucholtz JD. Metastatic epidural spinal cord compression. *Semin Oncol Nurs.* 1999;15(3):150–159.
64. McLinton A, Hutchison C. Malignant spinal cord compression: a retrospective audit of clinical practice at a UK regional cancer centre. *Br J Cancer.* 2006;94(4):486–491.
65. Quraishi NA, Ramoutar D, Sureshkumar D, et al. Metastatic spinal cord compression as a result of the unknown primary tumour. *Eur Spine J.* 2014;23(7):1502–1507.
66. Furstenberg CH, Wiedenhofer B, Gerner HJ, Putz C. The effect of early surgical treatment on recovery in patients with metastatic compression of the spinal cord. *J Bone Jt Surg Br.* 2009;91(2):240–244.
67. Chaichana KL, Woodworth GF, Sciubba DM, et al. Predictors of ambulatory function after decompressive surgery for metastatic epidural spinal cord compression. *Neurosurgery.* 2008;62(3):683–692. (discussion 683-692).
68. Bourassa-Moreau É, Versteeg A, Moskven E, et al. Sarcopenia, but not frailty, predicts early mortality and adverse events after emergent surgery for metastatic disease of the spine. *Spine J.* 2020;20(1):22–31.
69. Falicov A, Fisher CG, Sparkes J, et al. Impact of surgical intervention on quality of life in patients with spinal metastases. *Spine.* 2006;31:2849–2856.
70. Furlan JC, Chan KK, Sandoval GA, et al. The combined use of surgery and radiotherapy to treat patients with epidural cord compression due to metastatic disease: a cost-utility analysis. *Neuro Oncol.* 2012;14:631–640.
71. Thomas KC, Nosyk B, Fisher CG, et al. Cost-effectiveness of surgery plus radiotherapy versus radiotherapy alone for metastatic epidural spinal cord compression. *Int J Radiat Oncol Biol Phys.* 2006;66:1212–1218.
72. Tibbs MK. Wound healing following radiation therapy: a review. *Radiother Oncol.* 1997;42:99–106.
73. Payne WG, Naidu DK, Wheeler CK, et al. Wound healing in patients with cancer. *Eplasty.* 2008;8:e9.
74. Itshayek E, Yamada J, Bilsky M, et al. Timing of surgery and radiotherapy in the management of metastatic spine disease: a systematic review. *Int J Oncol.* 2010;36(3):533–544.

10

General Complications of Cervical Spine Surgery

PAUL D. MINETOS, RICK SASSO, AND MICHAEL H. MCCARTHY

CHAPTER OUTLINE

Preoperative Considerations

Prior to surgical intervention, a thorough multidisciplinary preoperative medical evaluation of the patient is imperative, as failure of preoperative medical optimization may contribute to negative outcomes. Comorbidities such as cardiovascular, pulmonary, and rheumatologic disorders can have a significant impact on preoperative decision making and risk assessment. Pulmonary circulation disorders are associated with an almost sevenfold increase in perioperative morbidity and 12-fold increase in mortality among patients undergoing surgery for cervical spondylotic myelopathy.[1] Coagulopathy (approximately 2× increase in morbidity and a 5× increase in mortality) and congestive heart failure (approximately 2× and 5×, respectively) are other factors to consider when determining patient candidacy for surgery.[1] Additionally, electrolyte imbalance has been found to be a significant predictor of major morbidity and mortality in patients undergoing cervical spine fusion.[1,2] Hyponatremia, considered to be preoperative serum sodium levels <135 mEq/L, increases risk of mortality, major morbidity, and prolonged hospitalization by 1.36×, 1.24×, and 1.13×, respectively.[2]

One major factor to consider when monitoring for potential sources of complications is positioning. While the anterior approach to the cervical spine allows for supine patient positioning, the prone position necessitated for posterior access has been associated with various complications. One complication of posterior spine surgery in the prone position is lateral femoral cutaneous nerve palsy, occurring in as many as 20% of patients.[3] Visual impairment is a known complication with general anesthesia and prone positioning and typically associated with prolonged surgical times, hypotension, and hypoxia that may lead to optic neuropathies. Other complications resulting from malpositioning include brachial plexopathy and injury to distal elements of the upper extremity, as well as pressure injury to the tongue, eyes, ears, and breasts.[4–8]

Complications may arise from the prone position even with anatomic patient positioning. For example, patients older than 70 years of age who are prone during cervical spine surgery develop hypertension and abnormal ECG and echocardiography findings more frequently than supine patients, even without prior cardiac risk factors.[9] Patients who are aged 70 years or older should therefore undergo cardiac assessment with ECG and echocardiography prior to elective posterior cervical spine surgery. Additionally, abdominal complications such as incarcerated bowel, while rare, have been reported among patients with a history of previous abdominal surgery undergoing lumbar spinal surgery in the prone position.[10] Care should be taken to determine patient candidacy and, if warranted, general surgery consultation obtained in patients with prior abdominal surgery before proceeding with posterior cervical spinal surgery.

Intraoperative Complications

Several important structures must be recognized when approaching the cervical spine. Anteriorly, the carotid sheath is one of the first major anatomic structures that should be avoided. While injury to the carotid artery, jugular vein, and vagus nerve could potentially result in catastrophic outcomes, carotid artery injury is extremely rare, occurring in less than 1 every 17,625 patients.[11]

Additionally, although vessel retraction can cause a decrease in cross-sectional area of the carotid artery of up to 70%, flow remains laminar and returns to baseline in the recovery room.[12]

Consideration should be taken to protect the esophagus during anterior cervical spine surgery as well. Almost one-fifth of esophageal injuries are intraoperative and are due to retraction or operative tools.[13] Previous history of anterior neck surgery, radiation to the neck, and extensive tobacco use have been found to increase the possibility of esophageal perforation.[13] Spontaneous healing of the esophagus is unlikely, and perforation can lead to issues with dysphagia and bacterial seeding of hardware. Despite the intraoperative risk of injuring the esophagus, a plurality of esophageal perforations following anterior cervical spine surgery occur secondary to hardware failure. The majority of all perforations are found outside the first 30 postoperative days, with average time to diagnosis approaching 2 years.[13]

Incidental durotomy is another intraoperative complication that may occur during either anterior or posterior approaches to the cervical spine. Incidental durotomy at the cervical level occurs at an overall rate of 0.6%, although this rate has been found to vary from 0.5% to 3.6%.[14–16] Dural tears occur almost twice as often when the anterior approach is used compared to the posterior approach. The most common level included in patients with dural tears is C5 followed by C6, with 92% and 87% of patients with an incidental durotomy undergoing surgery including each of these levels, respectively. Durotomy frequently occurs with dissection of tissue that adheres to the dura mater, so factors that increase the likelihood of tissue clinging to the anterior surface of the dura mater present a greater risk for dural tear. For example, ossification of the posterior longitudinal ligament is a well-known risk factor for intraoperative dural tear when approaching the cervical spine anteriorly.[17–19] Other significant risk factors for incidental durotomy at the cervical level include revision anterior surgery, corpectomy, and male gender.[20]

Dural tear is almost always managed primarily if the tear is recognized intraoperatively.[21] The exposure of the cervical spine when approached anteriorly typically precludes suture repair, and use of suture may also increase the size of the dural defect. Common initial management options include Gelfoam (Pfizer) as well as cellulose or a fibrin patch with fibrin glue.[21,22] A dural substitute or a muscular plug may also be used to repair the defect primarily.[21] While rare, repair of dural tears can lead to impingement of the thecal sac if prominent.[23] Lumbar drain placement may assist by providing cerebrospinal fluid diversion in the event that primary repair is determined to be insufficient, although risks for drain placement include deep vein thrombosis from decreased mobility, meningitis, and overdrainage leading to subdural hematoma.[19,24–28]

Iatrogenic injury to the vertebral artery is an uncommon but potentially catastrophic complication. The overall rate of vertebral artery injury is about 1.4%, although this rate varies by approach and spinal level given the anatomy of the vertebral arteries as they course superiorly.[29] The vertebral artery begins at the superior aspect of the subclavian artery and enters the C6 transverse foramen in 87% to 89% of patients.[30] At the level of C7, the vertebral artery lies approximately 17 mm anterior to the posterior cortex of the vertebral body and 17.5 mm lateral to midline, which places it at risk with lateral mass screws at the C7 level.[31] Lateral mass screws, however, have been shown to have a significantly smaller association with vertebral artery injury compared to pedicle screws, although injury resulting from either technique remains rare.[32] The anterior approach to the subaxial cervical spine has been found to place the vertebral arteries at the least risk of injury, with a rate of 0.3% to 0.5%.[33,34] The greatest risk of injury, at a rate of 4% to 8%, involves a posterior approach to the upper cervical spine with instrumentation.[35,36]

In the event of vertebral artery injury, the first step involves temporarily controlling hemorrhage, typically with digital pressure.[37] Large hemostatic agents such as oxidized cellulose may also assist with immediate control. Smaller particulate hemostatic agents, such as hemostatic gel or bone wax, have a risk of embolization and should be avoided. Prompt communication with the anesthesia team as well as a vascular surgery consultation are imperative, and intravenous access, if not already present, should be obtained for aggressive fluid resuscitation. Once immediate tamponade is achieved, tissue surrounding the artery should be dissected to identify the proximal and distal ends of the injured vessel. Temporary aneurysm clips may be applied to either end to assist with hemorrhagic control during primary repair or end-to-end anastomosis of the artery, typically with 8-0 Prolene (Ethicon, Somerville, NJ). It is important to keep the cervical spine in neutral rotation throughout the repair process, as axial rotation of the cervical spine significantly decreases vertebral artery perfusion.[38] Retrograde flow from the distal end of the artery indicates intact contralateral circulation; poor flow may indicate the need for bypass to avoid neurologic morbidity.[39,40] Vascular bypass can be performed if primary repair is determined to provide insufficient flow.[41] Finally, sacrifice of the artery is associated with suboptimal results and should only be performed in the absence of other suitable options. Following surgery, CT angiography should be performed to further characterize the extent of injury, determine patency of surgical repair, and to assess collateral circulation to the brain.[40]

Postoperative Complications

Neurologic Complications

Spinal Cord Injury

Iatrogenic injury to the spinal cord is a rare but devastating complication of surgery to the cervical spine. Overall, iatrogenic spinal cord injury (SCI) occurs at a rate of up to 0.24% of patients undergoing cervical spine surgery, although a variety of factors may impact the likelihood of SCI.[42] For example, as many as 13.5% of patients with cervical kyphotic deformity have neurologic complications, most often with dorsal osteotomy at the cervicothoracic junction.[43] Foraminotomy or single-level anterior cervical discectomy and fusion (ACDF), however, would be expected to have a lower rate of iatrogenic SCI. In fact, only 14% of all iatrogenic SCI at any level of the spine occur secondary to cervical degenerative disease.[44] If a postoperative SCI is detected, a cause should first be determined. Advanced imaging, including CT and/or MRI, should be obtained emergently to further characterize the injury, and the patient should return to the operating suite as soon as possible if a compressive pathology is found to be the source of injury. Subsequent management should focus on maintaining cord perfusion. Mean arterial pressure greater than 85 mmHg may be kept for as long as 7 days postoperatively and has been shown to improve motor function and bladder and bowel recovery after traumatic SCI.[45] Corticosteroid use has been shown to lack significant long-term benefit among patients with acute spinal cord injury and should be avoided.[42,46]

The role of intraoperative neuromonitoring to prevent neurologic complication is well defined for use in spinal deformity correction, although the role of neuromonitoring in routine cervical spine surgery is less clear.[47–50] While monitoring somatosensory- and motor-evoked potentials may clue the surgeon into immediate changes in neurologic status, the use of intraoperative neuromonitoring for surgical intervention at the cervical spine has been associated with increased time and healthcare costs, and patients undergoing ACDF without neuromonitoring do not have a higher rate of postoperative neurologic complication.[51,52] As such the utility of intraoperative neuromonitoring likely depends on the severity of spinal disease and is ultimately up to surgeon discretion.

Recurrent Laryngeal Nerve Palsy

The recurrent laryngeal nerve (RLN) is a unique anatomic structure that must be carefully avoided with anterior cervical spine surgery. Both the right and left RLN begin as branches off of the respective vagus nerves (CN X), traveling inferiorly next to the external carotid vasculature. On the right, the vagus nerve then tracks posterior to the right lung and gives off the right RLN, which traverses around the right subclavian artery and ascends superiorly in a lateral to medial manner. In contrast, the left RLN branches off of the left vagus nerve at the level of the aortic arch, looping inferior to the arch and then superiorly. Both nerves then ascend between the trachea and esophagus, innervating the intrinsic musculature of the larynx.[53]

Unilateral or bilateral injury to the RLN may result in dysphonia, dysphagia, or aspiration, and may occur secondary to direct ligation, traction injury, or entrapment between the endotracheal tube cuff and retractor blades.[54–58] Postoperative incidence of RLN palsy ranges from 0.6% to 2.9%, although the rate of vocal cord paralysis may be as high as 24% in the immediate postoperative period.[54,59] Among ACDF patients with RLN palsy, as many as 74% to 80% recover fully by the 12-month postoperative mark, with about 16% resolving with residual effects.[54,55] Because of the unique pathway that each RLN traverses, a left-sided approach to the anterior cervical spine provides a theoretical advantage of avoiding the RLN. While some studies have shown as much as half of the rate of postoperative RLN palsy when the spine is approached from the patient's left, others have failed to recreate these findings.[54,55,58,60,61] An additional consideration is the dominant hand of the surgeon, with an approach on the right side of the patient affording the right-handed surgeon a potentially easier approach technically. Regardless of initial approach, reoperation should occur on the ipsilateral side of the index procedure or the patient should be evaluated by ENT to assess vocal cord function. Reoperation has been associated with a significantly higher incidence of RLN palsy, and damage to the bilateral RLN may leave the patient without intrinsic laryngeal muscular innervation.[59,61,62]

C5 Palsy

C5 palsy may occur because of either anterior or posterior cervical spine surgery. Overall rates of C5 palsy vary drastically with surgical approach, disease, and definition of C5 palsy. While typically accepted as a decrease in one grade of deltoid and/or biceps muscle strength without associated myelopathic deterioration compared to preoperative function, other definitions include somatosensory disturbance or an overall deltoid and/or biceps score of 3 out of 5 following operative intervention.[63–68] Although the pathogenesis of C5 palsy is unclear, it may be related to inadvertent injury to the nerve root, traction on the nerve root via cord shift and "tethering" following decompression, ischemia secondary to decreased radicular artery perfusion, or reperfusion injury.[63] Regardless of etiology, factors that increase risk of developing C5 palsy include ossification of the posterior longitudinal ligament (OPLL) and spondylotic myelopathy. Patients with OPLL have a significantly greater risk of developing C5 palsy compared to spondylotic myelopathy, with as much as a 9× increased risk, while patients with spondylotic myelopathy develop C5 palsy at a greater rate than patients with radiculopathy from degenerative disease.[63,66,69–73] Additionally, the rate of C5 palsy is approximately 2-3× higher with a posterior approach, with a rate as high as 11% in posterior laminectomy and fusion patients and as high as 3% among ACDF patients.[72–74] Prophylactic foraminotomy has been theorized to prevent palsy although results are debatable, with potential for causing a palsy at the C5 level via iatrogenic injury, and most patients resolve by 6 months with conservative therapy.[63,64,66,75]

Horner Syndrome

Horner syndrome is an additional risk of anterior cervical spinal surgery, although this occurrence is rare, occurring in 0.06% of patients.[76] Injury to the sympathetic trunk, resulting in ptosis, miosis, and anhidrosis, occurs most commonly at the C5 and C6 levels. A midline surgical trajectory as well as subperiosteal retractor placement to avoid direct retraction of the longus colli muscle may help avoid iatrogenic injury to the sympathetic trunk. Most patients experience at least partial recovery without additional intervention.[76,77]

Gastrointestinal Complications

Dysphagia is the most common postoperative complication following anterior cervical spine surgery, with an incidence as high as 71% in the first 2 weeks of surgery.[78] The incidence of dysphagia decreases over time, with as many as 12.5% of patients having symptoms at 12 months postoperatively, and only about 5% complaining of moderate to severe symptoms at 6 months postoperatively.[79] Female gender and multiple surgical levels have been identified as risk factors for dysphagia, while the role of age, implant type, and operative levels are unclear.[78,80–83] Additionally, use of bone morphogenic protein has been associated with postoperative dysphagia in patients undergoing ACDF, which may be related to a higher rate of heterotopic ossification.[84] Preoperative tracheal and esophageal traction exercise, perioperative methylprednisolone, endotracheal tube cuff pressure monitoring, and the use of a low profile plate may decrease postoperative dysphagia rates.[85–89] Dysphagia is also less common in patients undergoing disc arthroplasty compared to ACDF with instrumentation.[90] Given the decrease in incidence over time and relatively benign nature of dysphagia, management is typically expectant with diet modification unless symptoms are persistent and severe.[91]

As previously mentioned, most esophageal perforations occur postoperatively, with a time to diagnosis of greater than 30 days in approximately 68% of perforations, and an average time to diagnosis of just over 1.5 years.[13] The most common etiology of perforation is a slow, erosive process related to hardware failure, which accounts for 41% of perforations, as well as prominent anterior instrumentation. Patients may report a history of multiple symptoms, with the most common being dysphagia or odynophagia, fever, neck swelling, and leakage from the neck wound. Complications from esophageal perforation typically involve bacterial contamination from the gastrointestinal tract, leading to pneumonia, mediastinitis, osteomyelitis, and sepsis. Diagnosis of perforation can be confirmed on Gastrografin swallow study, which is preferred over barium if perforation is suspected, and repair often involves sternocleidomastoid or other muscular flap. Secondary complications occur in just over 1 in 10 cases of esophageal repair, with average time to oral intake occurring at approximately 1 month.[13] Given the substantial risk of infectious sequelae, broad-spectrum antibiotics with anaerobic and gastrointestinal microbial coverage is imperative.

Hematoma and Infection

Hematoma may form in any invasive procedure involving the cervical spine and can form from direct arterial injury, such as to the superior thyroid artery during the anterior approach; inadequate hemostasis; increased blood pressure following anesthesia emergence; elevated venous pressure due to Valsalva after extubation and subsequent coughing; or coagulopathy.[92,93] The incidence of hematoma following an anterior approach is just under 1%, although this estimate may underrepresent the true incidence due to asymptomatic cases of hematoma formation.[94–97] Hematoma may form in any plane of the surgical approach, including at the epidural or retropharyngeal spaces, with sequelae depending on location. Epidural hematoma, typically resulting in neurologic compromise, occurs in approximately 1 in 1000 cervical spine procedures, although it may occur in up to 1.5% of patients undergoing posterior cervical spine surgery.[98,99] Anterior hematoma formation is particularly concerning because of its propensity to compromise the patient's airway. Retropharyngeal hematoma may cause loss of airway patency by directly compressing the trachea, although high extrinsic pressures are required to directly compress the cartilaginous trachea. A more likely etiology involves edema secondary to venous occlusion, resulting in swelling of supraglottic structures such as the epiglottis and arytenoids.[100]

Diagnosis of symptomatic hematoma is typically clinical.[101] In cases where the patient's airway is not compromised, prompt return to the operating suite for hematoma evacuation and hemostasis is warranted. A tracheostomy tray should be available in the event of rapid deterioration of the patient's airway status. If hematoma is accompanied by critical decline in respiratory status, the emergency response system should first be activated. A non-rebreather face mask administering 100% oxygen should be placed, followed by awake intubation and subsequent transfer to the operating suite for evacuation. In the event that immediate ventilation is unsatisfactory, the surgical wound should be opened emergently, and the hematoma evacuated, followed by repeat intubation attempt. Cricothyroidotomy should be performed if multiple attempts at establishing an airway fail.[101]

Overall rates of surgical site infection (SSI) range from 1% to 7%, although posterior infection rates exceed anterior rates, with an incidence as high as 18%.[102–108] Surgery at the level of the cervical spine, however, carries a decreased risk of infection compared to other locations.[109] Independent predictors of SSI include body mass index exceeding 35 kg/m^2, chronic steroid use, increased operative time, trauma, SCI, and thickness of subcutaneous fat.[105,108,110] Prevention of SSI involves optimizing patient nutritional status, smoking cessation, as well as common perioperative measures such as meticulous aseptic technique and prophylactic antibiotic administration prior to incision.[111,112] When SSI does occur, diagnosis includes a combination of clinical status, laboratory measures, and imaging. Patients with acute infection may present with constitutional symptoms such has fever, hypotension, and altered mental status, whereas chronic infections may lack these red flag symptoms. Laboratory tests should include white blood cell count, C-reactive protein, and erythrocyte sedimentation rate.[113] Wound cultures should be obtained when possible, especially when a return to the operating suite is warranted. Imaging should include plain film radiographs for macroscopic assessment of the spine and any implanted hardware. MRI with gadolinium enhancement provides the best view for determining marrow signal changes, rim-enhancing lesions, and fluid collection although MRI may be obscured by hardware. CT may also characterize bony destruction or implant loosening. Management depends on the acuity of the infection, but may involve any combination of acute and/or chronic culture-directed antibiotic administration, irrigation and debridement, and revision surgery.[114]

Mechanical Complications

Structural and mechanical complications involving the cervical spine may present regardless of approach. Mechanical measurements of the cervical spine, including segmental and global lordosis, sagittal vertical axis, and T1 slope, may be obtained with anteroposterior (AP), lateral, and lateral flexion/extension plain views, whereas advanced imaging is preferred for assessment of bony fusion.[115–117] Radiographic complications and their risk factors depend on several patient factors as well as the procedure performed. Common complications include pseudarthrosis, adjacent segment disease, and complications related to graft or hardware such as failure or subsidence. An important consideration when assessing structural complications involves determining whether clinical symptoms are present when radiographic evidence of pathology is apparent. For example, pseudarthrosis at the cervical spine is an undesirable complication, although radiographic evidence may not necessarily correlate with clinical outcomes and patient satisfaction.[84,118] Additionally, preoperative radiographic parameters within the native spine do not necessarily correlate with postoperative clinical outcomes, although they may guide treatment and help the surgeon anticipate potential complications.[119–122] As such, clinical findings should be confirmed prior to initiating additional treatment or revision.

Conclusion

Complications related to cervical spine surgery may be related to several modifiable or nonmodifiable factors and can present intraoperatively or postoperatively. A thorough medical evaluation involving a multidisciplinary team is imperative to risk-stratify patients and to anticipate potential negative outcomes. Anatomic structures should be recognized and carefully protected during intervention. The patient should be monitored in the immediate postoperative setting to ensure airway status, with prompt intervention in the event of respiratory decline. Postoperative care should include evaluation for neurologic, gastrointestinal, and infectious complications. Finally, structural and mechanical complications should be identified radiographically and addressed appropriately.

References

1. David Kaye I, Marascalchi BJ, Macagno AE, Lafage VA, Bendo JA, Passias PG. Predictors of morbidity and mortality among patients with cervical spondylotic myelopathy treated surgically. *Eur Spine J.* 2015;24(12):2910–2917. https://doi.org/10.1007/s00586-015-4010-2.
2. Pennington Z, Bomberger TT, Lubelski D, Benzel EC, Steinmetz MP, Mroz TE. Preoperative hyponatremia and perioperative complications in cervical spinal fusion. *World Neurosurg.* 2020;141:e864–e872. https://doi.org/10.1016/j.wneu.2020.06.068.
3. Mirovsky Y, Neuwirth M. Injuries to the lateral femoral cutaneous nerve during spine surgery. *Spine.* 2000;25(10):1266–1269. https://doi.org/10.1097/00007632-200005150-00011.
4. Goettler CE, Pryor JP, Reilly PM. Brachial plexopathy after prone positioning. *Crit Care Lond Engl.* 2002;6(6):540–542. https://doi.org/10.1186/cc1823.
5. Stevens WR, Glazer PA, Kelley SD, Lietman TM, Bradford DS. Ophthalmic complications after spinal surgery. *Spine.* 1997;22(12):1319–1324. https://doi.org/10.1097/00007632-199706150-00008.
6. Cheng MA, Todorov A, Tempelhoff R, McHugh T, Crowder CM, Lauryssen C. The effect of prone positioning on intraocular pressure in anesthetized patients. *Anesthesiology.* 2001;95(6):1351–1355. https://doi.org/10.1097/00000542-200112000-00012.
7. Burdet L, Liaudet L, Schaller MD, Broccard AF. Bilateral breast necrosis after prone position ventilation. *Intensive Care Med.* 2001;27(8):1435. https://doi.org/10.1007/s001340100990.
8. Sinha A, Agarwal A, Gaur A, Pandey CK. Oropharyngeal swelling and macroglossia after cervical spine surgery in the prone position. *J Neurosurg Anesthesiol.* 2001;13(3):237–239. https://doi.org/10.1097/00008506-200107000-00010.
9. Kumagai G, Takeuchi K, Aburakawa S, et al. Perioperative cardiopulmonary complications after cervical spine surgery in the prone position: the relationship between age and preoperative testing. *Arch Orthop Trauma Surg.* 2011;131(7):911–916. https://doi.org/10.1007/s00402-010-1234-9.
10. Shih P, Slimack NP, Roy A, Fessler RG, Koski TR. Abdominal complications following posterior spinal fusion in patients with previous abdominal surgeries. *Neurosurg Focus.* 2011;31(4):E16. https://doi.org/10.3171/2011.8.FOCUS11132.
11. Härtl R, Alimi M, Abdelatif Boukebir M, et al. Carotid artery injury in anterior cervical spine surgery: Multicenter cohort study and literature review. *Global Spine J.* 2017;7(1 Suppl):71S–75S. https://doi.org/10.1177/2192568216688192.
12. Pollard ME, Little PW. Changes in carotid artery blood flow during anterior cervical. *spine surgery. Spine.* 2002;27(2):152–155. https://doi.org/10.1097/00007632-200201150-00006.
13. Halani SH, Baum GR, Riley JP, et al. Esophageal perforation after anterior cervical spine surgery: a systematic review of the

literature. *J Neurosurg Spine*. 2016;25(3):285–291. https://doi.org/10.3171/2016.1.SPINE15898.

14. O'Neill KR, Fehlings MG, Mroz TE, et al. A multicenter study of the presentation, treatment, and outcomes of cervical dural tears. *Global Spine J*. 2017;7(1 Suppl):58S–63S. https://doi.org/10.1177/2192568216688186.
15. O'Neill KR, Neuman BJ, Peters C, Riew KD. Risk factors for dural tears in the cervical spine. *Spine*. 2014;39(17):E1015–1020. https://doi.org/10.1097/BRS.0000000000000416.
16. Bertalanffy H, Eggert HR. Complications of anterior cervical discectomy without fusion in 450 consecutive patients. *Acta Neurochir (Wien)*. 1989;99(1-2):41–50. https://doi.org/10.1007/BF01407775.
17. Lei T, Shen Y, Wang L-F, Cao J-M, Ding W-Y, Ma Q-H. Cerebrospinal fluid leakage during anterior approach cervical spine surgery for severe ossification of the posterior longitudinal ligament: Prevention and treatment. *Orthop Surg*. 2012;4(4):247–252. https://doi.org/10.1111/os.12007.
18. Epstein N. Anterior approaches to cervical spondylosis and ossification of the posterior longitudinal ligament: review of operative technique and assessment of 65 multilevel circumferential procedures. *Surg Neurol*. 2001;55(6):313–324. https://doi.org/10.1016/S0090-3019(01)00464-5.
19. Elder BD, Theodros D, Sankey EW, et al. Management of cerebrospinal fluid leakage during anterior cervical discectomy and fusion and its effect on spinal fusion. *World Neurosurg*. 2016;89:636–640. https://doi.org/10.1016/j.wneu.2015.11.033.
20. Hannallah D, Lee J, Khan M, Donaldson WF, Kang JD. Cerebrospinal fluid leaks following cervical spine surgery. *J Bone Joint Surg Am*. 2008;90(5):1101–1105. https://doi.org/10.2106/JBJS.F.01114.
21. Syre P, Bohman LE, Baltuch G, Le Roux P, Welch WC. Cerebrospinal fluid leaks and their management after anterior cervical discectomy and fusion: A report of 13 cases and a review of the literature. *Spine*. 2014;39(16):E936. https://doi.org/10.1097/BRS.0000000000000404.
22. Gazzeri R, Galarza M, Callovini G. Use of tissue sealant patch (TachoSil) in the management of cerebrospinal fluid leaks after anterior cervical spine discectomy and fusion. *Br J Neurosurg*. 2021:1–8. https://doi.org/10.1080/02688697.2021.1881444.
23. Thavarajah D, De Lacy P, Hussain R, Redfern RM. Postoperative cervical cord compression induced by hydrogel (DuraSeal): A possible complication. *Spine*. 2010;35(1):E25. https://doi.org/10.1097/BRS.0b013e3181b9fc45.
24. Kitchel SH, Eismont FJ, Green BA. Closed subarachnoid drainage for management of cerebrospinal fluid leakage after an operation on the spine. *J Bone Joint Surg Am*. 1989;71(7):984–987.
25. Macdonald RL, Fehlings MG, Tator CH, et al. Multilevel anterior cervical corpectomy and fibular allograft fusion for cervical myelopathy. *J Neurosurg*. 1997;86(6):990–997. https://doi.org/10.3171/jns.1997.86.6.0990.
26. Min JH, Jang JS, Lee SH. Clinical results of ossification of the posterior longitudinal ligament (OPLL) of the thoracic spine treated by anterior decompression. *Clin Spine Surg*. 2008;21(2):116–119. https://doi.org/10.1097/BSD.0b013e318060091a.
27. Mazur M, Jost GF, Schmidt MH, Bisson EF. Management of cerebrospinal fluid leaks after anterior decompression for ossification of the posterior longitudinal ligament: a review of the literature. *Neurosurg Focus*. 2011;30(3):E13. https://doi.org/10.3171/2010.12.FOCUS10255.
28. Weill-Engerer S, Meaume S, Lahlou A, et al. Risk factors for deep vein thrombosis in inpatients aged 65 and older: A case-control multicenter study. *J Am Geriatr Soc*. 2004;52(8):1299–1304. https://doi.org/10.1111/j.1532-5415.2004.52359.x.
29. Rampersaud YR, Moro ERP, Neary MA, et al. Intraoperative adverse events and related postoperative complications in spine surgery: Implications for enhancing patient safety founded on evidence-based protocols. *Spine*. 2006;31(13):1503–1510. https://doi.org/10.1097/01.brs.0000220652.39970.c2.
30. Argenson G, Sylla S, Dintimille H, Papasion S, DiMarino V. The vertebral arteries (segments V1 and V2). *Anat Clin*. 1980;2:29–41.
31. Xu R, Ebraheim NA, Tang G, Stanescu S. Location of the vertebral artery in the cervicothoracic junction. *Am J Orthop Belle Mead NJ*. 2000;29(6):453–456.
32. Yoshihara H, Passias PG, Errico TJ. Screw-related complications in the subaxial cervical spine with the use of lateral mass versus cervical pedicle screws: A systematic review. *J Neurosurg Spine*. 2013;19(5):614–623. https://doi.org/10.3171/2013.8.SPINE13136.
33. Smith MD, Emery SE, Dudley A, Murray KJ, Leventhal M. Vertebral artery injury during anterior decompression of the cervical spine. A retrospective review of ten patients. *J Bone Joint Surg Br*. 1993;75(3):410–415. https://doi.org/10.1302/0301-620X.75B3.8496209.
34. Burke JP, Gerszten PC, Welch WC. Iatrogenic vertebral artery injury during anterior cervical spine surgery. *Spine J Off J North Am Spine Soc*. 2005;5(5):508–514; discussion 514. https://doi.org/10.1016/j.spinee.2004.11.015.
35. Wright NM, Lauryssen C. Vertebral artery injury in C1-2 transarticular screw fixation: results of a survey of the AANS/CNS section on disorders of the spine and peripheral nerves. American Association of Neurological Surgeons/Congress of Neurological Surgeons. *J Neurosurg*. 1998;88(4):634–640. https://doi.org/10.3171/jns.1998.88.4.0634.
36. Madawi AA, Casey AT, Solanki GA, Tuite G, Veres R, Crockard HA. Radiological and anatomical evaluation of the atlantoaxial transarticular screw fixation technique. *J Neurosurg*. 1997;86(6):961–968. https://doi.org/10.3171/jns.1997.86.6.0961.
37. Golfinos JG, Dickman CA, Zabramski JM, Sonntag VKH, Spetzler RF. Repair of vertebral artery injury during anterior cervical decompression. *Spine*. 1994;19(22):2552–2556.
38. Mitchell JA. Changes in vertebral artery blood flow following normal rotation of the cervical spine. *J Manipulative Physiol Ther*. 2003;26(6):347–351. https://doi.org/10.1016/S0161-4754(03)00074-5.
39. Peng CW, Chou BT, Bendo JA, Spivak JM. Vertebral artery injury in cervical spine surgery: anatomical considerations, management, and preventive measures. *Spine J*. 2009;9(1):70–76. https://doi.org/10.1016/j.spinee.2008.03.006.
40. An TY, Kang DH, Kim DH. Anastomosis and endovascular treatment of iatrogenic vertebral artery injury. *Korean J Neurotrauma*. 2021;17(2):204–211. https://doi.org/10.13004/kjnt.2021.17.e28.
41. Devin CJ, Kang JD. Vertebral artery injury in cervical spine surgery. *Instr Course Lect*. 2009;58:717–728.
42. Daniels AH, Hart RA, Hilibrand AS, et al. Iatrogenic spinal cord injury resulting from cervical spine surgery. *Glob Spine J*. 2017;7(1 Suppl):84S–90S. https://doi.org/10.1177/2192568216688188.

43. Etame AB, Wang AC, Than KD, Marca FL, Park P. Outcomes after surgery for cervical spine deformity: review of the literature. *Neurosurg Focus.* 2010;28(3):E14. https://doi.org/10.3171/2010.1.FOCUS09278.
44. Montalva-Iborra A, Alcanyis-Alberola M, Grao-Castellote C, Torralba-Collados F, Giner-Pascual M. Risk factors in iatrogenic spinal cord injury. *Spinal Cord.* 2017;55(9):818–822. https://doi.org/10.1038/sc.2017.21.
45. Vale FL, Burns J, Jackson AB, Hadley MN. Combined medical and surgical treatment after acute spinal cord injury: results of a prospective pilot study to assess the merits of aggressive medical resuscitation and blood pressure management. *J Neurosurg.* 1997;87(2):239–246. https://doi.org/10.3171/jns.1997.87.2.0239.
46. Evaniew N, Belley-Côté EP, Fallah N, Noonan VK, Rivers CS, Dvorak MF. Methylprednisolone for the treatment of patients with acute spinal cord injuries: A systematic review and meta-analysis. *J Neurotrauma.* 2016;33(5):468–481. https://doi.org/10.1089/neu.2015.4192.
47. Ziewacz JE, Berven SH, Mummaneni VP, et al. The design, development, and implementation of a checklist for intraoperative neuromonitoring changes. *Neurosurg Focus.* 2012;33(5):E11. https://doi.org/10.3171/2012.9.FOCUS12263.
48. Vitale MG, Skaggs DL, Pace GI, et al. Best practices in intraoperative neuromonitoring in spine deformity surgery: Development of an intraoperative checklist to optimize response. *Spine Deform.* 2014;2(5):333–339. https://doi.org/10.1016/j.jspd.2014.05.003.
49. Vitale MG, Moore DW, Matsumoto H, et al. Risk factors for spinal cord injury during surgery for spinal deformity. *J Bone Joint Surg Am.* 2010;92(1):64–71. https://doi.org/10.2106/JBJS.H.01839.
50. Feng B, Qiu G, Shen J, et al. Impact of multimodal intraoperative monitoring during surgery for spine deformity and potential risk factors for neurological monitoring changes. *Clin Spine Surg.* 2012;25(4):E108. https://doi.org/10.1097/BSD.0b013e31824d2a2f.
51. Ajiboye RM, D'Oro A, Ashana AO, et al. Routine use of intraoperative neuromonitoring during ACDFs for the treatment of spondylotic myelopathy and radiculopathy is questionable. *Spine.* 2017;42(1):14–19. https://doi.org/10.1097/BRS.0000000000001662.
52. Traynelis VC, Abode-Iyamah KO, Leick KM, Bender SM, Greenlee JDW. Cervical decompression and reconstruction without intraoperative neurophysiological monitoring. *J Neurosurg Spine.* 2012;16(2):107–113. https://doi.org/10.3171/2011.10.SPINE11199.
53. Allen E, Minutello K, Murcek BW. Anatomy, head and neck, larynx recurrent laryngeal nerve. In: StatPearls. StatPearls Publishing; 2022. Accessed June 27, 2022. http://www.ncbi.nlm.nih.gov/books/NBK470179/
54. Gokaslan ZL, Bydon M, De la Garza-Ramos R, et al. Recurrent laryngeal nerve palsy after cervical spine surgery: A multicenter AOSpine Clinical Research Network Study. *Global Spine J.* 2017;7(1 Suppl):53S–57S. https://doi.org/10.1177/2192568216687547.
55. Morpeth JF, Williams MF. Vocal fold paralysis after anterior cervical diskectomy and fusion. *Laryngoscope.* 2000;110(1):43–46. https://doi.org/10.1097/00005537-200001000-00009.
56. Bulger RF, Rejowski JE, Beatty RA. Vocal cord paralysis associated with anterior cervical fusion: considerations for prevention and treatment. *J Neurosurg.* 1985;62(5):657–661. https://doi.org/10.3171/jns.1985.62.5.0657.
57. Yamada M, Hirano M, Ohkubo H. Recurrent laryngeal nerve paralysis. A 10-year review of 564 patients. *Auris Nasus Larynx.* 1983;10(Suppl:):S1–15. https://doi.org/10.1016/s0385-8146(83)80001-7.
58. Jung A, Schramm J. How to reduce recurrent laryngeal nerve palsy in anterior cervical spine surgery: a prospective observational study. *Neurosurgery.* 2010;67(1):10–15; discussion 15. https://doi.org/10.1227/01.NEU.0000370203.26164.24.
59. Tan TP, Govindarajulu AP, Massicotte EM, Venkatraghavan L. Vocal cord palsy after anterior cervical spine surgery: a qualitative systematic review. *Spine J Off J North Am Spine Soc.* 2014;14(7):1332–1342. https://doi.org/10.1016/j.spinee.2014.02.017.
60. Kilburg C, Sullivan HG, Mathiason MA. Effect of approach side during anterior cervical discectomy and fusion on the incidence of recurrent laryngeal nerve injury. *J Neurosurg Spine.* 2006;4(4):273–277. https://doi.org/10.3171/spi.2006.4.4.273.
61. Beutler WJ, Sweeney CA, Connolly PJ. Recurrent laryngeal nerve injury with anterior cervical spine surgery risk with laterality of surgical approach. *Spine.* 2001;26(12):1337–1342. https://doi.org/10.1097/00007632-200106150-00014.
62. Erwood MS, Hadley MN, Gordon AS, Carroll WR, Agee BS, Walters BC. Recurrent laryngeal nerve injury following reoperative anterior cervical discectomy and fusion: a meta-analysis. *J Neurosurg Spine.* 2016;25(2):198–204. https://doi.org/10.3171/2015.9.SPINE15187.
63. Sakaura H, Hosono N, Mukai Y, Ishii T, Yoshikawa H. C5 palsy after decompression surgery for cervical myelopathy: review of the literature. *Spine.* 2003;28(21):2447–2451. https://doi.org/10.1097/01.BRS.0000090833.96168.3F.
64. Kalisvaart MM, Nassr A, Eck JC. C5 palsy after cervical decompression procedures. *Neurosurg Q.* 2009;19(4):276–282. https://doi.org/10.1097/WNQ.0b013e3181bd47f8.
65. Currier BL. Neurological complications of cervical spine surgery: C5 palsy and intraoperative monitoring. *Spine.* 2012;37(5):E328–334. https://doi.org/10.1097/BRS.0b013e3182417276.
66. Bydon M, Macki M, Kaloostian P, et al. Incidence and prognostic factors of c5 palsy: a clinical study of 1001 cases and review of the literature. *Neurosurgery.* 2014;74(6):595–604; discussion 604–605. https://doi.org/10.1227/NEU.0000000000000322.
67. Eskander MS, Balsis SM, Balinger C, et al. The association between preoperative spinal cord rotation and postoperative C5 nerve palsy. *J Bone Joint Surg Am.* 2012;94(17):1605–1609. https://doi.org/10.2106/JBJS.K.00664.
68. Hasegawa K, Homma T, Chiba Y. Upper extremity palsy following cervical decompression surgery results from a transient spinal cord lesion. *Spine.* 2007;32(6):E197–202. https://doi.org/10.1097/01.brs.0000257576.84646.49.
69. Nakashima H, Imagama S, Yukawa Y, et al. Multivariate analysis of C-5 palsy incidence after cervical posterior fusion with instrumentation. *J Neurosurg Spine.* 2012;17(2):103–110. https://doi.org/10.3171/2012.4.SPINE11255.
70. Nakamae T, Tanaka N, Nakanishi K, et al. Investigation of segmental motor paralysis after cervical laminoplasty using intraoperative spinal cord monitoring with transcranial electric motor-evoked potentials. *J Spinal Disord Tech.* 2012;25(2):92–98. https://doi.org/10.1097/BSD.0b013e318211fc4e.

71. Wu FL, Sun Y, Pan SF, Zhang L, Liu ZJ. Risk factors associated with upper extremity palsy after expansive open-door laminoplasty for cervical myelopathy. *Spine J Off J North Am Spine Soc.* 2014;14(6):909–915. https://doi.org/10.1016/j.spinee.2013.07.445.
72. Thompson SE, Smith ZA, Hsu WK, et al. C5 palsy after cervical spine surgery: A multicenter retrospective review of 59 cases. *Global Spine J.* 2017;7(1 Suppl):64S–70S. https://doi.org/10.1177/2192568216688189.
73. Shou F, Li Z, Wang H, Yan C, Liu Q, Xiao C. Prevalence of C5 nerve root palsy after cervical decompressive surgery: a meta-analysis. *Eur Spine J.* 2015;24(12):2724–2734. https://doi.org/10.1007/s00586-015-4186-5.
74. Oh JK, Hong JT, Kang DH, et al. Epidemiology of C5 palsy after cervical spine surgery: A 21-center study. *Neurospine.* 2019;16(3):558–562. https://doi.org/10.14245/ns.1938142.071.
75. Imagama S, Matsuyama Y, Yukawa Y, et al. C5 palsy after cervical laminoplasty: a multicentre study. *J Bone Joint Surg Br.* 2010;92(3):393–400. https://doi.org/10.1302/0301-620X.92B3.22786.
76. Traynelis VC, Malone HR, Smith ZA, et al. Rare complications of cervical spine surgery: Horner's syndrome. *Global Spine J.* 2017;7(1 Suppl):103S–108S. https://doi.org/10.1177/2192568216688184.
77. Lubelski D, Pennington Z, Sciubba DM, Theodore N, Bydon A. Horner syndrome after anterior cervical discectomy and fusion: Case series and systematic review. *World Neurosurg.* 2020;133:e68–e75. https://doi.org/10.1016/j.wneu.2019.08.101.
78. Cho SK, Lu Y, Lee DH. Dysphagia following anterior cervical spinal surgery: a systematic review. *Bone Jt J.* 2013;95-B(7):868–873. https://doi.org/10.1302/0301-620X.95B7.31029.
79. Bazaz R, Lee MJ, Yoo JU. Incidence of dysphagia after anterior cervical spine surgery: a prospective study. *Spine.* 2002;27(22):2453–2458. https://doi.org/10.1097/00007632-200211150-00007.
80. Li Z, Li G, Chen C, et al. Risk factors for dysphagia after anterior cervical spine surgery. *Orthopedics.* 2018;41(1):e110–e116. https://doi.org/10.3928/01477447-20171213-04.
81. De La Garza-Ramos R, Xu R, Ramhmdani S, et al. Long-term clinical outcomes following 3- and 4-level anterior cervical discectomy and fusion. *J Neurosurg Spine.* 2016;24(6):885–891. https://doi.org/10.3171/2015.10.SPINE15795.
82. Fountas KN, Kapsalaki EZ, Nikolakakos LG, et al. Anterior cervical discectomy and fusion associated complications. *Spine.* 2007;32(21):2310–2317. https://doi.org/10.1097/BRS.0b013e318154c57e.
83. Riley LHI, Vaccaro AR, Dettori JR, Hashimoto R. Postoperative dysphagia in anterior cervical. *spine surgery. Spine.* 2010;35(9S):S76. https://doi.org/10.1097/BRS.0b013e3181d81a96.
84. Burkus JK, Dryer RF, Arnold PM, Foley KT. Clinical and radiographic outcomes in patients undergoing single-level anterior cervical arthrodesis: A prospective trial comparing allograft to a reduced dose of rhBMP-2. *Clin Spine Surg.* 2017;30(9):E1321–E1332. https://doi.org/10.1097/BSD.0000000000000409.
85. Chen Z, Wei X, Li F, et al. Tracheal traction exercise reduces the occurrence of postoperative dysphagia after anterior cervical. *spine surgery. Spine.* 2012;37(15):1292–1296. https://doi.org/10.1097/BRS.0b013e3182477f26.
86. Ratnaraj J, Todorov A, McHugh T, Cheng MA, Lauryssen C. Effects of decreasing endotracheal tube cuff pressures during neck retraction for anterior cervical spine surgery. *J Neurosurg.* 2002;97(2 Suppl):176–179. https://doi.org/10.3171/spi.2002.97.2.0176.
87. Vaidya R, Weir R, Sethi A, Meisterling S, Hakeos W, Wybo CD. Interbody fusion with allograft and rhBMP-2 leads to consistent fusion but early subsidence. *J Bone Joint Surg Br.* 2007;89(3):342–345. https://doi.org/10.1302/0301-620X.89B3.18270.
88. Pedram M, Castagnera L, Carat X, Macouillard G, Vital JM. Pharyngolaryngeal lesions in patients undergoing cervical spine surgery through the anterior approach: contribution of methylprednisolone. *Eur Spine J.* 2003;12(1):84–90. https://doi.org/10.1007/s00586-002-0495-6.
89. Lee MJ, Bazaz R, Furey CG, Yoo J. Influence of anterior cervical plate design on Dysphagia: a 2-year prospective longitudinal follow-up study. *J Spinal Disord Tech.* 2005;18(5):406–409. https://doi.org/10.1097/01.bsd.0000177211.44960.71.
90. McAfee PC, Cappuccino A, Cunningham BW, et al. Lower incidence of dysphagia with cervical arthroplasty compared with ACDF in a prospective randomized clinical trial. *J Spinal Disord Tech.* 2010;23(1):1–8. https://doi.org/10.1097/BSD.0b013e31819e2ab8.
91. Fogel GR, McDonnell MF. Surgical treatment of dysphagia after anterior cervical interbody fusion. *Spine J.* 2005;5(2):140–144. https://doi.org/10.1016/j.spinee.2004.06.022.
92. Yu NH, Jahng TA, Kim CH, Chung CK. Life-threatening late hemorrhage due to superior thyroid artery dissection after anterior cervical discectomy and fusion. *Spine.* 2010;35(15):E739–742. https://doi.org/10.1097/BRS.0b013e3181cf46b4.
93. Sethi R, Tandon MS, Ganjoo P. Neck hematoma causing acute airway and hemodynamic compromise after anterior cervical spine surgery. *J Neurosurg Anesthesiol.* 2008;20(1):69–70. https://doi.org/10.1097/ANA.0b013e318157f749.
94. Skeppholm M, Lindgren L, Henriques T, Vavruch L, Löfgren H, Olerud C. The Discover artificial disc replacement versus fusion in cervical radiculopathy--a randomized controlled outcome trial with 2-year follow-up. *Spine J Off J North Am Spine Soc.* 2015;15(6):1284–1294. https://doi.org/10.1016/j.spinee.2015.02.039.
95. Chong E, Mobbs RJ, Pelletier MH, Walsh WR. Titanium/polyetheretherketone cages for cervical arthrodesis with degenerative and traumatic pathologies: Early clinical outcomes and fusion rates. *Orthop Surg.* 2016;8(1):19–26. https://doi.org/10.1111/os.12221.
96. He S, Feng H, Lan Z, et al. A randomized trial comparing clinical outcomes between zero-profile and traditional multilevel anterior cervical discectomy and fusion surgery for cervical myelopathy. *Spine.* 2018;43(5):E259–E266. https://doi.org/10.1097/BRS.0000000000002323.
97. Bovonratwet P, Fu MC, Tyagi V, et al. Incidence, risk factors, and clinical implications of postoperative hematoma requiring reoperation following anterior cervical discectomy and fusion. *Spine.* 2019;44(8):543–549. https://doi.org/10.1097/BRS.0000000000002885.
98. Schroeder GD, Hilibrand AS, Arnold PM, et al. Epidural hematoma following cervical spine surgery. *Global Spine J.* 2017;7(1 Suppl):120S–126S. https://doi.org/10.1177/2192568216687754.
99. Goldstein CL, Bains I, Hurlbert RJ. Symptomatic spinal epidural hematoma after posterior cervical surgery: incidence and risk factors. *Spine J.* 2015;15(6):1179–1187. https://doi.org/10.1016/j.spinee.2013.11.043.

100. Carr ERM, Benjamin E. In vitro study investigating post neck surgery haematoma airway obstruction. *J Laryngol Otol.* 2009;123(6):662–665. https://doi.org/10.1017/S0022215108003423.
101. Palumbo MA, Aidlen JP, Daniels AH, Thakur NA, Caiati J. Airway compromise due to wound hematoma following anterior cervical spine surgery. *Open Orthop J.* 2012;6:108–113. https://doi.org/10.2174/1874325001206010108.
102. Olsen MA, Nepple JJ, Riew KD, et al. Risk factors for surgical site infection following orthopaedic spinal operations. *J Bone Joint Surg Am.* 2008;90(1):62–69. https://doi.org/10.2106/JBJS.F.01515.
103. Olsen MA, Mayfield J, Lauryssen C, et al. Risk factors for surgical site infection in spinal surgery. *J Neurosurg.* 2003;98(2 Suppl):149–155.
104. Watanabe M, Sakai D, Matsuyama D, Yamamoto Y, Sato M, Mochida J. Risk factors for surgical site infection following spine surgery: efficacy of intraoperative saline irrigation. *J Neurosurg Spine.* 2010;12(5):540–546. https://doi.org/10.3171/2009.11.SPINE09308.
105. Sebastian A, Huddleston P, Kakar S, Habermann E, Wagie A, Nassr A. Risk factors for surgical site infection after posterior cervical spine surgery: an analysis of 5,441 patients from the ACS NSQIP 2005–2012. *Spine J.* 2016;16(4):504–509. https://doi.org/10.1016/j.spinee.2015.12.009.
106. Kwon BK, Fisher CG, Boyd MC, et al. A prospective randomized controlled trial of anterior compared with posterior stabilization for unilateral facet injuries of the cervical spine. *J Neurosurg Spine.* 2007;7(1):1–12. https://doi.org/10.3171/SPI-07/07/001.
107. Xu R, Bydon M, Sciubba DM, et al. Safety and efficacy of rhBMP2 in posterior cervical spinal fusion for subaxial degenerative spine disease: Analysis of outcomes in 204 patients. *Surg Neurol Int.* 2011;2:109. https://doi.org/10.4103/2152-7806.83726.
108. Mehta AI, Babu R, Sharma R, et al. Thickness of subcutaneous fat as a risk factor for infection in cervical spine fusion surgery. *J Bone Joint Surg Am.* 2013;95(4):323–328. https://doi.org/10.2106/JBJS.L.00225.
109. Fei Q, Li J, Lin J, et al. Risk factors for surgical site infection after spinal surgery: A meta-analysis. *World Neurosurg.* 2016;95:507–515. https://doi.org/10.1016/j.wneu.2015.05.059.
110. Haddad S, Millhouse PW, Maltenfort M, Restrepo C, Kepler CK, Vaccaro AR. Diagnosis and neurologic status as predictors of surgical site infection in primary cervical spinal surgery. *Spine J Off J North Am Spine Soc.* 2016;16(5):632–642. https://doi.org/10.1016/j.spinee.2016.01.019.
111. Hampson F, Ridgway E. Prophylactic antibiotics in surgery. *Surg Oxf.* 2005;23(8):290–293. https://doi.org/10.1383/surg.2005.23.8.290.
112. Theiss SM, Lonstein JE, Winter RB. Wound infections in reconstructive spine surgery. *Orthop Clin North Am.* 1996;27(1):105–110. https://doi.org/10.1016/S0030-5898(20)32055-1.
113. Kang BU, Lee SH, Ahn Y, Choi WC, Choi YG. Surgical site infection in spinal surgery: detection and management based on serial C-reactive protein measurements. *J Neurosurg Spine.* 2010;13(2):158–164. https://doi.org/10.3171/2010.3.SPINE09403.
114. Hegde V, Meredith DS, Kepler CK, Huang RC. Management of postoperative spinal infections. *World J Orthop.* 2012;3(11):182–189. https://doi.org/10.5312/wjo.v3.i11.182.
115. Patel PD, Arutyunyan G, Plusch K, Jr AV, Vaccaro AR. A review of cervical spine alignment in the normal and degenerative spine. *J Spine Surg.* 2020;6(1):106–123. https://doi.org/10.21037/jss.2020.01.10.
116. Ouchida J, Yukawa Y, Ito K, et al. Functional computed tomography scanning for evaluating fusion status after anterior cervical decompression fusion. *Eur Spine J.* 2015;24(12):2924–2929. https://doi.org/10.1007/s00586-014-3722-z.
117. Riew KD, Yang JJ, Chang DG, et al. What is the most accurate radiographic criterion to determine anterior cervical fusion? *Spine J.* 2019;19(3):469–475. https://doi.org/10.1016/j.spinee.2018.07.003.
118. Crawford CH, Carreon LY, Mummaneni P, Dryer RF, Glassman SD. Asymptomatic ACDF nonunions underestimate the true prevalence of radiographic pseudarthrosis. *Spine.* 2020;45(13):E776–E780. https://doi.org/10.1097/BRS.0000000000003444.
119. Singh A, Crockard HA, Platts A, Stevens J. Clinical and radiological correlates of severity and surgery-related outcome in cervical spondylosis. *J Neurosurg.* 2001;94(2 Suppl):189–198. https://doi.org/10.3171/spi.2001.94.2.0189.
120. Suri A, Chabbra RPS, Mehta VS, Gaikwad S, Pandey RM. Effect of intramedullary signal changes on the surgical outcome of patients with cervical spondylotic myelopathy. *Spine J.* 2003;3(1):33–45. https://doi.org/10.1016/s1529-9430(02)00448-5.
121. Houten JK, Cooper PR. Laminectomy and posterior cervical plating for multilevel cervical spondylotic myelopathy and ossification of the posterior longitudinal ligament: effects on cervical alignment, spinal cord compression, and neurological outcome. *Neurosurgery.* 2003;52(5):1081–1087; discussion 1087–1088.
122. Huang S, Sun X, Chen L, et al. MRI T2WI high signal is a risk factor for perioperative complications in patients with cervical spondylosis with spinal cord compression: A propensity matching score analysis. *BioMed Res Int.* 2022;2022:8040437. https://doi.org/10.1155/2022/8040437.

11

Anterior Approach Related Complications

MARK J. LAMBRECHTS, GREGORY R. TOCI, MICHAEL V. CARTER, AND ALEXANDER R. VACCARO

CHAPTER OUTLINE

Introduction

Originally described by Smith and Robinson in the mid-1950s, their approach to the anterior cervical spine has become an indispensable tool for spine surgeons to maximize efficiency and minimize surgical risk during anterior cervical discectomy and fusion (ACDF) and cervical disc arthroplasty (CDA) procedures.[1] ACDFs are one of the most commonly performed spine procedures in the United States, and surgeons must be facile in the approach and understand any potential complications that could arise during the procedure.[2] The risk of experiencing intraoperative or postoperative complications following ACDF is believed to range from 13.2% to 19.3% with most complications related to postoperative dysphagia.[3,4] Generally, the risk for postoperative complications is greater for patients undergoing revision procedures due to scar tissue formation. Once structures become adherent, the degree of difficulty in safely isolating vulnerable structures and identifying anatomic variants like the recurrent laryngeal nerve, substantially increases.[5,6] For this reason, some surgeons may elect to proceed with an approach on the contralateral side from the index surgery; however, this is often done once the patient is confirmed to have bilateral functioning recurrent laryngeal nerves as determined by direct laryngoscopic examination. If there is a nonfunctioning or poorly functioning recurrent laryngeal nerve, the approach is often done on that side to avoid injury to the functioning nerve.[7]

Postoperative Dysphagia

Dysphagia is the most reported complication following anterior cervical spinal surgery. Incidence rates vary widely, with some studies indicating some form of dysphagia present in 71% of patients.[8] While this is likely an overestimation of the rate of clinically relevant dysphagia, it does illustrate the significant variability in dysphagia reporting. The variation in reported rates may be due to differences in defining postoperative dysphagia (relating to severity, length of time postoperatively, and number of dysphagic episodes) or differences in study methodology (e.g., retrospective studies limited to chart review compared to prospective barium swallow studies).[9,10] The most common method of diagnosis is the Bazaz Dysphagia Score, which assesses both the types of food that precipitate dysphagia, as well as the frequency of these dysphagic episodes.[11]

Although the underlying cause for the high incidence of postoperative dysphagia has not been clearly defined, it may be caused by indirect injury to the recurrent laryngeal nerve. Postoperative hematoma, edema, high endotracheal tube cuff pressures, increased number of levels fused, and prolonged surgical duration and retraction contribute to recurrent laryngeal nerve neuropraxia due to stretching of the expansive network of small recurrent laryngeal nerve branches immediately adjacent to the esophagus.[12,13] Instrumentation of the lower cervical spine with an anterior plate is also believed to carry a higher risk of postoperative dysphagia due to the closer proximity of the esophageal branches of the recurrent laryngeal nerve to the surgical field.[14] These risk factors may explain why both local infiltration and intravenous administration of corticosteroids improve dysphagia within the first 2 weeks of surgery.[15]

Additional risk factors for dysphagia may include female sex, greater age, and smoking status, but the exact mechanism and their overall contribution to postoperative dysphagia is ill-defined.[4,16–19] Further risk factors proposed include the use of larger cervical interbody spacers, which may stimulate bone growth around the esophageal tissue, and the use of bone morphogenic proteins (BMPs), which causes inflammation of the esophagus and surrounding soft tissues.[16,20]

Although postoperative dysphagia is usually temporary, with 93% of patients recovering completely within 1 year, some prophylactic measures to reduce the incidence of dysphagia have been proposed.[4,10] As previously discussed, the most promising option is methylprednisolone due to its ability to minimize the immune system's ability to induce secondary injury through proinflammatory pathways and due to its purported ability to enhance neurologic recovery.[21–23] Manual preoperative tracheal traction exercises have also been shown to decrease the rate of postoperative dysphagia in limited studies; however, these techniques have not gained widespread acceptance and the therapeutic benefit of this practice continues to remain questionable.[24,25]

Esophageal Injury

Damage to the esophagus is a relatively rare complication, with incidence rates estimated at 0.02% to 1.52%.[26] Early esophageal perforations, defined as injuries that occur within the first 30 postoperative days, are predominantly iatrogenic, resulting from intraoperative laceration or retractor-mediated damage.[27] The most commonly identified level for esophageal perforation is at C5-C6 due to the vulnerability of the cricoid muscles at this level.[28] Late esophageal perforations, which represent the majority of perforations, usually occur after instrumentation failure/loosening, whereby the adjacent cervical plates and/or screws either loosen and inflict mechanical damage to the esophagus or slowly erode into the esophageal wall.[26,27]

Early symptoms associated with esophageal perforation include dysphagia, odynophagia, fever, neck swelling, and wound drainage.[26] In severe cases, patients may develop mediastinal abscesses, sepsis, or esophageal mucosal necrosis, which can be fatal in up to 25% of cases.[27,29,30] Late esophageal perforations occur on average 2 years following the index surgery and may be misdiagnosed as an unrelated condition rather than a surgical complication, which can further complicate and delay treatment.[26,29] Patients should be educated on the related symptoms of esophageal perforation such that they can recognize them and disclose their past surgical history to emergency medical providers.[26]

Immediate surgical repair of the esophagus, if identified intraoperatively, is optimal for any patient with esophageal perforation.[29] For late perforations with migrated or loose instrumentation, repair of the esophagus can be performed at the time of surgery if the surgical bed is amenable to repair with consultation with an otolaryngologist or the esophagus can be bypassed with a feeding tube for a delayed reconstruction.[26,29] Outcomes of esophageal repair are generally favorable, with up to 91% of patients experiencing complete resolution of their symptoms postoperatively.[29]

One technical pearl to limit inadvertent esophageal injury (especially for an ACDF including the C5/6 level) is to place retractor blades posterior to the longus colli muscle when performing the fusion. This can prevent inadvertent retraction on Killian's triangle, which is located where the thyropharyngeus and cricopharyngeus muscles meet, and it is the weakest and most vulnerable area of the esophagus during the ACDF approach.[31]

Recurrent Laryngeal Nerve Injury/Vocal Cord Injury

Incidence of vocal cord palsy (VCP) following ACDF is estimated to occur in 2.3% to 24.2% of cases.[32] The most common injury mechanism results from damage to either the recurrent laryngeal nerve (innervates most intrinsic laryngeal muscles except for the cricothyroid) or the superior laryngeal nerve (innervates the cricothyroid). Injury to either nerve is common due to their immediate proximity to the esophagus, which increases their vulnerability to damage from retractors. However, since traction from retractors leads to a resultant stretch of the nerve by as much as 24%, most injuries are defined as neuropraxias and resolve over time.[14,33] As previously discussed in the risk factors for dysphagia, the use of high endotracheal tube cuff pressures can cause ischemic injury to the anterior branch of the recurrent laryngeal nerve, which supplies the lateral cricoarytenoid and thyroarytenoid muscles and results in postoperative dysphonia.[32,34] A recent prospective randomized controlled trial suggests that adjustment of endotracheal tube cuff pressures may decrease the incidence of dysphonia, although further research is required before definitive guidelines can be placed on cuff pressure maintenance throughout the procedure as an effective prophylactic measure.[12,35] While rare, complete transection of the recurrent laryngeal nerve can occur with separation of the carotid sheath from the visceral sheath (from the nearby trachea and esophagus), which most often occurs at the level of C7 on right-sided approaches.[36]

A technical note should be added due to the considerable debate over left-sided versus right-sided surgical approaches. Due to historical biases, most surgeons prefer to only perform approaches on the left side (the recurrent laryngeal nerve demonstrates a more reliable medial cranial ascent into the larynx since it is fixed to the ligamentum arteriosum and lies deep within the esophagotracheal groove), while the right recurrent laryngeal nerve is more variable in its lateral to medial ascent across the surgical field and it does not lie deep within the esophagotracheal groove.[36–38] However, to date, there is no evidence demonstrating that right- or left-sided surgical approaches independently predict lower rates of recurrent laryngeal nerve injury.[32] Therefore, the side of approach should be dictated by the surgeon unless the patient has had prior neck surgery.[38] In revision procedures, incidence of recurrent laryngeal nerve palsy rise to 14% and, the surgeon should consider using the contralateral side unless the patient has a documented recurrent laryngeal nerve injury on the original side of exposure on laryngoscopic examination.[7,38]

Superior laryngeal nerve palsy is a rarer condition, occurring in around 1.25% of patients.[5] The superior laryngeal nerve is typically located within the pretracheal fascia that covers the longus colli muscle, and superficial placement of retractors on the longus colli may lead to damage of this nerve.[5] The superior laryngeal nerve branches into internal and external branches in close proximity to the superior thyroid artery, which represents an additional location for injury.[5] Most cases of postoperative vocal cord palsy are subclinical and as a result go undiagnosed.[39] Fortunately, symptomatic cases are usually temporary with irreversible vocal cord paralysis only seen in approximately 2% of cases.[40] Although patients with an injury to the recurrent laryngeal nerve frequently exhibit hoarseness, dysphagia, or dysphonia, patients with an injury to the superior laryngeal nerve are usually asymptomatic.[5,41] Treatment of these injuries is supportive until patients experience spontaneous resolution of their symptoms.[4]

Thoracic Duct Injury

The thoracic duct drains lymphatic fluid from the entire left side of the body as well as the lower right quadrant of the body. It is the largest lymphatic vessel in the body, and it is generally located on the left side of the cervical spine, although right-sided variations have been reported.[42,43] Thoracic duct injury during cervical spine surgery is relatively infrequent when compared to thoracic and lumbar spine procedures, and only a handful of cases have been described in the literature.[44,45] In fact, one retrospective series of 9591 patients who underwent anterior cervical spine surgery only reported two thoracic duct injuries.[42] In one case, the duct was repaired intraoperatively without postoperative evidence of injury, while the thoracic duct injury that was not repaired resulted in a collection of chylous fluid 2 months postoperatively and required percutaneous aspiration. A separate case report of a thoracic duct injury described a variable ascent of the thoracic duct, with the duct extending to the superior thyroid cornu (far superior to its expected location near the clavicle), thereby predisposing the duct to injury.[44]

Damage to the thoracic duct can cause chylothorax, chyloretroperitoneum, or chylous fistula formation, which can in turn lead to difficulties with respiration, immune function, and nutrient absorption.[46] If undetected intraoperatively, the presence of chyle in either the postoperative drain or via aspiration of the neck can be used to make a diagnosis.[42] Treatment is dependent on the severity of the injury and can include supportive care, chest tube drainage, pharmacologic therapy, or surgical ligation of the duct.[42]

Horner Syndrome

Horner syndrome is classically defined as a triad of ptosis, miosis, and anhidrosis that often occurs following sympathetic denervation. It is usually seen following either iatrogenic laceration or due to traction of the longus colli muscles that run adjacent to these fibers.[47] Though an exceedingly rare complication of anterior cervical spine surgery (seen in only 0.45% of patients), incidence rates of Horner syndrome are highest amongst patients who undergo surgery at either C4-C5 or C5-C6; at these levels, ascending sympathetic fibers are significantly closer to the vertebrae than they are at higher levels, which puts them at greater risk of intraoperative injury.[47,48] Interestingly, the majority of Horner syndrome cases are seen on the left side of the body; whether this is due to more surgeons feeling comfortable with left-sided approaches due to consistent anatomy of the left recurrent laryngeal nerve is less clear.[47]

A technical pearl that will allow surgeons to minimize the risk of Horner syndrome is avoiding temptation to perform transverse incisions on the longus colli, as this places the sympathetic cervical trunk at increased risk for injury. Additionally, meticulous subperiosteal elevation of the longus colli must be ensured when attempting to gain additional exposure of the lateral vertebrae. After subperiosteal elevation of the longus colli, retractors can be safely placed posterior to the longus colli. If prolonged retraction is necessary for the procedure, periodic relaxation may minimize the risk of neuropraxic injury to the sympathetic trunk.[49]

Long-term outcomes of patients with postoperative Horner syndrome vary. While most patients see a reduction in Horner symptoms over the course of their postoperative recovery, only about 61% experience complete resolution.[47] Treatment for Horner syndrome is largely supportive, and there is currently no effective cure.

Hypoglossal Injury

Hypoglossal nerve palsy is an exceedingly rare complication of anterior cervical spine surgery (fewer than 10 cases have been currently described) due to its proximity to the mandibular angle.[50] Patients who experience this complication usually have an anatomical anomaly such that the hypoglossal nerve is displaced inferior relative to its expected location. During surgery, caudally located hypoglossal nerve anatomic variants can be further displaced inferiorly during endotracheal intubation, particularly in procedures involving the upper levels of the subaxial cervical spine.[51]

The hypoglossal nerve innervates the majority of the extrinsic and intrinsic muscles of the tongue and is responsible for tongue movement. As such, lesions to the hypoglossal nerve result in dysphagia, dysarthria, and deviation of the tongue toward the side of the lesion, which can result in chronic weight loss and recurrent aspiration pneumonia.[50] Long-term outcomes vary, as some patients experience complete resolution, while others remain symptomatic long term. Speech therapy and swallowing therapy may help some patients regain some tongue mobility, but their long-term improvement is often limited.[50]

Hematomas/Airway Compromise

Prevertebral hematomas are seen in up to 6% of patients undergoing anterior cervical spine surgery, and usually develop within the first 24 hours after surgery (Fig. 11.1).[3,52] In some cases, hematomas may form despite the use of postoperative drains and meticulous hemostasis. The main risk factor is oozing from small blood vessels in and around the longus colli muscle.[52] The excessive use of sharp tools (as opposed to blunt tools) during dissection also increases the risk of hematoma formation due to the increased likelihood of blood vessel damage.[4]

Patients with a hematoma may complain of a lump in their neck and may experience difficulty breathing or dysphagia if the hematoma obstructs the trachea or esophagus, respectively.[52,53] Approximately half of patients with postoperative hematomas undergo surgical evacuation, while the other half can effectively and safely be treated nonoperatively.[3,18,52] Hematomas requiring surgical intervention are typically seen in patients of male gender, a lower BMI, a history of anemia, and in patients who had a multilevel procedure.[3]

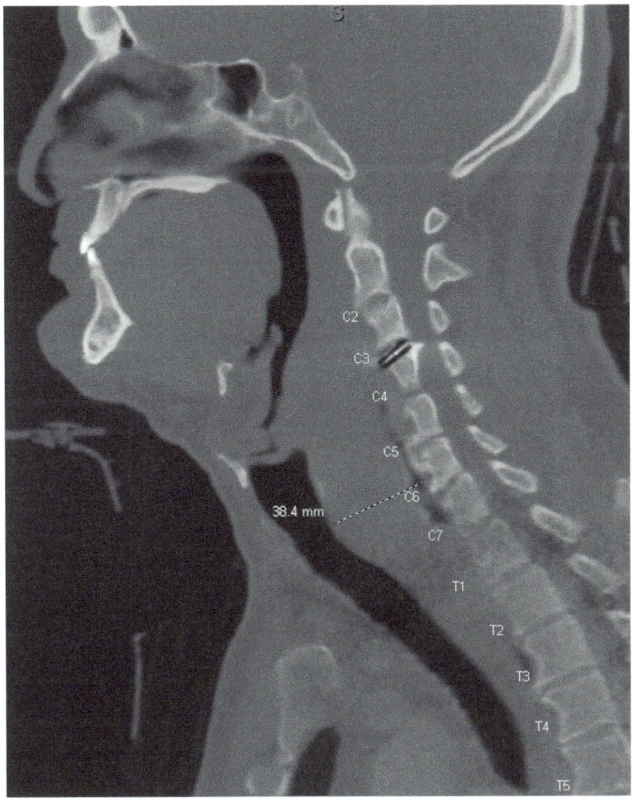

• **Fig. 11.1** Patient underwent a cervical disc arthroplasty from C3-C4 and anterior cervical discectomy and fusion from C4-C7. Patient developed a prevertebral hematoma adjacent to the surgical site, as seen on the lateral CT image of the cervical spine. Patient was emergently treated with irrigation and debridement of the hematoma due to difficulty breathing from the compromised airway.

Postoperative drains have historically been used for patients undergoing ACDFs. However, current literature suggests that drains are not only ineffective at reducing hematoma formation, but they increase the likelihood of postoperative blood transfusions 14-fold, while also increasing hospital length of stay twofold.[54] In fact, even when stratifying drain usage based on single-level versus multilevel surgery, there has been no evidence to support drain use prevents postoperative complications.[55] Based on current evidence, postoperative drain usage should be left to the discretion of the surgeon with the understanding that there is poor literature to support its efficacy.

Instrumentation Related Complications

ACDFs generally have a high success rate, with symptomatic pseudoarthrosis rates estimated to require revision in approximately 10% of patients.[56] In the setting of a pseudoarthrosis, instrumentation failure may occur due to loosening, fracture, and/or migration of the implants. Instrumentation failure is only identified in around 2% of all patients undergoing ACDF, although incidence rates are difficult to predict due to its predominant asymptomatic presentation.[53,57] Even if instrumentation failure occurs, it is estimated that only 5% of patients will experience clinical symptoms, such as esophageal perforation or injury to adjacent neurovascular structures.[57] In these patients, removal of implants and revision fusion is indicated (Fig. 11.2).

Unique instrumentation complications can be seen following CDA that are not associated with other anterior cervical spine procedures. Heterotopic ossification around the cervical implant is noted in approximately half of patients and is one of the most common complications of CDA.[58,59] While there is usually not enough bone deposition to cause symptoms, heterotopic ossification may cause the interspace to ultimately fuse. Osteolysis of the vertebral bodies is another common complication, and, while usually asymptomatic, it may cause severe vertebral collapse and localized kyphosis that also requires surgical treatment.[59,60] Rarer, but more serious complications of CDA include subsidence and vertebral body fractures, both of which often require surgical revision. Immune rejection of implants has been occasionally described in the literature but is rarely diagnosed due to a largely subclinical presentation.[59] Perhaps the most catastrophic complication after CDA is implant extrusion. This typically occurs in high demand individuals and should be immediately identified on radiographic imaging. If implant extrusion occurs, the CDA should be urgently removed, and the most reliable salvage procedure is fusion.[61]

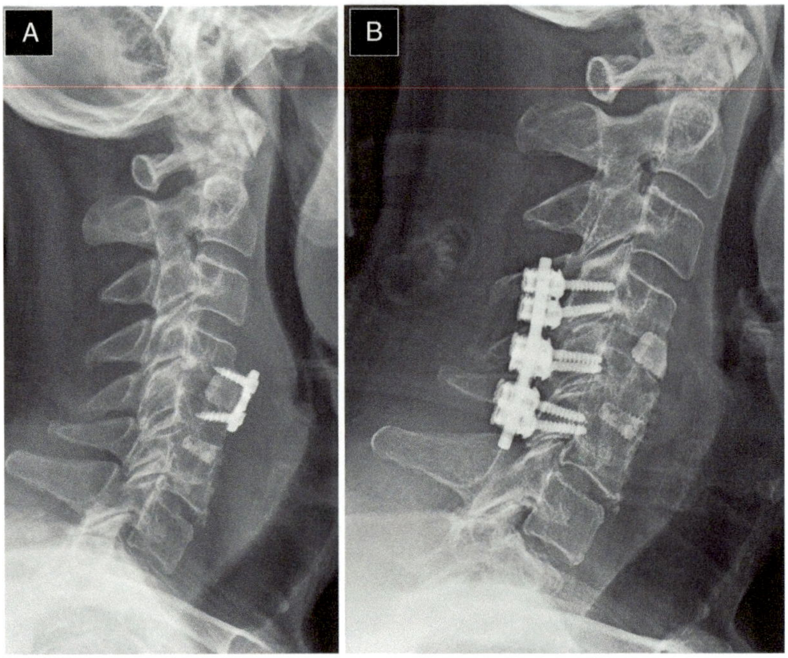

• **Fig. 11.2** Patient was indicated for surgery due to junctional stenosis from an anterior cervical discectomy and fusion from C5-C6. Patient underwent removal of the anterior cervical plate, exploration of fusion, and anterior cervical discectomy and fusion of C4-C5. The patient developed swallowing difficulties and was found to have migration of the anterior cervical plate, as seen on the lateral cervical spine radiograph (a). Patient underwent removal of the anterior cervical plate, partial corpectomy at C4, and placement of bone graft at C4-C5 followed by posterior cervical fusion with lateral mass instrumentation from C4-C6 with local bone graft from the C4 corpectomy, as seen on the lateral cervical spine radiograph (b).

Conclusion

Despite substantial advancements, anterior cervical spine surgery is not without risk. While many of the common complications are transient, others can result in lifelong impairment and can significantly alter a patient's quality of life. Knowledge of these risk factors and the pitfalls that cause them is important in minimizing the likelihood of these complications occurring.

References

1. Aronson N, Filtzer DL, Bagan M. Anterior cervical fusion by the Smith-Robinson approach. *J Neurosurg*. 1968;29:397–404. https://doi.org/10.3171/jns.1968.29.4.0397.
2. Saifi C, Fein AW, Cazzulino A, et al. Trends in resource utilization and rate of cervical disc arthroplasty and anterior cervical discectomy and fusion throughout the United States from 2006 to 2013. *Spine J*. 2018;18:1022–1029. https://doi.org/10.1016/j.spinee.2017.10.072.
3. Epstein NE. A review of complication rates for anterior cervical diskectomy and fusion (ACDF). *Surg Neurol Int*. 2019;10:100. https://doi.org/10.25259/sni-191-2019.
4. Fountas KN, Kapsalaki EZ, Nikolakakos LG, et al. Anterior cervical discectomy and fusion associated complications. *Spine*. 2007;32:2310–2317. https://doi.org/10.1097/brs.0b013e318154c57e.
5. Tempel ZJ, Smith JS, Shaffrey C, et al. A multicenter review of superior laryngeal nerve injury following anterior cervical spine surgery. *Global Spine J*. 2017;7:7S–11S. https://doi.org/10.1177/2192568216687296.
6. Thomas AM, Fahim DK, Gemechu JM. Anatomical variations of the recurrent laryngeal nerve and implications for injury prevention during surgical procedures of the neck. *Diagnostics*. 2020;10:670. https://doi.org/10.3390/diagnostics10090670.
7. Gowd A, Nazemi A, Carmouche J, Albert T, Behrend C. Indications for direct laryngoscopic examination of vocal cord function prior to anterior cervical surgery. *Geriatr Orthop Surg Rehabil*. 2016;8:54–63. https://doi.org/10.1177/2151458516681144.
8. Rihn JA, Kane J, Albert TJ, Vaccaro AR, Hilibrand AS. What is the incidence and severity of dysphagia after anterior cervical surgery? *Clin Orthop Relat Res*. 2011;469:658–665. https://doi.org/10.1007/s11999-010-1731-8.
9. Rosenthal BD, Nair R, Hsu WK, Patel AA, Savage JW. Dysphagia and dysphonia assessment tools after anterior cervical spine surgery. *Clin Spine Surg*. 2016;29:363–367. https://doi.org/10.1097/bsd.0000000000000373.
10. Shriver MF, Lewis DJ, Kshettry VR, Rosenbaum BP, Benzel EC, Mroz TE. Dysphagia rates after anterior cervical diskectomy and fusion: A systematic review and meta-analysis. *Global Spine J*. 2017;7:95–103. https://doi.org/10.1055/s-0036-1583944.
11. Anderson KK, Arnold PM. Oropharyngeal dysphagia after anterior cervical spine surgery: A Review. *Global Spine J*. 2013;03:273–286. https://doi.org/10.1055/s-0033-1354253.
12. Arts MP, Rettig TCD, de Vries J, Wolfs JFC, in't Veld BA. Maintaining endotracheal tube cuff pressure at 20 mm Hg to

prevent dysphagia after anterior cervical spine surgery; protocol of a double-blind randomised controlled trial. *BMC Musculoskelet Disord.* 2013;14:280. https://doi.org/10.1186/1471-2474-14-280.

13. Rajabian A, Quraishi NA. Is dysphagia after ACDF due to recurrent laryngeal nerve (RLN) neuropraxia? A fresh cadaveric study. *Spine J.* 2017;17:S13144. https://doi.org/10.1016/j.spinee.2016.12.042.
14. Fisahn C, Yilmaz E, Iwanaga J, et al. Avoiding the esophageal branches of the recurrent laryngeal nerve during retractor placement: Precluding postoperative dysphagia during anterior approaches to the cervical spine. *Global Spine J.* 2019;9:383–387. https://doi.org/10.1177/2192568218810198.
15. Jenkins TJ, Nair R, Bhatt S, et al. The effect of local versus intravenous corticosteroids on the likelihood of dysphagia and dysphonia following anterior cervical discectomy and fusion. *J Bone Jt Surg.* 2018;100:1461–1472. https://doi.org/10.2106/jbjs.17.01540.
16. Joaquim AF, Murar J, Savage JW, Patel AA. Dysphagia after anterior cervical spine surgery: a systematic review of potential preventative measures. *Spine J.* 2014;14:2246–2260. https://doi.org/10.1016/j.spinee.2014.03.030.
17. Siska PA, Ponnappan RK, Hohl JB, Lee JY, Kang JD, Donaldson WF. Dysphagia after anterior cervical. *spine surgery. Spine.* 2011;36:1387–1391. https://doi.org/10.1097/brs.0b013e31822340f2.
18. Kim S, Alan N, Sansosti A, Agarwal N, Wecht DA. Complications after 3- and 4-level anterior cervical diskectomy and fusion. *World Neurosurg.* 2019;130:e1105–1110. https://doi.org/10.1016/j.wneu.2019.07.099.
19. Liu F-Y, Yang D-L, Huang W-Z, et al. Risk factors for dysphagia after anterior cervical spine surgery. *Medicine.* 2017;96:e6267. https://doi.org/10.1097/md.0000000000006267.
20. Cho SK, Lu Y, Lee D-H. Dysphagia following anterior cervical spinal surgery: A systematic review. *Bone Jt J.* 2013;95-B:868–873. https://doi.org/10.1302/0301-620x.95b7.31029.
21. Coutinho AE, Chapman KE. The anti-inflammatory and immunosuppressive effects of glucocorticoids, recent developments and mechanistic insights. *Mol Cell Endocrinol.* 2011;335:2–13. https://doi.org/10.1016/j.mce.2010.04.005.
22. Adenikinju AS, Halani SH, Rindler RS, Gary MF, Michael KW, Ahmad FU. Effect of perioperative steroids on dysphagia after anterior cervical spine surgery: A systematic review. *Int J Spine Surg.* 2017;11:9. https://doi.org/10.14444/4009.
23. Lee S-H, Kim K-T, Suk K-S, Park K-J, Oh K-I. Effect of retropharyngeal steroid on prevertebral soft tissue swelling following anterior cervical discectomy and fusion. *Spine.* 2011;36:2286–2292.https://doi.org/10.1097/brs.0b013e318237e5d0.
24. Chen Z, Wei X, Li F, et al. Tracheal traction exercise reduces the occurrence of postoperative dysphagia after anterior cervical spine surgery. *Spine.* 2012;37:1292–1296. https://doi.org/10.1097/brs.0b013e3182477f26.
25. Chaudhary SK, Yu B, Pan F, et al. Manual preoperative tracheal retraction exercise decreases the occurrence of postoperative oropharyngeal dysphagia after anterior cervical discectomy and fusion. *J Orthop Surg (Hong Kong).* 2017;25:2309499017731446. https://doi.org/10.1177/2309499017731446.
26. Halani SH, Baum GR, Riley JP, Pradilla G, Refai D, Rodts GE, et al. Esophageal perforation after anterior cervical spine surgery: a systematic review of the literature. *J Neurosurg Spine.* 2016;25:285–291. https://doi.org/10.3171/2016.1.spine15898.
27. Ghirelli M, Molinari G, Rosini M, et al. Pharyngo-esophageal perforations after anterior cervical spine surgery: Management and outcomes. *World Neurosurg.* 2020;139:e463–473. https://doi.org/10.1016/j.wneu.2020.04.040.
28. Haku T, Okuda S, Kanematsu F, et al. Repair of cervical esophageal perforation using longus colli muscle flap: a case report of a patient with cervical spinal cord injury. *Spine J.* 2008;8:831–835. https://doi.org/10.1016/j.spinee.2007.06.017.
29. Bufkin BL, Miller JI, Mansour KA. Esophageal perforation: Emphasis on management. *Ann Thorac Surg.* 1996;61:1447–1452. https://doi.org/10.1016/0003-4975(96)00053-7.
30. Nanda A, Sharma M, Sonig A, Ambekar S, Bollam P. Surgical complications of anterior cervical diskectomy and fusion for cervical degenerative disk disease: A single surgeon's experience of 1576 patients. *World Neurosurg.* 2014;82:1380–1387. https://doi.org/10.1016/j.wneu.2013.09.022.
31. Hershman SH, Kunkle WA, Kelly MP, et al. Esophageal perforation following anterior cervical spine surgery: Case report and review of the literature. *Global Spine J.* 2017;7:28S–36S. https://doi.org/10.1177/2192568216687535.
32. Tan TP, Govindarajulu AP, Massicotte EM, Venkatraghavan L. Vocal cord palsy after anterior cervical spine surgery: a qualitative systematic review. *Spine J.* 2014;14:1332–1342. https://doi.org/10.1016/j.spinee.2014.02.017.
33. Weisberg NK, Spengler DM, Netterville JL. Stretch-induced nerve injury as a cause of paralysis secondary to the anterior cervical approach. *Otolaryngol Head Neck Surg.* 1997;116:317–326. https://doi.org/10.1016/s0194-59989770266-3.
34. Whited RE. A study of endotracheal tube injury to the subglottis. *Laryngoscope.* 1985;95:1216–1219. https://doi.org/10.1288/00005537-198510000-00014.
35. Sejkorová A, Bolcha M, Beneš J, Kalhous J, Sameš M, Vachata P. Intraoperative measurement of endotracheal tube cuff pressure and its change during surgery in correlation with recurrent laryngeal nerve palsies, hoarseness, and dysphagia after anterior cervical discectomy and fusion: A prospective randomized controlled trial. *Global Spine J.* 2021:219256822110468. https://doi.org/10.1177/21925682211046895.
36. Shan J, Jiang H, Ren D, Wang C. Anatomic relationship between right recurrent laryngeal nerve and cervical fascia and its application significance in anterior cervical spine surgical approach. *Spine.* 2017;42:E443–447. https://doi.org/10.1097/brs.0000000000001881.
37. Johnson MD, Matur AV, Asghar F, Nasser R, Cheng JS, Prestigiacomo CJ. Right versus left approach to anterior cervical discectomy and fusion: An anatomic versus historic debate. *World Neurosurg.* 2020;135:135–140. https://doi.org/10.1016/j.wneu.2019.12.052.
38. Erwood MS, Hadley MN, Gordon AS, Carroll WR, Agee BS, Walters BC. Recurrent laryngeal nerve injury following reoperative anterior cervical discectomy and fusion: a meta-analysis. *J Neurosurg Spine.* 2016;25:198–204. https://doi.org/10.3171/2015.9.spine15187.
39. Jung A, Schramm J, Lehnerdt K, Herberhold C. Recurrent laryngeal nerve palsy during anterior cervical spine surgery: a prospective study. *J Neurosurg Spine.* 2005;2:123–127. https://doi.org/10.3171/spi.2005.2.2.0123.
40. Cloward RB. New method of diagnosis and treatment of cervical disc disease. *Neurosurgery.* 1962;8:93–132. https://doi.org/10.1093/neurosurgery/8.cn_suppl_1.93.
41. Eckley CA, Sataloff RT, Hawkshaw M, Spiegel JR, Mandel S. Voice range in superior laryngealnerve paresis and paralysis.

J Voice. 1998;12:340–348. https://doi.org/10.1016/s0892-1997(98)80024-6.
42. Derakhshan A, Lubelski D, Steinmetz MP, et al. Thoracic duct injury following cervical spine surgery: A multicenter retrospective review. *Global Spine J*. 2017;7:115S–119S. https://doi.org/10.1177/2192568216688194.
43. Greenfield J, Gottlieb MI. Variations in the terminal portion of the human thoracic duct. *AMA Arch Surg*. 1956;73:955–959. https://doi.org/10.1001/archsurg.1956.01280060055012.
44. Hart AK, Greinwald JH, Shaffrey CI, Postma GN. Thoracic duct injury during anterior cervical discectomy: a rare complication. Case report. *J Neurosurg*. 1998;88:151–154. https://doi.org/10.3171/jns.1998.88.1.0151.
45. Klug T, Sebelik M, Shires CB. Chyloma formation after anterior cervical disc fusion. *Clin Case Reports*. 2020;8:2721–2724. https://doi.org/10.1002/ccr3.3274.
46. Riquet M, Badia A. Chirurgie des chylothorax. *Rev Pneumol Clin*. 2004;60:104–108. https://doi.org/10.1016/s0761-8417(04)73477-x.
47. Lubelski D, Pennington Z, Sciubba DM, Theodore N, Bydon A. Horner syndrome after anterior cervical discectomy and fusion: Case series and systematic review. *World Neurosurg*. 2020;133:e68–75. https://doi.org/10.1016/j.wneu.2019.08.101.
48. Ebraheim NA, Lu J, Yang H, Heck BE, Yeasting RA. Vulnerability of the sympathetic trunk during the anterior approach to the lower cervical. *spine. Spine*. 2000;25:1603–1606. https://doi.org/10.1097/00007632-200007010-00002.
49. Traynelis VC, Malone HR, Smith ZA, et al. Rare complications of cervical spine surgery: Horner's syndrome. *Global Spine J*. 2017;7:103S–108S. https://doi.org/10.1177/2192568216688184.
50. Colón LF, Isaza J, Katsuura Y, Nuss D. Hypoglossal nerve palsy after anterior cervical spine surgery: A case report and literature review. *JBJS Case Connect*. 2020;10:e0098. https://doi.org/10.2106/jbjs.cc.19.00098.
51. Ghedia R, Hughes J, Clarke P. Hypoglossal nerve identification during head and neck surgery. *Clin Otolaryngol*. 2016;41:202–203. https://doi.org/10.1111/coa.12412.
52. Razi A, Saleh H, DeLacure MD, Kim Y. Anterior approach to the subaxial cervical spine: Pearls and pitfalls. *J Am Acad Orthop Surg*. 2020;29:189–195. https://doi.org/10.5435/jaaos-d-17-00891.
53. Yee TJ, Swong K, Park P. Complications of anterior cervical spine surgery: a systematic review of the literature. *J Spine Surg*. 2020;6:302–322. https://doi.org/10.21037/jss.2020.01.14.
54. Adogwa O, Khalid SI, Elsamadicy AA, Voung VD, Lilly DT, Desai SA, et al. The use of subfascial drains after multi-level anterior cervical discectomy and fusion: does the data support its use. *J Spine Surg*. 2018;4:227–232. https://doi.org/10.21037/jss.2018.05.10.
55. Poorman CE, Passias PG, Bianco KM, Boniello A, Yang S, Gerling MC. Effectiveness of postoperative wound drains in one- and two-level cervical spine fusions. *Int J Spine Surg*. 2014;8:34. https://doi.org/10.14444/1034.
56. Buttermann GR. Anterior cervical discectomy and fusion outcomes over 10 years. *Spine*. 2018;43:207–214. https://doi.org/10.1097/brs.0000000000002273.
57. Lowery GL, McDonough RF. The significance of hardware failure in anterior cervical plate fixation. *Spine*. 1998;23:181–186. https://doi.org/10.1097/00007632-199801150-00006.
58. Chen J, Wang X, Bai W, Shen X, Yuan W. Prevalence of heterotopic ossification after cervical total disc arthroplasty: a meta-analysis. *Eur Spine J*. 2012;21:674–680. https://doi.org/10.1007/s00586-011-2094-x.
59. Price RL, Coric D, Ray WZ. Cervical total disc replacement: Complications and complication avoidance. *Neurosurg Clin N Am*. 2021;32:473–481. https://doi.org/10.1016/j.nec.2021.05.006.
60. Heo DH, Lee DC, Oh JY, Park CK. Bone loss of vertebral bodies at the operative segment after cervical arthroplasty: a potential complication? *Neurosurg Focus*. 2017;42:E7. https://doi.org/10.3171/2016.10.focus16393.
61. Niu T, Hoffman H, Lu D. Cervical artificial disc extrusion after a paragliding accident. *Surg Neurol Int*. 2017;8:138. https://doi.org/10.4103/sni.sni_386_15.

12

Posterior Approach Related Complications

ANH X. LE, BOBBY K-B TAY, AND ALEXANDER C. WULFF

CHAPTER OUTLINE

Introduction

The posterior approach is utilized to address numerous cervical pathologies ranging from simple degenerative conditions to complex deformities. It is versatile and offers surgeons access to the posterior spine from the occipito-cervical junction to the cervicothoracic junction. Surgical procedures performed using this approach range from minimally invasive foraminotomies to corrective osteotomies and instrumented fusion. The posterior approach avoids many of the approach-related morbidities of the anterior approach to the cervical spine such as dysphagia and vocal dysfunction. Despite these advantages, there are several challenges associated with the posterior approach including patient positioning, more disruptive soft tissue dissection, challenges with hardware placement, and increased postoperative pain and infection risk compared the to the anterior approach.[1] The higher surgical complication rate seen with posterior approaches to the cervical spine is frequently cited as the main concern when an alternative approach is chosen to address a certain type of spinal pathology.

The incidence of complications associated with posterior cervical spinal fusion is between 15% and 25% while that of anterior cervical spinal fusion is approximately 7.5%.[2] Generally, complications of posterior cervical spinal fusion are classified into two broad categories, immediate and long-term complications.[1,3] The reported long-term complications typically involve the untoward mechanical effects of cervical spinal fusion. Therefore, it is out of the scope of this chapter and addressed in a different section of this book.

In this chapter, we will discuss different challenges arising at the time of surgery and in the early postoperative period. Specifically, potential complications will be divided into three different subcategories: positioning complications, intraoperative complications, and postoperative complications.

Positioning Complications

Although suspension of the head during surgery reduces the incidence of postoperative blindness,[4] the use of three-pronged head holders carries its own complications. Comparing skull thickness in adults versus pediatric patients, the average thickness of the pediatric skulls is 3 mm thinner in both anterolateral and posterolateral locations,[5] predisposing them to increased risk of pin penetration. Therefore, complications such as skull fractures, intracranial hematoma, epidural hematoma, cerebrospinal fluid leak, venous air embolism, pin site infections, head slippage, and scalp lacerations have been reported predominantly in pediatric patients.[6] However, Furuya and colleagues reported a case of skull fractures and epidural hematoma associated with head clamp application in an adult patient who was on chronic hemodialysis.[7]

Placing the patient in reverse Trendelenburg or the seated position may be the preferred positions for posterior cervical approaches. These positions improve the venous drainage from the head and neck, reducing blood loss during surgery.[8] The main complications of these positions are hypotension and increased risk of venous air embolism.[8,9]

Intraoperative Complications

The posterior cervical spine is divided into three regions: the occipito-cervical junction, the sub axial cervical spine, and the cervicothoracic junction. Each of these regions has its own unique anatomy presenting different challenges for exposure and for internal fixation. The incidence of hardware-related complications for posterior cervical spinal operations ranges from 6.7% to 30%.[10–13] Although the advent of spinal navigation can improve the reliability, accuracy, and safety of screw placement, awareness of potential problems is still paramount to avoid hardware-related complications.

Occipito-cervical Junction

In cases where cervical occipital fusion is required, occipital plates are the preferred method of a fixation of the occiput. During the exposure of the superior arch of C1 and the posterior occiput, vertebral artery injury and dural tears can occur. The location for plate placement is typically in the area between the superior and inferior nuchal lines. The torcula is located inside the cranium at the level of the external occipital protuberance. Inappropriate screw insertion can cause occlusion of the torcula, leading to catastrophic vascular injury and even death.[14] Therefore, it is recommended that the occipital plate should be placed just below the external occipital protuberance using unicortical screws. Because the thickness of the skull in different locations is variable, preoperative planning with imaging is advisable for screw length selection.[15] Inappropriate screw length can also cause dural leakage at the drill site. In such situation, placement of screw tamponades the leakage. Hwang and colleagues reported two cases of cerebral spinal fluid (CSF) leakage and two cases of vigorous venous bleeding in a series of 20 patients.[16]

Another significant potential complication is damage to the cerebellar cortex from screw placement. Injury to the parenchyma can result in suboccipital hematoma. Such lesion can be fatal due to the limited space in the posterior fossa. Therefore, urgent computed tomography (CT) should be performed if there is suspicion of suboccipital hematoma.[17] One case of cerebellar abscess was also reported after poor placement of an occipital plate.[18] This patient was successfully treated with sequential external ventricular and abscess drainage. Injury to the dominant vertebral artery is the most devastating vascular complication that can occur during the exposure or instrumentation of the occipito-cervical junction. Historically, incidence of vertebral artery injury during the posterior exposure to the cervical spine was 11.7%.[19] During normal posterior exposure, injury to the vertebral arteries can occur if dissection of the superior arch of C1 is extended more than 1 cm from the midline. However, variations of the course of the vertebral artery at the occipital vertebral junction, such as the presence of a persistent first intersegmental artery, can lead to vertebral artery injury during routine dissection of C2[20,21] (Fig. 12.1). Magnetic resonance angiography has demonstrated a persistent intersegmental artery in 3.2% of normal patients and an overall prevalence of vertebral anomalies of 5%.[22] The Cervical Spine Research Society reported a 0.07% overall incidence of vertebral artery injury during surgery, and 20% of those injuries were related to an anomalous course of the vertebral artery.[23] Therefore, dedicated preoperative vertebral artery imaging should be considered prior to approaching the cranio-cervical junction, especially if the variations in the bony anatomy of C1 and C2 are observed.

Instrumentation of the cranio-cervical junction for the purpose of fusion is done predominantly through the posterior approach. The unique anatomy of the atlas and axis, as well as its intricate relationship with important vessels, such as the vertebral arteries posteriorly and the carotid arteries anteriorly, present challenges to screw placement. The two most popular techniques for atlantoaxial fixation are Harms' C1 lateral mass and C2 isthmus screws and Magerl's transarticular screws.

In the cranio-cervical junction, the internal carotid arteries (ICAs) have an intimate relationship to the anterior aspect of C1 lateral masses. Hoh and colleagues studied the position of the ICA in association with C 1 lateral mass by CT scanning and magnetic resonant imaging.[24] They found that the left and right ICAs are directly located in front of C1 lateral masses in 58% and 74%, respectively. Medial to the C1 lateral mass, the presence of the carotid arteries occurs in 1% of the cases. The mean distance of the ICA from the anterior cortex is 3.5 mm ± 1.5 mm for the left and 3.9 mm ± 1.6 mm for the right. Therefore, bicortical screw purchase, by over drilling and tapping of the anterior cortex, may lead to ICA injury.

The hypoglossal nerve lies vertically and anterior to the lateral portion of the C1 lateral mass at the C1-C2 facet joints, and therefore it is subjected to similar mechanism of injury. The incidence of hypoglossal nerve injury by bicortical screw purchase is approximately 0.6%.[25] The presenting symptoms for hypoglossal nerve injury are dysphasia, dysarthria, and ipsilateral tongue deviation. Fortunately, these neurological deficits tend to resolve after 2 months without the need for hardware revision.[26]

To mitigate the risks to the vertebral artery during instrumentation of the atlas and axis, Harms popularized Goel's technique on atlantoaxial screw fixation. In 2001, they described an atlantoaxial stabilization technique involving fixation of the C1 lateral masses and C2 isthmus using polyaxial screws.[27] Although the risk of vertebral artery injury is less, it can still occur during instrumentation of C1 and C2 using this technique. The incidence of vertebral artery injury during C1 lateral mass screw placement has been reported to be 0.58%.[28] Mueller and colleagues reported a high number (17%) of inaccurately placed C2 isthmus screws, seen on postoperative CT.[29] 44.6% of the errant screws breached the vertebral artery foramen. However, they did not cause injury to the vertebral arteries.

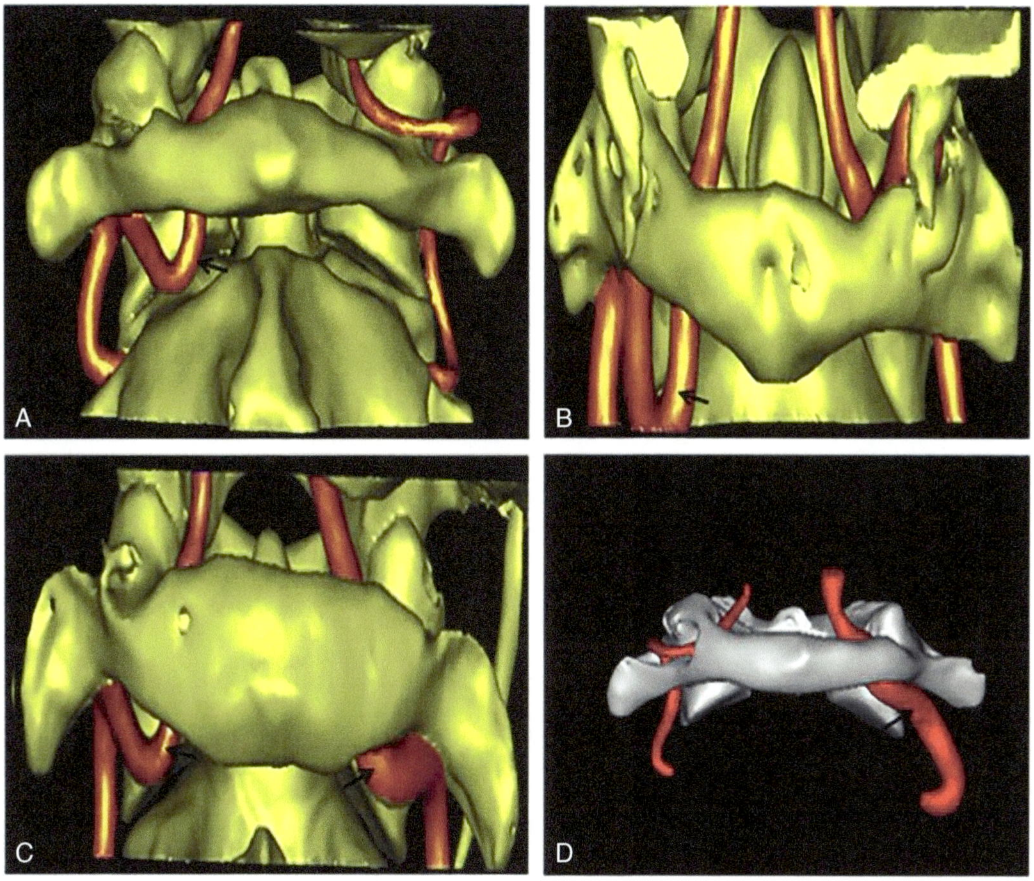

• **Fig. 12.1** Different variations of persistent first intersegmental artery (PFIA). The black arrows indicate different variations of PFIA. (A) Dorsal view of left unilateral PFIA. (B) Anterior view of right unilateral PFIA. (C) Dorsal view of bilateral PFIA. (D) Dorsal view of right dominant PFIA.

The posterior inferior cerebellar artery and the internal carotid artery are also at risk during placement of C1 lateral mass screws. The posterior inferior cerebellar artery (PICA) originates intracranially from the first branch of the vertebral artery. An anomalous PICA can originate extracranially from the foramen magnum in 5% to 20% of cases. In 1% of these anomalies, the origin of the PICA occurs at C1-C2, putting it at risk during screw placement. Lateral medullary syndrome has been reported in two cases after C1 lateral mass screw placement caused damage to an anomalous PICA.[30,31] Both patients were treated conservatively and achieved full recovery after 2 weeks.

Basede on the C1 anatomic discussion above, the proximity of the internal carotid artery and the hypoglossal nerve to C1 lateral mass make bicortical placement of C1 lateral mass screws dangerous to the ICA and hypoglossal nerve. Therefore, Murakami and colleagues recommended a 10 degree medial trajectory to avoid these complications.[32]

Another challenge to the Harms' technique is poor visualization of the C1 lateral mass due to the presence of the C2 nerve root and its surrounding venous plexus. It occupies the dorsal aspect of C1-C2 facet joint and obscures important landmarks for correct screw placement. The C2 nerve innervates the rectus capitis anterior, the rectus capitis lateralis muscles, and provides sensory branches to the trapezius. Therefore, damage to the C2 nerve root can cause occipital numbness and neuralgia. The incidence of occipital numbness ranges anywhere from 6.7% to 100% after atlantoaxial fusion.[33] However, C2 neuralgia is more problematic in postoperative patient management. For this reason, intraoperative resection of the C2 nerve root was implemented and studied.

Intraoperative neurolysis of C2 has been found to decrease the incidence of C1 screw malposition, intraoperative blood loss and operative time[34–37] (Fig. 12.2). Badhiwala and colleagues reported no difference in the incidence of postoperative C2 neuralgia in the resection and preservation groups.[33] Yamagata and colleagues[38] also reported no cases of C2 neuropathic pain after C2 nerve root resection. However, in a post hoc analysis, Yeom and colleagues reported 29% of patients complained of increased neuropathic pain after C2 resection.[34] Four out of seven patients continued to require daily pain medication 80 months after surgery. In the C2 nerve root preservation group, only 10% of patients reported increased postoperative neuropathic pain that subsided in all patients at 1-year follow-up. The

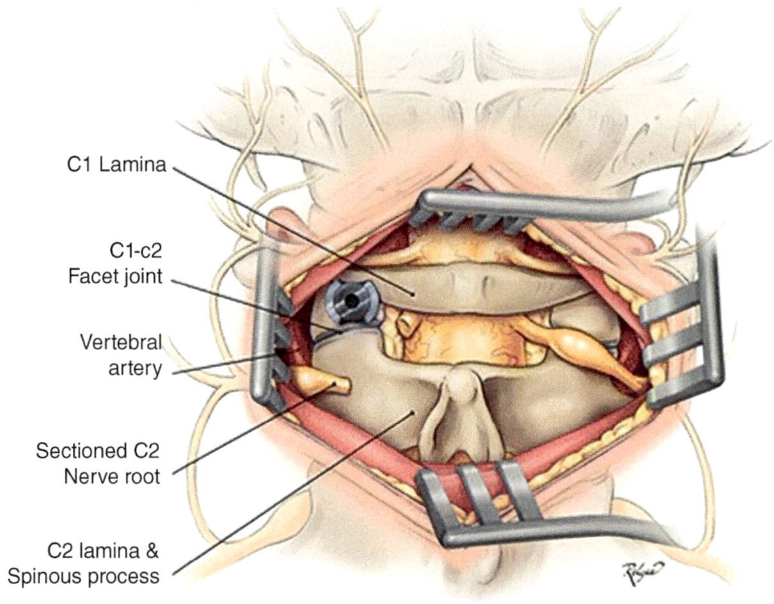

• **Fig. 12.2** Routine sectioning of the C2 nerve root and ganglion for placement of C1 lateral mass screws. (From Klepinowski T, Żyłka N, Pala B, Poncyljusz W, Sagan L: Prevalence of high-riding vertebral arteries and narrow C2 pedicles among Central-European population: a computed tomography-based study, *Neurosurg Rev.* 2021;44(6):3277–3282. https://doi.org/10.1007/s10143-021-01493-6.)

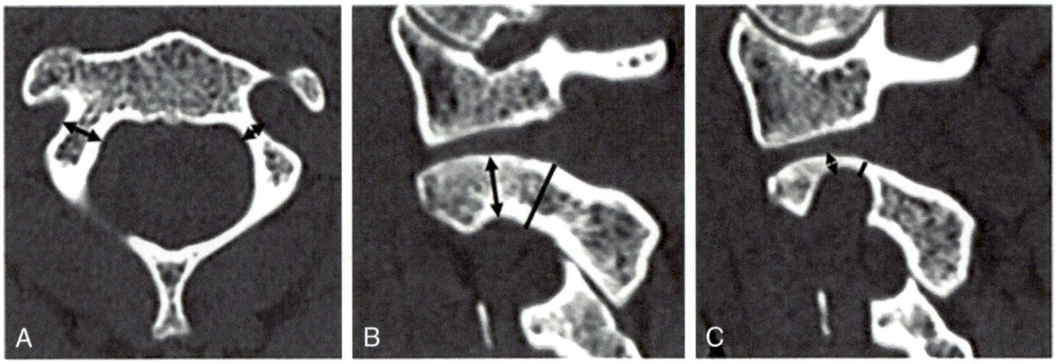

• **Fig. 12.3** Different variations of vertebral artery in the intertransverse foramen of C2 pedicles. (a) Variations of C2 pedicle width; normal pedicle width on the *right side*; narrow pedicle width on the *left side*. (b) Normal C2 isthmus height (solid line) and C2 internal height (arrow line). (c) High-riding vertebral artery with short C2 isthmus height (solid line) and short C2 internal height (arrow line).

controversial debate surrounding preservation versus sacrifice of C2 nerve root during C1 lateral mass screw placement continues to exist.

Placement of transarticular screws requires a steep trajectory putting the vertebral artery at risk as it exits from the transverse foramen of C2 and pursues an almost vertical course as far as the transverse process of the axis. In 18% of cases, transarticular screws cannot be safely placed due to the presence of high riding vertebral artery[35,36](Fig. 12.3). The reported incidence of vertebral artery injury associated with transarticular screw placement ranges anywhere from 2.4% to 8.2%%.[37,39–41] The unilateral injury to the vertebral artery appears to be well tolerated in the majority of the subjects as only 3.7% of those patients exhibited neurological deficits (symptoms related to cerebrovascular accident). However, bilateral vertebral artery injury can be fatal. The reported mortality rate of 0.1% associated with the placement of transarticular screws is related to one case of bilateral vertebral artery injuries.[40] In addition to vertebral artery injuries, other associated complications with transarticular screw placement include injuries to the internal carotid artery and the hypoglossal nerve (Fig. 12.4).

Subaxial Cervical Spine

In the subaxial cervical spine, the vertebral arteries are located ventral to the lateral mass, reducing the risks of vertebral artery injury during dissection. However, unusual

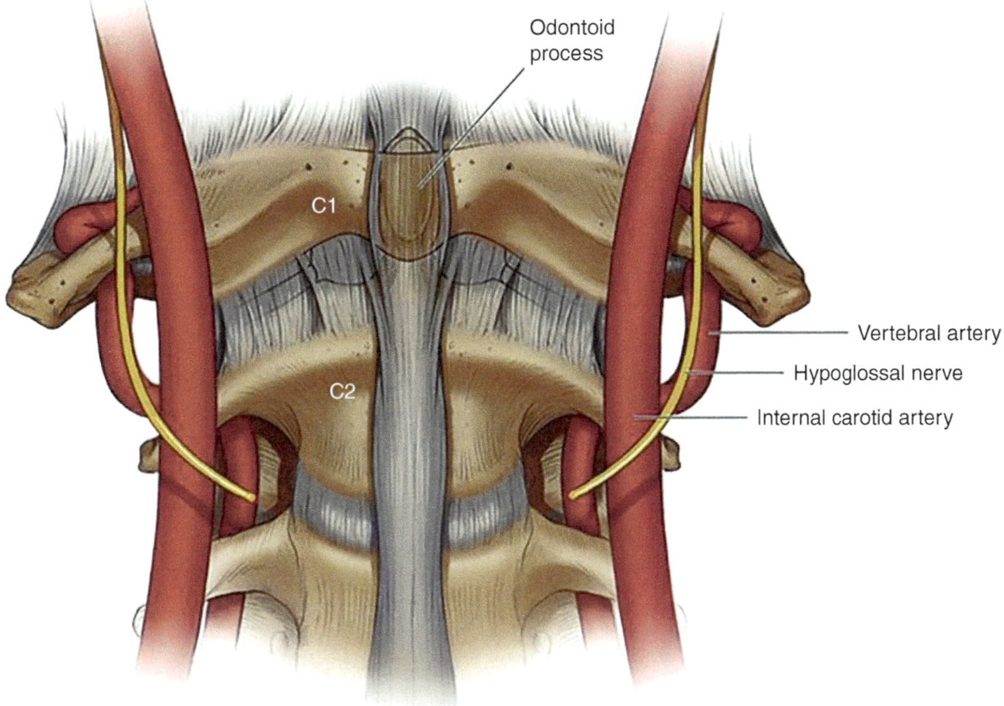

• **Fig. 12.4** Relationship of the hypoglossal nerve, vertebral artery and internal carotid artery to C1 and C2 vertebral bodies. (From Morrey BF, Morrey MC, editors: *Relevant surgical exposures: master techniques in orthopaedic surgery*, Philadelphia, 2007, Lippincott, Williams & Wilkins.)

course of the vertebral artery in relationship to the nerve root has been reported in the literature. In a cadaveric dissection study, the left vertebral artery was found passing underneath the left C5 nerve root in the fourth intertransverse space.[42] This finding raises concern for potential injury of the vertebral artery during lamino-foraminotomy. Ye and colleagues also reported a single case where the vertebral artery was injured during wide subaxial exposure.[43] Resection of the lateral mass was required to achieve control of the bleeding from the injured vessels.

The two most popular techniques to instrument the posterior cervical spine are lateral mass screws and cervical pedicle screws. The lateral mass screw fixation was first introduced by Roy-Camille in 1964. Currently the three commonly used techniques for lateral mass screw placement are the Roy-Camille technique, the Magerl technique, and the An technique. Although the starting points on the lateral mass are slightly different between the later two techniques, they share the same outward trajectory reducing the risks of injury to the spinal cord and the vertebral artery. The An technique is a modification of the Magerl technique. In the An technique, the entry point for screw insertion is located 1 mm medial to the midpoint of the lateral mass. Coe and colleagues[44] performed a systematic review of the literature and reported low complication rates from lateral mass screw insertion. The incidence of nerve root injury was 1%, and there was no vertebral artery injury.[44] In two other studies, there was no injury to the vertebral artery, exiting nerve root, or spinal cord associated with placement of 2687 lateral mass screws.[45,46]

In cases where the lateral masses are deficient (comminuted fracture, metastatic disease, osteoporosis, or revision surgery), cervical pedicle screws offer another alternative to gain fixation. In 1994, Abumi and colleagues introduced the technique of cervical pedicle screw placement using landmarks with C-arm guidance.[47] Since Abumi et al.'s introduction of the cervical pedicle screw, several modifications were developed to reduce the risk of vertebral artery and spinal cord injury. These modifications include using different surface landmarks, exposing the medial border of the pedicle through a laminotomy and employing intraoperative navigation.

The general trajectory of pedicle screws is lateral to medial, placing the vertebral artery, nerve roots, and spinal cord at risk for injury. Lateral breach can damage the vertebral artery. Medial breach can injure the spinal cord. Superior or inferior breach can injure the exiting nerve roots. The reported incidence of pedicle screw perforation ranges from 6.7% to 30%.[10] In most of these cases, the perforations occur at the lateral wall because it is the thinnest part of the pedicle. In addition, the spinal level also plays an important role in correct placement. Correct screw placement was found in 91% at C6 and only 48% at C4.[10] Differences in pedicle anatomy are responsible for these findings. The pedicles are smallest at C3 and C4 and have a high horizontal angulation. Despite high perforation rate, the incidence of neurovascular injury is relatively low. Out of 350 patients in 5 different studies, only 2 patients had vertebral artery injury and 5 had nerve root injury.[10] Patients with nerve root injury only exhibited temporary neurological deficits and were treated with conservative management. There was no cerebral ischemia or neurological deficits reported in patients with vertebral artery injury. In addition, no spinal cord injury was reported. The low rate of adverse clinical presentation associated with screw breach may be explained by the unique anatomy of the subaxial cervical spine. The vertebral artery only occupies 35% of the foramen transversarium and the distance between the vertebral artery to the lateral wall increases from C2-C7.[48] The exiting nerve roots occupy one-half of the inferior portion of the neuroforamen and lie nearly opposed to the superior part of the caudal pedicle.[49] The use of computer navigation to assist cervical pedicle screw placement has been shown to reduce the rate of perforation. Ludwig and colleagues reported 65% pedicle breach using surface landmarks alone, 39.5% with laminal foraminotomy and 10.5 % with computer navigation.[50] More recently, the reported range of screw breach for surface landmarks technique is from 3% to 8.6% and 1.2% to 3% for computer-navigated technique.[51,52]

Cervicothoracic Junction

In multilevel posterior cervical constructs, C7 is often the most caudal point of fixation and is, therefore, the site of highest stress concentration. The transitional anatomy of C7, from cervical to thoracic spine, presents challenges to placement of lateral mass screws. The lateral mass of C7 is thinner than those of other subaxial cervical vertebra. The C7 spinal nerve is relatively larger and lies closer to the anterior aspect of the lateral mass.[53] These anatomical features adversely affect the pullout strength of C7 lateral mass screw and increase the risk of C7 spinal nerve injury. Despite these concerns, a study has shown a low rate of screw loosening and high rate of fusion associated with C7 lateral masses and posterior cervical fusion.[54]

C7 pedicle screws are biomechanically more advantageous than C7 lateral mass screws. Their pullout strength is statistically much higher. Anatomically, the pedicles of C7 are relatively larger and the vertebral artery is present in the C7 transverse foramen in only 10% to 15% of cases. Clifton and colleagues reported an accuracy rate of 89% using a freehand technique.[55] Out of 36 placed screws only 4 presented with minor breach (less than 2 mm). There were no vascular or neurological complications associated with these breaches.

Intraoperative Dural Injury and Cerebral Spinal Fluid Leakage

The incidence of intraoperative dural tears is approximately 1%. Risk factors for intraoperative dural injuries are: older age, ossification of the posterior longitudinal ligament, cervical deformity, rheumatoid arthritis, larger number of surgical levels, corpectomy or revision laminectomy.[56] Direct suture repair, augmented repair with dural substitute materials (fat, muscle tissue, or fascia graft), and use of sealant/patch are common methods used to achieve dural closure. Lumbar drain may be used to reduce CSF pressure when watertight repair is not possible intraoperatively. Approximately 10% to 12% of the cases require additional treatment related to persistent CSF leakage beyond the index surgery.[57,58] In 93% of the cases, there are no associated clinical sequelae after successful repair.[57] However, severe complications from cervical dural tears have been documented. These complications include fistula formation, meningitis or life-threatening, intracranial pneumocephalus, subarachnoid hemorrhage, and acute subdural hematoma.[59] To avoid these potential severe complications, intraoperative dural tears should be identified and repaired expeditiously.

Postoperative Wound Complications

The reported incidence of wound infection within 30 days after surgery is between 2% to 10%. The rate of superficial infections and deep infections are similar, ranging from 1.5% to 2%.[60,61] Staphylococcus aureus, Staphylococcus epidermidis, and group A streptococcus are typical bacteria found in acute postoperative wound infections.[1] Less virulent bacteria such as Propionibacterium and gram-negative bacilli are found in latent wound infections.

Risk factors associated with postoperative wound infection are obesity, chronic steroid use, and diabetes. In obese patients, large body habitus creates challenges to surgical dissection requiring a longer incision and increased surgical time. The ratio of fat thickness to total thickness from the lamina to the skin was found to be associated with increased risk of infection.[62] Prolonged retraction negatively affects tissue perfusion causing tissue necrosis and wound infection. Chronic steroid use causes immunosuppression and impairs patients' immune system to fight pathogens. Specifically, patients with rheumatoid arthritis are at increased risk for postoperative wound infection after posterior cervical spinal fusion.[63]

In cases of postoperative wound infection, surgical wound debridement and prolonged systemic antibiotic therapy are typically required. These additional treatments significantly increase the cost of posterior cervical spinal fusion. Therefore, multiple strategies have been employed to reduce the rate of postoperative wound infection. Using alcohol foam to prepare the skin and placement of a superficial drain where the subcutaneous fat exceeds 2 cm have reduced the rate of wound infection to 0.3%. In addition, local application of vancomycin powder prior to wound closure may have significant effect. In 195 cases, use of vancomycin powder was found to reduce the rate of wound infection to zero.[63]

Postoperative C5 Palsy

The incidence of postoperative neurological deficits following posterior cervical fusion is approximately 8.5%.[64] The most common deficit is C5 palsy affecting 6.7% to 9.5% of patients following posterior cervical spinal fusion.[65] The physical manifestations of C5 palsy are weakness of biceps brachii and deltoid muscles. These patients may or may not have shoulder pain and sensory deficits.

The etiology of this complication is still unclear at this point. However, there are several proposed mechanisms that could account for C5 palsy. They range from the tethering effect on the C5 nerve caused by the posterior drift back of the spinal cord after decompression to reperfusion injury after spinal cord ischemia. Posterior drifting of the spinal cord can occur after wide laminectomies. In cases where intervertebral foraminal stenosis is present, posterior drifting of the spinal cord can further exacerbate this chronic compression. Perioperative intervertebral foraminal stenosis, where the diameter of the foramen is less than 2.3 mm, increases the risk of C5 palsy by threefold.[66] In addition, the presence of ossification of posterior longitudinal ligament (OPLL) can cause tethering of the nerve root after decompression.[67] Although there are recent studies that argue against the theory of posterior drifting of the spinal cord as the cause of C5 palsy, preventative foraminotomy is still being recommended to reduce this complication.[68,69]

Fortunately, the majority of patients with C5 palsy recover fully from this complication. Approximately 96% of patients with minor palsies and 71% with severe palsies achieve full recovery.[1] However, time to recovery is highly variable, ranging from 48 hours to 41 months.[65] In cases of prolonged recovery, C5 palsy impairs the patients' capacity for self-care and increases the overall cost of treatment per patient.[70]

Conclusion

Although the posterior approach to the cervical spine is versatile in treating numerous cervical pathologies, the complex vertebral anatomy, its intimate relationship to the vertebral arteries, and neurological structures increases the risk of complications. Vertebral artery anomalies frequently occur in the upper cervical spine; to that end, dedicated vertebral artery imaging prior to surgery is highly recommended.

The incidence of pedicle breach is quite high with subaxial pedicle screw placement. Fortunately, the associated neurovascular symptoms remain low. Computer-navigated screw placement has been shown to decrease the rate of pedicle breach.

Obesity and chronic steroid use are major factors that increase the rate of postoperative wound infection. Even though most cases of postoperative C5 palsy recover fully, it remains a dreaded and costly complication. Prophylactic foraminotomy may reduce the risk of C5 palsy.

References

1. Badiee RK, Mayer R, Pennicooke B, Chou D, Mummaneni PV, Tan LA. Complications following posterior cervical decompression and fusion: a review of incidence, risk factors, and prevention strategies. *J Spine Surg*. 2020;6(1):323–333. https://doi.org/10.21037/jss.2019.11.01.
2. Campbell PG, Yadla S, Malone J, et al. Early complications related to approach in cervical spine surgery: Single-center prospective study. *World Neurosurg*. 2010;74(2-3):363–368. https://doi.org/10.1016/j.wneu.2010.05.034.
3. Memtsoudis SG, Hughes A, Ma Y, Chiu YL, Sama AA, Girardi FP. Increased in-hospital complications after primary posterior versus primary anterior cervical fusion. *Clin Orthop Relat Res*. 2011;469(3):649–657. https://doi.org/10.1007/s11999-010-1549-4.
4. Baerts WDM, de Lange JJ, Booij LHDJ, Broere G. Complications of the Mayfield skull clamp. *Anesthesiology*. 1984;61(4):460. https://doi.org/10.1097/00000542-198410000-00017.
5. Chavasiri C, Chavasiri S. The thickness of skull at the halo pin insertion site. *Spine*. 2011;36(22):1819–1823. https://doi.org/10.1097/BRS.0b013e3181d3cfa3.
6. Lee M, Rezai AR, Chou J. Depressed skull fractures in children secondary to skull clamp fixation devices. *Pediatr Neurosurg*. 1994;21(3):174–178. https://doi.org/10.1159/000120830.
7. Furuya T, Yamazaki M, Nemoto T, Okawa A, Ohtori S. Skull fracture and epidural hematoma caused by use of a Mayfield skull clamp in an adult patient with chronic hemodialysis: a case report. *J Med Case Rep*. 2021;15:154. https://doi.org/10.1186/s13256-021-02776-8.
8. Knight DJ, Mahajan RP. Patient positioning in anaesthesia. *Continuing Education in Anaesthesia Critical Care & Pain*. 2004;4(5):160–163. https://doi.org/10.1093/bjaceaccp/mkh044.
9. Grinberg F, Slaughter TF, McGrath BJ. Probable venous air embolism associated with removal of the Mayfield skull clamp. *Anesth Analg*. 1995;80(5):1049–1050.
10. Ghori A, Le HV, Makanji H, Cha T. Posterior fixation techniques in the subaxial cervical spine. *Cureus*. 2015;7(10):e338. https://doi.org/10.7759/cureus.338.
11. Nakashima H, Yukawa Y, Imagama S, et al. Complications of cervical pedicle screw fixation for nontraumatic lesions: a multicenter study of 84 patients. *J Neurosurg Spine*. 2012;16(3):238–247. https://doi.org/10.3171/2011.11.SPINE11102.
12. Shimokawa N, Takami T. Surgical safety of cervical pedicle screw placement with computer navigation system. *Neurosurg Rev*. 2017;40(2):251–258. https://doi.org/10.1007/s10143-016-0757-0.
13. Soliman MAR, Khan S, Ruggiero N, et al. Complications associated with subaxial placement of pedicle screws versus lateral mass screws in the cervical spine: systematic review and meta-analysis comprising 1768 patients and 8636 screws. *Neurosurg Rev*. 2022;45(3):1941–1950. https://doi.org/10.1007/s10143-022-01750-2.
14. Joaquim AF, Osorio JA, Riew KD. Occipitocervical fixation: General considerations and surgical technique. *Global Spine J*. 2020;10(5):647–656. https://doi.org/10.1177/2192568219877878.
15. Batista UC, Joaquim AF, Fernandes YB, Mathias RN, Ghizoni E, Tedeschi H. Computed tomography evaluation of the normal craniocervical junction craniometry in 100 asymptomatic patients. *Neurosurg Focus*. 2015;38(4):E5. https://doi.org/10.3171/2015.1.FOCUS14642.
16. Hwang SW, Gressot LV, Chern JJ, Relyea K, Jea A. Complications of occipital screw placement for occipitocervical fusion in children: Clinical article. *J Neurosurg Pediatr*. 2012;9(6):586–593. https://doi.org/10.3171/2012.2.PEDS11497.

17. Macki M, Hamilton T, Pawloski J, Chang V. Occipital fixation techniques and complications. *J Spine Surg.* 2020;6(1):145–155. https://doi.org/10.21037/jss.2019.12.01.
18. Lee CC, Liu YT. Occipitocervical fusion complicated with cerebellar abscess: a case report. *BMC Musculoskelet Disord.* 2020;21(1):129. https://doi.org/10.1186/s12891-020-3157-0.
19. Hsu WK, Kannan A, Mai HT, et al. Epidemiology and outcomes of vertebral artery injury in 16582 cervical spine surgery patients: An AOSpine North America multicenter study. *Global Spine J.* 2017;7(1_suppl):21S–27S. https://doi.org/10.1177/2192568216686753.
20. Molinari RW, Chimenti PC, Molinari R, Gruhn W. Vertebral Artery Injury during Routine Posterior Cervical Exposure: Case Reports and Review of Literature. *Global Spine J.* 2015;5(6): 528–532. https://doi.org/10.1055/s-0035-1566225.
21. Zhang H, Chai W, Wang S, Wang Y, Li H. Persistent first intersegmental artery (PFIA) visualized by three-dimensional computed tomography angiography in Chinese population. *Int J Surg.* 2018;52:233–236. https://doi.org/10.1016/j.ijsu.2018.02.038.
22. Uchino A, Saito N, Takahashi M, Kurita H, Ishihara S. Cerebral arterial variations associated with Moyamoya disease diagnosed by MR angiography. *Neuroradiol J.* 2014;27(6):697–701. https://doi.org/10.15274/NRJ-2014-10093.
23. Lunardini DJ, Eskander MS, Even JL, et al. Vertebral artery injuries in cervical spine surgery. *Spine J.* 2014;14(8):1520–1525. https://doi.org/10.1016/j.spinee.2013.09.016.
24. Hoh DJ, Maya M, Jung A, Ponrartana S, Lauryssen CL. Anatomical relationship of the internal carotid artery to C-1: clinical implications for screw fixation of the atlas. *J Neurosurg Spine.* 2008;8(4):335–340. https://doi.org/10.3171/SPI/2008/8/4/335.
25. Grob D, Jeanneret B, Aebi M, Markwalder TM. Atlanto-axial fusion with transarticular screw fixation. *J Bone Joint Surg Br.* 1991;73(6):972–976. https://doi.org/10.1302/0301-620X.73B6.1955447.
26. Hong JT, Lee SW, Son BC, Sung JH, Kim IS, Park CK. Hypoglossal nerve palsy after posterior screw placement on the C-1 lateral mass. Case report. *J Neurosurg Spine.* 2006;5(1):83–85. https://doi.org/10.3171/spi.2006.5.1.83.
27. Harms J, Melcher RP. Posterior C1-C2 fusion with polyaxial screw and rod fixation. *Spine (Phila Pa 1976).* 2001;26(22):2467–2471. https://doi.org/10.1097/00007632-200111150-00014.
28. Lall R, Patel NJ, Resnick DK. A review of complications associated with craniocervical fusion surgery. *Neurosurgery.* 2010; 67(5):1396–1402; discussion 1402–1403. https://doi.org/10.1227/NEU.0b013e3181f1ec73.
29. Mueller CA, Roesseler L, Podlogar M, Kovacs A, Kristof RA. Accuracy and complications of transpedicular C2 screw placement without the use of spinal navigation. *Eur Spine J.* 2010;19(5): 809–814. https://doi.org/10.1007/s00586-010-1291-3.
30. Nassr AN, Swann PP, Huston J, Abdelfatah MM, Rose PS, Currier BL. Aberrant posterior inferior cerebellar artery injury with C1 lateral mass screw placement: a case report and review of the literature. *Spine J.* 2014;14(9):e7–e14. https://doi.org/10.1016/j.spinee.2014.02.024.
31. Won D, Lee JM, Park IS, et al. Posterior inferior cerebellar artery infarction originating at C1-2 after C1-2 fusion. *Korean J Neurotrauma.* 2019;15(2):192–198. https://doi.org/10.13004/kjnt.2019.15.e27.
32. Murakami S, Mizutani J, Fukuoka M, et al. Relationship between screw trajectory of C1 lateral mass screw and internal carotid artery. *Spine (Phila Pa 1976).* 2008;33(24):2581–2585. https://doi.org/10.1097/BRS.0b013e318186b2fd.
33. Badhiwala JH, Nassiri F, Witiw CD, Mansouri A, Almenawer SA, Fehlings MG. Does transection of the C2 nerve roots during C1 lateral mass screw placement for atlantoaxial fixation result in a superior outcome?: A systematic review of the literature and meta-analysis. *Spine (Phila Pa 1976).* 2017;42(18):E1067–E1076. https://doi.org/10.1097/BRS.0000000000002069.
34. Yeom JS, Buchowski JM, Kim HJ, Chang BS, Lee CK, Riew KD. Postoperative occipital neuralgia with and without C2 nerve root transection during atlantoaxial screw fixation: a post-hoc comparative outcome study of prospectively collected data. *Spine J.* 2013;13(7):786–795. https://doi.org/10.1016/j.spinee.2013.04.006.
35. Dunn R, Stander H. Atlanto-axial fusion: Magerl transarticular versus Harms instrumentation techniques. *SA Orthop J.* 2014;13:31–34.
36. Klepinowski T, Żyłka N, Pala B, Poncyljusz W, Sagan L. Prevalence of high-riding vertebral arteries and narrow C2 pedicles among Central-European population: a computed tomography-based study. *Neurosurg Rev.* 2021;44(6):3277–3282. https://doi.org/10.1007/s10143-021-01493-6.
37. Gluf WM, Brockmeyer DL. Atlantoaxial transarticular screw fixation: a review of surgical indications, fusion rate, complications, and lessons learned in 67 pediatric patients. *J Neurosurg Spine.* 2005;2(2):164–169. https://doi.org/10.3171/spi.2005.2.2.0164.
38. Yamagata T, Takami T, Naito K, Ohata K C2 nerve root resection to achieve safe and wide exposure of lateral atlantoaxial joints in posterior C1-2 instrumented fixation: technical note. Neurol Med Chir (Tokyo). 2013;53(12):914–919. https://doi.org/10.2176/nmc.tn2012-0288.
39. Barsa P, Buchvald P, Suchomel P, Lukás R. [Traumatic spondylolisthesis of L5-S1]. *Acta Chir Orthop Traumatol Cech.* 2003; 70(2):121–125.
40. Wright NM, Lauryssen C. Vertebral artery injury in C1-2 transarticular screw fixation: results of a survey of the AANS/CNS section on disorders of the spine and peripheral nerves. American Association of Neurological Surgeons/Congress of Neurological Surgeons. *J Neurosurg.* 1998;88(4):634–640. https://doi.org/10.3171/jns.1998.88.4.0634.
41. Chen Q, Brahimaj BC, Khanna R, et al. Posterior atlantoaxial fusion: a comprehensive review of surgical techniques and relevant vascular anomalies. *J Spine Surg.* 2020;6(1):164–180. https://doi.org/10.21037/jss.2020.03.05.
42. Nourbakhsh A, Yang J, Ziran B, Garges KJ. An unusual course of the vertebral artery posterior to the nerve root in the intertransverse space: a cadaveric study. *Patient Saf Surg.* 2015;9:19. https://doi.org/10.1186/s13037-015-0072-7.
43. Ye JY, Ayyash OM, Eskander MS, Kang JD. Control of the vertebral artery from a posterior approach: a technical report. *Spine J.* 2014;14(6):e37–41. https://doi.org/10.1016/j.spinee.2013.11.059.
44. Coe JD, Vaccaro AR, Dailey AT, et al. Lateral mass screw fixation in the cervical spine: a systematic literature review. *J Bone Joint Surg Am.* 2013;95(23):2136–2143. https://doi.org/10.2106/JBJS.L.01522.
45. Sekhon LHS. Posterior cervical lateral mass screw fixation: analysis of 1026 consecutive screws in 143 patients. *J Spinal Disord Tech.* 2005;18(4):297–303. https://doi.org/10.1097/01.bsd.0000166640.23448.09.
46. Katonis P, Papadakis SA, Galanakos S, et al. Lateral mass screw complications: analysis of 1662 screws. *J Spinal Disord Tech.* 2011;24(7):415–420. https://doi.org/10.1097/BSD.0b013e3182024c06.

47. Abumi K, Itoh H, Taneichi H, Kaneda K. Transpedicular screw fixation for traumatic lesions of the middle and lower cervical spine: description of the techniques and preliminary report. *J Spinal Disord.* 1994;7(1):19–28. https://doi.org/10.1097/00002517-199407010-00003.
48. Tomasino A, Parikh K, Koller H, et al. The vertebral artery and the cervical pedicle: morphometric analysis of a critical neighborhood. *J Neurosurg Spine.* 2010;13(1):52–60. https://doi.org/10.3171/2010.3.SPINE09231.
49. Xu R, Kang A, Ebraheim NA, Yeasting RA. Anatomic relation between the cervical pedicle and the adjacent neural structures. *Spine (Phila Pa 1976).* 1999;24(5):451–454. https://doi.org/10.1097/00007632-199903010-00008.
50. Ludwig SC, Kramer DL, Balderston RA, Vaccaro AR, Foley KF, Albert TJ. Placement of pedicle screws in the human cadaveric cervical spine: comparative accuracy of three techniques. *Spine (Phila Pa 1976).* 2000;25(13):1655–1667. https://doi.org/10.1097/00007632-200007010-00009.
51. Richter M, Cakir B, Schmidt R. Cervical pedicle screws: conventional versus computer-assisted placement of cannulated screws. *Spine (Phila Pa 1976).* 2005;30(20):2280–2287. https://doi.org/10.1097/01.brs.0000182275.31425.cd.
52. Kotani Y, Abumi K, Ito M, Minami A. Improved accuracy of computer-assisted cervical pedicle screw insertion. *J Neurosurg.* 2003;99(3 Suppl):257–263. https://doi.org/10.3171/spi.2003.99.3.0257.
53. Ebraheim N. Posterior lateral mass screw fixation: Anatomic and radiographic considerations. *University Pa Orthop J.* 1999;12:66–72.
54. Zhang C, Zhou Q, Arnold P. Safety and efficacy of lateral mass screws at C7 in the treatment of cervical degenerative disease. *Surg Neurol Int.* 2017;8(1):218. https://doi.org/10.4103/sni.sni_6_17.
55. Clifton W, Louie C, Williams DB, Damon A, Dove C, Pichelmann M. Safety and accuracy of the freehand placement of C7 pedicle screws in cervical and cervicothoracic constructs. *Cureus.* 11(8):e5304. https://doi.org/10.7759/cureus.5304.
56. O'Neill KR, Neuman BJ, Peters C, Riew KD. Risk factors for dural tears in the cervical. *spine. Spine.* 2014;39(17):E1015. https://doi.org/10.1097/BRS.0000000000000416.
57. O'Neill KR, Fehlings MG, Mroz TE, et al. A multicenter study of the presentation, treatment, and outcomes of cervical dural tears. *Global Spine J.* 2017;7(1 Suppl):58S–63S. https://doi.org/10.1177/2192568216688186.
58. Hannallah D, Lee J, Khan M, Donaldson WF, Kang JD. Cerebrospinal fluid leaks following cervical spine surgery. *J Bone Joint Surg Am.* 2008;90(5):1101–1105. https://doi.org/10.2106/JBJS.F.01114.
59. Al-Gethami H, Cenic A, Kachur E. Seizures following cervical laminectomy and lateral mass fusion: case report and review of the literature. *J Spine Surg.* 2021;7(3):445–455. https://doi.org/10.21037/jss-20-642.
60. Badiee RK, Chan AK, Rivera J, et al. Preoperative narcotic use, impaired ambulation status, and increased intraoperative blood loss are independent risk factors for complications following posterior cervical laminectomy and fusion surgery. *Neurospine.* 2019;16(3):548–557. https://doi.org/10.14245/ns.1938198.099.
61. Leckie S, Yoon ST, Isaacs R, et al. Perioperative complications of cervical spine surgery: Analysis of a prospectively gathered database through the Association for Collaborative Spinal Research. *Global Spine J.* 2016;6(7):640–649. https://doi.org/10.1055/s-0035-1570089.
62. Mehta AI, Babu R, Sharma R, et al. Thickness of subcutaneous fat as a risk factor for infection in cervical spine fusion surgery. *J Bone Joint Surg Am.* 2013;95(4):323–328. https://doi.org/10.2106/JBJS.L.00225.
63. Pahys JM, Pahys JR, Cho SK, et al. Methods to decrease postoperative infections following posterior cervical spine surgery. *J Bone Joint Surg Am.* 2013;95(6):549–554. https://doi.org/10.2106/JBJS.K.00756.
64. Dayananda S, Mehta A, Agarwal N, Nwachuku EL, Hamilton DK, Thirumala PD. Impact of perioperative neurologic deficits on clinical outcomes after posterior cervical fusion. *World Neurosurg.* 2018;119:e250–e261. https://doi.org/10.1016/j.wneu.2018.07.126.
65. Pan FM, Wang SJ, Ma B, Wu DS. C5 nerve root palsy after posterior cervical spine surgery. *J Orthop Surg (Hong Kong).* 2017;25(1): https://doi.org/10.1177/2309499016684502.2309499016684502.
66. Nakashima H, Imagama S, Yukawa Y, et al. Multivariate analysis of C-5 palsy incidence after cervical posterior fusion with instrumentation: Clinical article. *J Neurosurg Spine.* 2012;17(2):103–110. https://doi.org/10.3171/2012.4.SPINE11255.
67. Chen Y, Chen D, Wang X, Guo Y, He Z. C5 palsy after laminectomy and posterior cervical fixation for ossification of posterior longitudinal ligament. *J Spinal Disord Tech.* 2007;20(7):533–535. https://doi.org/10.1097/BSD.0b013e318042b655.
68. Pennington Z, Lubelski D, Westbroek EM, et al. Spinal cord float back is not an independent predictor of postoperative C5 palsy in patients undergoing posterior cervical decompression. *Spine J.* 2020;20(2):266–275. https://doi.org/10.1016/j.spinee.2019.09.017.
69. Ohashi M, Yamazaki A, Watanabe K, Katsumi K, Shoji H. Two-year clinical and radiological outcomes of open-door cervical laminoplasty with prophylactic bilateral C4-C5 foraminotomy in a prospective study. *Spine (Phila Pa 1976).* 2014;39(9):721–727. https://doi.org/10.1097/BRS.0000000000000251.
70. Miller JA, Lubelski D, Alvin MD, Benzel EC, Mroz TE. C5 palsy after posterior cervical decompression and fusion: cost and quality-of-life implications. *Spine J.* 2014;14(12):2854–2860. https://doi.org/10.1016/j.spinee.2014.03.038.

13

Long-Term Complications following Cervical Spine Surgery

MITCHELL S. FOURMAN, AND HAN JO KIM

CHAPTER OUTLINE

Introduction

More than 10% of patients require a revision procedure greater than 10 years after cervical spine surgery.[1] The meta-analysis by Loidolt et al.[2] reported acute/chronic adverse event rates following anterior cervical discectomy and fusion (ACDF) and cervical disc replacement (CDR) of 98.7% and 98.4%, respectively, which included rates of adjacent segment degeneration (ASD) > 20%, neurologic deficits > 40%, and chronic pain > 50%. Hirvonen et al.[3,4] published two works analyzing quality of life surveys distributed to patients treated over a 15-year period at a single European institution. They reported that patient surgical satisfaction was > 90%, with over two-thirds still working 12 to 28 years after surgery. However, younger patients (18–40 years old) who required a cervical spine procedure reported a lower quality of life, impaired mobility, and increased pain compared with the general population.

Complications such as distal junctional kyphosis (DJK) considerably increase the total cost of care, impacting cost efficacy versus clinical benefit arguments.[5] A particular challenge of cervical spine surgery, particularly for patients with myelopathy, is that outcomes are largely influenced by nonmodifiable patient and disease factors, such as poor preoperative functional outcome scores, male sex, and length of symptoms.[6] Minimizing surgical complications and the need for a revision procedure is therefore critical to preserving the best possible outcome for hosts with fixed vulnerabilities.

Long-term complications following cervical spine surgery that are of particular interest due to their high prevalence or potentially preventable nature include ASD, DJK, pseudoarthrosis of the fusion levels, adjacent level ossification development (ALOD), and heterotopic ossification (HO). Current evidence regarding the incidence of these events will be reviewed, and potential preventative and treatment strategies will be addressed.

Adjacent Segment Degeneration/Disease

ASD refers to the development of radiographic degenerative changes at levels adjacent to a spine fusion (Fig. 13.1). ASD is highly common and represents degenerative changes independent from those associated with aging alone.[7] While not always symptomatic, ASD can lead to myelopathy, focal neurologic deficits, and pain, mandating surgical revision.[8,9] ASD is multifactorial in nature, which makes it a challenge to anticipate and prevent.[10] While the exact etiology behind a specific patient's ASD is often impossible to identify, factors commonly implicated include altered motion and load across adjacent segments, abnormal postoperative sagittal alignment,[11] and preexisting degeneration.

Few patients with ASD require additional surgery, and more recent works have focused on predicting symptomatic disease (radiculopathy or myelopathy, also known as adjacent segment failure) rather than ASD. It is known that multilevel ACDF predisposes to ASD, with over 50% of 46 patients managed with a 3 or more level ACDF at a single center developing radiographic ASD.[12] However, only one (2.2% of total cohort) required further surgery. A meta-analysis of nine randomized controlled trials from 2010 to 2017 that compared single level ACDF and CDR over a minimum 4-year follow-up period reported that

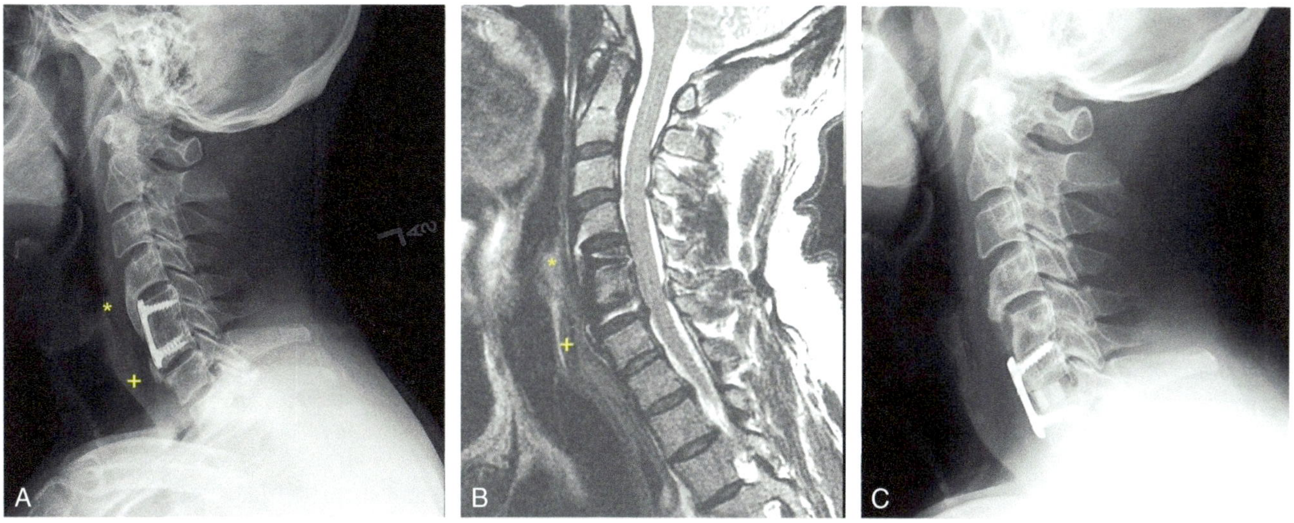

• **Fig. 13.1** The (A) lateral x-ray and (B) sagittal magnetic resonance imaging (MRI) of a patient who underwent a C5-C6 anterior cervical discectomy and fusion (ACDF) with a plate that extended proximally into the C4-C5 interspace, resulting in adjacent level ossification development (ALOD). The patient also presented with myelopathy secondary to adjacent segment disease at the C6-C7 level. (C) The patient was treated with an ACDF at C6-C7, excision of the heterotopic bone at C4-C5, and revision plate fixation. Yellow asterisks demonstrate two levels of adjacent level ossification development, and permit localization on both MRI scans in A and B.

patients who underwent CDR had a significantly lower incidence of symptomatic ASD that required revision surgery than ACDF (odds ratio 0.38, 95% confidence interval 0.27 to 0.53).[13] A subsequent meta-analysis that assessed both short- and long-term outcomes found no difference between ACDF and CDR 2 years after surgery but reported a divergence in outcomes that began approximately 5 years postoperatively.[14] This significance was found to persist up to at least 7 years after the procedure, which was the longest tested timepoint.[15–20]

A subject of notable prior debate was the need to include the cervicothoracic junction (C7-T1) in fusion constructs to prevent adjacent degeneration due to increased forces across the inflection between thoracic kyphosis and cervical lordosis. A small series of 58 patients with largely C2-C7 and C2-T1-3 constructs reported a significant increase in the need for revision surgery with lower instrumented vertebrae (LIV) C7 versus T1-3 (45.0% vs 5.3%, $P = 0.001$).[21] However, this concern has not been borne out by the larger body of literature.[22,23] A large retrospective analysis of 369 patients who underwent posterior cervical decompression and fusion to C3-C6, C3-C7, or C3-T1 found no difference in reoperation (2.6% C3-6, 8.2% C3-C7, 5.5% C3-T1) or complication rates, although blood loss increased with additional fusion levels.[24] This was reflective of a prior multicenter analysis that found that extending a posterior cervical fusion construct into the proximal thoracic spine improved pseudoarthrosis rates but had no impact on ASD, revision surgery rates, or functional outcome.[25]

Sagittal malalignment has largely not been associated with symptomatic ASD after cervical spine surgery, although one work found an association between ASD and occipitocervical angle (the angle formed by a line tangential to the posterior C4 vertebral body and a line connecting the most caudal point on the occipital bone and the posterior hard palate).[26] However, altered mechanics following a motion-altering cervical spine procedure can exacerbate preexisting degenerative changes at adjacent levels. Hilibrand et al.[9] reported that patients with no evidence of ASD at the time of an ACDF had a mean time until the development of symptomatic ASD of 7 years, with a strong inverse relationship observed between the degree of initial ASD and time until symptom onset. A finite element model analysis demonstrated that preexisting degenerative disc disease adjacent to an ACDF increased multidirectional stress across the disc by 5% to 7% and increased facet loading by 11%.[27] An in vivo analysis of healthy controls and patients treated with an ACDF or CDR reported that an ACDF increases the magnitude of intersegmental rotation and contact forces at adjacent levels while a CDR does not,[28] which may provide further understanding about the relative differences in symptomatic ASD between these procedures. Endplate abnormalities beyond typical Schmorl's nodes likely representative of focal degenerative change were also associated with operative ASD.[29] However, mild spondylolisthesis adjacent to a CDR was not associated with an increased risk of ASD over 5 years of follow-up.[30]

While it is easy to dwell on modifiable risk factors for ASD such as construct and level selection, the importance of host characteristics should not be ignored. A machine learning analysis of patients who developed ASD within 6 months of a 2-level ACDF identified paraspinal muscle cross-sectional area at C5 and C7 were predictive of early ASD,[31] a finding similar to what has been reported in the lumbar spine.[32] The incidence of symptomatic ASD was associated with the need for lumbar microdiscectomy or the need for appendicular joint (i.e., hip, knee, shoulder) arthroplasty, suggesting that hosts with symptomatic ASD may be globally predisposed to degenerative disease.[7]

Adjacent Level Ossification Development

ALOD, ossification of the disc space immediately above or below an anterior cervical fusion construct (Fig. 13.1) is a form of HO that occurs in over half (59%) of cephalad adjacent discs and 29% of caudal adjacent discs after ACDF[33] and after 6% to 24% of cervical disc replacements.[34] ALOD has been strongly associated with the placement of an anterior cervical plate too close to the adjacent disc.[35] A plate tip to disc distance of < 5 mm was associated with ALOD in 31% to 66% of cases, and encroachment of the adjacent disc space by the plate resulted in ALOD in up to 100% of cases.[36,37] Adjacent segment ossification can occur shortly after surgery, and radiographic ossification 3 to 12 months after surgery was predictive of advanced ossification 2 years postoperatively.[33] The stiffness imparted by advanced ALOD, defined as anterior osteophytes that traverse > 50% of the adjacent disc, significantly increases the range of motion (ROM) of the level beyond the one with ALOD, which can result in hypermobility at that level and long-term multilevel adjacent segment disease.[38] Management of ALOD is largely preventative as this is almost entirely an iatrogenic complication.[34] However, while maximizing the distance from the plate to the adjacent disc space will minimize ALOD, it does not impact ASD.[36]

Heterotopic Ossification after Cervical Disc Replacement

While HO has been reported after ACDF, particularly following the use of recombinant bone morphogenic protein-2 (rhBMP-2) in the anterior cervical spine, the clinical consequences of HO following anterior cervical fusions are unclear.[39] However, HO can also occur following up to 85% of cervical disc replacements,[40,41] which may have clinical consequences (Fig. 13.2). Factors that predispose to HO include kyphotic sagittal alignment (Sagittal Vertical Axis [SVA] > 2 cm), male sex, and preexisting HO at the surgical level, although some implant design-dependent factors such as sagittal endplate coverage by the implant may also exist.[42–45]

The clinical outcomes of patients with HO versus those without are largely equivalent when modest levels of HO are noted (nonbridging, nonankylosing bony overgrowth). However, more severe degrees of HO can severely or entirely restrict prosthesis ROM.[42] Despite this, the clinical impact of even severe HO following cervical disc replacement is unclear, and increased pain and worse functional outcome scores have been only inconsistently correlated with the patient's degree of HO and ROM restriction.[46] However, high grade HO has been associated with the eventual development of ASD (22.7% vs 11.1%).[47] At present there are no clear indications for revision of a cervical disc replacement due to HO, as ossification at this level appears to simply render the level fused, not compromised.[48]

Distal Junctional Kyphosis

DJK is the loss of normal sagittal alignment one or two levels below the lowest instrumented vertebra (Fig. 13.3). DJK is common after deformity correction procedures, occurring in 23.8% to 75% of cases within 1 year of surgery.[49,50] The causes of DJK are multifactorial, and multivariate modeling has identified comorbid hosts, more significant deformity correction, baseline neurologic impairment/hand muscle atrophy, and a combined front/back approach as predictive of DJK.[49,50]

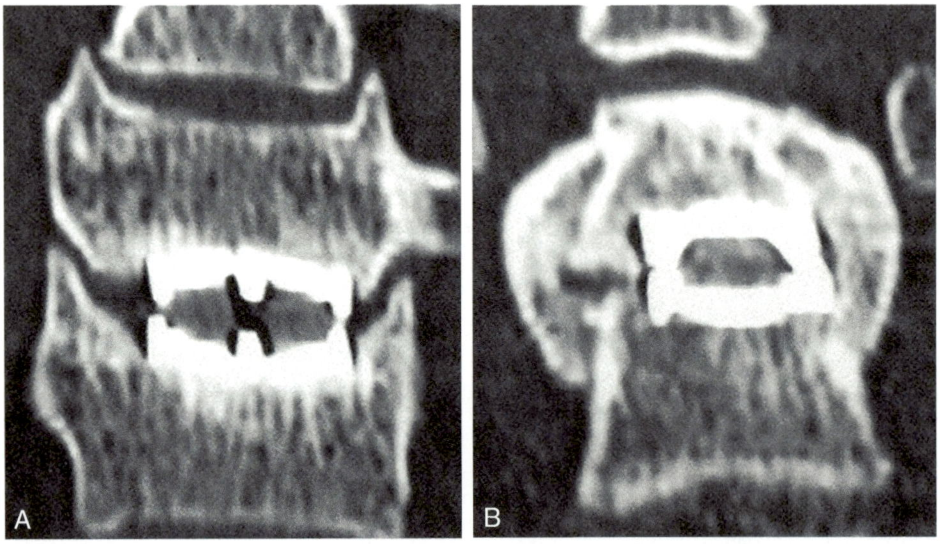

• **Fig. 13.2** Coronal CT scans depicting (A) incomplete and (B) complete ossification of a cervical disc replacement.

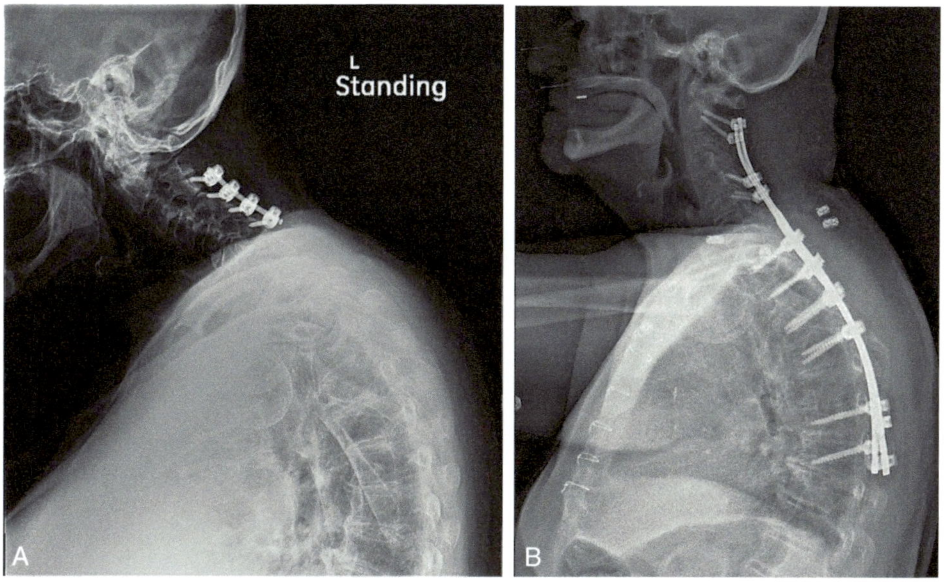

• **Fig. 13.3** (A) A lateral standing x-ray of a 76-year-old male who reported increased neck pain, progressive kyphosis, and the inability to hold his head up straight in the year since a C2-C7 laminectomy with unilateral C3-C6 lateral mass screws. His preoperative standing T1-T12 thoracic kyphosis was 80 degrees, his cervical lordosis was 0 degrees, and his T1-slope was 56 degrees. (B) The patient underwent a revision cervicothoracic fusion from C2-T8 with Smith Petersen osteotomies at C7-T4. His standing cervical lordosis is now 15 degrees and his T1-T12 thoracic kyphosis is 56 degrees. His horizontal gaze has significantly improved.

Patients who undergo more significant deformity corrections are more likely to develop DJK, a contributor that appears to be independent of the degree of under- versus overcorrection of their deformity or the location of the lowest instrumented vertebra.[51] Conditional Interference Decision Tree analysis of 101 patients from a prospective multicenter database found that patients with a preoperative thoracic kyphosis > 50.6°, a C2-C7 lordosis < –12°, a preoperative cervical SVA > 56.3 mm, and T1 slope – cervical lordosis > 36.4° were 5 to 6 times more likely to develop DJK due to increased shear stress along the distal aspect of the fusion construct.[50] The importance of shear stress as a predictor of junctional change in the cervical spine matches that reported to influence proximal junctional kyphosis (PJK) in the lumbar spine.[52] Notably, extension of the fusion construct across the cervicothoracic junction was not associated with a reduced incidence of DJK, although a greater magnitude of deformity correction was possible with constructs that included the proximal thoracic spine.[53] Similarly, the flexibility of the cervical deformity (change in cervical lordosis > 10° between flexion and extension radiographs) as measured in 127 patients included in a prospective multicenter cervical deformity database had no impact on the incidence of DJK.[54]

While DJK appears to be largely driven by deformity and fusion mechanics, intrinsic host qualities are also likely to play a role in the development of DJK. Neurologic comorbidities such as Parkinson's or neuromuscular disease increase the risk of DJK by 3.7 times,[50] likely secondary to the inability for the patient's surrounding musculature to adapt to the altered axial alignment imparted by the fusion construct and the patient's reduced baseline balance. Poor bone quality has been shown to increase the risk of PJK in the lumbar spine[55] and may also play a role in DJK, although current analyses to this end are underpowered.

Pseudoarthrosis

Only a fraction of patients with a pseudoarthrosis, or nonunion of a level of the spine that has been prepared for fusion (Fig. 13.4) become symptomatic. A retrospective analysis of participants in a prior randomized trial who underwent a single level ACDF reported that while the overall rate of pseudoarthrosis following this procedure was 13%, patient-reported outcomes between fused versus pseudoarthrosis 2 years after surgery were equivalent, and only one-fifth of those patients required a subsequent procedure 8 years postoperatively.[56] The incidence of pseudoarthrosis within multilevel anterior constructs approaches 40%, although again few are symptomatic.[57–59] It is therefore unclear to what degree pseudoarthroses impact clinical outcomes following either anterior or posterior fusion procedures.[60–62] However, those that become symptomatic are a source of significant functional disability[63] and are technically challenging to manage.

Few patient or technical factors have been associated with the development of a pseudoarthrosis in the cervical spine. Proton pump inhibitor use was associated with an increased risk of clinically symptomatic pseudoarthroses after ACDF, although a causal relationship was not

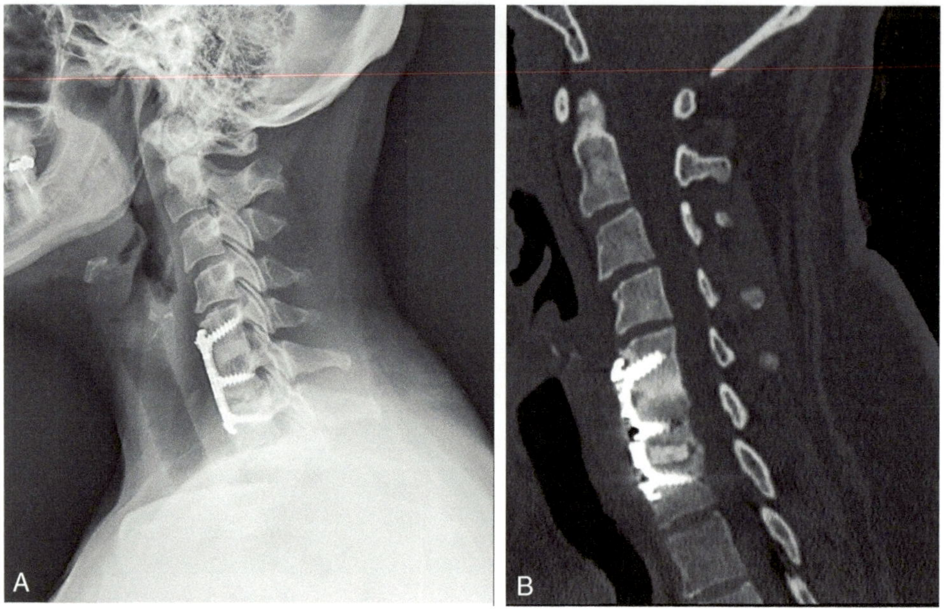

• **Fig. 13.4** Lateral Radiograph and Sagittal CT of the Cervical Spine Demonstrating Pseudoarthrosis (A) A lateral x-ray and (B) sagittal CT cut depicting a pseudoarthrosis at the C6-C7 level of a C5-C7 ACDF.

demonstrated.[64] Short ACDF screws that did not traverse > 75% of the vertebral body were associated with interspinous motion of ≥ 1 mm, a radiographic indicator of pseudoarthrosis, although no relationship with symptomatic pseudoarthrosis or revision surgery was observed.[65] A retrospective study of 122 patients who underwent at least a one-level ACDF for cervical radiculopathy reported an incidence of radiographic pseudoarthrosis of 19.7%, with a higher incidence in patients who underwent > 1 level ACDF (17/60, 28.3%) than after single level fusions (7/62, 11.3%, $P < 0.01$).[57] However, only 4 of 24 patients with pseudoarthroses were symptomatic enough to warrant surgical revision. An increased rate of symptomatic pseudoarthroses in patients with > 1 level ACDF when performed with stand-alone intervertebral cages without plate augmentation was reported in a single work, although this relationship was not statistically powered.[66] Anterior plate fixation significantly reduced the pseudoarthrosis rates of two- and three-level ACDF constructs from 25% and 37% without plating to 0% and 18% with a plate, respectively.[58,59] Implant choice may contribute to nonunions. The use of polyetheretherketone (PEEK) cages in multilevel ACDF constructs led to a reoperation rate for symptomatic pseudoarthrosis of 14% compared with 0% after the use of allograft,[67] although this difference was not shown when only one- to two-level constructs were evaluated.[68,69]

The use of low-dose rhBMP-2 during anterior cervical fusions in patients at risk for pseudoarthrosis, such as smokers or those undergoing multilevel surgeries, was well tolerated and yielded a fusion rate of 96% to 100%.[70,71] An increased incidence of dysphagia following the use of rhBMP-2 in one- or two-level ACDF constructs has been reported, although in > 2 level fusions dysphagia was equivalent regardless of rhBMP-2 use.[72] rhBMP-2 is presently not approved by the U.S. Food and Drug Administration (FDA) for use in the anterior cervical spine, and therefore such applications are off-label.

Priorities when revising a pseudoarthrosis are preparing or repreparing a good fusion bed, creating a stable fusion construct, and augmenting the fusion with bone graft or bone graft substitute as needed.[73] Revision surgery in the cervical spine requires careful anatomic consideration. Patients who have had a previous posterior decompression should be revised anteriorly if possible to avoid the risk of a durotomy and 30-day emergency department (ED) admission.[74] Patients with a prior anterior surgery should be fused posteriorly, which has shown to reliably yield successful fusion[75] with minimal risk for revision surgery[76] while avoiding the increased technical challenge and anatomic risk[77] of reaccessing the anterior cervical spine. Significant improvements in functional outcome scores and neck/arm pain in the 6 months following posterior revision of an ACDF pseudoarthrosis were reported, although these improvements plateaued thereafter.[78] Pseudoarthrosis with associated kyphotic deformity may warrant a combined anterior-posterior approach.[79]

Postdecompression Kyphosis after Posterior Cervical Decompression

Postdecompression kyphosis is common after posterior cervical decompression, particularly following a laminectomy. In a 6-year follow-up comparative study following posterior cervical decompression for myelopathy, 33% of patients who underwent a laminectomy developed a kyphotic "buckling" alignment compared with 6% of those after laminoplasty.[80] A 10-year follow-up study of 133 patients who underwent en bloc laminoplasty reported similarly low rates of postoperative kyphosis (8/133, 6%), although those who did become kyphotic had worse quality-of-life scores than those who maintained a lordotic or neutral cervical alignment.[81]

The tendency towards postoperative kyphosis after cervical laminectomy versus laminoplasty has been characterized biomechanically. Goats who underwent laminectomy had significant increased sagittal plane slack versus laminoplasty and were stiff in flexion while those who underwent laminoplasty were stiff in extension, leading to a 70% decrease in cervical curvature over 6 months.[82] The loads required to rotate the cervical spine 2.5 to 7.5 degrees were markedly lower after French open door, en bloc, or double-door laminoplasty.[83]

Preoperative sagittal alignment can predict postdecompressive kyphosis. Postlaminectomy kyphosis was only observed in patients with preoperative cervical lordosis of < 20° after 9 years of follow-up.[84] Increased T1 slope has been associated with increased C2-C7 SVA and thereby kyphosis due to the anterior shift in the postoperative center of gravity.[85] An association between postlaminectomy kyphosis and C5 palsy has also been reported.[86] A large retrospective study of 174 laminoplasty patients found a preoperative center of gravity of the head-C7 SVA > 42 mm and age ≥ 75 years to be predictive of kyphotic deformity after 1 year, with associated poor recovery of quality-of-life scores.[87]

Reduced extensibility, defined as the difference between the C2-C7 cobb angle measured on neutral versus extension cervical films and related to the integrity and function of the posterior neck muscular-ligament complex (PMLC), has been implicated in postlaminectomy kyphosis.[88] Compromise of the PMLC, specifically the muscular attachments of the C2 and C7 vertebrae during laminectomy or laminoplasty, can lead to postoperative cervical deformity rates as high as 26.7%.[86]

Kyphosis following laminectomy or laminoplasty in patients with ossification of the posterior longitudinal ligament (OPLL) is somewhat less common and appears to be less consequential. A mean 4.5-year follow-up study of 34 patients with OPLL who required a posterior cervical laminectomy found that only three (8.8%) had fallen into a kyphotic alignment (0% preoperatively).[89] A series of 64 patients with OPLL who underwent cervical laminoplasty reported that a higher T1 slope were more likely to lose some degree of cervical lordosis, but few patients drifted into frank kyphosis.[90] Loss of cervical lordosis after laminoplasty in patients with OPLL was also not associated with decreased functional outcome scores,[91] in contrast with those without OPLL.

Conclusions

Long-term complications following cervical spine surgery are functionally debilitating for the patient and technically challenging for the surgeon. While there will always be some risk of complication following surgical intervention, those after cervical spine surgery are largely iatrogenic. Continued development of superior implants and thoughtful indications and surgical technique can minimize the need for revision surgery and maximize the patient's long-term quality of life.

References

1. Kotkansalo A, Leinonen V, Korajoki M, Korhonen K, Rinne J, Malmivaara A. Occurrence, risk factors, and time trends for late reoperations due to degenerative cervical spine disease: A Finnish National Register Study of 19 377 patients operated on between 1999 and 2015. *Neurosurgery*. 2021;88(3):558–573. https://doi.org/10.1093/neuros/nyaa464.
2. Loidolt T, Kurra S, Riew KD, Levi AD, Florman J, Lavelle WF. Comparison of adverse events between cervical disc arthroplasty and anterior cervical discectomy and fusion: a 10-year follow-up. *Spine J*. 2021;21(2):253–264. https://doi.org/10.1016/j.spinee.2020.10.013.
3. Hirvonen T, Marjamaa J, Siironen J, Koskinen S, Niemelä M, Koski-Palkén A. Young adults undergoing ACDF surgery exhibit decreased health-related quality of life in the long term in comparison to the general population. *Spine J*. 2021;21(6):924–936. https://doi.org/10.1016/j.spinee.2021.01.021.
4. Hirvonen T, Siironen J, Marjamaa J, Niemelä M, Koski-Palkén A. Anterior cervical discectomy and fusion in young adults leads to favorable outcome in long-term follow-up. *Spine J*. 2020;20(7):1073–1084. https://doi.org/10.1016/j.spinee.2020.03.016.
5. Horn SR, Passias PG, Hockley A, et al. Cost-utility of revisions for cervical deformity correction warrants minimization of reoperations. *J Spine Surg*. 2018;4(4):702–711. https://doi.org/10.21037/jss.2018.10.02.
6. Khan O, Badhiwala JH, Akbar MA, Fehlings MG. Prediction of worse functional status after surgery for degenerative cervical myelopathy: A machine learning approach. *Neurosurgery*. 2021;88(3):584–591. https://doi.org/10.1093/neuros/nyaa477.
7. Burkhardt BW, Simgen A, Wagenpfeil G, Hendrix P, Reith W, Oertel JM. Adjacent segment disease following anterior cervical fusion and the presence of surgery for lumbar disc herniation and surgery at the musculoskeletal joints: are they related. *Spine J*. 2020;20(12):1925–1933. https://doi.org/10.1016/j.spinee.2020.07.008.
8. Hilibrand AS, Robbins M. Adjacent segment degeneration and adjacent segment disease: The consequences of spinal fusion? *Spine J*. 2004;4(6 SUPPL.). https://doi.org/10.1016/j.spinee.2004.07.007.
9. Hilibrand AS, Carlson GD, Palumbo MA, Jones PK, Bohlman HH. Radiculopathy and myelopathy at segments adjacent to the site of a previous anterior cervical arthrodesis. *J Bone Joint Surg Am*. 1999;81(4):519–528. https://doi.org/10.2106/00004623-199904000-00009.
10. Tobert DG, Antoci V, Patel SP, Saadat E, Bono CM. Adjacent segment disease in the cervical and lumbar spine. *Clin Spine Surg*. 2017;30(3):94–101. https://doi.org/10.1097/BSD.0000000000000442.
11. Katsuura A, Hukuda S, Saruhashi Y, Mori K. Kyphotic malalignment after anterior cervical fusion is one of the factors promoting the degenerative process in adjacent intervertebral levels. *Eur Spine J*. 2001;10(4):320–324. https://doi.org/10.1007/s005860000243.

12. Teo SJ, Goh GS, Yeo W, Chen JLT, Soh RCC. The relationship between cervical sagittal balance and adjacent segment disease after three-level anterior cervical discectomy and fusion. *Clin Spine Surg.* 2021;34(5):E264–E270. https://doi.org/10.1097/BSD.0000000000001135.
13. Deng Y, Li G, Liu H, Hong Y, Meng Y. Mid- To long-term rates of symptomatic adjacent-level disease requiring surgery after cervical total disc replacement compared with anterior cervical discectomy and fusion: A meta-analysis of prospective randomized clinical trials. *J Orthop Surg Res.* 2020;15(1):468. https://doi.org/10.1186/s13018-020-01957-3.
14. Delamarter RB, Zigler J. Five-year reoperation rates, cervical total disc replacement versus fusion, results of a prospective randomized clinical trial. *Spine (Phila Pa 1976).* 2013;38(9):711–717. https://doi.org/10.1097/BRS.0b013e3182797592.
15. Ghobrial GM, Lavelle WF, Florman JE, Riew KD, Levi AD. Symptomatic adjacent level disease requiring surgery: Analysis of 10-year results from a prospective, randomized, clinical trial comparing cervical disc arthroplasty to anterior cervical fusion. *Clin Neurosurg.* 2019;84(2):347–354. https://doi.org/10.1093/neuros/nyy118.
16. Badhiwala JH, Platt A, Witiw CD, Traynelis VC. Cervical disc arthroplasty versus anterior cervical discectomy and fusion: A meta-analysis of rates of adjacent-level surgery to 7-year follow-up. *J Spine Surg.* 2020;6(1):217–232. https://doi.org/10.21037/jss.2019.12.09.
17. Radcliff K, Davis RJ, Hisey MS, et al. Long-term evaluation of cervical disc arthroplasty with the Mobi-C© cervical disc: A randomized, prospective, multicenter clinical trial with seven-year follow-up. *Int J Spine Surg.* 2017;11(4):244–262. https://doi.org/10.14444/4031.
18. Phillips FM, Geisler FH, Gilder KM, Reah C, Howell KM, McAfee PC. Long-term outcomes of the US FDA IDE prospective, randomized controlled clinical trial comparing PCM cervical disc arthroplasty with anterior cervical discectomy and fusion. *Spine (Phila Pa 1976).* 2015;40(10):674–683. https://doi.org/10.1097/BRS.0000000000000869.
19. Burkus JK, Traynelis VC, Haid RW, Mummaneni PV. Clinical and radiographic analysis of an artificial cervical disc: 7-year follow-up from the Prestige prospective randomized controlled clinical trial. *J Neurosurg Spine.* 2014;21(4):516–528. https://doi.org/10.3171/2014.6.SPINE13996.
20. Loumeau TP, Darden BV, Kesman TJ, et al. A RCT comparing 7-year clinical outcomes of one level symptomatic cervical disc disease (SCDD) following ProDisc-C total disc arthroplasty (TDA) versus anterior cervical discectomy and fusion (ACDF). *Eur Spine J.* 2016;25(7):2263–2270. https://doi.org/10.1007/s00586-016-4431-6.
21. Scholz C, Klingler JH, Masalha W, et al. Long-term results after multilevel fusion of the cervical spine and the cervicothoracic junction: To bridge or not to bridge? *World Neurosurg.* 2021;148:e556–e564. https://doi.org/10.1016/j.wneu.2021.01.025.
22. Louie PK, Presciutti SM, Iantorno SE, et al. There is no increased risk of adjacent segment disease at the cervicothoracic junction following an anterior cervical discectomy and fusion to C7. *Spine J.* 2017;17(9):1264–1271. https://doi.org/10.1016/j.spinee.2017.04.027.
23. Kim HJ, Yao YC, Bannwarth M, et al. Cervicothoracic versus proximal thoracic lower instrumented vertebra have comparable radiographic and clinical outcomes in adult cervical deformity. *Glob Spine J.* 2023;13(4):1056–1063. https://doi.org/10.1177/21925682211017478.
24. Hines K, Wilt ZT, Franco D, et al. Long-segment posterior cervical decompression and fusion: Does caudal level affect revision rate? *J Neurosurg Spine.* 2021;35(1):1–7. https://doi.org/10.3171/2020.10.SPINE201385.
25. Truumees E, Singh D, Geck MJ, Stokes JK. Should long-segment cervical fusions be routinely carried into the thoracic spine? A multicenter analysis. *Spine J.* 2018;18(5):782–787. https://doi.org/10.1016/j.spinee.2017.09.010.
26. Yang X, Bartels RHMA, Donk R, Arts MP, Goedmakers CMW, Vleggeert-Lankamp CLA. The association of cervical sagittal alignment with adjacent segment degeneration. *Eur Spine J.* 2020;29(11):2655–2664. https://doi.org/10.1007/s00586-019-06157-0.
27. Li X-F, Lv Z-D, Yin H-L, Song X-X. Impact of adjacent pre-existing disc degeneration status on its biomechanics after single-level anterior cervical interbody fusion. *Comput Methods Programs Biomed.* 2021:209. https://doi.org/10.1016/j.cmpb.2021.106355.
28. Liu F, Cheng J, Komistek RD, Mahfouz MR, Sharma A. In vivo evaluation of dynamic characteristics of the normal, fused, and disc replacement cervical spines. *Spine (Phila Pa 1976).* 2007;32(23):2578–2584. https://doi.org/10.1097/BRS.0b013e318158cdf8.
29. Harada GK, Alter K, Nguyen AQ, et al. Cervical spine endplate abnormalities and association with pain, disability, and adjacent segment degeneration after anterior cervical discectomy and fusion. *Spine (Phila Pa 1976).* 2020;45(15):E917–E926. https://doi.org/10.1097/BRS.0000000000003460.
30. Kieser DC, Cawley DT, Roscop C, et al. Spondylolisthesis adjacent to a cervical disc arthroplasty does not increase the risk of adjacent level degeneration. *Eur Spine J.* 2018;27(6):1440–1446. https://doi.org/10.1007/s00586-018-5574-4.
31. Wong AYL, Harada G, Lee R, et al. Preoperative paraspinal neck muscle characteristics predict early onset adjacent segment degeneration in anterior cervical fusion patients: A machine-learning modeling analysis. *J Orthop Res.* 2021;39(8):1732–1744. https://doi.org/10.1002/jor.24829.
32. Kim JY, Ryu DS, Paik HK, et al. Paraspinal muscle, facet joint, and disc problems: risk factors for adjacent segment degeneration after lumbar fusion. *Spine J.* 2016;16(7):867–875. https://doi.org/10.1016/j.spinee.2016.03.010.
33. Park JB, Cho YS, Riew KD. Development of adjacent-level ossification in patients with an anterior cervical plate. *J Bone Jt Surg Am.* 2005;87(3):558–563. https://doi.org/10.2106/JBJS.C.01555.
34. Kim HJ, Kelly MP, Ely CG, Riew KD, Dettori JR. The risk of adjacent-level ossification development after surgery in the cervical spine: Are there factors that affect the risk? A systematic review. *Spine (Phila Pa 1976).* 2012;37(Suppl. 22). https://doi.org/10.1097/BRS.0b013e31826cb8f5.
35. Lee DH, Lee JS, Yi JS, Cho W, Zebala LP, Riew KD. Anterior cervical plating technique to prevent adjacent-level ossification development. *Spine J.* 2013;13(7):823–829. https://doi.org/10.1016/j.spinee.2013.03.009.
36. Yang H, Lu X, He H, et al. Longer plate-to-disc distance prevents adjacent-level ossification development but does not influence adjacent-segment degeneration. *Spine (Phila Pa 1976).* 2015;40(7):E388–E393. https://doi.org/10.1097/BRS.0000000000000800.
37. Huang C, Mobbs R, Selby M, Phan K, Rao P. Adjacent-level ossification development in single-level standalone anterior cervical discectomy and fusion versus anterior cervical discectomy and fusion with plate. *Glob Spine J.* 2021;11(3):292–298. https://doi.org/10.1177/2192568220902749.

38. Lee DH, Park S, Park JW, et al. Adjacent level ossification development following anterior cervical fusion: How does it affect the next level disc. *Spine (Phila Pa 1976)*. 2020;45(22):E1469–E1475. https://doi.org/10.1097/BRS.0000000000003656.
39. Arnold PM, Anderson KK, Selim A, Dryer RF, Burkus JK. Heterotopic ossification following single-level anterior cervical discectomy and fusion: Results from the prospective, multicenter, historically controlled trial comparing allograft to an optimized dose of rhBMP-2. *J Neurosurg Spine*. 2016;25(3):292–302. https://doi.org/10.3171/2016.1.SPINE15798.
40. Yang X, Donk R, Bartels RHMA, Arts MP, Depreitere B, Vleggeert-Lankamp CLA. Comparing heterotopic ossification in two cervical disc prostheses. *Spine (Phila Pa 1976)*. 2020;45(19):1329–1334. https://doi.org/10.1097/BRS.0000000000003537.
41. Chen J, Wang X, Bai W, Shen X, Yuan W. Prevalence of heterotopic ossification after cervical total disc arthroplasty: A meta-analysis. *Eur Spine J*. 2012;21(4):674–680. https://doi.org/10.1007/s00586-011-2094-x.
42. Yi S, Shin DA, Kim KN, et al. The predisposing factors for the heterotopic ossification after cervical artificial disc replacement. *Spine J*. 2013;13(9):1048–1054. https://doi.org/10.1016/j.spinee.2013.02.036.
43. Yi S, Kim KN, Yang MS, et al. Difference in occurrence of heterotopic ossification according to prosthesis type in the cervical artificial disc replacement. *Spine (Phila Pa 1976)*. 2010;35(16):1556–1561. https://doi.org/10.1097/BRS.0B013E3181C6526B.
44. Zeng J, Liu H, Chen H, et al. Effect of prosthesis width and depth on heterotopic ossification after cervical disc arthroplasty. *Spine (Phila Pa 1976)*. 2019;44(9):624–628. https://doi.org/10.1097/BRS.0000000000002915.
45. Xu S, Ou Y, Du X, He B, Li Y, Yu H. Heterotopic ossification after prestige-LP cervical disc arthroplasty is related to insufficient sagittal coverage of the endplate by the prosthesis. *Med Sci Monit*. 2021:27. https://doi.org/10.12659/MSM.929890.
46. Brenke C, Scharf J, Schmieder K, Barth M. High prevalence of heterotopic ossification after cervical disc arthroplasty: Outcome and intraoperative findings following explantation of 22 cervical disc prostheses - Clinical article. *J Neurosurg Spine*. 2012;17(2):141–146. https://doi.org/10.3171/2012.4.SPINE12223.
47. Wang H, Wang X, Liu H, Meng Y, Guo Y, Hong Y. Risk factors for high-grade heterotopic ossification after total disc replacement: A single-center experience of 394 cases. *Neurosurgery*. 2021;89(5):852–861. https://doi.org/10.1093/neuros/nyab298.
48. Marques C, MacDowall A, Skeppholm M, Canto Moreira N, Olerud C. Unintended fusion in cervical artificial disk replacement: a prospective study on heterotopic ossification, progression, and clinical outcome, with 5-year follow-up. *Eur Spine J*. 2021;30(6):1662–1669. https://doi.org/10.1007/s00586-021-06722-6.
49. Passias PG, Horn SR, Oh C, et al. Predicting the occurrence of postoperative distal junctional kyphosis in cervical deformity patients. *Neurosurgery*. 2020;86(1):E38–E46. https://doi.org/10.1093/neuros/nyz347.
50. Passias PG, Vasquez-Montes D, Poorman GW, et al. Predictive model for distal junctional kyphosis after cervical deformity surgery. *Spine J*. 2018;18(12):2187–2194. https://doi.org/10.1016/j.spinee.2018.04.017.
51. Passias P, Horn S, Lafage V, et al. Effect of age-adjusted alignment goals and distal inclination angle on the fate of distal junctional kyphosis in cervical deformity surgery. *J Craniovertebr Junction Spine*. 2021;12(1):65–71. https://doi.org/10.4103/jcvjs.jcvjs_170_20.
52. Kim HJ, Iyer S. Proximal junctional kyphosis. *J Am Acad Orthop Surg*. 2016;24(5):318–326. https://doi.org/10.5435/JAAOS-D-14-00393.
53. Bortz C, Passias PG, Pierce KE, et al. Radiographic benefit of incorporating the inflection between the cervical and thoracic curves in fusion constructs for surgical cervical deformity patients. *J Craniovertebral Junction Spine*. 2020;11(2):131. https://doi.org/10.4103/JCVJS.JCVJS_57_20.
54. Protopsaltis TS, Stekas N, Smith JS, et al. Surgical outcomes in rigid versus flexible cervical deformities. *J Neurosurg Spine*. 2021;34(5):716–724. https://doi.org/10.3171/2020.8.SPINE191185.
55. Cho SK, Shin JI, Kim YJ. Proximal junctional kyphosis following adult spinal deformity surgery. *Eur Spine J*. 2014;23(12):2726–2736. https://doi.org/10.1007/s00586-014-3531-4.
56. Crawford CH, Carreon LY, Mummaneni P, Dryer RF, Glassman SD. Asymptomatic ACDF nonunions underestimate the true prevalence of radiographic pseudarthrosis. *Spine (Phila Pa 1976)*. 2020;45(13):E776–E780. https://doi.org/10.1097/BRS.0000000000003444.
57. Bohlman HH, Emery SE, Goodfellow DBJP. Robinson anterior cervical discectomy and arthrodesis for cervical radiculopathy. Long-term follow-up of one hundred and twenty-two patients. *J Bone Jt Surg Am*. 1993;75(9):1298–1307.
58. Wang JC, McDonough PW, Kanim LEA, Endow KK, Delamarter RB. Increased fusion rates with cervical plating for three-level anterior cervical discectomy and fusion. *Spine (Phila Pa 1976)*. 2001;26(6):643–646. https://doi.org/10.1097/00007632-200103150-00015.
59. Wang JC, McDonough PW, Endow KK, Delamarter RB. Increased fusion rates with cervical plating for two-level anterior cervical pas and fusion. *Spine (Phila Pa 1976)*. 2000;25(1):41–45. https://doi.org/10.1097/00007632-200001010-00009.
60. Kaiser MG, Mummaneni PV, Matz PG, et al. Management of anterior cervical pseudarthrosis. *J Neurosurg Spine*. 2009;11(2):228–237. https://doi.org/10.3171/2009.2.SPINE08729.
61. Lee CJ, Boody BS, Demeter J, Smucker JD, Sasso RC. Long-term radiographic and functional outcomes of patients with absence of radiographic union at 2 years after single-level anterior cervical discectomy and fusion. *Global Spine J*. 2020;10(6):741–747. https://doi.org/10.1177/2192568219874768.
62. Couch BK, Wawrose RA, LeVasseur CM, et al. Residual motion and graft type do not influence patient-reported outcomes following one- or two-level anterior cervical discectomy and fusion. *Spine (Phila Pa 1976)*. 2021;46(15):E817–E825. https://doi.org/10.1097/BRS.0000000000003918.
63. Pennington Z, Mehta VA, Lubelski D, et al. Quality of life and cost implications of pseudarthrosis after anterior cervical discectomy and fusion and its subsequent revision surgery. *World Neurosurg*. 2020;133:e592–e599. https://doi.org/10.1016/j.wneu.2019.09.104.
64. Mangan JJ, Divi SN, McKenzie JC, et al. Proton pump inhibitor use affects pseudarthrosis rates and influences patient-reported outcomes. *Global Spine J*. 2020;10(1):55–62. https://doi.org/10.1177/2192568219853222.
65. Lee NJ, Vulapalli M, Park P, et al. Does screw length for primary two-level ACDF influence pseudarthrosis risk. *Spine J*. 2020;20(11):1752–1760. https://doi.org/10.1016/j.spinee.2020.07.002.

66. Iunes EA, Barletta EA, Belsuzarri TAB, et al. Pseudarthrosis in anterior cervical discectomy and fusion with a self-locking, stand-alone cage filled with hydroxyapatite: A retrospective study with clinical and radiological outcomes of 98 levels with a minimum 2-year follow-up. *J Neurosurg Spine.* 2020;33(6): 717–726. https://doi.org/10.3171/2020.4.SPINE20357.
67. Teton ZE, Cheaney B, Obayashi JT, Than KD. PEEK interbody devices for multilevel anterior cervical discectomy and fusion: Association with more than 6-fold higher rates of pseudarthrosis compared to structural allograft. *J Neurosurg Spine.* 2020;32 (5):696–702. https://doi.org/10.3171/2019.11.SPINE19788.
68. Buyuk AF, Onyekwelu I, Gaffney CJ, et al. Symptomatic pseudarthrosis requiring revision surgery after 1-or 2-level acdf with plating: Peek versus allograft. *J Spine Surg.* 2020;6(4):670–680. https://doi.org/10.21037/jss-19-419.
69. Wang M, Chou D, Chang CC, et al. Anterior cervical discectomy and fusion performed using structural allograft or polyetheretherketone: Pseudarthrosis and revision surgery rates with minimum 2-year follow-up. *J Neurosurg Spine.* 2020;32(4): 562–569. https://doi.org/10.3171/2019.9.SPINE19879.
70. Mendenhall SK, Priddy BH, Mobasser JP, Potts EA. Safety and efficacy of low-dose rhBMP-2 use for anterior cervical fusion. *Neurosurg Focus.* 2021;50(6):1–5. https://doi.org/10.3171/2021 .3.FOCUS2171.
71. Tumialán LM, Pan J, Rodts GE, Mummaneni PV. The safety and efficacy of anterior cervical discectomy and fusion with polyetheretherketone spacer and recombinant human bone morphogenetic protein-2: A review of 200 patients. *J Neurosurg Spine.* 2008;8(6):529–535. https://doi.org/10.3171/SPI/2008/8/6/529.
72. Lu DC, Tumialán LM, Chou D. Multilevel anterior cervical discectomy and fusion with and without rhBMP-2: A comparison of dysphagia rates and outcomes in 150 patients - Clinical article. *J Neurosurg Spine.* 2013;18(1):43–49. https://doi.org/ 10.3171/2012.10.SPINE10231.
73. Rihn JA, Harrod C, Albert TJ. Revision cervical spine surgery. *Orthop Clin North Am.* 2012;43(1):123–136. https://doi. org/10.1016/j.ocl.2011.09.001.
74. Martini ML, Baron RB, Gal JS, et al. Comparison of cost and perioperative outcome profiles for primary and revision posterior cervical fusion procedures. *Spine (Phila Pa 1976).* 2021;46(19):1295–1301. https://doi.org/10.1097/brs.000000 0000004019.
75. Elder BD, Sankey EW, Theodros D, et al. Successful anterior fusion following posterior cervical fusion for revision of anterior cervical discectomy and fusion pseudarthrosis. *J Clin Neurosci.* 2016;24:57–62. https://doi.org/10.1016/j.jocn.2015.07.019.
76. Carreon L, Glassman SD, Campbell MJ. Treatment of anterior cervical pseudoarthrosis: Posterior fusion versus anterior revision. *Spine J.* 2006;6(2):154–156. https://doi.org/10.1016/j. spinee.2005.07.003.
77. Ji H, Liu D, You W, Zhou F, Liu Z. Success in esophageal perforation repair with open-wound management after revision cervical spine surgery: A case report. *Spine (Phila Pa 1976).* 2015;40(3):E183–E185. https://doi.org/10.1097/BRS. 0000000000000712.
78. Steinhaus ME, York PJ, Bronheim RS, Yang J, Lovecchio F, Kim HJ. Outcomes of revision surgery for pseudarthrosis after anterior cervical fusion: Case series and systematic review. *Global Spine J.* 2020;10(5):559–570. https://doi.org/10.1177/ 2192568219863808.
79. Verla T, Xu DS, Davis MJ, et al. Failure in cervical spinal fusion and current management modalities. *Semin Plast Surg.* 2021;35(1):10–13. https://doi.org/10.1055/s-0041-1722853.
80. Matsunaga S, Sakou T, Nakanisi K. Analysis of the cervical spine alignment following laminoplasty and laminectomy. *Spinal Cord.* 1999;37(1):20–24. https://doi.org/10.1038/sj.sc.3100749.
81. Kawaguchi Y, Kanamori M, Ishihara H, Ohmori K, Nakamura H, Kimura T. Minimum 10-year followup after en bloc cervical laminoplasty. *Clin Orthop Relat Res.* 2003;411:129–139. https:// doi.org/10.1097/01.blo.0000069889.31220.62.
82. Baisden J, Voo LM, Cusick JF, Pintar FA, Yoganandan N. Evaluation of cervical laminectomy and laminoplasty: A longitudinal study in the goat model. *Spine (Phila Pa 1976).* 1999;24(13):1283–1289. https://doi.org/10.1097/00007632-199907010-00003.
83. Hashiguchi A, Kanchiku T, Nishida N, Taguchi T. Biomechanical study of cervical posterior decompression. *Asian Spine J.* 2018;12(23):391–397. https://doi.org/10.4184/asj. 2018.12.3.391.
84. van Geest S, de Vormer AMJ, Arts MP, Peul WC, Vleggeert-Lankamp CLA. Long-term follow-up of clinical and radiological outcome after cervical laminectomy. *Eur Spine J.* 2015;24(2): 229–235. https://doi.org/10.1007/s00586-013-3089-6.
85. Lee JS, Son DW, Lee SH, Kim DH, Lee SW, Song GS. The predictable factors of the postoperative kyphotic change of sagittal alignment of the cervical spine after the laminoplasty. *J Korean Neurosurg Soc.* 2017;60(5):577–583. https://doi.org/10.3340/ jkns.2017.0505.007.
86. Oe S, Kurosu K, Hasegawa T, et al. Risk factors for cervical deformity after posterior cervical decompression surgery: A multicenter study. *Global Spine J.* Published online. 2021. https://doi. org/10.1177/21925682211036660.
87. Sakai K, Yoshii T, Hirai T, et al. Cervical sagittal imbalance is a predictor of kyphotic deformity after laminoplasty in cervical spondylotic myelopathy patients without preoperative kyphotic alignment. *Spine (Phila Pa 1976).* 2016;41(4):299–305. https:// doi.org/10.1097/BRS.0000000000001206.
88. Jeon H, Kim HC, Kim TW, et al. Prediction of angular kyphosis after cervical laminoplasty using radiologic measurements. *J Clin Neurosci.* 2021;85:13–19. https://doi.org/10.1016/j.jocn. 2020.12.002.
89. Lee SE, Chung CK, Jahng TA, Kim HJ. Long-term outcome of laminectomy for cervical ossification of the posterior longitudinal ligament. *J Neurosurg Spine.* 2013;18(5):465–471. https:// doi.org/10.3171/2013.1.SPINE12779.
90. Kim B, Yoon DH, Ha Y, et al. Relationship between T1 slope and loss of lordosis after laminoplasty in patients with cervical ossification of the posterior longitudinal ligament. *Spine J.* 2016;16(2):219–225. https://doi.org/10.1016/j.spinee.2015. 10.042.
91. Miyazaki M, Ishihara T, Notani N, Kanezaki S, Tsumura H. Relationship of T1 slope with loss of lordosis and surgical outcomes after laminoplasty for cervical ossification of the posterior longitudinal ligament. *Clin Neurol Neurosurg.* 2018;164:19–24. https://doi.org/10.1016/j.clineuro.2017.11.007.

14

Complications of Posterior Minimally Invasive Surgery of the Cervical Spine

MARK BASILIOUS, ROGER HÄRTL, AND IBRAHIM HUSSAIN

CHAPTER OUTLINE

Introduction

The field of spine surgery has evolved dramatically over the last several decades, with greater emphasis being placed on the development of surgical techniques that minimize collateral damage, preserve as much normal anatomy as possible, and reduce the total physical stress placed on the patient's body.[1] Minimally invasive approaches to lumbar and thoracic spinal pathology have been rapidly adopted by the field, offering patients improved outcomes and a reduced risk of complications. The adoption of these techniques, however, has not been as rapid in cervical spine surgery. Cervical pathology has historically been viewed as higher risk, largely owing to the perceived danger of devastating cervical spinal cord and vascular injury. The smaller operating window, density of the surrounding neck anatomy, and risk of injury to vascular structures in close proximity represent unique challenges in cervical spine surgery that have contributed to this slower adoption of minimally invasive techniques.[2]

Despite these perceived barriers, several approaches to minimally invasive surgery in the cervical spine have evolved and demonstrated similar benefits to their thoracolumbar counterparts. In addition to better functional outcomes for patients, minimally invasive approaches in cervical pathology have been associated with shorter hospital stays, less blood loss, and reduced postoperative opiate use.[3] The risk and etiology of complications associated with minimally invasive surgery (MIS) in the cervical spine vary dramatically by indication, procedure, surgical approach utilized, and the ultimate goal of surgery. In this chapter we will discuss some of the more frequently encountered complications seen in cervical MIS procedures, in addition to incidence, risk factors, and optimal management strategies (Table 14.1).

MIS Posterior Cervical Procedures

Posterior Cervical Foraminotomy

Cervical radiculopathy as a result of foraminal stenosis or secondary to a herniation of a far lateral disc is likely to resolve with conservative, nonoperative management.[4] In patients with persistent radiculopathy symptoms that are refractory to conservative treatment, surgical intervention is indicated. Anterior and posterior approaches have been described for the treatment of cervical foraminal stenosis. With the expansion of minimally invasive techniques in the cervical spine, tubular and endoscopic posterior cervical foraminotomies are increasingly being performed. The perceived benefits of a posterior cervical foraminotomy over an anterior cervical decompression and fusion (ACDF) or anterior cervical disc arthroplasty (ACDA) for the treatment of cervical radiculopathy include a lower risk of anterior approach related morbidities such as dysphagia or hoarseness postoperatively (from esophageal retraction and recurrent laryngeal nerve injury, respectively). Likewise, the risk of adjacent segment disease, implant-related complications, and pseudarthrosis are all mitigated when utilizing a posterior cervical foraminotomy.[5] Posterior cervical foraminotomy is, however, associated with its own set of complications. Serious ones are rare, but some of the more commonly reported complications include transient dermatome hypesthesia, cerebrospinal fluid (CSF) leak, hematoma, and radiculitis, which usually do not require additional surgical intervention.[6,7]

TABLE 14.1 **Commonly reported complications of each surgical technique described in this chapter.**

Procedure	Complication	Incidence	Risk Factors
Posterior Cervical Foraminotomy	C5 palsy	1.4%–8.6% (higher if operating on C4-C5)	Male sex, bony stenosis with longitudinal ligament ossification, preoperative C4-C5 hypersensitivity, preoperative myelomalacia at C4-C5
Cervical Unilateral Laminotomy for Bilateral Decompression	Spinal cord injury, incidental durotomy	0%–6% (all complications)	Endoscopic: Endoscope angle of trajectory, irrigation pressure, use of open techniques Tubular: Tight stenosis is a risk factor for incidental durotomy
Percutaneous Cervical Pedicle Screw Stabilization	Screw mispositioning	11%–19.5%	Preoperative cervical spine instability
Percutaneous Cervical Intrafacet Stabilization	Unilateral fracture of the facet during implantation, superficial infection of the surgical wound	1.7% Unilateral fracture rate 5.7% Superficial infection rate*	

*Retained suture in the posterior wound was cited as the leading reason for infection

Another consideration is that a minimally invasive posterior cervical foraminotomy may be a destabilizing procedure causing a predisposition to progressive kyphosis. This is especially true of the patients presenting with degenerative scoliosis or spondylolisthesis.[8] More aggressive foraminotomy is associated with an increased risk of progressive instability or slippage.[9] Some texts recommend limiting facetectomy to no more than one-third of the facet joint and preserving the pars interarticularis whenever possible, and single-sided foraminotomies are typically limited to two to three levels, with more extensive procedures carrying a substantial risk of destabilization (Fig. 14.1).[8] As a result, a subset of patients may require a subsequent reoperation and fusion to stabilize the cervical spine at the incident or adjacent level. In trials limited to minimally invasive posterior cervical foraminotomy, the rate of reoperation with fusion is still relatively low at 5% within 5 years.[10] Patients with bilateral foraminal stenosis are generally not candidates for a bilateral foraminotomy, and these cases should be considered for ACDF or ACDA.[11]

A more common complication that may be associated with the minimally invasive posterior foraminotomy procedure specifically at the C4/5 level is C5 palsy. A C5 nerve palsy can present in varying ways, but most typically involves diminished muscular power of the deltoid or biceps brachii without an impact on lower muscle function.[12] This complication can have a substantial impact on a patient's quality of life and autonomy. While a nerve palsy at other levels during a posterior cervical foraminotomy is possible, these are much rarer than a C5 nerve palsy and are scarcely reported. The exact etiology of this complication remains controversial, but it is possible that the C5 nerve root is most vulnerable because it is shorter and due to its anatomic positioning across the intervertebral disc at a relatively sharp angle.[13]

Estimates for the incidence of C5 palsy across cohorts including both open and minimally invasive posterior cervical foraminotomies are highly variable, with trials reporting rates from 1.4% to 8.6%, with the risk following operation on the C4-C5 level reaching as high as 11.6%.[13–15] Risk factors associated with the development of a postoperative C5 palsy include male sex, bony stenosis with longitudinal ligament ossification, preoperative C4-C5 hypersensitivity, and preoperative myelomalacia at C4-5.[15,16]

The risk of C5 palsy in minimally invasive posterior cervical foraminotomy is believed to lower, with some large studies not reporting a single event.[10] There are, however, case reports of this complication occurring with a minimally invasive approach.[17] Large studies evaluating tubular posterior cervical foraminotomy reported complication and reoperation rates of 2.2% and 3.7%, respectively, as compared to open techniques reporting an overall complication rate up to 5.3% and reoperation rates ranging from 1% to 14%.[18] Fewer data points are currently available for totally endoscopic posterior cervical foraminotomy, but a recent study reported no incidence of C5 palsy and no reoperations in a short-term follow-up period.[19] Additionally, the application of intraoperative neuromonitoring can further reduce the risk of nerve damage and C5 palsy.[20]

Importantly, the majority of patients who develop a postoperative C5 palsy have a good prognosis with conservative management. It has been reported that more than 70% of patients experiencing this complication will make a full recovery within 6 months; however, up to 20% of patients still report residual pain or neurological deficit at that point. Given the impact of this complication, it is important for the surgeon to consider each patient's risk when considering a minimally invasive posterior cervical foraminotomy.[21]

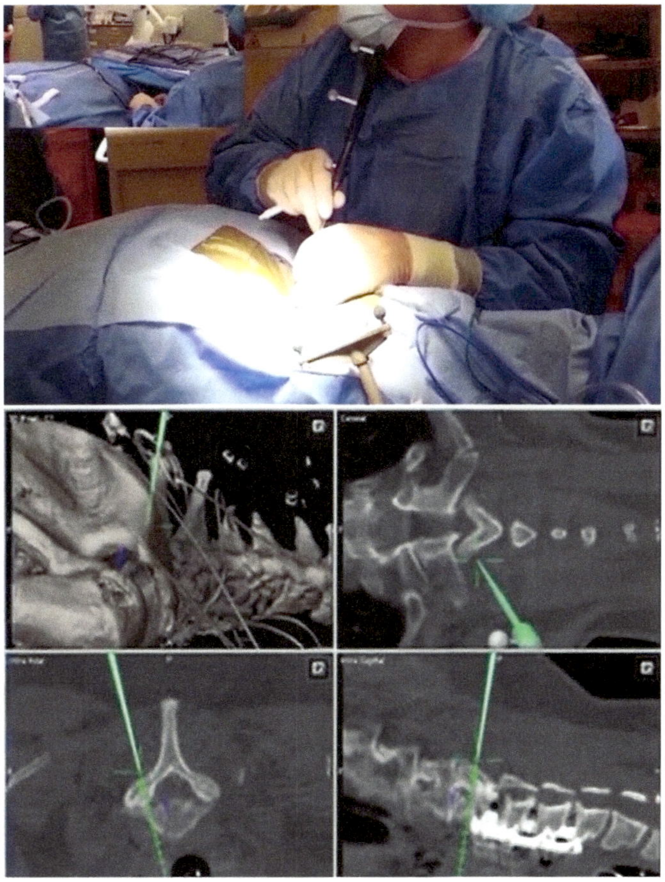

• **Fig. 14.1** The utilization of 3D navigation technology for performing minimally invasive posterior cervical foraminotomy and maximal lateral extent of facet resection to avoid instability.

Cervical Laminectomy

Traditional open cervical laminectomy for decompression of central stenosis requires disruption of the interspinous ligamentous structure and extensive soft tissue dissection depending on the number of levels requiring treatment.[22] These maneuvers can result in long-term neck pain and progressive kyphotic deformity (when performed without fusion) despite adequate decompression of the spinal canal.[23] The unilateral laminotomy for bilateral decompression (ULBD), first described in the lumbar spine, is a technique that allows surgeons to achieve bilateral decompression through a single incision often in an ambulatory setting, while preserving the posterior tension band. Having found consistent success in the lumbar spine while achieving decompression and/or fusion through an ultraminimally invasive incision, recent adoption of this technique to the cervical spine has been described.[24] Cervical ULBD can be performed in a minimally invasive fashion via a tubular or endoscopic technique for the treatment of cervical myelopathy in patients without evidence of instability (Fig. 14.2).[25,26] As with other minimally invasive procedures of the cervical spine, the primary benefits associated with this approach are reductions in blood loss, hospital stay, and postoperative narcotic utilization.[24] This approach also requires less bony removal and muscle disruption, which is perceived to lower the risk of postlaminectomy kyphosis and deformity.[27]

The primary complication risk associated with MIS cervical ULBD is spinal cord injury resulting in transient or permanent neurological deficit. Neurological deficit secondary to spinal cord injury can often be first identified intraoperatively using electrophysiological neuromonitoring.[25] While not standard of care, intraoperative neuromonitoring has been demonstrated to reduce the general risk of postoperative myelopathy in spine surgery.[28–30] However, studies evaluating the use of intraoperative neurophysiological monitoring during cervical laminectomy found that while monitoring was highly effective in detecting patients who would develop a C5 nerve palsy, it was rarely possible to prevent postoperative deltoid weakness with subsequent foraminotomy.[31] In the few incidences reported in the literature, these neurological deficits tend to improve with time, with many patients experiencing a full recovery of neurological function in just a few months.[25]

The use of an endoscope in cervical ULBD is associated with certain complications specific to endoscopy that warrant consideration. The angle of trajectory chosen for the endoscope can increase the risk for spinal cord injury. If a contralateral trajectory is used in order to spare the interspinous ligament, as opposed to a midline approach, the risk of spinal cord injury is greater in the event of ventral

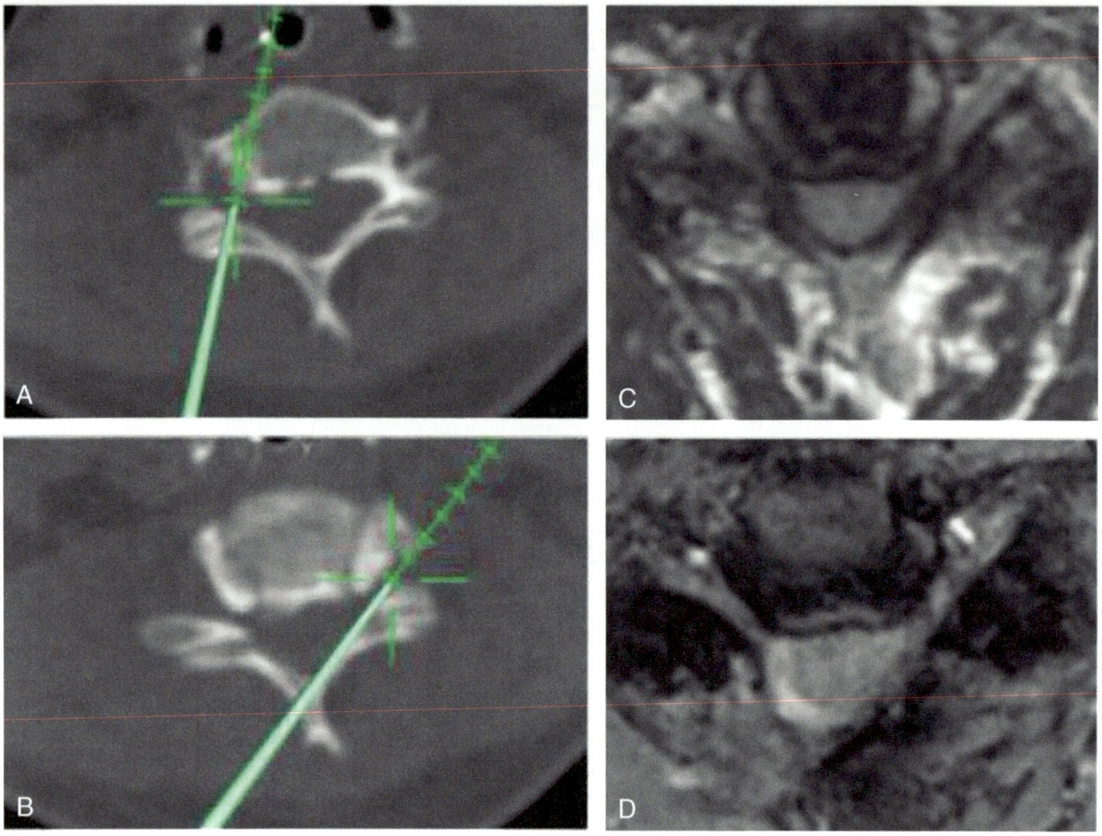

• **Fig. 14.2** Endoscopic or tubular unilateral laminotomy for bilateral decompression (ULBD) can achieve adequate decompression of the spinal cord through a minimally invasive corridor. 3D-computer navigation is useful for defining the trajectory and determining when the contralateral extent has been reached (A and B). (C) Axial T2 MRI demonstrating loss of CSF signal around the cord in a patient with cervical myelopathy. (D) Postoperative MRI demonstrating the right-sided approach for MIS ULBD with undercutting of the contralateral lamina to achieve bilateral decompression.

misplacement of the surgical instruments.[24,25] Endoscopic surgery also requires constant irrigation of the surgical field to maintain adequate visibility and remove debris. In endoscopic cervical MIS ULBD, care must be taken to limit the amount of irrigation in order to prevent injury to the spinal cord or vascular structures from excessive water pressure.[24] It has been recommended that continuous water pressure not exceed 40 mmHg, while adequately undercutting the spinous process can also provide another barrier against direct irrigation onto the spinal cord while maintaining enough of an opening for instruments to be used without applying unnecessary pressure to the dorsal surface of the spinal cord.[24,25]

While well tolerated in most cases with appropriately selected patients,[26] the overall complication rate observed in minimally invasive cervical ULBD, whether performed tubular or endoscopically, ranges from 0% to 6%.[32–36] In addition to the risk of spinal cord injury, incidental durotomy has been reported.[32–36] Larger trials comparing minimally invasive ULBD in the lumbar and thoracic spine to their open counterparts have consistently reported lower complication rates associated with the minimally invasive approach.[37,38]

Percutaneous Pedicle Screw Stabilization

Posterior stabilization of the subaxial cervical spine is indicated for several pathologies, including trauma, tumor, pseudoarthrosis, and deformity. This is traditionally performed via lateral mass instrumentation with or without decompression when required. While pedicle screws offer superior fixation and biomechanical strength, they are often deferred for a number of reasons.[39–41] First, they require more extensive dissection of paraspinal musculature to reach the starting point to achieve their lateral to medial trajectory.[42] Second, cervical pedicles may vary in width and thus are at higher risk for breach.[43] With the very close proximity to the vertebral artery and spinal cord, the risk of injury often dissuades their use, though this risk can be mitigated to some degree with intraoperative sonography.[44,45] Third, freehand and fluoroscopic guidance are not as reliable as they are in the thoracolumbar spine. The advent of intraoperative 3D navigation, however, has significantly increased the reliability of safely placing cervical pedicle screws, offering a much more viable option for posterior fixation.[46,47]

Given the extreme lateral starting point, medialized trajectory, and computer navigation, percutaneous insertion of

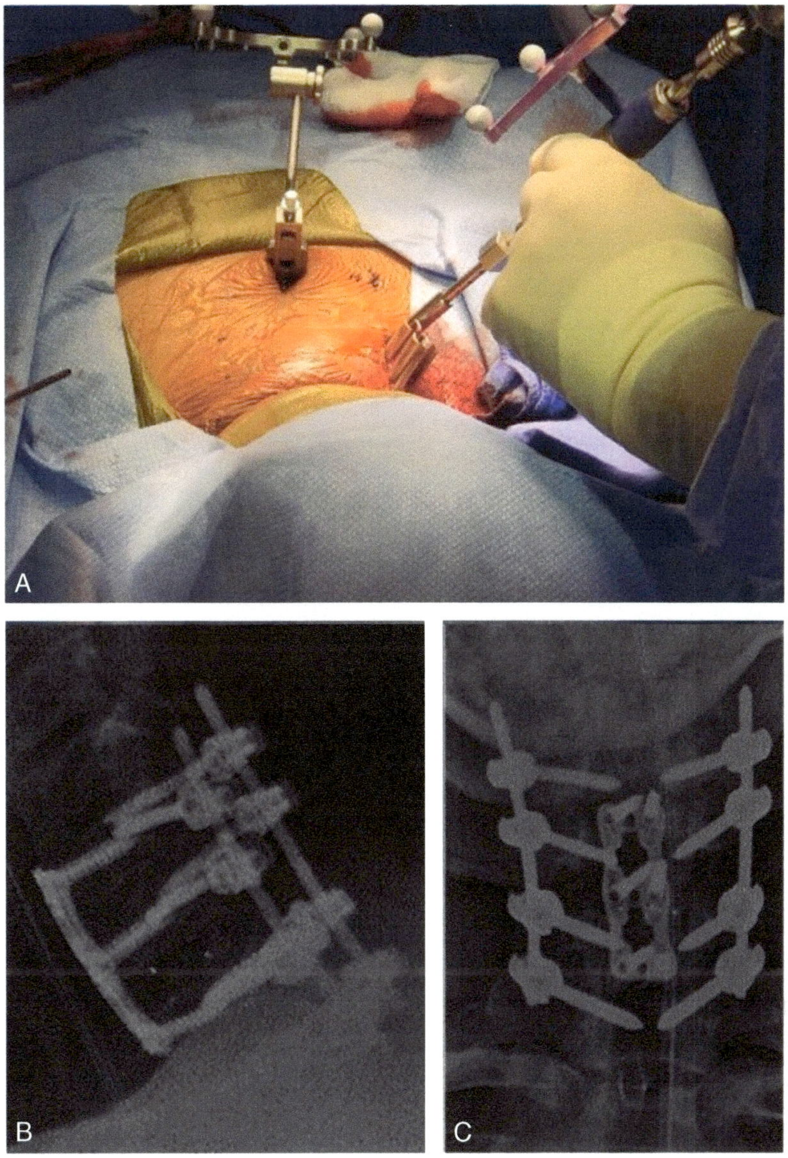

• **Fig. 14.3** (A) Surgical insertion of percutaneous pedicle screws. (B, C) Lateral and AP postoperative radiographs showing the placement of these screws with an extreme lateral to medial trajectory. (Photo courtesy Vincent Rossi, MD, MBA and Domagoj Coric, MD.)

cervical pedicle screws has been described.[48] Indications are limited and include those that have amenable anatomy and do not require a concomitant decompression.[49] The most common complication associated with percutaneous cervical pedicle screw fixation is screw malpositioning.[50] The severity of cervical pedicle screw malplacement is classified as Grade I if less than half of the screw is outside of the pedicle or Grade II if greater than half of the screw is outside of the pedicle.[51] Estimates of the incidence of malpositioned cervical pedicle screws range from 11% to 19.5%, with most malplacements categorized as Grade I.[51] Another important consideration is that malplaced screws are significantly more likely to deviate laterally than medially, which could potentially compromise the foramen transversarium and result in vertebral artery injury.[52,53] Notably, superior or inferior deviations are far less common due to the anatomic nature of the cervical pedicles: their narrow structure makes deviations in the medial-lateral plane much more likely[52] (Fig. 14.3).

The primary risk factor identified in the malplacement of cervical pedicle screws is the presence of preoperative cervical spine instability, particularly at the level of screw placement. To date, no other statistically significant risk factors have been identified for complications in the absence of screw malplacement, such as neurological deficit from spinal cord, nerve root, or vertebral artery injury.[52] Few studies have reported on hardware-related failures and infection in cervical pedicle screw fixation but reported rates of instrumentation failure range from 4.2% to 13.1% and a deep wound infection rate of 1.0% to 1.2%.[52,54] One study found a pseudoarthrosis rate of 1.2%.[52] While no suitable studies comparing the fusion rates of percutaneous versus open

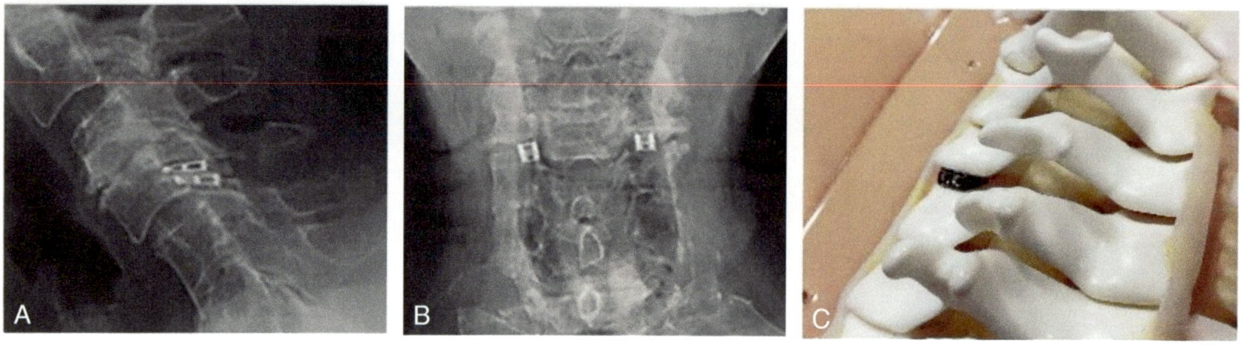

• **Fig. 14.4** Example of a percutaneous placed intrafacet joint cage. (A) Lateral x-ray, (B) AP x-ray, and (C) actual cage inserted into a spinal model.

cervical pedicle screw placement were identified, there is believed to be a theoretical higher risk of nonfusion with the percutaneous approach owing the lack of access to drill into the joints and pack with bone graft to promote arthrodesis.

The diagnosis of cervical pedicle screw malplacement and sequelae center around intraoperative and postoperative imaging. The utilization of intraoperative 3D navigation can help surgeons better plan the trajectory of the screw and monitor placement. Final confirmatory intraoperative imaging can often reveal suboptimal screw placement that can be revised before the conclusion of the operation. If there is a reasonable index of suspicion that the screw has compromised the foramen transversarium, mean arterial pressures should be maintained, the screw should be left in place, and immediate endovascular evaluation should be sought.[55,56] It is critical that screws are put in one side at a time to avoid the risk of bilateral vascular injury. Serial postoperative radiographs are also important to monitor for hardware fracture, migration, or pull-out.[52,53] Postoperative nerve root injuries are rare and typically present immediately after surgery with motor deficits and/or pain.[52] These patients should be evaluated with CT radiography and additional treatment. Patients with postoperative motor deficiencies secondary to pedicle screw misplacement may require revision surgery with screw removal.[57] Generally, these patients' symptoms will resolve within the first postoperative year.

Percutaneous Cervical Intrafacet Stabilization

Cervical intrafacet spacers or cages are a more recent advancement in the treatment of cervical radiculopathy refractory to conservative management. By achieving a distraction facet joint, these percutaneous implants can increase foraminal height and volume to achieve an indirect decompression of the exiting nerve root.[58,59] The utilization of percutaneous cervical intrafacet stabilization as an alternative or complement to ACDF is suggested to achieve cervical decompression and arthrodesis with fewer procedure-related morbidities.[60] This involves deploying a cage system through a minimally invasive approach and distracting the facet, ultimately achieving decompression and fusion.[61] The procedure is conducted utilizing a series of tools through a singular small percutaneous incision. First, a shim is inserted that takes advantage of the natural inclination of the cervical facet joint in the transverse plane to open up the neural foramina.[62] The facet is then stabilized with instrumented distraction utilizing a cage system. A decorticator then is used to promote definitive bone healing and arthrodesis. This percutaneous approach with a shim prevents the removal of tissue from the patient and the procedure is less invasive than other surgical techniques.[63] As such, the purported benefits of this procedure include a minimally invasive approach and deployment, decreasing the operative time and related morbidities and complications[60] (Fig. 14.4).

The incidence of significant neurological or vascular injury or complications associated with percutaneous cervical intrafacet stabilization is believed to be exceedingly rare, with several studies reporting no incidences of major complications or reoperations in the perioperative period.[60] The most common surgical complications reported were unilateral fracture of the facet during implantation and superficial infection of the surgical wound.[62,64] McCormack et al. reported an incidence rate of unilateral facet fracture of 1.7%.[62] These fractures were typically identified via intraoperative radiography and were managed by utilizing a unilateral stabilization as opposed to bilateral implants. Notably, each patient who experienced a unilateral facet fracture went on to achieve radiographic fusion and had a good clinical outcome. Subsequent modifications in the instrumentation used, including switching to a chisel with a flat leading edge, led to no further fractures in the McCormack et al. study.[62] The incidence of superficial wound infection was estimated in another study to be 5.7%.[64] Overall, the risk of complications associated with percutaneous cervical intrafacet stabilization is considered to be much lower than the risk associated with ACDF.[60,62–64] By comparison, neurologic complications reportedly occur in 4.81% of ACDF procedures (range 0%–32%) and in 9.89% of posterior lateral mass screw procedures (range, 0%–20.3%).[65–71] In general, the reported rates of fusion in the cervical spine utilizing percutaneous posterior intrafacet stabilization are high, ranging from 93% to 100%.[60,72,73] In utilizing the posterior percutaneous approach to deploy cervical cages directly into the facet joints, vascular complications and vertebral artery injury are likely avoided because ventral overadvancement into the foramen transversarium is obstructed by the cephalic cervical pedicle. In fact, the use of percutaneous cervical intrafacet stabilization in combination with ACDF may reduce the risk of pseudarthrosis in high-risk patients with comorbidities or extensive procedures.[64]

Conclusion

Minimally invasive approaches for posterior cervical spine surgery will continue to evolve concomitant with advances with 3D computer navigation, and advanced techniques utilizing tubular and endoscopic technology. In this regard, the procedures mentioned in this chapter including posterior endoscopic and tubular cervical foraminotomy, unilateral laminotomy for bilateral decompression, percutaneous pedicle screw stabilization, and percutaneous posterior cervical intrafacet fusion represent the newest iterations of minimally invasive posterior cervical procedures aiming to achieve these goals. The preservation of the posterior tension band while minimizing muscle dissection provides opportunities for mitigation of long-term complications relevant to instability as well as accelerating patient recovery postoperatively as has been witnessed in the lumbar spine. Nonetheless, most of these procedures are still in their relative infancy and therefore require larger studies and longer-term outcomes to justify their utility more fully.

References

1. Yoon JW, Wang MY. The evolution of minimally invasive spine surgery. *J Neurosurg Spine*. 2019;30(2):149–158. https://doi.org/10.3171/2018.11.SPINE181215.
2. Skovrlj B, Qureshi SA. Minimally invasive cervical spine surgery. *J Neurosurg Sci*. 2017;61(3):325–334. https://doi.org/10.23736/S0390-5616.16.03906-0.
3. Fessler RG, Khoo LT. Minimally invasive cervical microendoscopic foraminotomy: an initial clinical experience. *Neurosurgery*. 2002;51(5 Suppl):S37–S45.
4. Saal JS, Saal JA, Yurth EF. Nonoperative management of herniated cervical intervertebral disc with radiculopathy. *Spine*. 1996;21(16):1877–1883. https://doi.org/10.1097/00007632-199608150-00008.
5. van Geest S, Kuijper B, Oterdoom M, et al. CASINO: surgical or nonsurgical treatment for cervical radiculopathy, a randomised controlled trial. *BMC Musculoskelet Disord*. 2014;15:129. https://doi.org/10.1186/1471-2474-15-129.
6. Jagannathan J, Sherman JH, Szabo T, Shaffrey CI, Jane JA. The posterior cervical foraminotomy in the treatment of cervical disc/osteophyte disease: a single-surgeon experience with a minimum of 5 years' clinical and radiographic follow-up. *J Neurosurg Spine*. 2009;10(4):347–356. https://doi.org/10.3171/2008.12.SPINE08576.
7. Ruetten S, Komp M, Merk H, Godolias G. Full-endoscopic cervical posterior foraminotomy for the operation of lateral disc herniations using 5.9-mm endoscopes: a prospective, randomized, controlled study. *Spine*. 2008;33(9):940–948. https://doi.org/10.1097/BRS.0b013e31816c8b67.
8. Miele VF, Vadera S, Benzel EC. Spinal stenosis with spondylolisthesis. In: *The Comprehensive Treatment of the Aging Spine (Minimally Invasive and Advanced Techniques)*. 2011.
9. Buraimoh M, Ansok C, Pawloski J, Jung EK, Bartol S. Facet sparing foraminal decompression using the flexible shaver foraminotomy system: nerve safety, pain relief, and patient satisfaction. *Int J Spine Surg*. 2018;12(2):92–97. https://doi.org/10.14444/5015.
10. Skovrlj B, Gologorsky Y, Haque R, Fessler RG, Qureshi SA. Complications, outcomes, and need for fusion after minimally invasive posterior cervical foraminotomy and microdiscectomy. *Spine J*. 2014;14(10):2405–2411. https://doi.org/10.1016/j.spinee.2014.01.048.
11. Nguyen J, Chu B, Kuo CC, Leasure JM, Ames C, Kondrashov D. Changes in foraminal area with anterior decompression versus keyhole foraminotomy in the cervical spine: a biomechanical investigation. *J Neurosurg Spine*. 2017;27(6):620–626. https://doi.org/10.3171/2017.2.SPINE141237.
12. Jack A, Ramey WL, Dettori JR, et al. Factors associated with C5 palsy following cervical spine surgery: A systematic review. *Global Spine J*. 2019;9(8):881–894. https://doi.org/10.1177/2192568219874771.
13. Choi K-C, Ahn Y, Kang B-U, Ahn S-T, Lee S-H. Motor palsy after posterior cervical foraminotomy: anatomical consideration. *World Neurosurg*. 2013;79(2):405. https://doi.org/10.1016/j.wneu.2011.03.043.e1-4.
14. Bydon M, Macki M, Kaloostian P, et al. Incidence and prognostic factors of c5 palsy: a clinical study of 1001 cases and review of the literature. *Neurosurgery*. 2014;74(6):595–604. https://doi.org/10.1227/NEU.0000000000000322.discussion 604.
15. Liu B, Chu Y, Ma J, et al. Analysis of risk factors for C5 nerve root paralysis after posterior cervical decompression. *BMC Musculoskelet Disord*. 2021;22(1):614. https://doi.org/10.1186/s12891-021-04434-y.
16. Houten JK, Buksbaum JR, Collins MJ. Patterns of neurological deficits and recovery of postoperative C5 nerve palsy. *J Neurosurg Spine*. 2020:1–9. https://doi.org/10.3171/2020.5.SPINE20514.
17. Wu Z, Wu H, Wang H, et al. Clinical quiz: A rare complication after minimally invasive posterior cervical laminoforaminotomy. *J Musculoskelet Neuronal Interact*. 2016;16(2):172–173.
18. Branch BC, Hilton DL, Watts C. Minimally invasive tubular access for posterior cervical foraminotomy. *Surg Neurol Int*. 2015;6:81. https://doi.org/10.4103/2152-7806.157308.
19. Dinh SN, Dinh HT. The first experience with fully endoscopic posterior cervical foraminotomy and discectomy for radiculopathy performed in Viet Duc University Hospital. *Sci Rep*. 2022;12(1):8314. https://doi.org/10.1038/s41598-022-12493-x.
20. Barak U, Sheinis D, Sidon E, Shemesh S, Amitai A, Ohana N. C5 palsy following cervical spine decompression. *Isr Med Assoc J*. 2021;23(8):521–525.
21. Currier BL. Neurological complications of cervical spine surgery: C5 palsy and intraoperative monitoring. *Spine*. 2012;37(5):E328–E334. https://doi.org/10.1097/BRS.0b013e3182417276.
22. Geck MJ, Eismont FJ. Surgical options for the treatment of cervical spondylotic myelopathy. *Orthop Clin North Am*. 2002;33(2):329–348. https://doi.org/10.1016/s0030-5898(02)00002-0.
23. Oppenheimer JH, DeCastro I, McDonnell DE. Minimally invasive spine technology and minimally invasive spine surgery:

a historical review. *Neurosurg Focus.* 2009;27(3):E9. https://doi.org/10.3171/2009.7.FOCUS09121.

24. Hussain I, Hofstetter CP, Wang MY. Innovations in spinal endoscopy. *World Neurosurg.* 2022;160:138–148. https://doi.org/10.1016/j.wneu.2021.11.099.
25. Carr DA, Abecassis IJ, Hofstetter CP. Full endoscopic unilateral laminotomy for bilateral decompression of the cervical spine: surgical technique and early experience. *J Spine Surg.* 2020;6(2):447–456. https://doi.org/10.21037/jss.2020.01.03.
26. Hernandez RN, Wipplinger C, Navarro-Ramirez R, et al. Ten-step minimally invasive cervical decompression via unilateral tubular laminotomy: Technical note and early clinical Experience. *Oper Neurosurg (Hagerstown).* 2020;18(3):284–294. https://doi.org/10.1093/ons/opz156.
27. Kirnaz S, Wipplinger C, Wong T, Schmidt FA, Nangunoori R, Härtl R. Less invasive cervical decompression via unilateral tubular laminotomy using 3-dimensional total navigation: 2-dimensional operative video. *Oper Neurosurg (Hagerstown).* 2020;19(4):E418. https://doi.org/10.1093/ons/opaa059.
28. Nuwer MR, Dawson EG, Carlson LG, Kanim LE, Sherman JE. Somatosensory evoked potential spinal cord monitoring reduces neurologic deficits after scoliosis surgery: results of a large multicenter survey. *Electroencephalogr Clin Neurophysiol.* 1995;96(1):6–11.
29. Holland NR. Intraoperative electromyography. *J Clin Neurophysiol.* 2002;19(5):444–453. https://doi.org/10.1097/00004691-200210000-00007.
30. Wang Y-B, Zhao X-B, Geng B, et al. Application of triggered EMG in the intraoperative neurophysiological monitoring of posterior percutaneous endoscopic cervical discectomy. *Orthop Surg.* 2021;13(8):2236–2245. https://doi.org/10.1111/os.13092.
31. Ando M, Tamaki T, Matsumoto T, et al. Can postoperative deltoid weakness after cervical laminoplasty be prevented by using intraoperative neurophysiological monitoring. *J Clin Monit Comput.* 2019;33(1):123–132. https://doi.org/10.1007/s10877-018-0141-4.
32. Dahdaleh NS, Wong AP, Smith ZA, Wong RH, Lam SK, Fessler RG. Microendoscopic decompression for cervical spondylotic myelopathy. *Neurosurg Focus.* 2013;35(1):E8. https://doi.org/10.3171/2013.3.FOCUS135.
33. Abbas SF, Spurgas MP, Szewczyk BS, Yim B, Ata A, German JW. A comparison of minimally invasive posterior cervical decompression and open anterior cervical decompression and instrumented fusion in the surgical management of degenerative cervical myelopathy. *Neurosurg Focus.* 2016;40(6):E7. https://doi.org/10.3171/2016.3.FOCUS1650.
34. Hur J-W, Kim J-S, Shin M-H, Ryu K-S. Minimally invasive posterior cervical decompression using tubular retractor: The technical note and early clinical outcome. *Surg Neurol Int.* 2014;5:34. https://doi.org/10.4103/2152-7806.128915.
35. Vergara P. Minimally invasive microscopic posterior cervical decompression: simple, safe, and effective. *J Neurol Surg A Cent Eur Neurosurg.* 2017;78(5):440–445. https://doi.org/10.1055/s-0037-1598051.
36. Minamide A, Yoshida M, Simpson AK, et al. Microendoscopic laminotomy versus conventional laminoplasty for cervical spondylotic myelopathy: 5-year follow-up study. *J Neurosurg Spine.* 2017;27(4):403–409. https://doi.org/10.3171/2017.2.SPINE16939.
37. Takahashi H, Aoki Y, Saito J, et al. Unilateral laminectomy for bilateral decompression improves low back pain while standing equally on both sides in patients with lumbar canal stenosis: analysis using a detailed visual analogue scale. *BMC Musculoskelet Disord.* 2019;20(1):100. https://doi.org/10.1186/s12891-019-2475-6.
38. Thomé C, Zevgaridis D, Leheta O, et al. Outcome after less-invasive decompression of lumbar spinal stenosis: a randomized comparison of unilateral laminotomy, bilateral laminotomy, and laminectomy. *J Neurosurg Spine.* 2005;3(2):129–141. https://doi.org/10.3171/spi.2005.3.2.0129.
39. Jones EL, Heller JG, Silcox DH, Hutton WC. Cervical pedicle screws versus lateral mass screws. Anatomic feasibility and biomechanical comparison. *Spine.* 1997;22(9):977–982. https://doi.org/10.1097/00007632-199705010-00009.
40. Johnston TL, Karaikovic EE, Lautenschlager EP, Marcu D. Cervical pedicle screws vs. lateral mass screws: uniplanar fatigue analysis and residual pullout strengths. *Spine J.* 2006;6(6):667–672. https://doi.org/10.1016/j.spinee.2006.03.019.
41. Yan L, He B, Liu T, Yang L, Hao D. A prospective, double-blind, randomized controlled trial of treatment of atlantoaxial instability with C1 posterior arches >4 mm by comparing C1 pedicle with lateral mass screws fixation. *BMC Musculoskelet Disord.* 2016;17:164. https://doi.org/10.1186/s12891-016-1017-8.
42. Farshad M, Spirig JM, Winkler E, et al. Template guided cervical pedicle screw instrumentation. *N Am Spine Soc J.* 2022;10:100120. https://doi.org/10.1016/j.xnsj.2022.100120.
43. Mao JZ, Soliman MAR, Karamian BA, et al. Anatomical and technical considerations of robot-assisted cervical pedicle screw placement: A cadaveric study. *Global Spine J.* 2022 https://doi.org/10.1177/21925682211068410.21925682211068410.
44. Lee SH, Park J-H, Lee JB, et al. Safety and efficacy of intraoperative Doppler sonography-assisted cervical pedicle screw fixation-A retrospective comparison with conventional pedicle screw implantation. *Global Spine J.* 2022. https://doi.org/10.1177/21925682211041965.21925682211041965.
45. Yang J, Li T, Wang Q, et al. Morphological characteristics of subaxial cervical pedicles and surrounding critical structures in patients with vertebral artery dominance - an anatomical study based on computed tomographic imaging. *BMC Musculoskelet Disord.* 2022;23(1):306. https://doi.org/10.1186/s12891-022-05264-2.
46. Zhang K, Chen H, Chen K, Yang P, Yang H, Mao H. O-arm navigated cervical pedicle screw fixation in the treatment of lower cervical fracture-dislocation. *Orthop Surg.* 2022;14(6):1135–1142. https://doi.org/10.1111/os.13227.
47. Shin HK, Jeon SR, Roh SW, Park JH. Benefits and pitfalls of O-arm navigation in cervical pedicle screw. *World Neurosurg.* 2022;159:e460–e465. https://doi.org/10.1016/j.wneu.2021.12.077.
48. Perna A, Smakaj A, Vitiello R, et al. Posterior percutaneous pedicle screws fixation versus open surgical instrumented fusion for thoraco-lumbar spinal metastases palliative management: A systematic review and meta-analysis. *Front Oncol.* 2022;12:884928. https://doi.org/10.3389/fonc.2022.884928.
49. Coric D, Rossi V. Percutaneous posterior cervical pedicle instrumentation (C1 to C7) with navigation guidance: early series of 27 cases. *Global Spine J.* 2022;12(2_suppl):27S–33S. https://doi.org/10.1177/21925682211029215.
50. Cong T, Sivaganesan A, Mikhail CM, et al. Facet violation with percutaneous pedicle screw placement: impact of 3D navigation and facet orientation. *HSS J.* 2021;17(3):281–288. https://doi.org/10.1177/15563316211026324.
51. Yamada T, Hasegawa T, Yamato Y, et al. Characteristics of pedicle screw misplacement using freehand technique in

degenerative scoliosis surgery. *Arch Orthop Trauma Surg.* 2023;143(4):1861–1867. https://doi.org/10.1007/s00402-022-04380-x.
52. Nakashima H, Yukawa Y, Imagama S, et al. Complications of cervical pedicle screw fixation for nontraumatic lesions: a multicenter study of 84 patients. *J Neurosurg Spine.* 2012;16(3):238–247. https://doi.org/10.3171/2011.11.SPINE11102.
53. Coric D, Rossi VJ, Peloza J, Kim PK, Adamson TEPercutaneous. navigated minimally invasive posterior cervical pedicle screw fixation. *Int J Spine Surg.* 2020;14(s3):S14–S21. https://doi.org/10.14444/7122.
54. Yukawa Y, Kato F, Yoshihara H, Yanase M, Ito K. Cervical pedicle screw fixation in 100 cases of unstable cervical injuries: pedicle axis views obtained using fluoroscopy. *J Neurosurg Spine.* 2006;5(6):488–493. https://doi.org/10.3171/spi.2006.5.6.488.
55. Lunardini DJ, Eskander MS, Even JL, et al. Vertebral artery injuries in cervical spine surgery. *Spine J.* 2014;14(8):1520–1525. https://doi.org/10.1016/j.spinee.2013.09.016.
56. Schroeder GD, Hsu WK. Vertebral artery injuries in cervical spine surgery. *Surg Neurol Int.* 2013;4(Suppl 5):S362–S367. https://doi.org/10.4103/2152-7806.120777.
57. Takemitsu M, Cheung KMC, Wong YW, Cheung W-Y, Luk KDK. C5 nerve root palsy after cervical laminoplasty and posterior fusion with instrumentation. *J Spinal Disord Tech.* 2008;21(4):267–272. https://doi.org/10.1097/BSD.0b013e31812f6f54.
58. Goel A, Shah A. Facetal distraction as treatment for single- and multilevel cervical spondylotic radiculopathy and myelopathy: a preliminary report. *J Neurosurg Spine.* 2011;14(6):689–696. https://doi.org/10.3171/2011.2.SPINE10601.
59. Tan LA, Gerard CS, Anderson PA, Traynelis VC. Effect of machined interfacet allograft spacers on cervical foraminal height and area. *J Neurosurg Spine.* 2014;20(2):178–182. https://doi.org/10.3171/2013.11.SPINE131.
60. Laratta JL, Gupta K, Smith WD. Tissue-sparing posterior cervical fusion with interfacet cages: A systematic review of the literature. *Global Spine J.* 2020;10(2):230–236. https://doi.org/10.1177/2192568219837145.
61. Leasure JM, Buckley J. Biomechanical evaluation of an interfacet joint decompression and stabilization system. *J Biomech Eng.* 2014;136(7). https://doi.org/10.1115/1.4026363.
62. McCormack BM, Bundoc RC, Ver MR, Ignacio JMF, Berven SH, Eyster EF. Percutaneous posterior cervical fusion with the DTRAX Facet System for single-level radiculopathy: results in 60 patients. *J Neurosurg Spine.* 2013;18(3):245–254. https://doi.org/10.3171/2012.12.SPINE12477.
63. Yazdanshenas H, Osias E, Hwang R, Park DY, Lord E, Shamie AN. Retrospective evaluation of cervical fusion with DTRAX (R) cervical cage. *J Craniovertebr Junction Spine.* 2022;13(1):48–54. https://doi.org/10.4103/jcvjs.jcvjs_150_21.
64. Kramer S, Albana MF, Ferraro JB, Shah RV. Minimally invasive posterior cervical fusion with facet cages to augment high-risk anterior cervical arthrodesis: A case series. *Global Spine J.* 2020;10(2 Suppl):56S–60S. https://doi.org/10.1177/2192568220911031.
65. Guo Q, Bi X, Ni B, et al. Outcomes of three anterior decompression and fusion techniques in the treatment of three-level cervical spondylosis. *Eur Spine J.* 2011;20(9):1539–1544. https://doi.org/10.1007/s00586-011-1735-4.
66. Uribe JS, Sangala JR, Duckworth EAM, Vale FL. Comparison between anterior cervical discectomy fusion and cervical corpectomy fusion using titanium cages for reconstruction: analysis of outcome and long-term follow-up. *Eur Spine J.* 2009;18(5):654–662. https://doi.org/10.1007/s00586-009-0897-9.
67. Song K-J, Lee K-B, Song J-H. Efficacy of multilevel anterior cervical discectomy and fusion versus corpectomy and fusion for multilevel cervical spondylotic myelopathy: a minimum 5-year follow-up study. *Eur Spine J.* 2012;21(8):1551–1557. https://doi.org/10.1007/s00586-012-2296-x.
68. Lin Q, Zhou X, Wang X, Cao P, Tsai N, Yuan W. A comparison of anterior cervical discectomy and corpectomy in patients with multilevel cervical spondylotic myelopathy. *Eur Spine J.* 2012;21(3):474–481. https://doi.org/10.1007/s00586-011-1961-9.
69. Pateder DB, Carbone JJ. Lateral mass screw fixation for cervical spine trauma: associated complications and efficacy in maintaining alignment. *Spine J.* 2006;6(1):40–43. https://doi.org/10.1016/j.spinee.2005.04.010.
70. Sekhon LHS. Posterior cervical lateral mass screw fixation: analysis of 1026 consecutive screws in 143 patients. *J Spinal Disord Tech.* 2005;18(4):297–303. https://doi.org/10.1097/01.bsd.0000166640.23448.09.
71. Al Barbarawi MM, Allouh MZ. Cervical lateral mass screw-rod fixation: Surgical experience with 2500 consecutive screws, an analytical review, and long-term outcomes. *Br J Neurosurg.* 2015;29(5):699–704. https://doi.org/10.3109/02688697.2015.1026798.
72. Siemionow K, Janusz P, Phillips FM, et al. Clinical and radiographic results of indirect decompression and posterior cervical fusion for single-level cervical radiculopathy using an expandable implant with 2-year follow-up. *J Neurol Surg A Cent Eur Neurosurg.* 2016;77(6):482–488. https://doi.org/10.1055/s-0036-1584210.
73. Siemionow K, Monsef JB, Janusz P. Preliminary analysis of adjacent segment degeneration in patients treated with posterior cervical cages: 2-year follow-up. *World Neurosurg.* 2016;89:730 https://doi.org/10.1016/j.wneu.2016.01.053.e1-7.

15

When to Operate on the Thoracic Spine

STANLEY KISINDE, JOSEPH L. ALBANO, DAVID GEOFFREY BARNES, ALEXANDER M. SATIN, AND ISADOR H. LIEBERMAN

CHAPTER OUTLINE

Thoracic spine surgery is indicated for conditions deemed not amenable to improvement with nonoperative modalities.[1,2] Although there may be differing opinions on the timing of surgery and optimal surgical approach,[1,3,4] there is agreement on the primary goals of surgery—maintenance or restoration of spinal alignment and stability, preservation of neurologic function, and relief from pain.[2,5–7] Here we review the considerations and indications for thoracic spine surgery.

Metastatic Spine Tumors

Spinal metastases occur in approximately 20% of patients with cancer.[8,9] The goal of treatment in these instances is generally palliative—relief from pain, maintain or recover neurologic function, achieve local durable tumor control, restore or maintain spinal stability, and provide the patients with an improved quality of life. Radiation and surgery remain the most effective treatment modalities for spinal metastases. However, recent advancements in radiation technology, surgical techniques, and medical treatments have led to the evolution of treatment recommendations for spinal metastases.[7]

The NOMS framework[7] is a landmark clinical decision framework for the management of metastatic spine disease (Table 15.1). It emphasizes four vital assessment parameters: neurologic (N), oncologic (O), mechanical stability (M), and systemic disease (S) in order to determine the role of surgery and other treatment modalities. Furthermore, it incorporates the latest surgical techniques, radiation and medical oncology, and interventional radiology procedures in order to achieve optimal and standardized outcomes in patients with spinal metastases.

Neurologic Indications

The neurologic assessment focuses on the degree of spinal cord compromise as observed on imaging as well as the clinical assessment of myelopathy and/or radiculopathy. In the majority of patients with spinal metastases, radiographic evidence of epidural spinal cord compression (ESCC) is directly proportional to the exhibition of neurologic deficits attributable to the epidural tumor.

The Spine Oncology Study Group (SOSG) designed and validated a 6-point grading system[11] that uses axial T2-weighted images at the site of most severe compression to describe the degree of ESCC (Figs. 15.1 and 15.2).

TABLE 15.1 The Current NOMS Decision Framework

Neurologic	Oncologic	Mechanical	Systemic	Decision
ESCC grade ± Myelopathy	***Radio sensitivity***	***Stability***	***Ability to tolerate surgery***	
Low-grade ESCC with no myelopathy	Radiosensitive	Stable	–	cEBRT
	Radiosensitive	Unstable	–	Stabilization followed by cEBRT
	Radioresistant	Stable	–	SRS
	Radioresistant	Unstable	–	Stabilization followed by SRS
High grade ESCC with/without myelopathy	Radiosensitive	Stable	–	cEBRT
	Radiosensitive	Unstable	–	Stabilization followed by cEBRT
	Radioresistant	Stable	Able to tolerate surgery	Decompression Stabilization followed by SRS
	Radioresistant	Unstable	Unable to tolerate surgery	cEBRT
	Radioresistant	Stable	Able to tolerate surgery	Decompression Stabilization followed by SRS
	Radioresistant	Unstable	Unable to tolerate surgery	Stabilization followed by cEBRT

Adapted from Laufer I, Rubin DG, Lis E, et al. The NOMS framework: approach to the treatment of spinal metastatic tumors, *Oncologist*. 2013; 18(6):744–751. Low-grade ESCC is defined as grade 0 or 1 on Spine Oncology Study Group scoring system[7,10]. High-grade ESCC is defined as grade 2 or 3 on the ESCC scale[7,10]. Stabilization options include percutaneous cement augmentation; percutaneous pedicle screw instrumentation, and open instrumentation. For patients with significant systemic comorbidities that affect the ability to tolerate open surgery, stabilization may be limited to cement augmentation and/or percutaneous screw augmentation.*cEBRT*, Conventional external beam radiation; *ESCC*, epidural spinal cord compression; *NOMS*, neurologic, oncologic, mechanical, and systemic; *SRS*, stereotactic radiosurgery.

Grades 2 and 3 represent high grade ESCC, requiring surgical decompression prior to radiation therapy unless the tumor is highly radiosensitive. Grades 0, 1a, and 1b are considered for initial treatment with radiation provided there is no evidence of spinal instability. Grade 1c epidural tumors are considered indeterminate, requiring further individualized patient assessment to determine the role of surgical or radiosurgery intervention.[7]

Oncologic Indications

The responsiveness of a tumor to currently available nonsurgical treatment modalities defines its oncologic response in terms of sensitivity or resistance. The treatment modality that provides the yardstick for local tumor control is radiation, as this represents the least invasive yet most effective modality of treatment. Tumors are therefore defined as sensitive or resistant to radiation based on their response to conventional external beam radiation therapy (cEBRT), which is delivered in one or two radiation beams without precise conformal techniques. Tumor histology is a very important factor in determining the response to cEBRT.

Almost all authors classify lymphoma, seminoma, and myeloma as radiosensitive histologies, while there is some variation in reference to radiosensitive solid tumor histologies including breast, prostate, ovarian, and neuroendocrine carcinomas.[10,12–19] Inclusion in this class (radiosensitive) supports the use of cEBRT in the treatment of these tumors, regardless of the degree of ESCC or neurologic deficit. cEBRT is able to cause sufficient mitotic cell death within the tumor and subsequently spinal cord decompression,[20,21] thereby providing both symptomatic relief and satisfactory/durable local control in these patients, without causing damage to surrounding neurologic and other vital tissues. This often obviates the need for surgical intervention. Radiosensitive solid tumors may also be treated with stereotactic radiosurgery (SRS).

Renal, thyroid, hepatocellular, colon, nonsmall cell lung carcinomas, sarcoma, and melanoma represent radioresistant tumors.[10,12–19] These radioresistant tumor histologies do not have acceptable response rates to cEBRT. This is due to the fact that cEBRT is limited in delivering tumoricidal radiation doses to these tumors without a high risk of toxicity to the spinal cord or adjacent vital organs within the radiation field.

One of the recent technological advancements in the fields of radiation oncology and interventional radiology is image-guided radiation therapy (IGRT). IGRT allows for the delivery of conformal high doses of radiation with high spatial precision to the tumor, thereby maintaining acceptable radiation exposure to the spinal cord and other adjacent vital structures.

Patients with radioresistant tumors and ESCC grades 0, 1a, and 1b can be treated with IGRT, again obviating the need for surgical decompression. This is in contrast to previous treatment algorithms in which these patients were often initially offered excisional surgery due to the historically poor responses to cEBRT. The SRS, offered as an outpatient

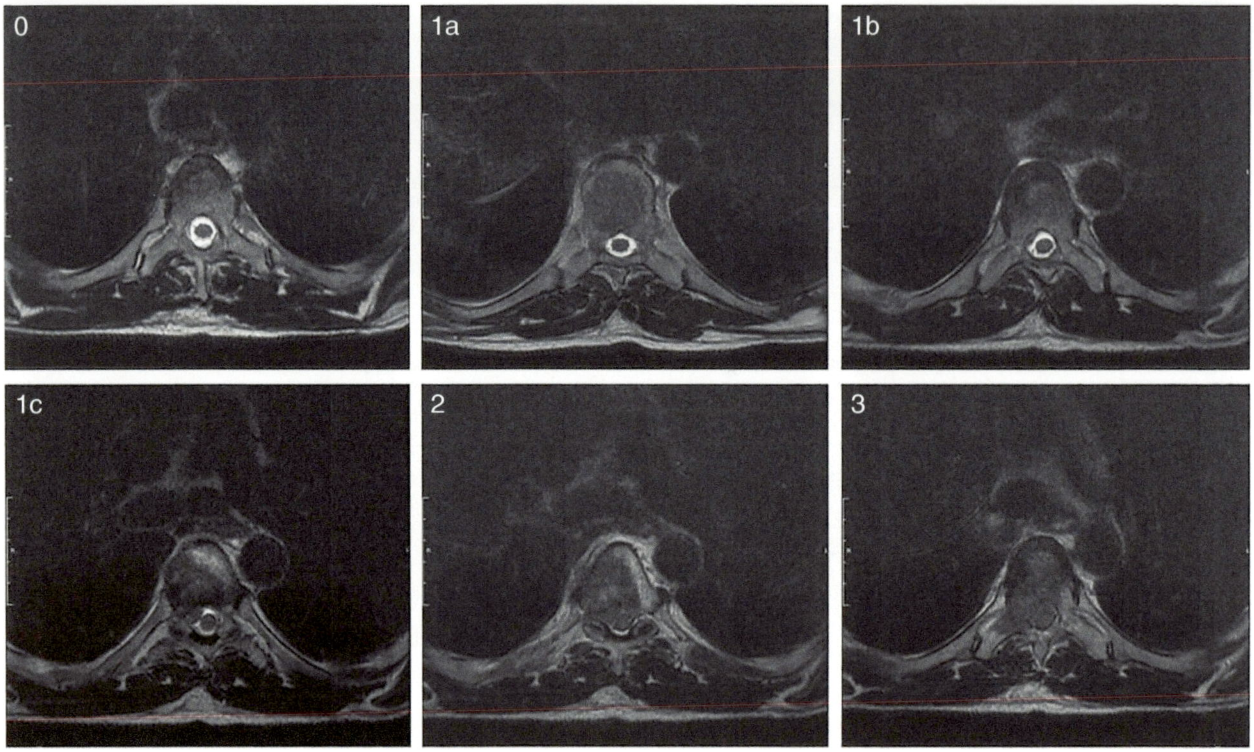

• **Fig. 15.1** Six-point ESCC grading scale system by the SOSG Group[11]: Grade 0 – disease confined to only bone; 1 – tumor extension into the epidural space but without deformation of the spinal cord; 1a – epidural impingement but without deformation of the thecal sac; 1b – deformation of the thecal sac but without spinal cord abutment; 1c – deformation of the thecal sac with spinal cord abutment, but without spinal cord compression; 2 – spinal cord compression, but with cerebrospinal fluid visible around the cord; and 3 – spinal cord compression without visible cerebrospinal fluid around the spinal cord.

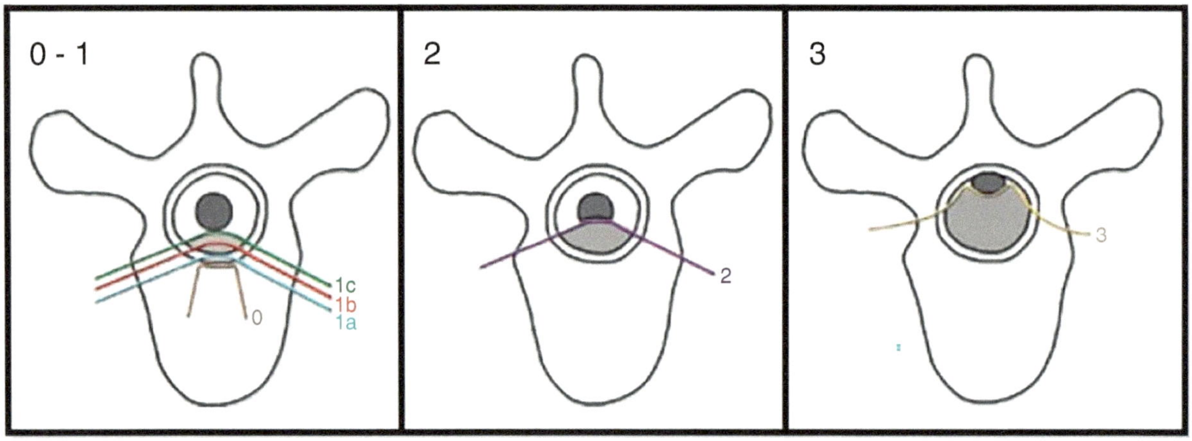

• **Fig. 15.2** Schematic images representing the progressive grades of epidural spinal cord compression. (With permission from Bilsky, M. H. et al., (2010). Reliability analysis of the epidural spinal cord compression scale: Clinical article. *Journal of Neurosurgery*: Spine SPI, 13(3), 324–328. https://doi.org/10.3171/2010.3.SPINE09459.)

procedure, is a better first-line treatment modality compared to extensive surgical resection, with fewer and milder complications. Radiation-induced spinal cord injury and delayed vertebral body fracture are rare complications.

Patients with radioresistant tumors and ESCC grades 2 and 3 require surgical decompression and stabilization prior to IGRT. However, the ability to deliver tumoricidal doses safely and effectively to gross residual tumor volumes while controlling for spinal cord toxicity with SRS has in effect changed the goals of surgery. Currently, the primary goals of surgery are preservation or restoration of mechanical stability and circumferential decompression of the spinal cord or "separation surgery." Separation surgery involves creating a small (2 mm) separation between the tumor and the spinal cord to preserve neurologic function and allow delivery of tumoricidal radiation doses to the entire tumor volume while controlling for toxicity to the spinal cord. In separation surgery, only minimal tumor resection, just enough to separate the tumor margin from the spinal cord, is carried out while the bulk of the tumor mass is left to be treated with radiation.

Mechanical Indications

According to the SOSG, spinal instability is defined as the "loss of spinal integrity as a result of a neoplastic process that is associated with movement-related pain, symptomatic or progressive deformity, and/or neural compromise under physiologic loads."[22] It is assessed on the basis of both clinical and radiographic criteria (The Spinal Instability Neoplastic Score [SINS]—Table 15.2).

Clinically, patients with spinal instability present with severe movement-related pain that is characteristic of the specific spinal level involved. Instability pain must be clearly distinguished from biologic pain.[23,24] In the thoracic spine, instability pain is often elicited with extension.

Patients may present with mechanical radiculopathy—severe radicular pain upon standing—due to collapse of the neural foramen when standing and subsequent compression of the exiting nerve root. This rarely occurs in the thoracic spine because of the reinforcement provided by the intact rib cage and sternum.

A general consensus is that mechanical instability serves as an independent indication for surgical stabilization or percutaneous cement augmentation. Although effective for local tumor control, radiation has no impact on spinal stability, and mechanical pain does not improve with steroid therapy. Patients with intermediate SINS tumors require further assessment to determine the need for surgery.

The development of segmental instability following radiotherapy is also considered an indication for surgical treatment.[25]

Systemic Indications

Assessment of systemic disease in terms of systemic medical comorbidities, tumor burden, and tumor histology can help determine which interventions the patient can tolerate physiologically. This involves metastatic staging workup and a surgical risk stratification to determine the appropriateness of the proposed intervention strategies in terms of acceptable risk to the patient.

Metastatic invasion of the spine by certain tumor histologies precludes benefit from certain interventions, especially in association with shortened survival. In such cases, for example, patients with aggressive tumors like nonsmall cell lung carcinoma, colon carcinoma, and carcinoma of unknown primary origin have median survival rates of approximately 4 months from the time of surgery.[26] As a result, these patients may not necessarily benefit from extensive interventions that require prolonged hospital stays or intensive physical therapy.

In cases where the complication risk secondary to systemic comorbidities and/or tumor characteristics preclude surgical intervention, radiation, and medical therapeutics can often be administered to patients, even in significantly advanced stages of their illness.

TABLE 15.2 The Spinal Instability Neoplastic Score (SINS) Classification

	Score
Location	
Junctional (occiput-C2, C7-T2, TI1-LI, L5-S1)	3
Mobile spine (C3-C6, L2-L4)	2
Semirigid (T3-T10)	1
Rigid (S2-S5)	0
Pain*	
Yes	0
Occasional pain but not mechanical	1
Pain-free lesion	0
Bone Lesion	
Lytic	2
Mixed (lytic/blastic)	1
Blastic	0
Radiographic spinal alignment	
Subluxation translation present	4
De novo deformity (kyphosis scoliosis)	2
Normal alignment	0
Vertebral body collapse	
> 50% collapse	3
< 50% collapse	2
No collapse with > 50% body involved	1
None of the above	0
Posterolateral involvement of spinal elements#	
Bilateral	3
Unilateral	1
None of the above	0
IMPLICATION	**TOTAL**
Stable	0-6
Indeterminate	7–12
Unstable	13–18

Adapted from Laufer I, Rubin DG, Lis E, et al. The NOMS framework: approach to the treatment of spinal metastatic tumors. *Oncologist*. 2013; 18(6):744–751 and Fisher CG, DiPaola CP, Ryken TC, et al. A novel classification system for spinal instability in neoplastic disease: an evidence-based approach and expert consensus from the Spine Oncology Study Group. *Spine. (Phila Pa 1976)*, 2010; 35(22):E1221–1229.
†Facet, pedicle, or costovertebral joint fracture or replacement with tumor.
*Pain improvement with recumbency and/or pain with movement/loading of spine.

Although prognostic scoring systems may help to determine appropriateness of the patient's surgical candidacy, they frequently tend to overestimate the expected survival time.[7] Additionally, the always-evolving armamentarium of anticancer pharmacotherapy continuously alters survival expectations. It is instead preferable to consider each patient's prognosis on a case-to-case basis.

Diagnostic Indications

A tumor tissue sample is usually obtained to establish a histopathologic diagnosis through percutaneous or minimally invasive means via either computed tomography (CT) guidance or fluoroscopy. In cases where these modes fail to provide adequate results, a surgical biopsy may be indicated. The surgical approach would depend on the location of the tumor.[25,27–29]

Conclusion

Presently, patients with radioresistant tumors with high grade ESCC require surgical intervention prior to radiation therapy. Surgery can be avoided in other cases unless there is progression of the tumor or neurologic deficits during radiation therapy or spinal instability. Mechanical spinal instability represents an independent indication for surgical stabilization or percutaneous cement augmentation. All treatment decisions are predicated on the patient's ability to tolerate the proposed intervention based on the extent of systemic comorbidities, tumor burden, and tumor histology. Separation surgery is the major aim of modern surgery for spinal metastases.

Trauma

In the setting of thoracic spine trauma, the surgeon must consider the patient's neurological status, spinal stability, the degree of deformity, and canal compromise within the injured spine segment in addition to injuries involving other regions of the spine or body. Generally, the accepted absolute indications for surgical decompression, reduction, and stabilization treatment in thoracic spinal fractures are included below (Table 15.3).[25,30]

Instability

Mechanical stability of the spine relates to the inherent structural integrity of the spinal column to resist physiologic loads without progressive deformity or damage to the neural elements.[31] On the other hand, neurologic stability of the spine denotes the presence or absence of neurologic deficits.[6] Since 1949, when the concept of stability in spinal injuries was first introduced by Nicoll (Mansfield, UK),[32] spinal injury classification systems have aimed to differentiate between stable and unstable fractures. In 1983, Francis Denis (Saint Paul, MN, USA) introduced the three-column spine concept (Fig. 15.3) to aid in the classification of thoracolumbar spine

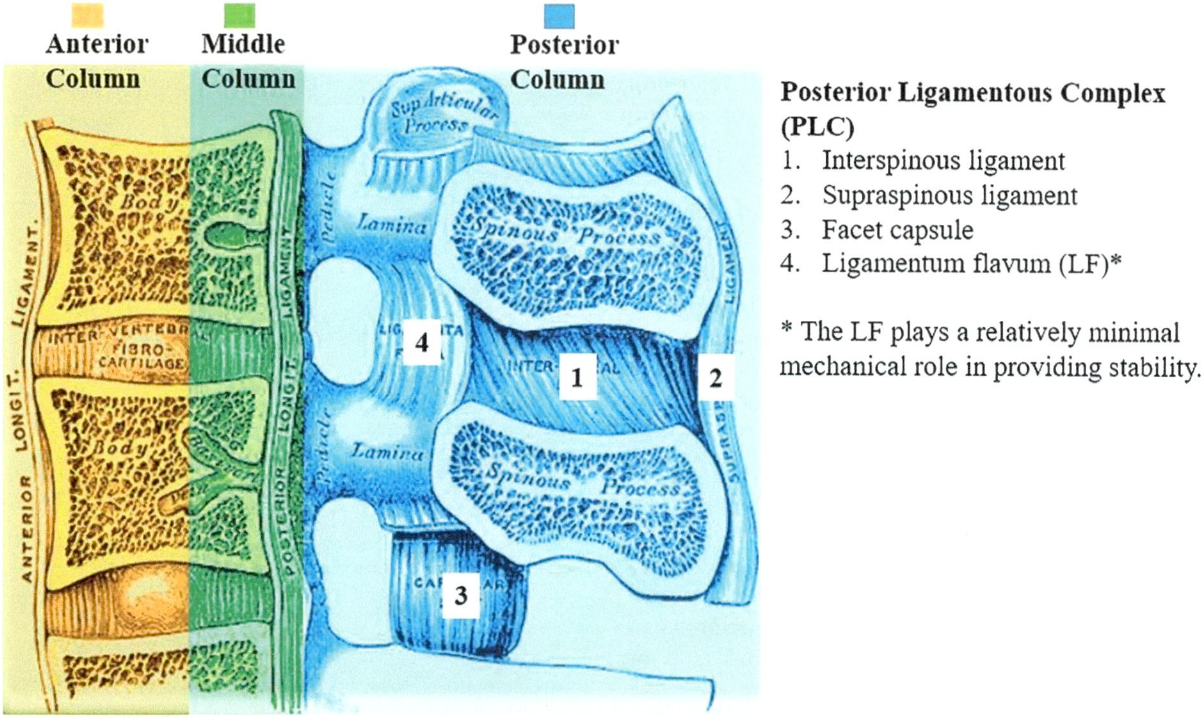

• **Fig. 15.3** Denis' three-column concept of thoracolumbar spinal fractures. Adapted from Gray H, Lewis WH. 1918, p. 288.[36] Inspired by[37].

TABLE 15.3 Indications for Surgical Treatment in Thoracic Trauma Patients

Absolute*	Relative
Unstable fracture patterns	*Purely osseous lesions*
TLICS ≥ 5	*Desire to return to regular activities early*
Presence of an incomplete or progressive neurologic deficit	*Prevention of secondary kyphosis*
Spinal cord compression with neurologic deficit	*Enabling nursing in paraplegic patients*
Significant segmental deformity > 30°	–
Junctional injuries - CTJ, TLJ	–
Concomitant injuries (cerebral, thoracic, long bone fractures, abdominal, and contiguous and noncontiguous spine injuries)	–

*Most investigators agree on absolute indications for surgery while relative indications are debatable. *CTJ*, Cervicothoracic junction; TLJ, thoracolumbar junction. Adapted from Heinzelmann M, Wanner GA. Thoracolumbar spinal injuries. In: Boos N, Aebi M, eds, *Spinal Disorders: Fundamentals of Diagnosis and Treatment*, Berlin/Heidelberg, 2008, Springer.

fractures.[33] He divided the spinal motion segment into three vertical parallel columns based on a retrospective review of biomechanical studies on spinal instability related to trauma.[33–35] The anterior column comprises the anterior longitudinal ligament (ALL) and the anterior two-thirds of the vertebral body and intervertebral disc (annulus fibrosus); the middle column comprises the posterior one-third of the vertebral body and intervertebral disc (annulus fibrosus), and the posterior longitudinal ligament (PLL); and the posterior column comprises everything posterior to the PLL, that is, the pedicles, facet joints and articular processes, ligamentum flavum, the neural arch and interconnecting ligaments, and the posterior ligamentous complex (PLC).[36,37] Denis considered injury to the middle column as the critical criterion for instability given that the bony part of this column resists compression forces while the ligamentous part, the PLL, resists distraction forces. Therefore, involvement of two contiguous columns by the injuries, either anterior and middle or middle and posterior, or a three-column injury indicates instability (Table 15.4).

Unstable spinal fractures are treated operatively.[35,38] Surgical stabilization of these injuries allows for early mobilization, helps control pain, avoids later neurological complications, facilitates nursing care (particularly in polytrauma patients) and has been associated with an earlier return to work.[39]

TABLE 15.4 Denis' Classification of Spinal Trauma Major Injuries*

Compression fracture *(failure of anterior column; middle column intact; there may be partial failure of posterior column)*
Type A - involvement of both endplates
Type B - involvement of superior endplate
Type C - inferior endplate
Type D - buckling of anterior cortex with both endplates intact
Burst fracture *(bone is retropulsed into the canal)*
Type A: Fracture of both endplates
Type B: Fracture of the superior endplate
Type C: Fracture of the inferior endplate
Type D: Burst rotation
Type E: Burst lateral flexion
Seat-belt (flexion-distraction) type
One-level injury
Through bone (Chance fracture)
Ligamentous disruption (PLC) and intervertebral disc
Two-level injury
Through either **bone** or **disc** at one level then **ligaments** at second level
Fracture-dislocation *(failure of all three columns under compression, tension, rotation, or shear)*
Flexion-rotation type
Flexion-distraction type
Shear type
Posteroanterior shear
Anteroposterior shear

Minor injuries†
Transverse processes fracture
Articular process fracture
Pars interarticularis fracture
Spinous process fracture

Adapted from Denis F. The three column spine and its significance in the classification of acute thoracolumbar spinal injuries. *Spine. (Phila Pa 1976)*. 1983; 8(8):817–831; Denis F. Spinal instability as defined by the three-column spine concept in acute spinal trauma. *Clin Orthop Relat Res*. 1984; (189):65–76; Denis F, Armstrong GW, Searls K, Matta L. Acute thoracolumbar burst fractures in the absence of neurologic deficit. A comparison between operative and nonoperative treatment. *Clin Orthop Relat Res*. 1984; (189):142–149.
*Each type of major fracture is further subdivided based on the severity of the damage. In terms of instability, the order of the major fracture types from most to least stable is wedge/compression > burst > seat-belt type > fracture-dislocation.
†Minor injuries involve only a part of the posterior column and do not lead to acute instability.

Thoracolumbar Injury Classification and Severity Score

The Spine Trauma Study Group (STSG) in 2005 conceptualized and proposed the Thoracolumbar Injury Classification and Severity Score (TLICS) (Table 15.5). TLICS assesses three major characteristics: morphology of the injury, integrity of the PLC, and neurological status of the patient. These characteristics are assessed in isolation, then after summation the final description of the injury as well as the injury severity score are used to guide treatment.[40,41]

TABLE 15.5 The Thoracolumbar Injury Classification and Severity Score (TLICS)

Category	Score
Injury Morphology	
Compression fracture	1
Burst fracture	2
Translational/rotational	3
Distraction	4
Posterior Ligamentous Complex Integrity	
Intact	0
Injury suspected/determinant	2
Injured	3
Neurologic Involvement	
Intact	0
Nerve root	2
Cord, conus medullaris	–
Complete injury	2
Incomplete injury	3
Cauda equina syndrome	3
Management According to TLICS Score*	**Total†**
Nonoperative	0–3
Indeterminate (Nonoperative or Operative)	4
Operative	≥ 5

Adapted from Vaccaro AR, Lehman RA, Jr., Hurlbert RJ, et al. A new classification of thoracolumbar injuries: the importance of injury morphology, the integrity of the posterior ligamentous complex, and neurologic status, *Spine (Phila Pa 1976)*, 30(20):2325–2333, 2005; Vaccaro AR, Zeiller SC, Hulbert RJ, et al. The thoracolumbar injury severity score: a proposed treatment algorithm. *J Spinal Disord Tech*. 2005; 18(3):209–215; Lee JY, Vaccaro AR, Lim MR, et al. Thoracolumbar injury classification and severity score: a new paradigm for the treatment of thoracolumbar spine trauma. *J Orthop Sci*, 2005; 10(6):671–675; Ratliff J, Anand N, Vaccaro AR, et al. Regional variability in use of a novel assessment of thoracolumbar spine fractures: United States versus international surgeons. *World J Emerg Surg*, 2007; 2:24.
*The TLICS score is only designed as a guideline BUT NOT as an absolute decision-making tool.
†The total score is a sum of the individual values in each category.

In scoring the injury morphology, one of the caveats to scoring distraction is that the PLC injury must be determinate. This is determined either clinically by the presence of a palpable gap between the spinous processes or radiologically through evidence of interspinous widening on plain radiographic or CT scan images, or hypersensitivity of the posterior ligamentous apparatus on fat-suppressed T2-weighted magnetic resonance imaging (MRI) images. Patients with an incomplete spinal cord injury or cauda equina syndrome are assigned three points versus two for complete spinal cord injury owing to the relative importance of surgical decompression in this neurologic subgroup.[42]

Patients with a TLICS score ≤ 3 total points are regarded as stable and may be considered for nonoperative treatment, whereas patients with a score ≥ 5 (unstable burst fractures [Fig. 15.4], burst fractures with neurological deficits, or distraction/rotational injuries) are regarded as unstable and thus are operative candidates. Patients with a total score equal to 4 fall into the indeterminate category and either operative or nonoperative treatment may be considered depending on surgeon's judgement.[42] TLICS, however, may not necessarily reflect culture- or region-specific issues, local surgical preferences, or even the most rational approach to treatment.[43]

Neurological Deficit

It is critical to perform and properly document a complete, accurate, well-detailed neurologic examination in a sequential and systematic manner. Clear documentation of subsequent variations of the patient's neurologic deficit is equally important to enable accurate assessment of neurologic deterioration or recovery. Two commonly used neurologic injury classification systems are the American Spinal Injury Association (ASIA score, preferred) classification and Frankel's classification. Both systems classify five distinct categories of neurological compromise below the level of the injury, with "A" and "E" describing complete paralysis and normal function, respectively, while "B to D" describe grades involving incomplete neurologic injury with some spared sensory or motor function (Table 15.6).[44–46] These systems help to guide treatment in that early surgical decompression and stabilization is recommended in patients with an incomplete spinal cord injury and evidence of persistent compression of neurogenic structures.

Traumatic Deformity

Patients presenting with severe segmental kyphosis (> 30°) at the fractured area are considered surgical candidates, as this is particularly associated with poor functional tolerance. Additionally, this is usually associated with severe pain due to canal or neuroforaminal compromise with or without peripheral symptoms, focal instability, muscle spasm, and adjacent painful compensatory deformity.[47]

Timing of Surgery

Early, versus late, stabilization of thoracic fractures is recommended.[48] The former is associated with reduced respiratory morbidity, reduced mean number of days on ventilator support, reduced number of days required in the intensive care unit, and overall reduction in the length of hospital stay.[49]

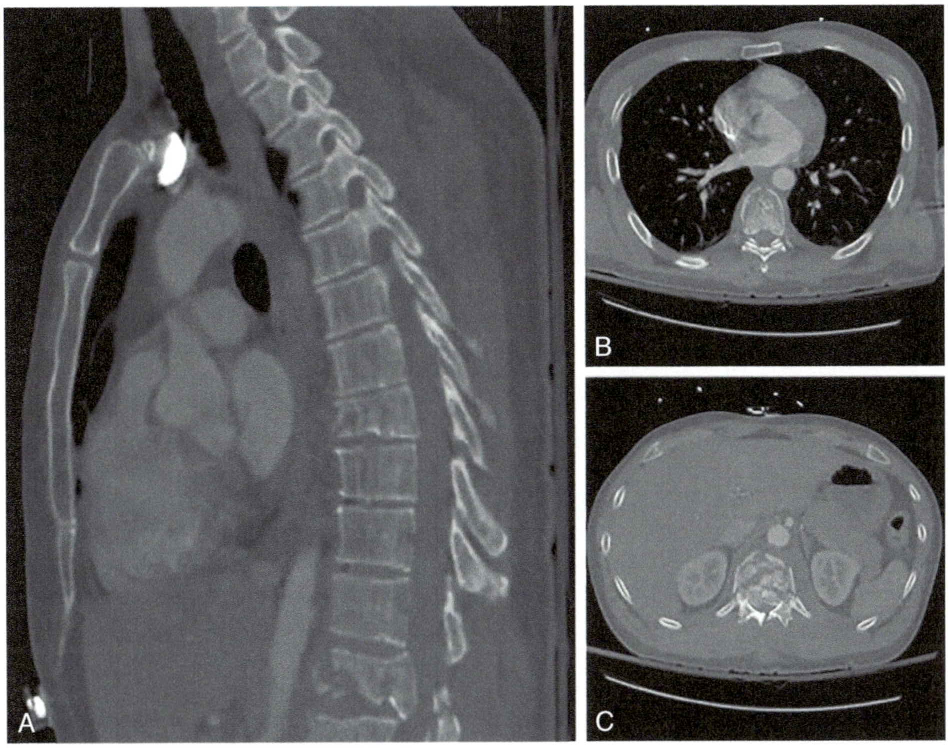

• **Fig. 15.4** (A) Midsagittal CT scan image showing concomitant burst fractures at the T8 and T12 vertebral bodies. (B) Axial CT scan image through the T8 vertebral body demonstrating the T8 burst fracture extending to the posterior aspect of the vertebral body. (C) Axial CT scan image through the T12 vertebral body demonstrating the T12 burst fracture with extrusion in the spinal canal causing severe central stenosis.

TABLE 15.6 **Neurological Injury Severity Classification Systems**

		American Spinal Injury Association Impairment Scale	Frankel Scale
A	Complete	No motor or sensory function is preserved in the sacral segments S4-S5.	No motor or sensory function below level of lesion.
B	Incomplete (Sensory only)	Sensory, but not motor, function is preserved below the neurological level and includes the sacral segments S4-S5.	No motor function, but some sensation preserved below level of lesion.
C	Incomplete (Motor useless/ nonfunctional)	Motor function is preserved below the neurological level, and more than half of key muscle below the neurological level have a muscle grade less than 3.	Some motor function without practical application.
D	Incomplete (Motor useful / fair-to-good function)	Motor function is preserved below the neurological level, and at least half of key muscles below the neurological level have a muscle grade of 3 or more.	Useful motor function below level of lesion.
E	Normal	Motor and sensory function are normal.	Normal motor and sensory function; may have reflex abnormalities.

Adapted from Waring WP, Biering-Sorensen F, Burns S, et al. 2009 Review and revisions of the International Standards for the Neurological Classification of Spinal Cord Injury. *J Spinal Cord Med*. 2010; 33(4):346–352; Van Middendorp JJ, Goss B, Urquhart S, Atresh S, Williams RP, Schuetz M. Diagnosis and prognosis of traumatic spinal cord injury. *Global Spine J*. 2011; 1(1):1–8; Roberts TT, Leonard GR, Cepela DJ. Classifications in brief: American Spinal Injury Association (ASIA) impairment scale. *Clin Orthop Relat Res*. 2017; 475(5):1499–1504.
NOTE: The neurological status is considered as the function below the injury level.

While some studies show no benefit of early decompression,[50] particularly in patients with complete traumatic spinal cord injury,[51] other recent series suggest that early decompression within 8 hours can be safely performed and is beneficial in terms of neurologic improvement.[52] In their meta-analysis on the same issue, La Rosa et al.[53] showed that early decompression within 24 hours resulted in statistically better outcomes compared to delayed compression (> 24 hrs) and conservative management. Other series have also shown improvement with early decompression within 24 hours,[50,54] better outcomes with indirect decompression within 48 hours.[55–58] There are no significant reports documenting adverse effects of early decompression.[39] A caveat to this, however, is that the potential benefit of early decompression must be weighed against other factors, such as medical optimization, management of coexisting injuries, and operating room conditions. For example, availability of neurophysiologic monitoring and the appropriate anesthesia team and operating room personnel are key to successful treatment and may be a reason for a small delay.[6]

Conclusion

Unstable thoracic spine fractures should be treated surgically. Patients with incomplete spinal cord injuries or progressive neurological deficits should be taken to surgery as soon as possible. The goals of surgical treatment should be to achieve anatomic reduction, provide sufficient stability to allow for early mobilization, achieve neural element decompression, avoid complications, and to proceed within the most appropriate time frame.

Thoracic Stenosis

The surgical decompression of thoracic stenosis is indicated for patients presenting with myelopathy and/or progressive neurological deficits. Neurological symptoms include impaired balance and ambulation; lower extremity weakness or paralysis; bowel, bladder and sexual dysfunction; and radicular pain.[59] Of note, the majority (77%) of patients presenting with thoracic radicular symptoms improve after a course of physical therapy.[60] As it pertains to myelopathy, it has been demonstrated that even chronic, severe symptoms can be reversed after decompression.[61] The most common causes of thoracic stenosis include thoracic disc herniation (TDH), ossified ligamentum flavum (OLF), and ossification of the posterior longitudinal ligament (OPLL).

When approaching decompression in the thoracic spine, avoidance of spinal cord manipulation is of paramount importance. There are many techniques and approaches available to safely decompress the thoracic spine. The optimal treatment method considers the clinical presentation and location of the lesion.

Thoracic Disc Herniations

While TDHs can be present in up to 15% of individuals, only between 0.15% to 4% are symptomatic.[59,62,63] The thoracolumbar segments tend to be the most involved due to the unique biomechanical environment, with T11/12 implicated in approximately 26% to 50% of all TDHs.[59,64]

While degeneration is the leading cause of symptomatic TDHs, trauma is also a cause, particularly in younger patients. Most disc herniations are posterolateral (~80%), with 5% to 11% demonstrating erosion through the dura.[65–67]

Patients with TDHs can present with myelopathy or predominantly lower extremity motor and sensory symptoms. Bowel, bladder, and sexual dysfunction can also occur.[59] In a large series of TDHs that were operatively treated, pain (radicular, localized, or axial) was the most common symptom followed by weakness and/or sensory deficits, hyperreflexia/spasticity, and bladder dysfunction.[68] A number of studies have reported on TDH presenting with unusual symptoms including abdominal pain,[69] nausea/vomiting,[70] and flank pain,[71] suggesting a high index of suspicion is needed to make the diagnosis.

TDH causing thoracic myelopathy was first described by Key in 1838.[72] The first documented treatment via laminectomy and discectomy was reported in 1922 by Adson and soon thereafter by Mixter and Barr.[73] The initial treatment of thoracic disc disease was laminectomy and discectomy, adopted from the standard treatment for lumbar disease. However, manipulation of the thoracic cord frequently resulted in significant neurologic morbidity (75% paraplegia) and even death (50% mortality).[73] As new techniques became available, such as costotransversectomy and transthoracic approaches, the mortality and morbidity rates for the surgical treatment of TDHs improved drastically.[74–79] The management of thoracic disc herniations continues to improve with new technology. For example, the use of endoscopic approaches to treat TDHs has increased significantly in recent years.

The gold standard for diagnosis of TDH is a noncontrast MRI of the thoracic spine (Fig. 15.5). In patients with contraindications to MRI, a CT myelogram may be used; however, significant stenosis may prevent contrast flow, negatively impacting image quality. Retrospective studies have been unable to differentiate image findings of asymptomatic versus symptomatic herniated nucleus pulposus (HNP), suggesting that the appearance of the herniation should not be the sole criteria used to indicate operative treatment.[65]

Little characterization has been done on the natural history of symptomatic thoracic HNP due to the rarity of the condition. One study by Brown et al. found that, in a series of 55 patients with symptomatic thoracic HNP who were treated conservatively, 77% had symptomatic improvement, allowing them to return to their baseline level of activity, and only 23% required operative intervention.[60]

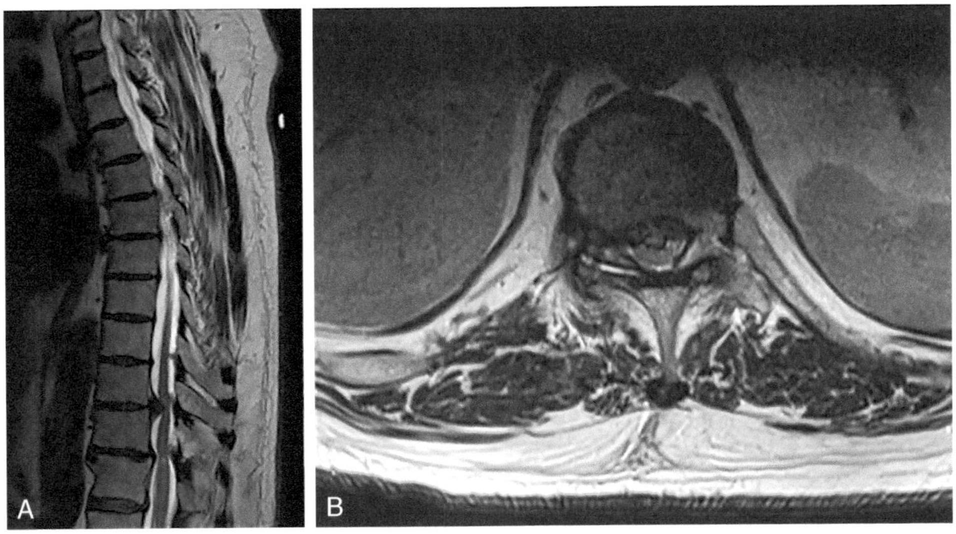

• **Fig. 15.5** (A) T2-weighted sagittal image of the thoracic spine showing a large disc herniation at T10/11. (B) T2-weighted axial image of a T10/11 thoracic disc herniation showing a large central disc herniation causing dorsal displacement of the spinal cord.

Moreover, studies on the outcomes of patients treated with discectomy for TDH tend to show that patients with more severe symptoms at initial presentation have the best outcomes with operative intervention.[80] These data seem to suggest that, especially in patients who present with mild symptoms, particularly axial or radicular pain alone, conservative management plays an important role. However, for patients who present with myelopathic symptoms, in particular weakness and/or bowel or bladder dysfunction, early operative intervention is typically recommended in order to prevent persistent neurologic deficits.

Ossified Ligamentum Flavum

OLF is an uncommon cause of thoracic myelopathy that occurs more frequently than TDH but less common than OPLL.[81] OLF was historically considered a condition of the Japanese population; however, more recently it has been described throughout all of Asia and the rest of the world.[81] The incidence has been described as high as 4.5% to 20%, with a higher incidence in individuals over 55.[81,82] A combination of factors including genetic and external stresses as caused by tensile stretch, in particular from prolonged squatting positions, has been shown to lead to OLF.[81] The tension imparted on the ligamentum flavum can lead to an increase in growth factors and the recruitment of fibroblasts causing endochondral ossification.[81,83]

CT scan is the primary means of classification and diagnosis (Fig. 15.6), but OLF can also be diagnosed on plain x-rays.[82] However, MRI is a useful tool to evaluate the extent of neural compression.[82]

Typical presentation of OLF includes back pain, stiffness of the back muscles, pain with motion, lower extremity muscle weakness, gait disturbances, and bowel/bladder issues. Depending on the level and proximity to the conus medullaris, one can also experience conus medullaris syndrome. OLF is most common in the lower thoracic spine.[82]

Due to its posterior anatomic location and resultant spinal cord compression, loss of proprioception and vibration tend to develop earlier with losses in the lateral corticospinal tracts developing later causing spastic paralysis.[81] As the ossification enlarges, the lateral spinothalamic tracts become compressed leading to loss of sensation.[81] Early surgical intervention is recommended in the face of spastic gait, severe muscle strength, bowel or bladder disturbance, or OLF with combined OPLL.[82] Notwithstanding early intervention, lower extremity symptoms including numbness and spastic gait tend to remain.[82]

OLF can be classified into five categories; lateral, extended, enlarged, fused, and tuberous. In the lateral, extended, and enlarged types, the bilateral ossifications of each individual ligament are unfused.[82] Fused and tuberous types are fused at midline, and tuberous spreads cranially and caudally to multiple locations.[82,83]

Due to the dorsal compression, surgical management of symptomatic OLF consists of a laminectomy with or without fusion. Generally speaking, fusion is required if the extent of the decompression renders the spine unstable. With a unilateral decompression, including hemilaminectomy, facetectomy, or unilateral costotransversectomy, studies do not show significant changes in intrinsic or global range of motion in the upper or lower thoracic spine, as the rib cage provides intrinsic stability in all planes of motion.[84,85]

Ossification of the Posterior Longitudinal Ligament

OPLL is the pathologic ectopic ossification of the posterior longitudinal ligament, which typically presents in the fifth or sixth decade of life.[86,87] OPLL had an estimated overall

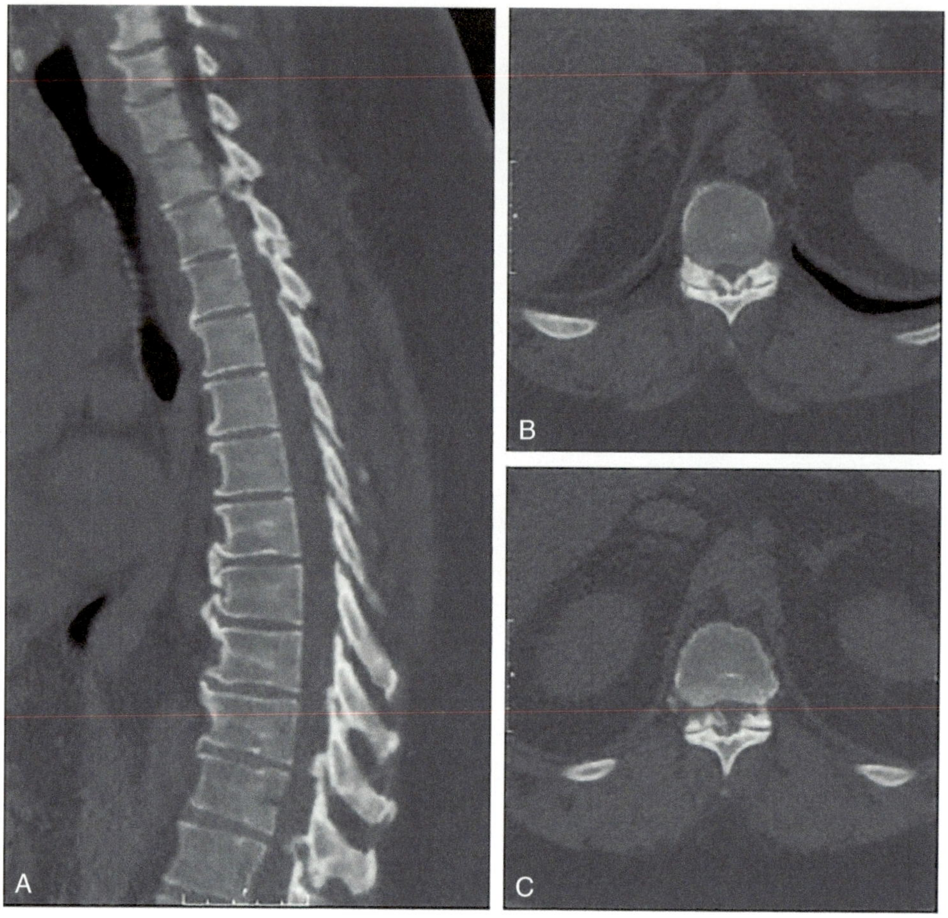

• **Fig. 15.6** (A) Sagittal CT scan of the thoracic spine showing ossified ligamentum flavum at the T10/11 and T11/12 levels. (B) Axial CT scan through the T10/11 disc space demonstrating ossified ligamentum flavum causing severe central stenosis. (C) Axial CT scan through the T11/12 disc space demonstrating right-sided ossified ligamentum flavum causing central stenosis and left-sided displacement of the spinal cord.

prevalence of 0.01% to 2% in the general population but has a higher incidence in the Japanese population with an estimated prevalence of 2% to 4%.[86] OPLL is approximately four times more common in the cervical spine than the thoracic spine (15% vs 70%).[86,87] There is a male preponderance of 2:1.[86]

Some studies suggest OPLL is a variant of diffuse idiopathic skeletal hyperostosis (DISH), but the pathogenesis is not well understood. There appear to be both environmental and genetic components, with the *HAO1A* gene stimulating endochondral ossification promotion.[86] Additionally, systemic factors such as hypertension and diabetes (33% prevalence) have been implicated as causative agents for OPLL.[87] To this point, some studies have also suggested an increase in bone mineral density in patients with OPLL.[86]

OPLL of the thoracic spine can be classified as either "flat" with continuous or a segmental conformation or "beaked" with a sharp protrusion behind the disc space.[86] Like other stenotic conditions of the thoracic spine, OPLL can have a variety of presentations including myelopathy, radiculopathy, or myeloradiculopathy.[86,88] Approximately 5% of diagnosed OPLL cases are asymptomatic.[86] CT scan is the best means of visualization and characterization of OPLL owing to its sclerotic nature. However, MRI is also essential in the workup for evaluation of the spinal cord in terms of swelling, myelomalacia, or gliosis.[87]

As with all thoracic stenosis surgeries, the decompressive approach for OPLL should be chosen based on the location of the lesion. Despite the body of literature pertaining to thoracic OPLL, there remains no consensus on the standard of treatment. Similar to other compressive thoracic lesions, the kyphotic thoracic spine, vulnerable cord, and tenuous blood supply make decompression challenging.[87] Surgical intervention is usually indicated in the face of clinically significant presentations.[86] Operative intervention of thoracic myelopathy from OPLL has shown favorable outcomes in severe cases. However, when presenting with mild myelopathic symptoms, the outcomes are equivalent to medical management, demonstrating that nonoperative management may play a role in this pathology.[88]

Surgical options vary based on the location of the lesion and include laminoplasty, anterior and/or posterior decompression through anterior and/or posterior approaches, and laminectomy with or without fusion.[86] For middle or lower thoracic OPLL at a single level, anterolateral or posterolateral decompression can be appropriate.[89] For short segment, multilevel disease, a posterior decompression with or without fusion is a reasonable choice.[89] If the OPLL is flat in nature, then a posterior decompression, with an additional segment decompressed cranially and caudally, may allow for adequate decompression of the lesion. Contrarily, if the lesion is raised and causing posterior migration of the spinal cord, it may necessitate posterior and anterior decompression.[89] The anterior decompression can be accomplished via a dorsal approach (Ohtsuka method) or a combined anterior and posterior approach (Tomita method). Anterior-based decompression of OPLL is associated with higher rates of complication and is much more technically demanding.[90] It has also been demonstrated that while some patients improve with anterior approaches, a significant percentage do not.[90]

Spinal Deformity

Adult spinal deformity (ASD) encompasses a wide range of etiologies including denovo scoliosis, progressive adolescent idiopathic scoliosis in adulthood, hyperkyphosis, iatrogenic sagittal deformity, focal deformity due to multiple degenerative disc disease with global deformity, and posttraumatic spinal deformity.[91] As such, there is no definite algorithmic management for ASD, and surgical treatment demands meticulous planning and careful patient selection.[92] Indications for operative care are not absolute; however, they should be considered in the context of patient-specific factors. Primary indications for surgical treatment of ASD include deformity progression, neurological dysfunction, pain, and functional limitations unresponsive to medical interventions.[92]

Nonoperative treatment of adult spinal deformity should be focused on improving quality of life by decreasing pain and disability. Conservative treatment is poorly defined but generally consists of physical therapy, chiropractic manipulation, epidural steroid injections, acupuncture, massage, water therapy, pharmacotherapy to include NSAIDs, nerve stabilizers, and narcotics.[93] Multiple studies have shown that improvements in pain or disability are unlikely in patients with ASD undergoing nonoperative treatments. If a patient expects significant improvements in pain and disability, operative management is preferred.[94–96]

The surgical treatment of ASD is complex and surgical planning must integrate regional, global, and pelvic compensatory/morphologic parameters to adequately correct deformity and ultimately provide pain relief and improvements in function.[97,98] Patient-specific radiological alignment criteria based on the Scoliosis Research Society (SRS)–Schwab Classification should be used for surgical planning in order to set targets for preventing undercorrection or overcorrection.[91,92] Several factors are crucial for structural decision-making, as follows: identification of deformity drivers, setting of alignment target, and determination of flexibility.

Several variables may necessitate operative intervention in the thoracic spine due to regional deformity or as part of a longer fusion construct to correct a global spinal malalignment. Regional indications include pain and neurologic dysfunction caused by progressive thoracic kyphosis, a thoracic deformity greater than 75 degrees or thoracolumbar deformity greater than 40 degrees. The accepted ideal sagittal/coronal spinopelvic parameters include a sagittal vertical axis (SVA) of less than 50 mm, a T1 pelvic angle (TPA) less than 0 degrees, a pelvic tilt less than 20 degrees, and lumbar lordosis (LL) within about 10 degrees of the pelvic incidence (PI) or LL = PI + 9 degrees (+/–9 degrees). Large deviations from these global alignment targets may be considered for surgical correction in order to improve health-related quality of life.[91,99] Also, age-appropriate parameters should be considered when planning the amount of correction needed.[100]

In summary, management of adult spinal deformity is complex, and surgical intervention must be individually tailored based on each patient's specific spinal pathology.

Infection

Thoracic spine infections include infectious diseases affecting the vertebral body, the intervertebral disc, and/or adjacent paraspinal tissue. Spinal infections are generally classified by their location; intraspinal (intramedullary abscess, subdural empyema, and epidural abscess/empyema), bone (osteomyelitis or spondylitis), disc (discitis or spondylodiscitis), disc and bone (spondylodiscitis), and paraspinal infection (i.e., psoas abscess).[101–103] Indications for the surgical treatment of thoracic spinal infections include acute or progressive neurological deficits, significant bony destruction causing spinal instability, intraspinal lesions with mass effect, inability to obtain cultures via needle biopsy, and failure of conservative therapy.[101,103]

The primary goals of surgical management include early decompression of the spinal canal, stabilization of unstable vertebral segments, aggressive tissue debridement to promote healing, and obtaining samples for microbiological and histological analysis to direct antimicrobial treatment.[102,103]

Intraspinal Infections

Intramedullary abscesses are scarcely reported in the literature and therefore there is no specific treatment algorithm. In general, early drainage and rapid administration of intravenous (IV) antibiotics have better neurological outcomes than conservative treatment or delayed drainage.[104] Subdural infection also requires prompt surgical drainage and administration of IV antibiotics as this represents a neurosurgical emergency. This may also require laminectomy at one or more levels depending on the extent of the lesion.[101]

The thoracic spine is the second most common site (31%) of spinal epidural abscesses (SEAs) (Fig. 15.7); however,

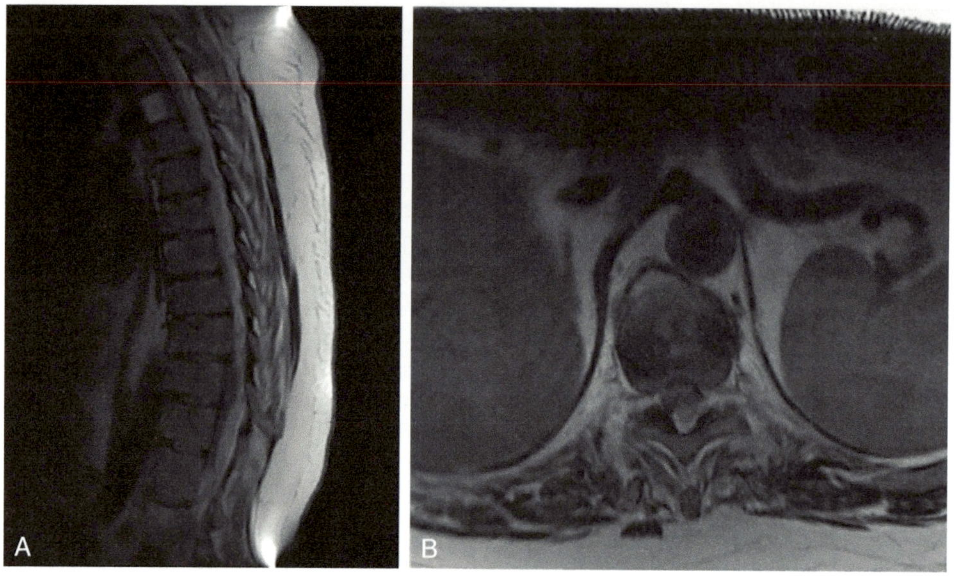

• **Fig. 15.7** (A) T2-weighted midsagittal MRI image of the thoracic spine demonstrating epidural abscess extending from the dorsal aspect of the T10 vertebral body to L1 vertebral body. (B) T2-weighted axial MRI image through T10/11 showing the epidural abscess with moderate to severe central stenosis and dorsal displacement of the spinal cord.

they often involve multiple spinal regions (20%).[105] Gold standard treatment consists of surgical decompression combined with systemic IV antibiotics.[101] There are a few circumstances in which conservative management may be considered. These include patients with severe comorbidities that limit surgical options, holospinal SEA whereby surgery may not be feasible, when the SEA is detected early and patients suffer from no neurologic deficits, or when the patient presents with complete paralysis for more than 72 hours.[106] It should be noted that the mortality of epidural abscess is reported to be 5% to 20%,[101] and up to 49% of patients initially treated conservatively still show progression of neurologic deficits.[107] Due to this, some authors recommend more aggressive surgical treatment in the presence of epidural abscess even without associated neurological deficits, especially at cord levels.[103,108] Patients considered to be at high risk for failure with medical management alone include patients older than 65 years of age with diabetes, MRSA infections, and neurologic compromise.[109]As such, surgical treatment should be the treatment of choice in any case of doubt.

Spondylodiscitis

Spondylodiscitis is defined as an infection of the disc and the adjacent vertebrae.[101] Conservative management is the treatment of choice in the early stages of spondylodiscitis without neurologic deficits or advanced collapse rendering the spine unstable. Obtaining adequate cultures is paramount to directing antimicrobial therapy. As such, surgical intervention may be necessary if blood cultures and CT biopsy do not yield positive cultures. Surgery should be considered when conservative treatment has failed or when patients present with neurologic deficits, progressive sepsis, and/or instability or deformity. Surgical options may include debridement, corpectomy, anterior reconstruction, posterior stabilization, or a combination of anterior and posterior reconstruction and stabilization.[101–103]

Paraspinal Abscesses

Generally, antibiotic treatment reaches the paraspinal tissue easier than the nonvascularized disc space. As a result, the recommended first-line therapy for paraspinal abscesses is broad-spectrum antibiotic therapy. Percutaneous CT or ultrasound-guided drainage may be attempted for larger collections. Surgical management is reserved for refractory cases or if surgical debridement of spondylodiscitis is required.[101,110,111]

Conclusion

Surgery is indicated for conditions involving the thoracic spine that are deemed unamenable to improvement with nonoperative modalities, including metastatic tumors, trauma, stenosis, and spinal deformity. The primary goals of surgical intervention are maintenance or restoration of spinal alignment and stability, preservation of neurologic function, and relief from pain. Overall, the management of thoracic spine conditions should be tailored to each individual patient's specific pathology and goals, instituted within an appropriate time frame, and in tandem with the latest available technologies and scientific information.

References

1. Aoude A, Nooh A, Fortin M, et al. Incidence, predictors, and postoperative complications of blood transfusion in thoracic and lumbar fusion surgery: An analysis of 13,695 patients from the American College of Surgeons National Surgical Quality Improvement Program Database. *Global Spine J*. 2016;6(8):756–764.
2. Yoon WW, Koch J. Herniated discs: when is surgery necessary? *EFORT Open Rev*. 2021;6(6):526–530.
3. Gonschorek O, Hauck S, Weiß T, Bühren V. Frakturen der Brust- und Lendenwirbelsäule. *Der Chirurg*. 2015;86(9):901–916.
4. Landi A, Delfini R, Ricci A, Barbanera A, Anichini G, Brogna C. New trends in instrumentation and complex techniques in spine surgery. *Biomed Res Int*. 2015;2015:1–3.
5. Pishnamaz M, Lichte P, Sellei RM, Pape HC, Kobbe P. Perkutane dorsale Stabilisierung der Brust- und Lendenwirbelsäule mit aktiver intraoperativer Repositionsmöglichkeit. *Oper Orthop Traumatol*. 2015;27(5):439–447.
6. Gjolaj JP, Williams SK. Thoracic and lumbar spinal injuries. In: Garfin SR, Eismont FJ, Bell GR, Bono CM, Fischgrund J, eds. *Rothman-Simeone The Spine E-Book*. Elsevier Health Sciences; 2017:1333–1363.
7. Laufer I, Rubin DG, Lis E, et al. The NOMS framework: approach to the treatment of spinal metastatic tumors. *Oncologist*. 2013;18(6):744–751.
8. Cobb 3rd CA, Leavens ME, Eckles N. Indications for nonoperative treatment of spinal cord compression due to breast cancer. *J Neurosurg*. 1977;47(5):653–658.
9. Walsh GL, Gokaslan ZL, McCutcheon IE, et al. Anterior approaches to the thoracic spine in patients with cancer: Indications and results. *Ann Thorac Surg*. 1997;64(6):1611–1618.
10. Bilsky MH, Laufer I, Fourney DR, et al. Reliability analysis of the epidural spinal cord compression scale. *J Neurosurg Spine*. 2010;13(3):324–328.
11. Gerszten PC, Mendel E, Yamada Y. Radiotherapy and radiosurgery for metastatic spine disease: what are the options, indications, and outcomes? *Spine (Phila Pa 1976)*. 2009;34(22 Suppl):S78–S92.
12. Gilbert RW, Kim JH, Posner JB. Epidural spinal cord compression from metastatic tumor: diagnosis and treatment. *Ann Neurol*. 1978;3(1):40–51.
13. Maranzano E, Bellavita R, Rossi R, et al. Short-course versus split-course radiotherapy in metastatic spinal cord compression: results of a phase III, randomized, multicenter trial. *J Clin Oncol*. 2005;23(15):3358–3365.
14. Maranzano E, Latini P, Perrucci E, Beneventi S, Lupattelli M, Corgna E. Short-course radiotherapy (8 Gy x 2) in metastatic spinal cord compression: an effective and feasible treatment. *Int J Radiat Oncol Biol Phys*. 1997;38(5):1037–1044.
15. Katagiri H, Takahashi M, Inagaki J, et al. Clinical results of nonsurgical treatment for spinal metastases. *Int J Radiat Oncol Biol Phys*. 1998;42(5):1127–1132.
16. Rades D, Fehlauer F, Schulte R, et al. Prognostic factors for local control and survival after radiotherapy of metastatic spinal cord compression. *J Clin Oncol*. 2006;24(21):3388–3393.
17. Rades D, Fehlauer F, Stalpers LJA, et al. A prospective evaluation of two radiotherapy schedules with 10 versus 20 fractions for the treatment of metastatic spinal cord compression. *Cancer*. 2004;101(11):2687–2692.
18. Rades D, Karstens JH, Alberti W. Role of radiotherapy in the treatment of motor dysfunction due to metastatic spinal cord compression: comparison of three different fractionation schedules. *Int J Radiat Oncol Biol Phys*. 2002;54(4):1160–1164.
19. Rades D, Huttenlocher S, Bajrovic A, et al. Surgery followed by radiotherapy versus radiotherapy alone for metastatic spinal cord compression from unfavorable tumors. *Int J Radiat Oncol Biol Phys*. 2011;81(5):e861–e868.
20. Maranzano E, Latini P. Effectiveness of radiation therapy without surgery in metastatic spinal cord compression: final results from a prospective trial. *Int J Radiat Oncol Biol Phys*. 1995;32(4):959–967.
21. Bilsky MH, Lis E, Raizer J, Lee H, Boland P. The diagnosis and treatment of metastatic spinal tumor. *Oncologist*. 1999;4(6):459–469.
22. Fisher CG, DiPaola CP, Ryken TC, et al. A novel classification system for spinal instability in neoplastic disease: an evidence-based approach and expert consensus from the Spine Oncology Study Group. *Spine (Phila Pa 1976)*. 2010;35(22):E1221–E1229.
23. Posner JB. Back pain and epidural spinal cord compression. *Med Clin North Am*. 1987;71(2):185–205.
24. Bates DW, Reuler JB. Back pain and epidural spinal cord compression. *J Gen Intern Med*. 1988;3(2):191–197.
25. Abraham DJ, Herkowitz HN, Katz JN. Indications for thoracic and lumbar spine fusion and trends in use. *Orthop Clin North Am*. 1998;29(4):803.
26. Wang JC, Boland P, Mitra N, et al. Single-stage posterolateral transpedicular approach for resection of epidural metastatic spine tumors involving the vertebral body with circumferential reconstruction: results in 140 patients. Invited submission from the Joint Section Meeting on Disorders of the Spine and Peripheral Nerves, March 2004. *J Neurosurg Spine*. 2004;1(3):287–298.
27. Mazel C, Balabaud L, Bennis S, Hansen S. Cervical and thoracic spine tumor management: surgical indications, techniques, and outcomes. *Orthop Clin North Am*. 2009;40(1):75–92. vi-vii.
28. Missenard G, Bouthors C, Fadel E, Court C. Surgical strategies for primary malignant tumors of the thoracic and lumbar spine. *Orthop Traumatol Surg Res*. 2020;106(1):S53–S62.
29. Ciftdemir M, Kaya M, Selcuk E, Yalniz E. Tumors of the spine. *World J Orthop*. 2016;7(2):109.
30. Rajasekaran S, Kanna RM, Shetty AP. Management of thoracolumbar spine trauma: An overview. *Indian J Orthop*. 2015;49(1):72–82.
31. White AA, Panjabi MM. *Clinical Biomechanics of the Spine*. Lippincott; 1978.
32. Nicoll EA. Fractures of the dorso-lumbar spine. *J Bone Joint Surg Br*. 1949;31b(3):376–394.
33. Denis F. The three column spine and its significance in the classification of acute thoracolumbar spinal injuries. *Spine (Phila Pa 1976)*. 1983;8(8):817–831.
34. Denis F. Spinal instability as defined by the three-column spine concept in acute spinal trauma. *Clin Orthop Relat Res*. 1984(189):65–76.
35. Denis F, Armstrong GW, Searls K, Matta L. Acute thoracolumbar burst fractures in the absence of neurologic deficit. A comparison between operative and nonoperative treatment. *Clin Orthop Relat Res*. 1984(189):142–149.
36. Gray H, Lewis WH. Articulations of the vertebral column. In: Lewis WH, ed. *Anatomy of the Human Body*. 20 ed. Philadelphia and New York: Lea & Febiger; 1918:287–289.
37. Forsthoefel C., Moore D.W. Thoracolumbar burst fractures. https://www.orthobullets.com/spine/2022/thoracolumbar-

burst-fractures. Published 2021. Updated 11/07/2021. Accessed 11/10/2021, 2021.
38. Gertzbein SD. Scoliosis Research Society. Multicenter spine fracture study. *Spine (Phila Pa 1976)*. 1992;17(5):528–540.
39. Heinzelmann M, Wanner GA. Thoracolumbar spinal injuries. In: Boos N, Aebi M, eds. *Spinal Disorders: Fundamentals of Diagnosis and Treatment*. Springer Berlin Heidelberg; 2008.
40. Vaccaro AR, Lehman Jr. RA, Hurlbert RJ, et al. A new classification of thoracolumbar injuries: the importance of injury morphology, the integrity of the posterior ligamentous complex, and neurologic status. *Spine (Phila Pa 1976)*. 2005;30(20):2325–2333.
41. Vaccaro AR, Zeiller SC, Hulbert RJ, et al. The thoracolumbar injury severity score: a proposed treatment algorithm. *J Spinal Disord Tech*. 2005;18(3):209–215.
42. Lee JY, Vaccaro AR, Lim MR, et al. Thoracolumbar injury classification and severity score: a new paradigm for the treatment of thoracolumbar spine trauma. *J Orthop Sci*. 2005;10(6):671–675.
43. Ratliff J, Anand N, Vaccaro AR, et al. Regional variability in use of a novel assessment of thoracolumbar spine fractures: United States versus international surgeons. *World J Emerg Surg*. 2007;2:24.
44. Waring WP, Biering-Sorensen F, Burns S, et al. 2009 Review and revisions of the International Standards for the Neurological Classification of Spinal Cord Injury. *J Spinal Cord Med*. 2010;33(4):346–352.
45. Van Middendorp JJ, Goss B, Urquhart S, Atresh S, Williams RP, Schuetz M. Diagnosis and prognosis of traumatic spinal cord injury. *Global Spine J*. 2011;1(1):1–8.
46. Roberts TT, Leonard GR, Cepela DJ. Classifications in brief: American Spinal Injury Association (ASIA) impairment scale. *Clin Orthop Relat Res*. 2017;475(5):1499–1504.
47. Munting E. Surgical treatment of post-traumatic kyphosis in the thoracolumbar spine: indications and technical aspects. *Eur Spine J*. 2010;19(S1):S69–S73.
48. Qadir I, Riew KD, Alam SR, Akram R, Waqas M, Aziz A. Timing of surgery in thoracolumbar spine injury: Impact on neurological outcome. *Global Spine J*. 2020;10(7):826–831.
49. Rudol G, Gummerson NW. (ii) Thoracolumbar spinal fractures: review of anatomy, biomechanics, classification and treatment. *Orthop Trauma*. 2014;28(2):70–78.
50. Dvorak MF, Noonan VK, Fallah N, et al. The influence of time from injury to surgery on motor recovery and length of hospital stay in acute traumatic spinal cord injury: An observational Canadian cohort study. *J Neurotrauma*. 2015;32(9):645–654.
51. Rahimi-Movaghar V. Efficacy of surgical decompression in the setting of complete thoracic spinal cord injury. *J Spinal Cord Med*. 2005;28(5):415–420.
52. Lee D-Y, Park Y-J, Kim H-J, Ahn H-S, Hwang S-C, Kim D-H. Early surgical decompression within 8 hours for traumatic spinal cord injury: Is it beneficial? A meta-analysis. *Acta Orthop Traumatol Turc*. 2018;52(2):101–108.
53. La Rosa G, Conti A, Cardali S, Cacciola F, Tomasello F. Does early decompression improve neurological outcome of spinal cord injured patients? Appraisal of the literature using a meta-analytical approach. *Spinal Cord*. 2004;42(9):503–512.
54. Wilson JR, Singh A, Craven C, et al. Early versus late surgery for traumatic spinal cord injury: the results of a prospective Canadian cohort study. *Spinal Cord*. 2012;50(11):840–843.
55. Edwards CC, Levine AM. Early rod-sleeve stabilization of the injured thoracic and lumbar spine. *Orthop Clin North Am*. 1986;17(1):121–145.
56. Crutcher Jr. JP, Anderson PA, King HA, Montesano PX. Indirect spinal canal decompression in patients with thoracolumbar burst fractures treated by posterior distraction rods. *J Spinal Disord*. 1991;4(1):39–48.
57. Doerr TE, Montesano PX, Burkus JK, Benson DR. Spinal canal decompression in traumatic thoracolumbar burst fractures: posterior distraction rods versus transpedicular screw fixation. *J Orthop Trauma*. 1991;5(4):403–411.
58. Harrington RM, Budorick T, Hoyt J, Anderson PA, Tencer AF. Biomechanics of indirect reduction of bone retropulsed into the spinal canal in vertebral fracture. *Spine (Phila Pa 1976)*. 1993;18(6):692–699.
59. Arce CA, Dohrmann GJ. Thoracic disc herniation. Improved diagnosis with computed tomographic scanning and a review of the literature. *Surg Neurol*. 1985;23(4):356–361.
60. Brown CW, Deffer Jr. PA, Akmakjian J, Donaldson DH, Brugman JL. The natural history of thoracic disc herniation. *Spine (Phila Pa 1976)*. 1992;17(6 Suppl):S97–S102.
61. Chang U, Choe W, Chung C, Kim H. Surgical treatment for thoracic spinal stenosis. *Spinal Cord*. 2001;39(7):362–369.
62. Alvarez O, Roque CT, Pampati M. Multilevel thoracic disk herniations: CT and MR studies. *J Comput Assist Tomogr*. 1988;12(4):649–652.
63. Russell T. Thoracic intervertebral disc protrusion: experience of 67 cases and review of the literature. *Br J Neurosurg*. 1989;3(2):153–160.
64. Radecki J, Feinberg JH, Zimmer ZR. T1 radiculopathy: electrodiagnostic evaluation. *HSS J*. 2009;5(1):73–77.
65. Awwad EE, Martin DS, Smith Jr. KR, Baker BK. Asymptomatic versus symptomatic herniated thoracic discs: their frequency and characteristics as detected by computed tomography after myelography. *Neurosurgery*. 1991;28(2):180–186.
66. Love JG, Schorn VG. Thoracic-disk protrusions. *JAMA*. 1965;191:627–631.
67. Epstein NE, Syrquin MS, Epstein JA, Decker RE. Intradural disc herniations in the cervical, thoracic, and lumbar spine: report of three cases and review of the literature. *J Spinal Disord*. 1990;3(4):396–403.
68. Stillerman CB, Chen TC, Couldwell WT, Zhang W, Weiss MH. Experience in the surgical management of 82 symptomatic herniated thoracic discs and review of the literature. *J Neurosurg*. 1998;88(4):623–633.
69. Chirchiglia D, Della Torre A, Stroscio CA, Vescio G, Lavano A. Intervertebral thoracic herniation disc presenting as acute abdomen. *J Neurosurg Sci*. 2018;62(4):522–523.
70. Rohde RS, Kang JD. Thoracic disc herniation presenting with chronic nausea and abdominal pain. A case report. *J Bone Joint Surg Am*. 2004;86(2):379–381.
71. Ozturk C, Tezer M, Sirvanci M, Sarier M, Aydogan M, Hamzaoglu A. Far lateral thoracic disc herniation presenting with flank pain. *Spine J*. 2006;6(2):201–203.
72. Key C. On Paraplegia: Depending on disease of the ligaments of the spine. *Guys Hospital Rep*. 1838;3:17–24.
73. Mixter WJ, Barr JS. Rupture of the intervertebral disc with involvement of the spinal canal. *N Engl J Med*. 1934;211(5):210–215.
74. Hodgson AR, Stock FE. Anterior spinal fusion. A preliminary communication on the radical treatment of Pott's disease and Pott's paraplegia. 1956. *Clin Orthop Relat Res*. 1994(300):16–23.
75. Crafoord C, Hiertonn T, Lindblom K, Olsson SE. Spinal cord compression caused by a protruded thoracic disc; report of a case treated with antero-lateral fenestration of the disc. *Acta Orthop Scand*. 1958;28(2):103–107.

76. Perot Jr. PL, Munro DD. Transthoracic removal of midline thoracic disc protrusions causing spinal cord compression. *J Neurosurg*. 1969;31(4):452–458.
77. Ransohoff J, Spencer F, Siew F, Gage Jr. L. Transthoracic removal of thoracic disc. Report of three cases. *J Neurosurg*. 1969; 31(4):459–461.
78. Carson J, Gumpert J, Jefferson A. Diagnosis and treatment of thoracic intervertebral disc protrusions. *J Neurol Neurosurg Psychiatry*. 1971;34(1):68–77.
79. Patterson Jr. RH, Arbit E. A surgical approach through the pedicle to protruded thoracic discs. *J Neurosurg*. 1978;48(5):768–772.
80. Anand N, Regan JJ. Video-assisted thoracoscopic surgery for thoracic disc disease: Classification and outcome study of 100 consecutive cases with a 2-year minimum follow-up period. *Spine (Phila Pa 1976)*. 2002;27(8):871–879.
81. Ahn DK, Lee S, Moon SH, Boo KH, Chang BK, Lee JI. Ossification of the ligamentum flavum. *Asian Spine J*. 2014;8(1):89.
82. Hirabayashi S. Ossification of the ligamentum flavum. *Spine Surg Relat Res*. 2017;1(4):158–163.
83. Christiano LD, Assina R, Goldstein IM. Ossification of the ligamentum flavum: a unique report of a Hispanic woman. *Neurosurg Focus*. 2011;30(3):E15.
84. Lubelski D, Healy AT, Mageswaran P, Benzel EC, Mroz TE. Biomechanics of the lower thoracic spine after decompression and fusion: a cadaveric analysis. *Spine J*. 2014;14(9):2216–2223.
85. Watkins Rt, Watkins 3rd R, Williams L, et al. Stability provided by the sternum and rib cage in the thoracic spine. *Spine (Phila Pa 1976)*. 2005;30(11):1283–1286.
86. Abiola R, Rubery P, Mesfin A. Ossification of the posterior longitudinal ligament: Etiology, diagnosis, and outcomes of nonoperative and operative management. *Global Spine J*. 2016; 6(2):195–204.
87. Kalb S, Martirosyan NL, Perez-Orribo L, Kalani MYS, Theodore N. Analysis of demographics, risk factors, clinical presentation, and surgical treatment modalities for the ossified posterior longitudinal ligament. *Neurosurg Focus*. 2011;30(3):E11.
88. Barrios-Anderson A, Wang EJ, Sastry R, Fridley JS. Ossification of the posterior longitudinal ligament in the cervical, thoracic, and lumbar spine. *Cureus*. 2021;13(3):e14041.
89. Chen Z-Q, Sun C-G. Clinical guideline for treatment of symptomatic thoracic spinal stenosis. *Orthop Surg*. 2015;7(3): 208–212.
90. Min JH, Jang JS, Lee SH. Clinical results of ossification of the posterior longitudinal ligament (OPLL) of the thoracic spine treated by anterior decompression. *J Spinal Disord Tech*. 2008;21(2):116–119.
91. Diebo BG, Shah NV, Boachie-Adjei O, et al. Adult spinal deformity. *Lancet*. 2019;394(10193):160–172.
92. Kim HJ, Yang JH, Chang DG, et al. Adult spinal deformity: Current concepts and decision-making strategies for management. *Asian Spine J*. 2020;14(6):886–897.
93. Garfin SR, Eismont F. *Rothman-Simeone and Herkowitz's The Spine*. Vol 2. 7 ed. Elsevier; 2018:1248–1249.
94. Glassman SD, Carreon LY, Shaffrey CI, et al. The costs and benefits of nonoperative management for adult scoliosis. *Spine (Phila Pa 1976)*. 2010;35(5):578–582.
95. Kelly MP, Lurie JD, Yanik EL, et al. Operative versus non-operative treatment for adult symptomatic lumbar scoliosis. *J Bone Joint Surg Am*. 2019;101(4):338–352.
96. Liu S, Diebo BG, Henry JK, et al. The benefit of nonoperative treatment for adult spinal deformity: identifying predictors for reaching a minimal clinically important difference. *Spine J*. 2016;16(2):210–218.
97. Bess S, Protopsaltis TS, Lafage V, et al. Clinical and radiographic evaluation of adult spinal deformity. *Clin Spine Surg*. 2016;29(1):6–16.
98. Smith JS, Bess S, Shaffrey CI, et al. Dynamic changes of the pelvis and spine are key to predicting postoperative sagittal alignment after pedicle subtraction osteotomy: a critical analysis of preoperative planning techniques. *Spine (Phila Pa 1976)*. 2012;37(10):845–853.
99. Schwab F, Patel A, Ungar B, Farcy JP, Lafage V. Adult spinal deformity-postoperative standing imbalance: how much can you tolerate? An overview of key parameters in assessing alignment and planning corrective surgery. *Spine (Phila Pa 1976)*. 2010;35(25):2224–2231.
100. Lafage R, Schwab F, Glassman S, et al. Age-adjusted alignment goals have the potential to reduce PJK. *Spine (Phila Pa 1976)*. 2017;42(17):1275–1282.
101. Lener S, Hartmann S, Barbagallo GMV, Certo F, Thomé C, Tschugg A. Management of spinal infection: a review of the literature. *Acta Neurochir (Wien)*. 2018;160(3):487–496.
102. Sobottke R, Seifert H, Fätkenheuer G, Schmidt M, Gossmann A, Eysel P. Current diagnosis and treatment of spondylodiscitis. *Dtsch Arztebl Int*. 2008;105(10):181–187.
103. Duarte RM, Vaccaro AR. Spinal infection: state of the art and management algorithm. *Eur Spine J*. 2013;22(12):2787–2799.
104. Iwasaki M, Yano S, Aoyama T, Hida K, Iwasaki Y. Acute onset intramedullary spinal cord abscess with spinal artery occlusion: a case report and review. *Eur Spine J*. 2011;20 Suppl 2(Suppl 2): S294–S301.
105. Arko Lt, Quach E, Nguyen V, Chang D, Sukul V, Kim BS. Medical and surgical management of spinal epidural abscess: a systematic review. *Neurosurg Focus*. 2014;37(2):E4.
106. Reihsaus E, Waldbaur H, Seeling W. Spinal epidural abscess: a meta-analysis of 915 patients. *Neurosurg Rev*. 2000;23(4): 175–204. discussion 205.
107. Curry Jr. WT, Hoh BL, Amin-Hanjani S, Eskandar EN. Spinal epidural abscess: clinical presentation, management, and outcome. *Surg Neurol*. 2005;63(4):364–371. discussion 371.
108. Darouiche RO. Spinal epidural abscess. *N Engl J Med*. 2006; 355(19):2012–2020.
109. Kim SD, Melikian R, Ju KL, et al. Independent predictors of failure of nonoperative management of spinal epidural abscesses. *Spine J*. 2014;14(8):1673–1679.
110. Mückley T, Schütz T, Kirschner M, Potulski M, Hofmann G, Bühren V. Psoas abscess: the spine as a primary source of infection. *Spine (Phila Pa 1976)*. 2003;28(6):E106–E113.
111. Yacoub WN, Sohn HJ, Chan S, et al. Psoas abscess rarely requires surgical intervention. *Am J Surg*. 2008;196(2):223–227.

16

Minimally Invasive Lateral Approach Related Complications

LAUREN E. STONE, JAY I. KUMAR, MD, AND ROBERT K. EASTLACK

CHAPTER OUTLINE

Introduction

The mini-open lateral approach to the thoracic spine evolved as a means to provide targeted access to the anterior spinal elements, while reducing the likelihood of damage to local structures.[1–3] Historically, large anterior thoracotomies and wide posterior resections provided access around the ribs and neurovascular bundles, great vessels, heart, lungs, and neural elements, but carried significant risk of multisystem complications.[1–6] Retropleural corridors for nonspinal pathology were published as early as the 1920s, but the technology necessary to stabilize a corridor to the spine had not yet been developed.[7–9] The advent and popularization of minimally invasive lateral access in the lumbar spine would provide the impetus for thoughtful experimentation in the thoracic spine. Surgeons hoped to apply the favorable minimally invasive surgery (MIS) complication profile to this more constrained region.[10,11] These attempts resulted in early reports of thoracic lateral interbody fusion, later modified and termed the "mini-open" approach, as described by multiple groups.[3,4,12]

The mini-open approach has since come into its own as a viable thoracic access corridor with an estimated major complication rate of 6.5% to 13.5%—a small percentage of these being neurologic deficit.[1,2] The potential complications are inherent to regional anatomy and perceived limitations of MIS techniques and require thoughtful management if confronted. In this chapter, we discuss the most common and feared iatrogenic complications associated with minimally invasive lateral access to the thoracic spine (Table 16.1).

Brief Considerations

Technical notes for the mini-open technique have been published by multiple groups.[2,3,6,13,14] Detailed discussion of indications for this approach is beyond the scope of this chapter. Briefly, mini-open lateral approaches are typically used for anterior spinal pathology between T6 at the scapula, and, if the diaphragm is crossed, the L4-5 disk space. Patient-specific factors mitigate ease of access, as obesity, new or old thoracic trauma, or pleural disruption may limit ease of access.[13] Additionally, the posterior elements cannot be accessed via the lateral mini-open corridor.

Variations in technique exist due to available technology, pathology characteristics, and surgeon familiarity. For example, rib resection may be necessary for wider exposure or retropleural access[2,6,15] whereas transpleural access between ribs is also viable.[16] Pertinent complications associated with all variations will be discussed.

This chapter also acknowledges that specific characteristics of the addressed pathology can significantly influence the complication profile. For example, calcified discs are more commonly associated with durotomy than a compressive vertebral body mass, as discussed below.[17] Thoughtful case preparation with appropriate advanced imaging (such as a computed tomography [CT] scan in the setting of a thoracic disc herniation) assists both surgical planning and complication avoidance.

The thoracic spine, especially the mid-thoracic spine, poses greater localization challenges than the cervical and lumbar spine. Wrong level surgery is not unique to lateral approaches, but this less familiar vector can confound orientation, and thus lead to errors. Preoperatively placed fiducials, intraoperative radiographic evaluation, and navigation technologies can be utilized to localize levels more

TABLE 16.1 Mini-open lateral thoracic approach complications.

Intercostal Neuralgia
Pulmonary
Pleural effusion
Pneumothorax
Hemothorax
Duropleural fistula
Durotomy
Cerebrospinal fluid leak
Diaphragm Injury

precisely, while experience with the approach can also mitigate risk.[18–20]

Lastly, this review is limited to intraoperative complications associated uniquely with the mini-open approach and is not meant to comprehensively compare alternative approaches. All spinal surgeries risk neural damage, the risk of which will only be discussed as it relates to distinctive elements of the mini-open approach. We do not discuss intraoperative neuromonitoring, although it is worth noting that (1) the thoracic spinal cord is delicate, and a "sick" cord may not tolerate complex maneuvers, such as distraction or retraction, and (2) vascular infarcts at the ventral spinal cord will evade dorsal column monitoring (standard somatosensory evoked potentials) or present in a delayed fashion.[21] Postoperatively acquired complications, such as graft subsidence, are similarly not discussed.

Complications Overview

When choosing a surgical approach, a defensive mindset helps protect critical structures. Lateral approaches contend with the chest wall (with risk of intercostal neuralgia), retropleural space (with multiple consequences to the lung and surrounding thoracic cavity), vascular structures (the aorta and its branches), the diaphragm, and the thoracic neural elements.

Complications associated with the above will be discussed here, including the likely timing of such encounters during the procedure workflow, prevention, and management strategies. Pulmonary complications are combined for simplicity, while others are discussed in kind with their local anatomy.

Intercostal Neuralgia

Intercostal neuralgia (IN) is a well-reported but poorly understood complication of thoracic access. Patients describe a sharp and/or burning pain radiating in the distribution of the affected intercostal nerve. Estimates in the mini-open literature place incidence between 0% and 6%, which is lower than the suggested incidence for open approaches (4.3%–50%).[22–24]

The intercostal nerve and neurovascular bundle typically—but not always—follow the anteroinferior margin of the rib body. It is encountered during initial access to the thoracic cavity and remains at risk until closure from both direct and indirect manipulation.[25] Techniques for handling the neurovascular bundle during rib resection have been published, describing careful subperiosteal dissection and confirmed visualization of the bundle to decrease the likelihood of direct damage.[26]

If the rib is not resected, damage to the nerve can occur by other means. Zhang et al.'s animal model study demonstrated that stretch from excessive intercostal retraction resulted in time-dependent deficits in intercostal neuromonitoring, detectable up to 30 minutes after retractor removal.[27] In clinical settings, others have found that retractors, often angled towards the rib and opened widely, can directly compress the neurovascular bundle against the rib, crushing and damaging the nerve.[16,28] While intraoperative neuromonitoring for intercostal nerve integrity is not routinely performed, careful positioning and conservative widening of the retractor may mitigate damage.

Closure technique can decrease risk of IN, especially if a rib is resected. Muscular re-approximation should be free of tension to avoid strangulating the bundle.[18] For open thoracotomies, multiple randomized control trials have suggested that use of intracostal sutures, placed into the adjacent rib, decrease rates of IN by diffusing the tension load. While the exposure for this is not usually obtained for a mini-open approach, tension should be minimized regardless of closure technique.[29–31]

Should a patient awake with IN, targeted intercostal nerve blocks as well as oral neuropathic medications may reduce pain. Some authors perform blocks routinely upon entry or closure.[1,32] Should IN persist, treatment with antidepressants, radiofrequency ablation, rhizotomy, ganglionectomy, and neurectomies have been reported, with variable success.[32–38]

The long-term outcomes for patients with IN in mini-open literature is unknown. In open reviews, 5% to 10% of patients with postoperative IN experience debilitating pain years after their procedure.[22,39,40]

Pulmonary

Most MIS techniques require the surgeon to become facile with traversing a previously unfamiliar plane with limited to no visualization. Mini-open lateral procedures include an approach through the retropleural space, which allows for access to the spine, while the lung remains inflated. This requires careful dissection between the parietal pleura and endothoracic fascia for safe passage to the thoracic spine.[5] While the retropleural approach avoids pulmonary compromise associated with lung deflation/single-lumen ventilation, mechanical damage or irritation of the pleura can result in several pulmonary complications, including pneumothorax, hemothorax, and pulmonary effusion. The combined incidence of these complications is estimated between 0% and 10.2%.[41]

Effusions occur when liquid collects in the retropleural space. Soda et al. reported 5.2% incidence of pulmonary effusion in their series, although none required subsequent drainage.[17] Uribe et al. reported one case (1.7% incidence) of postoperative chest tube placement for a symptomatic effusion after a transpleural approach.[2] The incidence is likely somewhere between these reports, although it may be higher near the thoracolumbar junction due to pleural adherence to the diaphragm and local structures.[2,4,17,24,42]

Damage to the pleura can result in air escaping into the retropleural space, the most dangerous outcome being a tension pneumothorax. The incidence of minor pneumothoraces is not always reported, but likely similar to that of pleural effusions (between 0%–9.7%).[2,17,24,42] Should a small pleural defect occur, quick maneuvers can prevent evolution into a major complication. A small piece of gelatin sponge over the site is usually sufficient to block air outflow. Bleeding is usually minor; cautery should be avoided to prevent more pleural damage. Some authors advocate for temporary placement of a drain or catheter in the retropleural space at the moment of detected damage. This serves as a makeshift chest tube with the exiting end placed in a fluid bath that serves as a water seal. Should an air leak exist after a Valsalva by the end of the case, a real chest tube can be placed.[6] Most surgeons routinely leave some form of pleural drain in place, regardless of observed pleural damage.[32,43]

The incidence of hemothorax in the mini-open approach is unknown and likely rare. Baaj et al. reported a single case of hemothorax in an 80-patient trauma cohort; this ultimately required evacuation, although no causal artery was found (Fig. 16.1).[24] Arterial bleeding sources in this corridor are limited. The segmental arteries at the vertebral border are usually well visualized. Gentle retraction and/or careful coagulation of the arteries is sufficient for

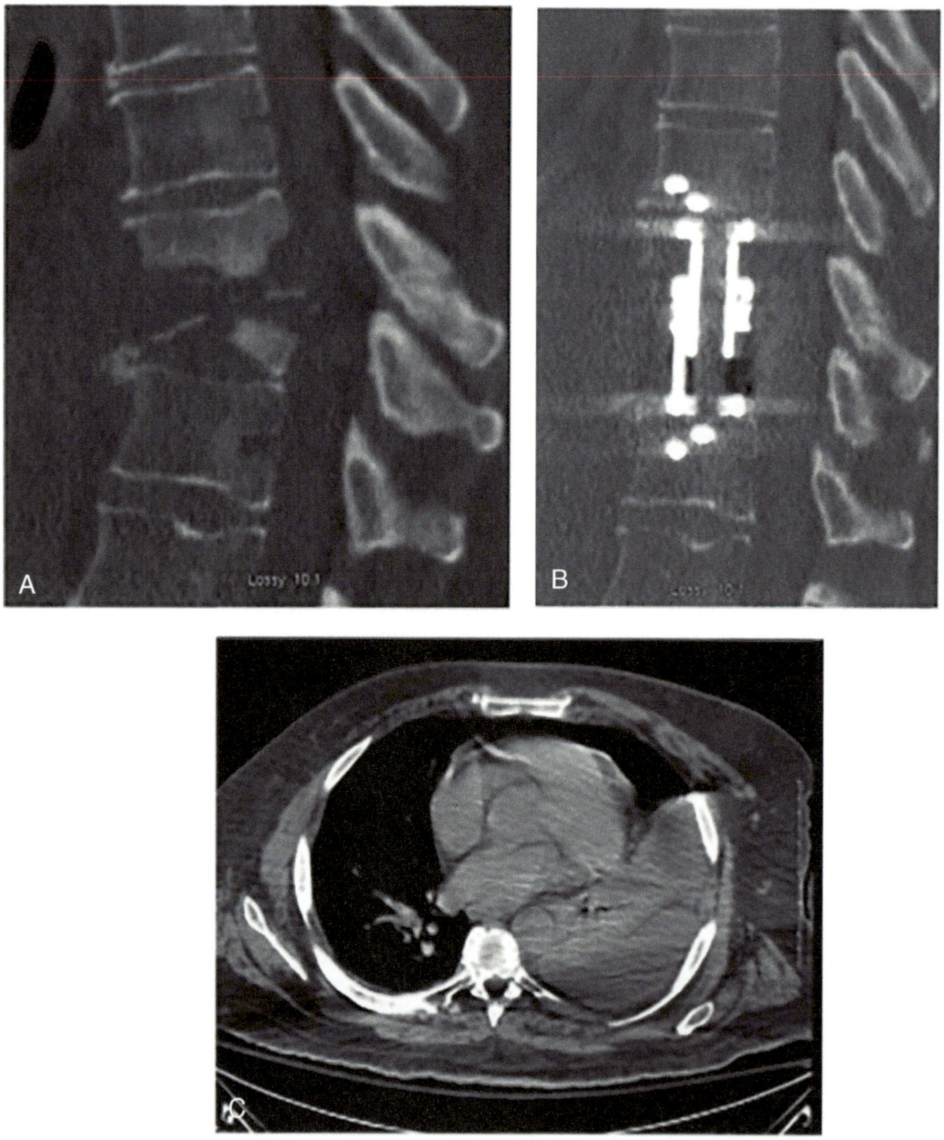

• **Fig. 16.1** Axial CT scan of the thoracic spine after myelogram revealing a fistulous connection **(thick black arrows)** between the spinal canal and the pleural space **(white arrows)**.

hemostasis, although bony bleeding may be harder to control. Neurologic deficits associated with segmental artery sacrifice are rare, especially when limited to a few unilateral vessels, but have been reported.[44,45] Intercostal artery injury, while possible, has not been reported. Great vessel injury has not been reported, although the position of the aorta can be directly in the operative vector in regions of the upper thoracic spine or in the direct contralateral pathway.[18] Careful review of preoperative imaging is necessary to avoid vascular injury or suggest planning a different approach. Should an issue be encountered intraoperatively, packing, vascular consultation, and anesthetic hemodynamic support are warranted.

Postoperative chest radiograph after all mini-open lateral cases can detect the majority of pulmonary complications. Many also advocate an additional radiograph 2 days after surgery, and another after chest tube/drain removal.[2]

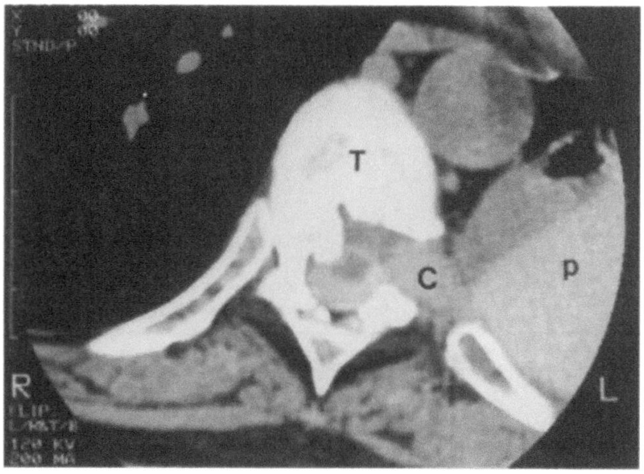

• **Fig. 16.2** Coronal CT scan of the thoracic spine after myelogram again demonstrating a fistulous connection between the spinal canal and pleural space.

Durotomy

The frequency of dural tears in mini-open lateral cases varies by pathology. Overall incidence is reported between 0% and 11.7%.[2,3,23,42,43] Calcified discs are notoriously adherent or infiltrating, resulting in a higher risk of durotomy with a reported incidence of 1.2% to 18% in all approaches to the thoracic spine.[17] Sharp, traumatic bony fragments may also pierce the dura, plugging a leak that becomes evident once the thecal sac is decompressed.[46] As such, durotomies may be unavoidable, but also more difficult to visualize and manage in the mini-open approach. Cadaveric or simulated practice sewing through a mini-open approach is not feasible for all surgeons, although this practice is anecdotally helpful. Careful evaluation of preoperative imaging is recommended to increase the surgeon's index of suspicion before the procedure.

Durotomies are most often encountered during dissection of the posterior longitudinal ligament (PLL) from an adherent, and occasionally confluent, thecal sac. Small, low-flow pinhole rents may respond better to intraoperative management than large, irregular high-flow tears. If the tear is accessible, primary closure with a 4-0 to 6-0 suture should be attempted, followed with a hydrophobic material (i.e., fat, muscle) and sealant (i.e., fibrin glue).[16,17,43] If the leak is accessible and sufficiently low flow, a thin layer of collagen matrix can be tented over top with dural tack-ups or allowed to adhere via surface tension.[47]

If a high-flow cerebrospinal fluid (CSF) leak is encountered or a tear is sufficiently irregular, multiple management options exist. Conversion to an open approach can be considered if expanded visualization and maneuverability is needed. Otherwise, a thin gelatin sponge onlay with local blood may form a rudimentary "blood patch" and a lumbar drain can **diver** cerebrospinal fluid. Placement of a local drain within the wound bed is not universally performed, but if done, must be carefully monitored for excessive output. Alternatively, the drain can be placed on gravity suction only in order to avoid creating a siphoning effect that disrupts the CSF repair site. If a corpectomy is being performed, placement of a lateral plate may hold the repair materials in place enough to mitigate recurrent CSF leaking and promote healing.[14]

Postoperative bedrest with careful neurologic monitoring is warranted. Serial physical exams can detect signs or symptoms suggestive of significant overdrainage (e.g., headache when sitting upright) or underdrainage (e.g., wound leakage, new regional neurologic defect from spinal cord compression).[47] Should wound leakage develop, administration of antibiotics beyond perioperative care is controversial but typically avoided in the absence of overt signs of infection.[48,49]

Most leaks resolve. For those that persist despite lumbar drainage, permanent CSF diversion (i.e., lumboperitoneal shunt) can be considered.[16,47] There are also reports of complex omental vascularized flaps as last attempt efforts, although these are not routine.[47]

Of note, if concurrent suspicion for pleural damage is high, there is a chance of forming a duropleural fistula, which may require chest tube placement or more invasive measures should respiratory status become compromised (Fig. 16.2).[50] The chest tube should be set to water seal to avoid further decreasing intrathoracic pressure and provoking the CSF leak.[6] Trials with noninvasive positive airway pressure have been suggested to **meliorate** the fistula flow rate enough for primary healing, although reoperation and tissue graft sealing is definitive treatment.[51,52] This is a serious, though rare complication of retropleural access whose incidence in mini-open cases is unknown.

Diaphragm Injury

Diaphragmatic injury is also rare. Our review found no description of the incidence in mini-open approaches, although it is hinted as "the diaphragm problem" by Von **Glinske's** discussion of MIS thoracolumbar access.[15] The discussion of diaphragm management is sourced from the lateral lumbar literature, although surgeons attempting to access the penultimate thoracic segments are required to have a working understanding of both the anatomy of and manipulation tolerated by this structure to avoid injury.

The diaphragm typically attaches between the 10th and 12th ribs, craniocaudally dividing the retropleural and retroperitoneal corridors. At the most posteroinferior margin of the 12th rib, the lateral arcuate ligament can be sectioned from its diaphragmatic connection, revealing the quadratus lumborum, which can be followed medially to the medial arcuate ligament. Once sectioned, the L1 transverse process is revealed, followed by the medial crus of the diaphragm and the anterolateral vertebral body.[5,6,53]

The union between the parietal pleura and diaphragm offers unique opportunities to damage both structures, possibly accounting for some reports of higher pleural injury after thoracolumbar approaches.[15] Should the diaphragm be damaged or intentionally incised to gain more caudal exposure, a large, nonabsorbable suture line in parallel to the muscle fiber's radial vector is advised to maximize muscle function.[54] Postoperative identification of a diaphragmatic injury is often subtle, usually not complete, and may present as subtle respiratory complaints. A high index of suspicion is required for diagnosis.

Future Directions

The role for navigation in complication mitigation is a new topic gaining interest.[55] Few reports describing utilization of these platforms with mini-open lateral approaches exist. Shabani et al. discuss a workflow for localization, trajectory planning, and real-time anatomy review for mini-open approaches.[18] In our review, no report directly examined complication rate reduction as a result of employing navigation.

Enabling technologies, such as robotics and augmented reality, have not been discussed in the mini-open literature, although are viable considerations for future exploration.

Conclusions

Mini-open lateral access to the thoracic spine is well tolerated overall, with a favorable complication profile. Mitigation of unique complications requires an index of suspicion in advance and knowledge of maneuvers to prevent or limit associated, undesirable outcomes. As with all MIS procedures, familiarity flattens the learning curve, improving efficiency in this corridor to ultimately yield effective results for patients with diverse pathologies.

References

1. Smith WD, Dakwar E, Le TV, Christian G, Serrano S, Uribe JS. Minimally invasive surgery for traumatic spinal pathologies: a mini-open, lateral approach in the thoracic and lumbar spine. *Spine (Phila Pa 1976)*. 2010;35(26 Suppl):S338–S346. https://doi.org/10.1097/BRS.0b013e3182023113.
2. Uribe JS, Smith WD, Pimenta L, et al. Minimally invasive lateral approach for symptomatic thoracic disc herniation: initial multicenter clinical experience. *J Neurosurg Spine*. 2012;16(3):264–279. https://doi.org/10.3171/2011.10.SPINE11291.
3. Uribe JS, Dakwar E, Le TV, Christian G, Serrano S, Smith WD. Minimally invasive surgery treatment for thoracic spine tumor removal: a mini-open, lateral approach. *Spine (Phila Pa 1976)*. 2010;35(26 Suppl):S347–S354. https://doi.org/10.1097/BRS.0b013e3182022d0f.
4. Meredith DS, Kepler CK, Huang RC, Hegde VV. Extreme lateral interbody fusion (XLIF) in the thoracic and thoracolumbar spine: Technical report and early outcomes. *HSS J*. 2013;9(1):25–31. https://doi.org/10.1007/s11420-012-9312-x.
5. Huangxs S, Christiansen PA, Tan H, et al. Mini-open lateral corpectomy for thoracolumbar junction lesions. *Oper Neurosurg (Hagerstown)*. 2020;18(6):640–647. https://doi.org/10.1093/ons/opz298.
6. Christiansen PA, Huang S, Smith JS, Shaffrey ME, Uribe JS, Yen C. Mini-open lateral retropleural/retroperitoneal approaches for thoracic and thoracolumbar junction anterior column pathologies. *Neurosurg Focus*. 2020;49(3):E13. https://doi.org/10.3171/2020.6.FOCUS20360.
7. Fey B. L'abord du rein voie thoraco-abodominale. *Urologicale Clin Necker*. 1925(5):169–178.
8. Francioli P. Ways of approach in lumbar and lumbothoracic sympathectomies. *Helv Chir Acta*. 1951;18:536–556.
9. Moskovich R, Benson D, Zhang ZH, Kabins M. Extracoelomic approach to the spine. *J Bone Joint Surg Br*. 1993;75:886–893.
10. Ozgur BM, Aryan HE, Pimenta L, Taylor WR. Extreme lateral interbody fusion (XLIF): a novel surgical technique for anterior lumbar interbody fusion. *Spine J*. 2006;6(4):435–443. https://doi.org/10.1016/j.spinee.2005.08.012.
11. Mayer HM. A new microsurgical technique for minimally invasive anterior lumbar interbody fusion. *Spine (Phila Pa 1976)*. 1997;22(6):691–699; discussion 700.
12. Karikari IO, Nimjee SM, Hardin CA, et al. Extreme lateral interbody fusion approach for isolated thoracic and thoracolumbar spine diseases: initial clinical experience and early outcomes. *J Spinal Disord Tech*. 2011;24(6):368–375. https://doi.org/10.1097/BSD.0b013e3181ffefd2.
13. Walker CT, Xu DS, Godzik J, Turner JD, Uribe JS, Smith WD. Minimally invasive surgery for thoracolumbar spinal trauma. *Ann Transl Med*. 2018;6(6):102. https://doi.org/10.21037/atm.2018.02.10.
14. Uribe JS, Katsevman GA, Morgan CD, Paisan GM, Snyder LA. Mini-open lateral retropleural thoracic discectomy approach. *Neurosurgical Focus: Video*. 2022;7(1):V2. https://doi.org/10.3171/2022.3.FOCVID2217.
15. Von Glinski A, Elia CJ, Takayanagi A, et al. Extreme Lateral Interbody Fusion for Thoracic and Thoracolumbar Disease: The Diaphragm Dilemma. *Global Spine J*. 2021;11(4):515–524. https://doi.org/10.1177/2192568220914883.
16. Strom RG, Mathur V, Givans H, Kondziolka DS, Perin NI. Technical modifications and decision-making to reduce morbidity in thoracic disc surgery: An institutional experience and treatment algorithm. *Clin Neurol Neurosurg*. 2015;133:75–82. https://doi.org/10.1016/j.clineuro.2015.03.014.
17. Soda C, Faccioli F, Marchesini N, et al. Trans-thoracic versus retropleural approach for symptomatic thoracic disc herniations: comparative analysis of 94 consecutive cases. *Br J Neurosurg*. 2021;35(2):195–202. https://doi.org/10.1080/02688697.2020.1779660.

18. Shabani S, Mummaneni PV, Chan A, et al. Management of thoracic disc pathology via the lateral approach: Advances using the minimally invasive approach and navigation. *Int J Spine Surg.* 2022;16(S1):S44–S52. https://doi.org/10.14444/8235.
19. Sclafani JA, Kim CW. Complications associated with the initial learning curve of minimally invasive spine surgery: A systematic review. *Clin Orthop Relat Res.* 2014;472:1711–1717. https://doi.org/10.1007/s11999-014-3495-z.
20. Madaelil TP, Long JR, Wallace AN, et al. Preoperative fiducial marker placement in the thoracic spine: A technical report. *Spine (Phila Pa 1976).* 2017;42(10):E624–E628. https://doi.org/10.1097/BRS.0000000000001890.
21. Minahan RE, Sepkuty JP, Lesser RP, Sponseller PD, Kostuik JP. Anterior spinal cord injury with preserved neurogenic 'motor' evoked potentials. *Clin Neurophysiol.* 2001;112(8):1442–1450. https://doi.org/10.1016/s1388-2457(01)00567-3.
22. Rogers ML, Duffy JP. Surgical aspects of chronic post-thoracotomy pain. *Eur J Cardiothorac Surg.* 2000;18(6):711–716. https://doi.org/10.1016/s1010-7940(00)00569-8.
23. Oltulu I, Cil H, Ulu MO, Deviren V. Clinical outcomes of symptomatic thoracic disk herniations treated surgically through minimally invasive lateral transthoracic approach. *Neurosurg Rev.* 2019;42(4):885–894. https://doi.org/10.1007/s10143-018-01064-2.
24. Baaj AA, Dakwar E, Le TV, et al. Complications of the mini-open anterolateral approach to the thoracolumbar spine. *J Clin Neurosci.* 2012;19(9):1265–1267. https://doi.org/10.1016/j.jocn.2012.01.026.
25. Schalow G, Aho A, Lang G. Microanatomy and number of nerve fibres of the lower intercostal nerves with respect to a nerve anastomosis. Donor nerve analysis. I. (IV). *Electromyogr Clin Neurophysiol.* 1992;32(4-5):171–185.
26. Li B, Kuzmik GA, Shabani S, et al. Short segment rib resection to mitigate risk of pleural violation during retropleural lateral thoracic interbody fusion. *Neurosurg Focus Video.* 2022;7(1):V4. https://doi.org/10.3171/2022.3.FOCVID21138.
27. Zhang R, Schwabe K, Krüger M, Haverich A, Krauss JK, Alam M. Electro-physiological evidence of intercostal nerve injury after thoracotomy: an experimental study in a sheep model. *J Thorac Dis.* 2017;9(8):2461–2465. https://doi.org/10.21037/jtd.2017.07.10.
28. Deviren V, Kuelling FA, Poulter G, Pekmezci M. Minimal invasive anterolateral transthoracic transpleural approach: a novel technique for thoracic disc herniation. A review of the literature, description of a new surgical technique and experience with first 12 consecutive patients. *J Spinal Disord Tech.* 2011;24(5):E40–E48. https://doi.org/10.1097/BSD.0b013e318220af6f.
29. Cerfolio RJ, Price TN, Bryant AS, Sale Bass C, Bartolucci AA. Intracostal sutures decrease the pain of thoracotomy. *Ann Thorac Surg.* 2003;76(2):407–412. https://doi.org/10.1016/s0003-4975(03)00447-8.
30. Bayram AS, Ozcan M, Kaya FN, Gebitekin C. Rib approximation without intercostal nerve compression reduces post-thoracotomy pain: a prospective randomized study. *Eur J Cardiothorac Surg.* 2011;39:570–574.
31. Sakakura N, Usami N, Taniguchi T, Kawaguchi K, Okagawa T, Yokoyama M, et al. Assessment of long-term postoperative pain in open thoracotomy patients: pain reduction by the edge closure technique. *Ann Thorac Surg.* 2010;89:1064–1070.
32. Ahmadian A, Uribe JS. Mini-open lateral retro-pleural thoracic corpectomy for osteomyelitis. *Neurosurg Focus.* 2013;35(2 Suppl). https://doi.org/10.3171/2013.V2.FOCUS13221.
33. Bajwa ZH, Sami N, Warfield CA, Wootton J. Topiramate relieves refractory intercostal neuralgia. *Neurology.* 1999;52(9):1917. https://doi.org/10.1212/wnl.52.9.1917.
34. Williams EH, Williams CG, Rosson GD, Heitmiller RF, Dellon AL. Neurectomy for treatment of intercostal neuralgia. *Ann Thorac Surg.* 2008;85(5):1766–1770. https://doi.org/10.1016/j.athoracsur.2007.11.058.
35. Finnerup NB, Attal N, Haroutounian S, et al. Pharmacotherapy for neuropathic pain in adults: a systematic review and meta-analysis. *Lancet Neurol.* 2015;14(2):162–173. https://doi.org/10.1016/S1474-4422(14)70251-0.
36. Abd-Elsayed A, Lee S, Jackson M. Radiofrequency Ablation for Treating Resistant Intercostal Neuralgia. *Ochsner J.* 2018 Spring; 18(1):91–93.
37. Wilkinson HA, Chan AS. Sensory ganglionectomy: theory, technical aspects, and clinical experience. *J Neurosurg.* 2001 Jul; 95(1):61–66.
38. Dorsi MJ, Lambrinos G, Dellon AL, Belzberg AJ. Dorsal rhizotomy for treatment of bilateral intercostal neuralgia following augmentation mammaplasty: case report and review of the literature. *Microsurgery.* 2011 Jan;31(1):41–44.
39. Gupta R, Van de Ven T, Pyati S. Post-Thoracotomy Pain: Current Strategies for Prevention and Treatment. *Drugs.* 2020;80(16):1677–1684. https://doi.org/10.1007/s40265-020-01390-0.
40. Sabanathan S. Has postoperative pain been eradicated? *Ann R Coll Surg Engl.* 1995;77(3):202–209.
41. Kasliwal MK, Deutsch H. Minimally invasive retropleural approach for central thoracic disc herniation. *Minim Invasive Neurosurg.* 2011;54(4):167–171. https://doi.org/10.1055/s-0031-1284400.
42. Noureldine MHA, Pressman E, Krafft PR, et al. Management of thoracic disc herniation using the mini-open retropleural approach: Technique illustration and clinical outcomes of 33 patients from a single academic center. *Oper Neurosurg (Hagerstown).* 2020;19(5):567–581. https://doi.org/10.1093/ons/opaa228.
43. Nacar OA, Ulu MO, Pekmezci M, Deviren V. Surgical treatment of thoracic disc disease via minimally invasive lateral transthoracic trans/retropleural approach: analysis of 33 patients. *Neurosurg Rev.* 2013;36(3):455–465. https://doi.org/10.1007/s10143-013-0461-2.
44. Leung YL, Grevitt M, Henderson L, Smith J. Cord monitoring changes and segmental vessel ligation in the "at risk" cord during anterior spinal deformity surgery. *Spine.* 2005;30:1870–1874.
45. Orchowski J, Bridwell KH, Lenke LG. Neurological deficit from a purely vascular etiology after unilateral vessel ligation during anterior thoracolumbar fusion of the spine. *Spine (Phila Pa 1976).* 2005;30(4):406–410. https://doi.org/10.1097/01.brs.0000153391.55608.72.
46. Carl AL, Matsumoto M, Whalen JT. Anterior dural laceration caused by thoracolumbar and lumbar burst fractures. *J Spinal Disord.* 2000;5:399–403.
47. Fang Z, Tian R, Jia YT, Xu TT, Liu Y. Treatment of cerebrospinal fluid leak after spine surgery. *Chin J Traumatol.* 2017;20(2):81–83. https://doi.org/10.1016/j.cjtee.2016.12.002.
48. Liu Y, Tan Q, Qin J, et al. Prophylactic use of antibiotics for fever after drainage removal following a dural tear during lumbar spinal surgery: A retrospective study. *Med Sci Monit.* 2022;28:e936652. https://doi.org/10.12659/MSM.936652.
49. Baker GA, Cizik AM, Bransford RJ, et al. Risk factors for unintended durotomy during spine surgery: A multivariate analysis. *Spine J.* 2012;12(2):121–126.

50. Monla-Hassan J, Eichenhorn M, Spickler E, Talati S, Nockels R, Hyzy R. Duropleural fistula manifested as a large pleural transudate: an unusual complication of transthoracic diskectomy. *Chest*. 1998;114(6):1786–1789. https://doi.org/10.1378/chest.114.6.1786.
51. Schlag HR, Muquit S, Hristov TB, Morassi G, Boszczyk BM, Shafafy M. Subarachnoidal pleural fistula after resection of intradural thoracic disc herniation and multimodal treatment with non-invasive positive pressure ventilation (NPPV. *Eur Spine J*. 2016; 25(1):155–159. https://doi.org/10.1007/s00586-015-4137-1.
52. Hentschel SJ, Rhines LD, Wong FC, Gokaslan ZL, McCutcheon IE. Subarachnoid-pleural fistula after resection of thoracic tumors. *J Neurosurg*. 2004;100(4 Suppl Spine):332–336. https://doi.org/10.3171/spi.2004.100.4.0332.
53. Dakwar E, Ahmadian A, Uribe JS. The anatomical relationship of the diaphragm to the thoracolumbar junction during the minimally invasive lateral extracoelomic (retropleural/retroperitoneal) approach. *J Neurosurg Spine*. 2012;16(4):359–364. https://doi.org/10.3171/2011.12.SPINE11626.
54. Baaj AA, Papadimitriou K, Amin AG, Kretzer RM, Wolinsky JP, Gokaslan ZL. Surgical anatomy of the diaphragm in the anterolateral approach to the spine: a cadaveric study. *J Spinal Disord Tech*. 2014;27(4):220–223. https://doi.org/10.1097/BSD.0b013e3182a18125.
55. Farber SH, Pacult MA, Godzik J, et al. Robotics in Spine Surgery: A Technical Overview and Review of Key Concepts. *Front Surg*. 2021;8:578674. Published 2021 Feb 23. https://doi.org/10.3389/fsurg.2021.578674.

17

Complications of the Posterior Approach in Thoracic Spine Surgery

DANYAL A. QURAISHI, MARK BASILIOUS, JACOB L. GOLDBERG, ROGER HÄRTL, AND IBRAHIM HUSSAIN

CHAPTER OUTLINE

Introduction

Disease processes that impact the thoracic spinal column include cancer, degenerative processes, fractures, and infections.[1] Proper care and surgical intervention is critical to these pathologies to prevent or treat nerve injury, spinal cord compression, or both, which can cause radiculopathy or myelopathy.[1] Surgical approaches to the thoracic spine have been constantly evolving in order to provide the optimal trajectory to treat the pathology at hand while minimizing collateral damage to surrounding structures or reducing complication risk to the spinal cord. Anterior approaches to the thoracic spine carry inherent morbidity associated with the mobilization of the lungs, great vessels, and other vital structures within the thoracic cavity.[1]

Posterior approaches to the thoracic spine including laminectomies have been extensively described and considered the workhorse for the treatment of compressive thoracic pathologies.[2–5] However, with lateral and ventral pathologies within the thoracic canal, laminectomy only can be associated with poor neurological outcomes and morbidity rates ranging from 24% to 75%.[2–4,6] Such outcomes are largely due to the mechanical manipulation of the spinal cord to access the ventral spine, potentially interfering with spinal cord blood supply and ischemic injury.[2,3,7] Consequently, alternative approaches to the ventral region of the thoracic spine from the posterior approach have been developed and popularized over the last several decades, including circumferential posterior approaches such as costotransversectomy and transpedicular routes (Fig. 17.1).[3–5,8,9] These approaches have been proposed to have exceptional functional outcomes with lower complication rates when compared to laminectomy methods only or ventrolateral approaches.[4,6] Their method and mode of access allow treatment of multiple spinal levels all in a single-stage surgery.[10,11] Other benefits include avoiding the violation of the pleura and facilitating instrumented stabilization through the same incision.[12] However, these approaches still pose a smaller but relevant risk of neurologic injury from potential manipulation of the thecal sac to obtain adequate access to the vertebral body.[11] In this review, we summarize approach-related complications associated with the costotransversectomy and transpedicular routes, as well as pathologic-related complications that may occur when performing these posterior approaches.

Costotransversectomy Approach

Generally speaking, posterior approaches to the thoracic spine can often yield similar postoperative complication profiles. The thoracic spine in particular poses unique challenges due to the biomechanical intricacies associated with the rib cage.[11] Many retrospective studies analyzing postoperative complications of the posterior approach in the thoracic spine also report occurrences of hardware failure, pneumonia, and superficial wound infection.[9,13,14]

The costotransversectomy approach was first described by Menard and Larson in order to manage Pott's paraplegia.[15,16] This method allows surgeons to visualize the ventral

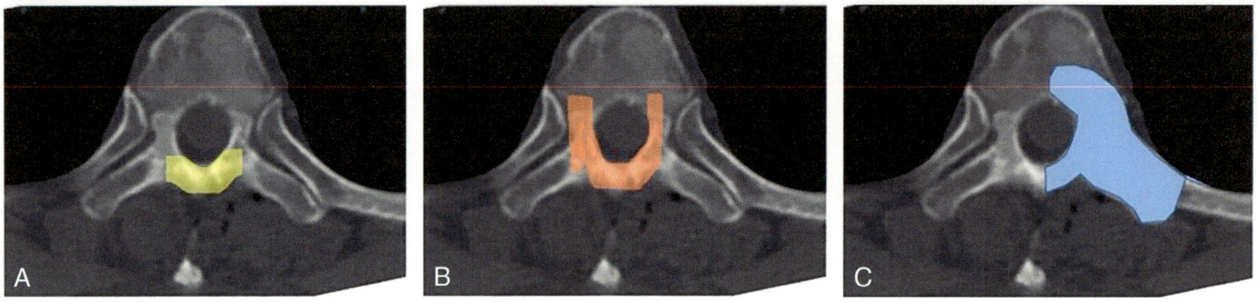

• **Fig. 17.1** Posterior approaches for thoracic spine pathologies. (A) Dorsal laminectomy. (B) Transpedicular approach (bilateral depicted). (C) Costotransversectomy (unilateral approach depicted).

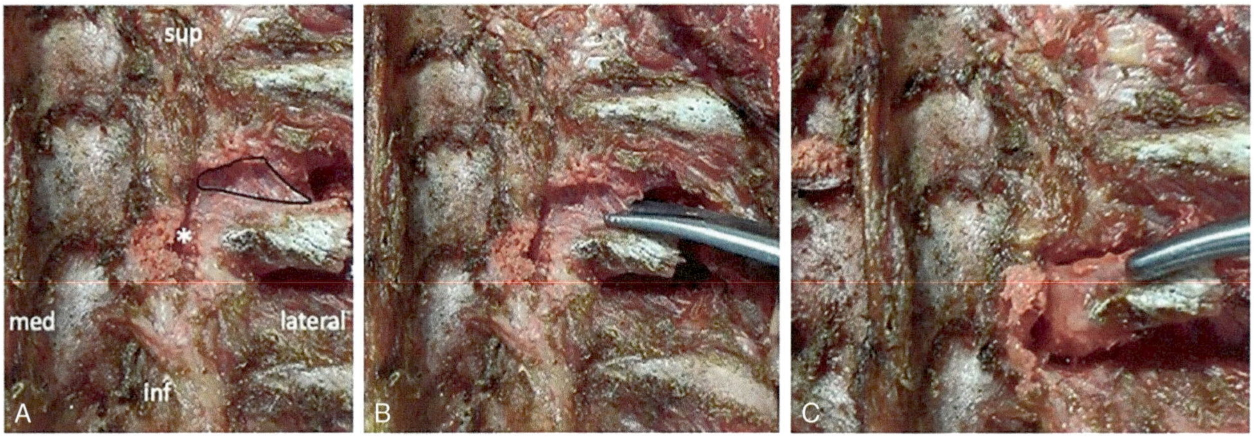

• **Fig. 17.2** Cadaveric dissection of anatomic landmarks in costotransversectomy. (A) Represents the view after the intercostal muscles have been dissected and the transverse process resected. The white asterix is the costovertebral joint and the black outline is the superior costotransverse ligament. This area is sharply cut (B) and allows removal of the rib head (C). (From Seung Jin Lee et al., An Anatomical Method for Rib Disconnection During Posterior Costotransversectomy for Paravertebral Access to the Ventral Thoracic Spine, *World Neurosurgery*, 164, 2022, 367–373, https://doi.org/10.1016/j.wneu.2022.03.099.)

thoracic spine through a primarily dorsal approach through tissue dissection as well as removal of the pedicle, transverse process, and rib head (Fig. 17.2).[6,8,14,17] Doing so provides simultaneous access to dorsal and ventral regions of the thoracic spine, providing an improved level of access and visibility of the thoracic spinal cord.[3,18] The costotransversectomy approach is quite versatile and can be used in a wide variety of pathologies such as metastatic tumors, disc herniations, traumatic lesions, and infections.[6,14,18,19]

However, the costotransversectomy approach carries unique risks for iatrogenic neurologic injury due to greater muscle and thoracic rib dissection.[3,20] Morbidities associated with costotransversectomies include pulmonary complications, chronic intercostal neuralgia, denervation of the paraspinal muscles, pneumothorax, and pleural effusion.[9,17] In a retrospective review of 164 patients undergoing costotransversectomy, Lubelski et al. found a mean complication rate of 15%, with the most common complications being wound infections (3.7%) and deep vein thrombosis/pulmonary embolism (3.7%).[14]

Particularly speaking, intercostal neuralgia is not uncommon in procedures where the anatomy of the rib is disrupted.[3,5] This is a predominantly transient complication and can oftentimes be treated with neuropathic pain medications.[5] Intercostal neuralgia tends to resolve within a few months and is more evidently seen in anterior approaches.[9] In a retrospective review of treatment in thoracic disc herniations, Strom et al. found a 5% and 0% rate of chronic intercostal neuralgia persisting greater than 3 months within patients undergoing an anterior or posterolateral approach, respectively.[9] In order to avoid injury to the intercostal nerve bundle, careful subperiosteal dissection is important when resecting the rib segment in a costotransversectomy approach.[9,21]

Costotransversectomy modifications are frequently described.[1,18,22,23] These modifications span from conservative adjustments such as paraspinal muscle preservation[23] to more intrusive measures such as additional rib resection,[18] all in hopes of enhancing visibility and reducing possible complications. Pei et al. performed a modified costotransversectomy through a posterior midline covered incision, which keeps the paraspinal muscle intact, facilitates control of bleeding, and allows more direct visualization of circumferential spinal cord decompression.[23] They found this modification to significantly alleviate initial symptoms in all study subjects, making it a reasonable alternative treatment option for thoracic myelopathy caused by single-level thoracic disc herniations between T10–L1.[23] Conversely, Chandra et al. found success through an extended costotransversectomy approach, which advocates for additional rib resection when encountering pathologies causing thoracic instability.[18] For example, a standard costotransversectomy requires removal of the rib head, neck, and tubercle, which collectively can provide up to 5 to 6 cm of bone for potential bone graft.[12] An extended costotransversectomy calls for 10 to 12 cm of the rib to be excised, which is later replaced with a titanium miniplate after the surgical procedure.[18] They proposed that this modification provides better exposure to the anterior border of the vertebral body, making the approach optimal to deal with both neoplastic and nonneoplastic pathologies.[18] Chandra et al. found this extended approach to hold adequate safety and efficacy for several different pathologies, stating pain improved in all cases and spinal stability was also achieved in all the treated cases.[18] Notable complications within this retrospective review of 46 patients include pleural tears (13%), pneumonitis (6.5%), pneumothorax (6.5%), and deep vein thrombosis (4.3%).[18]

Transpedicular Approach

Early descriptions of the transpedicular approach were introduced by Patterson and Arbit in the 1970s.[24] This surgical method allows anterolateral access to the dura after removal of the facet joint and pedicle ipsilateral to the lesion (Fig. 17.3).[6] Preservation of the rib head and avoidance of pleural exposure provides a more conservative surgical option than costotransversectomy and is a viable approach for patients with relative contraindications for more aggressive approaches.[8,25,26] The transpedicular approach has been shown to produce satisfactory outcomes for the treatment of metastatic spinal tumors, spinal infections, circumferential decompression, anterior reconstruction, and burst fractures.[8]

Although less invasive than its costotransversectomy counterpart, the transpedicular approach yields less visibility of the midline anterior spinal canal, providing opportunities for other complications to occur such as spinal cord injury and spinal fluid leaks.[3,27] Cerebral spinal fluid (CSF) leaks have been reported in up to 16% of patients undergoing a transpedicular approach.[26] Additionally, when performing anterior reconstruction following corpectomy, introducing interbody titanium cages through a limited access point provides its own disadvantages.[17] Removal of the pedicle also provides the opportunity for potential instability.[23] Other complications noted with a transpedicular approach include dural injury and blood loss.[27] Overall, the complication rates reported in the literature using the transpedicular approach range from 11% to 48%.[26] In a study involving 140 patients undergoing a transpedicular approach for resection of thoracolumbar metastatic tumors, Wang et al. reported a 30-day major complication rate of 14.3% and a mortality rate of 4.3%.[27]

Posterior Approach for Thoracic Corpectomy

During standard transpedicular corpectomies, large incisions with extensive stripping of the paraspinal muscles

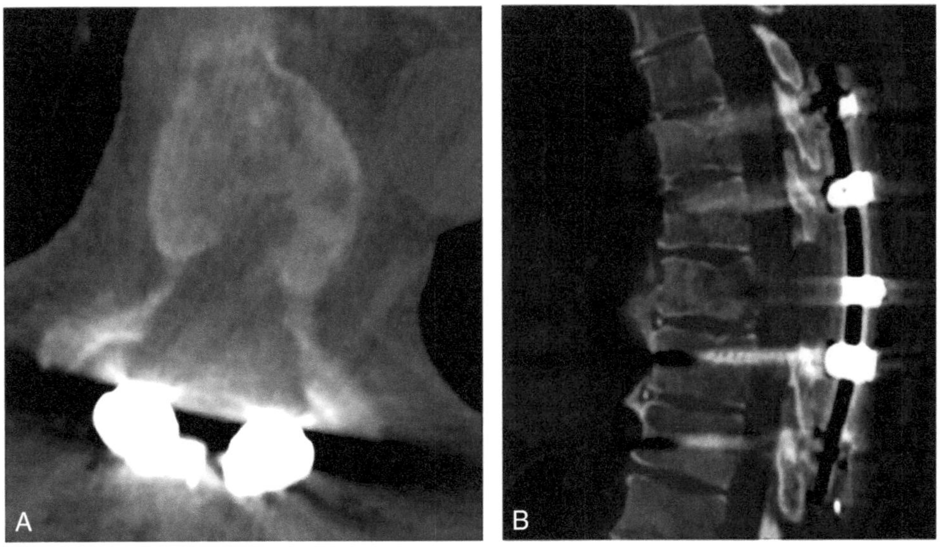

• **Fig. 17.3** Example of a transpedicular resection. (A) Axial CT scan demonstrating bilateral transpedicular resection. Of note, the medial wall of the pedicle is the most important to provide a working corridor, the lateral wall of the pedicle does not always have to be resected to achieve lateral spinal canal decompression or access to ventral pathology. (B) Lateral CT scan demonstrating the laminectomy and pedicular resection. With bilateral approaches, stabilization should be performed with minimum 2 points of fixation above and below.

may occur. In order to tackle this, one proposed modification is the utilization of minimally invasive surgery (MIS), which has been shown to yield less blood loss, shorter hospitalization, and lower infection rates than open approaches.[10,28,29] Authors have cited the use of MIS in diseases that hold more variability in the spinal location such as metastatic tumors, where traditional docking points may not be ideal.[10,29,30] Lau and Chou compared a mini-open approach to an open approach for posterior thoracic corpectomies for spinal metastases.[10] The mini-open approach consisted of preservation of the fascia, rostral placement of percutaneous pedicle screw, mini-opening of the corpectomy site, and a trapdoor rib head osteotomy. This comparative study found the mini-approach to result in less blood loss, a shorter hospital stay, and a tendency toward a lower perioperative complication rate and infection rate.[10] Additionally, retrospective reviews performed by Shedid et al. and Cho et al. found utility in a minimally invasive transpedicular technique when facing thoracic disc herniations.[31,32] This minimally invasive technique involves an oblique paraspinal approach using a tubular retractor. While Cho et al. found utility in this approach with paramedian soft thoracic herniations, Shedid et al. also reported great promise in its success with centrally calcified thoracic disc herniations.[31,32] Shedid et al. found this technique to be safe with no increased risk of neurological deterioration and no increased rate of dural tears as well as decreased blood loss and operating times.[31]

Pathology-Specific Complications from Posterior Approaches

Thoracic Disc Herniations

First reported by Mixter and Barr, thoracic disc herniation (TDH) may present with axial or abdominal pain, followed by myelopathy, radiculopathy, or a combination of the these.[2,4,6,33] Due to a smaller canal, attenuated blood supply, and an obligate anterior positioned thoracic spinal cord, a TDH is more serious than cervical or lumbar disc herniation.[9,21,33] Additionally, their frequent central location further limits the surgical corridor for safe removal.[34] TDHs tend to occur in the caudal segments of the thoracic spine and comprise 0.15% to 4% of all disc herniations.[4,7] Giant TDHs are defined as herniations occupying 40% of the anteroposterior diameter of the spinal cord and are known to cause functionally worse outcomes than smaller TDHs.[33]

Surgery for TDH is reserved for individuals with symptoms resistant to more conservative treatment or those presenting with progressive myelopathy.[7] Between 70% to 95% of patients present with myelopathy in giant, calcified TDHs, and surgical intervention is commonly implemented.[21,33] Approaches include anterior methods such as thoracotomy and thoracoscopy, as well as posterior methods such as costotransversectomy and transpedicular approaches. Most studies affirm that choice of approach is dependent on the size and location of the herniated disc, the general health of the patient, the underlying disease, and the surgeon's experience.[2,6,7,9,34]

Overall, TDH is associated with a complication rate ranging from 20% to 30%.[9,21] Complications associated with TDH surgeries include neurologic deterioration (motor or sensory pain), surgical site complications (wound infection), medical complications (pulmonary embolisms or deep vein thrombosis), and CSF-related complications (CSF leak or CSF-pleural fistula).[2–7,9,33,34] TDH's high tendency to erode dura and become transdural causes repair difficulty as well as increased complications for neurological impairment and CSF-pleural fistulas.[33,34] Neurologic injury represents the most common complication in TDH surgery, with rates reported as high as 75%.[5,9] Recent studies reported neurologic injury between 2% and 5% with no significant increased risk based on approach.[5]

Incidences of CSF leakage in thoracic disc surgery range from 0% to 15%.[3,5] Complications such as dural breaches presented by giant TDHs are often compounded by their calcified nature, which may lead to adherence to the thecal sac.[5,9,21] This is evident when comparing studies treating thoracic discs that are and are not calcified. A study conducted by Arts and Bartels found a 0% CSF leakage when performing a transpedicular approach towards a largely noncalcified cohort of 44 patients.[2] Conversely, Gong et al. experienced a 7% incidental durotomy for 15 patients who underwent a posterolateral approach, all of which were giant calcified TDHs.[33] McCormick et al. reported a 12% intradural TDH, with the majority of cases being densely calcified.[3] Court et al. report that intradural extension is only present in 0.26% to 0.3% of all disc herniations while it is present in 15% to 70% of giant calcified TDHs.[21] With a 70% to 100% calcification rate for giant thoracic discs, it is recommended that magnetic resonance imaging or a computerized tomography scan be used to identify the possible presence of calcification, which further heightens the risk for cerebrospinal fluid leakage.[2,3,5,9,33,34] Additionally, increasing the intrathoracic pressure to 40 cm H_2O before closure can ensure that there are no occult CSF leaks.[26] In the case that a CSF leak has been repaired intraoperatively, thrombin glue may be placed over the repair, and drains are routinely placed above the fasciae and not in the epidural space.[26]

Due to the high variation of herniated disc state, there is no gold standard in surgical approach for TDH. Selection of an approach remains a challenge due to the vulnerable thoracic cord and high incidence of dural adhesion from giant calcified TDHs.[33] However, there is some consensus on which approach should be used for certain circumstances. Generally speaking, a posterolateral approach such as costotransversectomy and transpedicular approach is recommended for paracentral TDHs or a subset of central TDHs that were both small and soft.[2,5,9,21,34] A more anterior approach is recommended for large, calcified TDHs that are more centrally located.[2,5,9]

Metastatic Tumors

Due to a gradually increasing population age, the prevalence and incidence of spinal metastases continue to grow.[17] With approximately 80% of spinal metastases involving the vertebral bodies, the spine is the third most common location for metastatic disease after the lung and liver.[19,35] Symptomatic spinal metastases are most commonly found in the thoracic spine, with a higher prevalence in lower thoracic regions (T9-T12) compared to higher thoracic regions (T1-T4).[8] This is most likely due to the thoracic region holding the most number of spinal segments, its kyphotic state, and its proximity to common sources of metastatic cancer such as the breast or kidney.[8] Spinal metastatic tumors are most commonly identified by local pain, radicular pain radiating in the distribution of the nerve root at the involved level, and neurological compromise.[36]

Although radiation therapy is an effective first-line therapy for spinal metastases, surgical intervention of spinal metastatic tumors is warranted when presented with neurologic deficits, instability, painful deformity, or radioresistant tumor progression with impending cord compression.[8,19,27,36] With evidence supporting surgical treatment improving clinical outcomes, surgeons have utilized methods such as the costotransversectomy and transpedicular methods when debulking tumor mass and restoring stability.[8,17,19,27,37] Such posterolateral methods are recommended when dealing with more laterally based lesions.[36] The transpedicular approach is cited as effective palliation for patients with spinal metastases and is often implemented due to the oncologic status of the patient.[26,27] Previous studies suggest that the major complication in posterior metastatic surgery is wound-related, which is most likely due to radiation, steroid use, poor nutritional status, and medical comorbidities of the patient.[8,27] In a retrospective review of 90 patients undergoing either transpedicular or costotransversectomy corpectomy for spinal metastases, Zhou et al. found a 4.44% complication rate for wound infection and CSF leak, the two highest complication rates in the study.[8]

Spinal Infections

Bacterial spinal infections include spinal tuberculosis, vertebral osteomyelitis, and epidural abscess. These infections are most commonly caused by pyogenic bacteria such as *Staphylococcus aureus.*[13,38,39] Typical teaching for the treatment of skeletal infections includes intravenous antibiotics, debridement of all purulent tissue, and spinal reconstruction as needed. When it comes to surgery, previous ideology avoided any thought of instrumentation due to fear of a recurrent infection; however, published data suggest that instrumentation does not increase the rate of recurrent infections in vertebral osteomyelitis.[13,38,39] Bydon and colleagues have noted similar rates of recurrent infection in a comparison of 118 patients undergoing debridement of spinal infections with or without instrumentation (8.3% for debridement and 9.8% for debridement with instrumentation).[40] Rayes et al. noted a low recurrent infection rate of 1.74% across 689 cases in a literature review of overall spinal infections.[41] Mohamed et al. advocates for acute instrumentation when prompted for spinal infections, as the acutely instrumented patients were less likely to require additional surgery than patients who were not treated with spinal instrumentation.[13]

Due to its narrowness and poor vasculature, the thoracic spinal cord is highly vulnerable to complications; thus proper surgical approach selection is of the utmost importance.[42,43] The best location and type of instrumentation for spinal infections is still debated. Bacterial spinal infections generally affect the anterior vertebral elements, thereby making the anterior surgical approach a more direct intervention to debride the infection.[13] However, the posterior approach is associated with earlier mobilization, more rapid rehabilitation, and higher fusion rates for infected patients.[13] Mohamed et al. found that their patient cohort of 14 patients undergoing posterior long-segment fixation, without formal debridement, resulted in resolution of bacterial spinal infection in all cases.[13] However, Lee et al. advised against a posterior approach in cases of severe bony destruction because posterior instrumentation may need to be extended over longer segments.[44]

Pott's Disease

Popularly known as Pott's disease, spinal tuberculosis is an infectious disease known to cause spinal instability, kyphosis deformity, and compression of the spinal cord that may cause neurological deficits such as paraplegia.[42,43,45] Pott's paraplegia is a particularly distinct case that arises from anterior pathologic compression either due to abscess extension or kyphotic collapse of the vertebrae.[39] Cited as one of the most common extrapulmonary sites of tuberculosis, spinal tuberculosis has also been linked with other infectious complications such as discitis, osteomyelitis, and epidural abscess.[10,42] With classic destruction of disk space and other spinal elements, spinal tuberculosis warrants prompt antituberculosis treatment.[45] Compared to other bacterial infections, spinal tuberculosis displays a greater risk for thoracic spine involvement, deformity, and significant neurologic deficits.[39] Garg and Somvanshi reported that 82% to 95% of patients with spinal tuberculosis respond well to medical treatment, with reports of pain relief, decrease in neurological deficit, and even slight correction of spinal deformity.[45]

Surgical intervention is an option in cases where severe kyphosis, abscess formation, paraplegia, and spinal instability become issues.[42,43,45,46] These concerns have the potential to become even more pronounced in spinal tuberculosis, as the possibility of adjacent multisegmented disease can cause even further risk for severe kyphosis and spinal cord compression.[39] Typical spinal tuberculosis surgery involves either debridement of the infected material or debridement with additional stabilization of the spine through bone grafts.[45] Historically, surgical approaches include anterior, posterior, or a combination of the two such as posterior instrumentation and anterior debridement.[42,43] Recent studies have begun comparing these three approaches when determining a surgical approach for spinal tuberculosis.[43,46] In a multicenter retrospective study of 394 patients undergoing thoracic spinal tuberculosis surgery, Wu et al. compared three divisional approaches: anterior (such as the transthoracic) approach, combined posterior instrumentation and anterior debridement, and a transpedicular posterior approach.[46] Wu et al. found their study to advise against the use of the anterior-only method, as the posterior-only method can achieve a similar result with fewer complications and operational risk.[46] They also found the posterior method to not be suitable in cases of large migrating abscesses, masses of dead bone, and multisegmented destruction, and a combined approach is suggested instead.[46] Overall, the posterior-only method is regarded as a simple, less traumatic surgical method for thoracic spinal tuberculosis.[46] The transpedicular method is capable of complete debridement, interbody fusion, and anterior spinal reconstruction in a single incision with little to no involvement with lung functionality.[46] To better understand long-term outcomes, Wang et al. conducted a 5-year follow-up of three surgical approaches similar to Wu et al. in patients with thoracic spinal tuberculosis.[43] In this single-center review of 185 thoracic spinal tuberculosis patients, overall complication rates for anterior, anterior-posterior combined, and posterior were 28.1%, 40%, and 12.9% respectively.[43] Complications seen in all three groups included superficial wound infections, water–electrolyte imbalance, and cerebrospinal fluid leakage.[43] Complications seen only in groups involving an anterior approach included pneumothorax, vascular injury, and pleural effusion.[43] The one complication seen in the only posterior group was a refractory intercostal neuralgia.[43] Overall, results showed that the operative time, blood loss, and rate of complications for the posterior group were significantly less than both the anterior and anterior-posterior groups.[43] However, a posterior approach should be avoided in patients who have more than three damaged vertebrae and in patients with an extensive tuberculosis abscess.[43] With this in mind, Wang et al. concluded that a posterior approach can achieve good results with reduced complications, operative time, and blood loss.[43]

Vertebral Osteomyelitis

Vertebral osteomyelitis is characterized by an acute or recurrent infection of the spine, followed by inflammatory destruction of bone.[47] Vertebral osteomyelitis is an infrequent disease, with the incidence ranging from 2.2 to 2.4 per 100,000 population with a higher incidence in older adults.[38] Leading risk factors for the development of vertebral osteomyelitis include diabetes mellitus, intravenous drug abuse, immunosuppression, alcoholism, rheumatological diseases, renal failure, and previous spinal disease or surgery.[38,44,47] Accounting for half of all cases, *Staphylococcus aureus* is most commonly responsible for vertebral osteomyelitis.[38] With a relatively high mortality rate of 2% to 17%, vertebral osteomyelitis is a condition that warrants prompt treatment.[48] Conservative treatment such as long-term antibiotic therapy has been a mainstay first-line of defense against vertebral osteomyelitis.[38,47,48] Similar to other bacterial infections, vertebral osteomyelitis instrumentation is not severely prone to recurrent infections; in a solely vertebral osteomyelitis cohort, Heary et al. noted a 7% recurrent infection rate in their cohort of 30 vertebral osteomyelitis patients undergoing pedicle screw fixation in the thoracic area.[38]

A surgical approach to vertebral osteomyelitis becomes a necessity in a minority of patients. In a retrospective cohort study performed by Miller et al., they found that out of 360 patients diagnosed with vertebral osteomyelitis, 310 (86%) were managed conservatively and 50 (14%) were managed surgically.[47] Surgery is considered more often when a patient presents with epidural abscess, severe neurological deficit, mechanical instability, severe kyphosis, or negligence of treatment.[38,47–49] Overall surgical goals include decompression, debridement, and reconstruction of the anterior column that can be done through anterior, posterior, or a combination of the two approaches.[39,48,49] Some studies point to the primary clinical benefit of vertebral osteomyelitis surgery with regard to long-term neurologic function and ambulatory status.[13,47,49] Despite a widely reported clinical improvement, reoperation, neurologic complications, and mortality are relatively common in the postoperative period.[47] Within a postoperative clinical course of 30 days or less, Miller et al. report an overall 48% complication rate within their surgical vertebral osteomyelitis cohort of 50 patients, the most common being wound infection (10%), instrumentation failure (6%), and superficial infection requiring incision and drainage (4%).[47]

Epidural Abscess

Spinal epidural abscess (SEA) is a serious, increasingly frequent pyogenic infection between the spinal dura mater and the vertebral periosteum.[50] This pyogenic infection enters the epidural space either through direct extension from a contiguous infection (such as spinal tuberculosis and vertebral osteomyelitis), hematogenous seeding from a remote site, or local invasion from prior surgical procedures.[51,52] Although a relatively rare occurrence, incidence numbers have doubled from 0.2 to 1.2 cases per 10,0000 to more than 2 cases per 10,000 admissions.[53–55] Possible sources for the increase in spinal epidural space infections include a widespread increase in intravenous drug abuse, an ever-aging population, and the increased prevalence of spinal implants and chronic vascular access.[53,55]

With the risk of neurologic injury, mechanical instability, and possible negligence to nonoperative management, surgical intervention is a common approach when necessary.[39,56] Most recent studies on SEA propose decompressive surgery, prompt surgical drainage, and systemic antibiotics as the gold standard in most circumstances.[51,56] Surgical approach depends on the location of the abscess, the presence of neurologic deficits, and the degree of spinal instability.[56] When treating SEA, Yao et al. found that a combined anterior and posterior approach is a significant risk factor for residual neurological deficit after surgical treatment.[56] Tan et al. reported a case review of ventral thoracic SEA that was successfully treated via minimally invasive transpedicular approach.[57] The patient had immediate and dramatic symptomatic improvement and was ambulatory on postoperative Day 1.[57] This case review concluded that the transpedicular approach can be used to drain the epidural abscess and excise disc and vertebral tissue affected by the infection and was considered safer than the anterior approach.[57]

Timing is of the essence when surgically managing SEA. Many studies have demonstrated the risk of delayed treatment, evoking complications such as paraplegia, incontinence, and even death.[58,59] Misdiagnosis compounds these effects, with up to 75% of cases misdiagnosed within initial healthcare encounters due to nonspecific symptoms.[52,59] A retrospective review by Davis et al. investigated the impact of diagnostic delays (admission to emergency department and greater than 24 hours without diagnosis) of SEA. They found a significantly higher incidence of residual motor weakness for SEA diagnostic delays: of the patients with a delay to diagnosis, 45% had residual weakness at discharge versus only 13% of patients without a delay.[60] Although Ghobrial et al. found no significant difference in the evacuation of SEA within 24 hours over delayed surgical treatment, the small sample size and significant differences in surgery time and patient age pose as possible confounders.[61] Overall, the early diagnosis of SEA is important to avoid any progression of potentially irreversible neurologic deficits.

Conclusion

Posterior approaches to the thoracic spine can achieve decompression objectives with less morbidity than anterior or lateral approaches. However, significant complications can still occur by virtue of less direct corridors to ventral pathologies. While dorsal laminectomy can be used for the vast majority of thoracic lesions, transpedicular and costotransversectomy approaches can also be leveraged when trying to achieve lateral and ventral decompression, including for partial corpectomy or for significant central calcified pathologies such as disc herniations. In addition to degenerative pathologies, metastatic tumors and infections are commonly seen in this region, which can be adequately addressed using posterior-only methods. While complications including the CSF leak, spinal cord injury, neuropathic pain, and iatrogenic instability can occur, these complications can be mitigated with adequate patient selection, approach selection, and surgical technique.

References

1. Lau D, Song Y, Guan Z, Sullivan S, La Marca F, Park P. Perioperative characteristics, complications, and outcomes of single-level versus multilevel thoracic corpectomies via modified costotransversectomy approach. *Spine (Phila Pa 1976)*. 2013;38(6):523–530. https://doi.org/10.1097/BRS.0b013e318273ab87.
2. Arts MP, Bartels RH. Anterior or posterior approach of thoracic disc herniation? A comparative cohort of mini-transthoracic versus transpedicular discectomies. *Spine J*. 2014;14(8):1654–1662. https://doi.org/10.1016/j.spinee.2013.09.053.
3. McCormick WE, Will SF, Benzel EC. Surgery for thoracic disc disease. Complication avoidance: overview and management. *Neurosurg Focus*. 2000;9(4):e13.. https://doi.org/10.3171/foc.2000.9.4.13.
4. Kerezoudis P, Rajjoub KR, Goncalves S, et al. Anterior versus posterior approaches for thoracic disc herniation: Association with postoperative complications. *Clin Neurol Neurosurg*. 2018;167:17–23. https://doi.org/10.1016/j.clineuro.2018.02.009.
5. Robinson WA, Nassr AN, Sebastian AS. Thoracic disc herniation, avoidance, and management of the surgical complications. *Int Orthop*. 2019;43(4):817–823. https://doi.org/10.1007/s00264-018-04282-x.
6. Fessler RG, Sturgill M. Review: complications of surgery for thoracic disc disease. *Surg Neurol*. 1998;49(6):609–618. https://doi.org/10.1016/s0090-3019(97)00434-5.
7. Brotis AG, Tasiou A, Paterakis K, Tzerefos C, Fountas KN. Complications associated with surgery for thoracic disc herniation: A systematic review and network meta-analysis. *World Neurosurg*. 2019;132:334–342. https://doi.org/10.1016/j.wneu.2019.08.202.
8. Zhou RP, Mummaneni PV, Chen KY, et al. Outcomes of posterior thoracic corpectomies for metastatic spine tumors: An analysis of 90 patients. *World Neurosurg*. 2019;123:e371–e378. https://doi.org/10.1016/j.wneu.2018.11.172.
9. Strom RG, Mathur V, Givans H, Kondziolka DS, Perin NI. Technical modifications and decision-making to reduce morbidity in thoracic disc surgery: An institutional experience and treatment algorithm. *Clin Neurol Neurosurg*. 2015;133:75–82. https://doi.org/10.1016/j.clineuro.2015.03.014.
10. Lau D, Chou D. Posterior thoracic corpectomy with cage reconstruction for metastatic spinal tumors: comparing the mini-open approach to the open approach. *J Neurosurg Spine*. 2015;23(2):217–227.https://doi.org/10.3171/2014.12.SPINE14543.
11. Chiu RG, Hobbs J, Esfahani DR, et al. Anterior versus posterior approach for thoracic corpectomy: An analysis of risk factors, outcomes, and complications. *World Neurosurg*. 2018;116:e723–e732. https://doi.org/10.1016/j.wneu.2018.05.074.
12. Lee SJ, Damon A, Pichelmann MA, et al. Anatomical method for rib disconnection during posterior costotransversectomy for paravertebral access to the ventral thoracic spine. *World Neurosurg*. 2022;164:367–373. https://doi.org/10.1016/j.wneu.2022.03.099.
13. Mohamed AS, Yoo J, Hart R, et al. Posterior fixation without debridement for vertebral body osteomyelitis and discitis. *Neurosurg Focus*. 2014;37(2):E6.. https://doi.org/10.3171/2014.6.FOCUS14142.
14. Lubelski D, Abdullah KG, Steinmetz MP, et al. Lateral extracavitary, costotransversectomy, and transthoracic thoracotomy approaches to the thoracic spine: review of techniques and

complications. *J Spinal Disord Tech.* 2013;26(4):222–232. https://doi.org/10.1097/BSD.0b013e31823f3139.
15. Menard V. Causes de la paraplegie dans le maladie de Pott, son traitment chirurgical par l'ouverture directe du foyer tuberculeux des vertebres. *Rev Orthop.* 1894;5:47–64.
16. Larson SJ, Holst RA, Hemmy DC, Sances Jr. A. Lateral extracavitary approach to traumatic lesions of the thoracic and lumbar spine. *J Neurosurg.* 1976;45(6):628–637. https://doi.org/10.3171/jns.1976.45.6.0628.
17. Metcalfe S, Gbejuade H, Patel NR. The posterior transpedicular approach for circumferential decompression and instrumented stabilization with titanium cage vertebrectomy reconstruction for spinal tumors: consecutive case series of 50 patients. *Spine (Phila Pa 1976).* 2012;37(16):1375–1383. https://doi.org/10.1097/BRS.0b013e318250a172.
18. Chandra SP, Ramdurg SR, Kurwale N, et al. Extended costotransversectomy to achieve circumferential fusion for pathologies causing thoracic instability. *Spine J.* 2014;14(9):2094–2101. https://doi.org/10.1016/j.spinee.2013.12.028.
19. Wiggins GC, Mirza S, Bellabarba C, West GA, Chapman JR, Shaffrey CI. Perioperative complications with costotransversectomy and anterior approaches to thoracic and thoracolumbar tumors. *Neurosurg Focus.* 2001;11(6):e4.. https://doi.org/10.3171/foc.2001.11.6.5.
20. Naga ANE, Tavolaro C, Agel J, Zhou H, Bellabarba C, Bransford RJ. Incidence and degrees of neurologic decline following thoracic costotransversectomy. *Spine J.* 2021;21(6):937–944. https://doi.org/10.1016/j.spinee.2021.01.008.
21. Court C, Mansour E, Bouthors C. Thoracic disc herniation: Surgical treatment. *Orthop Traumatol Surg Res.* 2018;104(1S): S31–S40. https://doi.org/10.1016/j.otsr.2017.04.022.
22. Cybulski GR, Stone JL, Opesanmi O. Spinal cord decompression via a modified costotransversectomy approach combined with posterior instrumentation for management of metastatic neoplasms of the thoracic spine. *Surg Neurol.* 1991;35(4):280–285. https://doi.org/10.1016/0090-3019(91)90005-t.
23. Pei B, Sun C, Xue R, et al. Circumferential decompression via a modified costotransversectomy approach for the treatment of single level hard herniated disc between T10 -L1. *Orthop Surg.* 2016;8(1):34–43. https://doi.org/10.1111/os.12223.
24. Patterson Jr. RH, Arbit E. A surgical approach through the pedicle to protruded thoracic discs. *J Neurosurg.* 1978;48:768–772. https://doi.org/10.3171/jns.1978.48.5.0768.
25. Lu DC, Lau D, Lee JG, Chou D. The transpedicular approach compared with the anterior approach: an analysis of 80 thoracolumbar corpectomies. *J Neurosurg Spine.* 2010;12(6):583–591. https://doi.org/10.3171/2010.1.SPINE09292.
26. Bilsky MH, Boland P, Lis E, Raizer JJ, Healey JH. Single-stage posterolateral transpedicle approach for spondylectomy, epidural decompression, and circumferential fusion of spinal metastases. *Spine (Phila Pa 1976).* 2000;25(17):2240–2249. discussion 250. https://doi.org/10.1097/00007632-200009010-00016.
27. Wang JC, Boland P, Mitra N, et al. Single-stage posterolateral transpedicular approach for resection of epidural metastatic spine tumors involving the vertebral body with circumferential reconstruction: results in 140 patients. Invited submission from the Joint Section Meeting on Disorders of the Spine and Peripheral Nerves, March 2004. *J Neurosurg Spine.* 2004;1(3):287–298. https://doi.org/10.3171/spi.2004.1.3.0287.
28. Chou D, Lu DC. Mini-open transpedicular corpectomies with expandable cage reconstruction. Technical note. *J Neurosurg Spine.* 2011;14(1):71–77. https://doi.org/10.3171/2010.10.SPINE091009.
29. Lu DC, Chou D, Mummaneni PV. A comparison of mini-open and open approaches for resection of thoracolumbar intradural spinal tumors. *J Neurosurg Spine.* 2011;14(6):758–764. https://doi.org/10.3171/2011.1.SPINE09860.
30. Charles YP, Schuller S, Sfeir G, Steib JP. Mini open tumor resection and percutaneous instrumentation for T11 renal cell carcinoma metastasis. *Eur Spine J.* 2013;22(6):1440–1442. https://doi.org/10.1007/s00586-013-2814-5.
31. Shedid D, Wang Z, Najjar A, Yuh SJ, Boubez G, Sebaaly A. Posterior minimally invasive transpedicular approach for giant calcified thoracic disc herniation. *Global Spine J.* 2021;11(6):918–924. https://doi.org/10.1177/2192568220933275.
32. Cho JY, Lee SH, Jang SH, Lee HY. Oblique paraspinal approach for thoracic disc herniations using tubular retractor with robotic holder: a technical note. *Eur Spine J.* 2012;21(12):2620–2625. https://doi.org/10.1007/s00586-012-2438-1.
33. Gong M, Liu G, Guan Q, Li L, Xing F, Xiang Z. Surgery for giant calcified herniated thoracic discs: A systematic review. *World Neurosurg.* 2018;118:109–117. https://doi.org/10.1016/j.wneu.2018.06.232.
34. Kapoor S, Amarouche M, Al-Obeidi F, UK-I JM, Thomas N, Bell D. Giant thoracic discs: treatment, outcome, and follow-up of 33 patients in a single centre. *Eur Spine J.* 2018;27(7):1555–1566. https://doi.org/10.1007/s00586-017-5192-6.
35. Witham TF, Khavkin YA, Gallia GL, Wolinsky JP, Gokaslan ZL. Surgery insight: current management of epidural spinal cord compression from metastatic spine disease. *Nat Clin Pract Neurol.* 2006;2(2):87–94. quiz 116. https://doi.org/10.1038/ncpneuro0116.
36. Jacobs WB, Perrin RG. Evaluation and treatment of spinal metastases: an overview. *Neurosurg Focus.* 2001;11(6):e10.. https://doi.org/10.3171/foc.2001.11.6.11.
37. Ge L, Arul K, Mesfin A. Spinal cord injury from spinal tumors: Prevalence, management, and outcomes. *World Neurosurg.* 2019;122:e1551–e1556. https://doi.org/10.1016/j.wneu.2018.11.099.
38. Heary RF, Agarwal N, Agarwal P, Goldstein IM. Surgical treatment with thoracic pedicle screw fixation of vertebral osteomyelitis with long-term follow-up. *Oper Neurosurg (Hagerstown).* 2019;17(5):443–451. https://doi.org/10.1093/ons/opy398.
39. Boody BS, Tarazona DA, Vaccaro AR. Evaluation and management of pyogenic and tubercular spine infections. *Curr Rev Musculoskelet Med.* 2018;11(4):643–652. https://doi.org/10.1007/s12178-018-9523-y.
40. Bydon M, De la Garza-Ramos R, Macki M, et al. Spinal instrumentation in patients with primary spinal infections does not lead to greater recurrent infection rates: an analysis of 118 cases. *World Neurosurg.* 2014;82(6):e807–e814. https://doi.org/10.1016/j.wneu.2014.06.014.
41. Rayes M, Colen CB, Bahgat DA, et al. Safety of instrumentation in patients with spinal infection. *J Neurosurg Spine.* 2010;12(6):647–659. https://doi.org/10.3171/2009.12.SPINE09428.
42. Li W, Liu Z, Xiao X, Zhang Z, Wang X. Comparison of anterior transthoracic debridement and fusion with posterior transpedicular debridement and fusion in the treatment of mid-thoracic spinal tuberculosis in adults. *BMC Musculoskelet Disord.* 2019;20(1):570.. https://doi.org/10.1186/s12891-019-2945-x.

43. Wang LJ, Zhang HQ, Tang MX, Gao QL, Zhou ZH, Yin XH. Comparison of three surgical approaches for thoracic spinal tuberculosis in adult: Minimum 5-year follow up. *Spine (Phila Pa 1976)*. 2017;42(11):808–817. https://doi.org/10.1097/BRS.0000000000001955.
44. Lee MC, Wang MY, Fessler RG, Liauw J, Kim DH. Instrumentation in patients with spinal infection. *Neurosurg Focus*. 2004;17(6):E7.. https://doi.org/10.3171/foc.2004.17.6.7.
45. Garg RK, Somvanshi DS. Spinal tuberculosis: a review. *J Spinal Cord Med*. 2011;34(5):440–454. https://doi.org/10.1179/2045772311Y.0000000023.
46. Wu W, Lyu J, Liu X, et al. Surgical treatment of thoracic spinal tuberculosis: A multicenter retrospective study. *World Neurosurg*. 2018;110:e842–e850. https://doi.org/10.1016/j.wneu.2017.11.126.
47. Miller JA, Achey RL, Derakhshan A, Lubelski D, Benzel EC, Mroz TE. Neurologic complications, reoperation, and clinical outcomes after surgery for vertebral osteomyelitis. *Spine (Phila Pa 1976)*. 2016;41(4):E197–E204. https://doi.org/10.1097/BRS.0000000000001157.
48. Gorensek M, Kosak R, Travnik L, Vengust R. Posterior instrumentation, anterior column reconstruction with single posterior approach for treatment of pyogenic osteomyelitis of thoracic and lumbar spine. *Eur Spine J*. 2013;22(3):633–641. https://doi.org/10.1007/s00586-012-2487-5.
49. Menon VK, Kumar KM, Al Ghafri K. One-stage biopsy, debridement, reconstruction, and stabilization of pyogenic vertebral osteomyelitis. *Global Spine J*. 2014;4(2):93–100. https://doi.org/10.1055/s-0034-1370789.
50. Arko Lt, Quach E, Nguyen V, Chang D, Sukul V, Kim BS. Medical and surgical management of spinal epidural abscess: a systematic review. *Neurosurg Focus*. 2014;37(2):E4.. https://doi.org/10.3171/2014.6.FOCUS14127.
51. Akhondi H, Baker MB Epidural Abscess. [Updated 2023 May 1]. In: StatPearls [Internet]. Treasure Island (FL): StatPearls Publishing; 2023. Available from: https://www.ncbi.nlm.nih.gov/books/NBK535450/
52. Bond A, Manian FA. Spinal epidural abscess: A review with special emphasis on earlier diagnosis. *Biomed Res Int*. 2016;2016:1614328.. https://doi.org/10.1155/2016/1614328.
53. Connor DE Jr, Chittiboina P, Caldito G, Nanda A. Comparison of operative and nonoperative management of spinal epidural abscess: a retrospective review of clinical and laboratory predictors of neurological outcome. *J Neurosurg Spine*. 2013;19(1):119–127. https://doi.org/10.3171/2013.3.SPINE12762.
54. Patel AR, Alton TB, Bransford RJ, Lee MJ, Bellabarba CB, Chapman JR. Spinal epidural abscesses: risk factors, medical versus surgical management, a retrospective review of 128 cases. *Spine J*. 2014;14(2):326–330. https://doi.org/10.1016/j.spinee.2013.10.046.
55. Eltorai AEM, Naqvi SS, Seetharam A, Brea BA, Simon C. Recent developments in the treatment of spinal epidural abscesses. *Orthop Rev (Pavia)*. 2017;9(2):7010.. https://doi.org/10.4081/or.2017.7010.
56. Yao YC, Lin HH, Chou PH, Wang ST, Liu CL, Chang MC. Risk factors for residual neurologic deficits after surgical treatment for epidural abscess in the thoracic or lumbar spine. *Spine J*. 2020;20(10):1638–1645. https://doi.org/10.1016/j.spinee.2020.05.001.
57. Tan LA, Takagi I, Deutsch H. Minimally invasive transpedicular approach for evacuation of epidural abscess and debridement of disc space in a patient with discitis in the thoracic spine. *Neurosurg Focus*. 2013;35(2 Suppl): Video 6. https://doi.org/10.3171/2013.V2.FOCUS13192.
58. Rigamonti D, Liem L, Sampath P, et al. Spinal epidural abscess: contemporary trends in etiology, evaluation, and management. *Surg Neurol*. 1999;52(2):189–196. discussion 197. https://doi.org/10.1016/s0090-3019(99)00055-5.
59. Tetsuka S, Suzuki T, Ogawa T, Hashimoto R, Kato H. Spinal epidural abscess: A review highlighting early diagnosis and management. *JMA J*. 2020;3(1):29–40. https://doi.org/10.31662/jmaj.2019-0038.
60. Davis DP, Wold RM, Patel RJ, et al. The clinical presentation and impact of diagnostic delays on emergency department patients with spinal epidural abscess. *J Emerg Med*. 2004;26(3):285–291. https://doi.org/10.1016/j.jemermed.2003.11.013.
61. Ghobrial GM, Beygi S, Viereck MJ, et al. Timing in the surgical evacuation of spinal epidural abscesses. *Neurosurg Focus*. 2014;37(2):E1.. https://doi.org/10.3171/2014.6.FOCUS14120.

18

Long-term Complications of Thoracic Spine Surgery

JENS CHAPMAN, YEVGENIY FREYVERT, AND ROD J. OSKOUIAN

CHAPTER OUTLINE

Overview

The thoracic spine offers a unique set of considerations to the spine surgeon. The proximity of the thoracic cavity, close apposition of the great vessels, and presence of the ribs alter the ease and risk profile of various approaches and procedures compared to analogous interventions elsewhere in the spinal column. Moreover, the tenuous vascular supply to the thoracic spinal cord renders it potentially more susceptible to injury and delayed recovery. As thoracic spine surgery is less common than its lumbar and cervical counterparts, fewer reliable studies are generally available for surgeon reference,[1] and thus fewer experiences are available in training to prepare practitioners for complications. Loss to follow-up further compounds the difficulty of reducing the rate of long-term complications as well as evaluating and improving long-term outcomes. Such factors are essential considerations in preoperative and intraoperative decision-making even in relatively routine thoracic spinal procedures.

While many postoperative spinal complications are not necessarily restricted to the thoracic spine, their incidence and management are altered by the distinct anatomy of this region. In this chapter, we explore common long-term complications resulting from thoracic spine surgery. We also explore potential chronic sequelae of shorter-term complications in the thoracic spine and conclude with a discussion of recent developments in the mitigation of long-term complications.

Post-laminectomy Thoracic Kyphosis

Kyphosis after thoracic decompressive surgery is an acknowledged but controversial phenomenon. The semi-rigid nature of the thoracic spine is thought to compensate for disruption to the posterior tension band inherent to most posterior decompressive procedures, facilitating decompression without fusion when compared to other more mobile spinal regions. However, despite favorable anatomic and biomechanical factors, progressive kyphosis after laminectomy in the thoracic spine is still well-documented.[2] Moreover, at least one study has demonstrated that thoracic laminectomy, while less kyphogenic than cervical laminectomy, actually predisposes patients to a higher risk of kyphosis than lumbar laminectomy.[3] Nonetheless, direct comparison is challenging given the differences in common pathologies and thus surgical indications among spinal regions.

Patient factors and comorbidities can alter the likelihood of kyphotic changes after decompressive surgery. It is well established that younger patients and especially patients who are not yet skeletally mature are more prone to developing kyphosis after decompressive surgery.[3] While multiple studies have failed to correlate patient gender with likelihood of kyphosis after laminectomy, the combination of female gender and long-segment laminectomy may increase the risk of kyphosis.[2] In achondroplasia, decompressive procedures involving the distal thoracic spine and lumbar spine are associated with significant increases in kyphotic deformity and often require revision surgery.[4] The development of postoperative kyphotic deformity is also frequently reported in the setting of surgery and radiation for pediatric spinal tumors, although radiation as an independent risk factor for kyphosis has not been isolated.[5]

Surgical intervention involving segments adjacent to or crossing the cervicothoracic and thoracolumbar junctions is identified as carrying a higher risk profile for subsequent kyphosis and consequently merits greater consideration for accompanying fusion. Larger decompressions have been correlated with increased likelihood of kyphosis in some cases, but this is not a consistent finding.[2,6] Some surgical variations on simple laminectomy have been proposed to have a lower rate of kyphogenesis. Hemilaminectomy, when possible, has been associated with lower rates of postoperative kyphosis.[7] Although thoracic laminoplasty represents a potentially motion-sparing alternative, evidence for the efficacy and durability of this procedure is limited and postlaminoplasty kyphosis can still occur.[8] Moreover, thoracic laminoplasty in adults is comparatively rare when compared to cervical laminoplasty, further reducing the availability of high-quality evidence.

While postlaminectomy thoracic kyphosis can be a clinically silent incidental finding on postoperative imaging, the associated alignment change can precipitate back pain and, in more severe instances, neurological deficits requiring further surgical intervention.[8,9] As of yet, a formal set of guidelines does not exist to dictate the type of revision surgery or threshold for operative intervention in the setting of this condition.

Thoracic Pseudoarthrosis

Although pseudoarthrosis is a common complication after spinal fusion and a frequent cause of postoperative morbidity and reoperation, it is not consistently defined in the existing literature. The most frequent descriptions of pseudoarthrosis center around evidence of continued instability or failed fusion at least 1 year after attempted spinal fusion surgery. Thoracic pseudoarthrosis after spinal fusion is rarely analyzed in isolation with many existing studies tending to pool lumbar and thoracic pseudoarthrosis for subsequent analysis.[10]

Reported rates of thoracic pseudoarthrosis tend to be below 10% in the existing smaller scale studies isolated to the thoracic spine.[11,12] This compares favorably to reported pseudoarthrosis rates after lumbar spine fusion which vary from 8% to 32%.[13,14] As surgical techniques and approaches vary between the lumbar and thoracic spine, it is unclear if any potential difference is the result of differing technique or other intrinsic factors.

While risk factors for thoracic pseudoarthrosis have not been independently defined, global considerations are likely to translate from other spinal regions. Nonsteroidal antiinflammatory drugs (NSAIDs) have been previously identified as a potential contributing factor to delayed osseous fusion in certain circumstances. Nonetheless, there is no conclusive evidence that short courses of NSAIDs at routine doses are likely to alter rates of pseudoarthrosis.[15] Smoking is more firmly associated with increased rates of pseudoarthrosis in many cases,[14,16] although the link between smoking and pseudoarthrosis is not always significant when scrutinized.[17] Multiple studies have identified rheumatoid arthritis as a potential risk factor for pseudoarthrosis in all spinal regions.[18,19] Studies focusing on other spinal regions have failed to isolate whether it is the disease process itself or the associated therapies that are ultimately responsible for increased rates of pseudoarthrosis,[20] and similar analyses are not available for the thoracic spine in isolation.

Surgical factors predisposing patients to pseudoarthrosis appear to mirror risk factors elsewhere in the spine. Posterior-only fusions are more likely to result in pseudoarthrosis when compared to circumferential thoracolumbar procedures, which appear to be protective.[14] Longer thoracolumbar fusion constructs are also associated with greater rates of pseudoarthrosis.[17] Whether this finding is a function of increased mechanical forces associated with a longer fusion segment, increased probability of failure due to the presence of more failure points, or a combination of factors has not yet been established. There is also evidence that incomplete operative correction of spinal alignment reduces the rate of successful fusion.[21]

Thoracic pseudoarthrosis is treated similarly to pseudoarthrosis elsewhere in the spinal column with surgical intervention typically offered when sufficiently disruptive symptoms arise. Such symptoms commonly include mechanical or radicular pain but may also include myelopathic findings in more severe cases. Radiographic pseudoarthrosis in the absence of clinical symptoms is not typically considered as an indication for surgical revision although it may be a harbinger of eventual hardware failure. While there is no standardized protocol for surgical treatment of pseudoarthrosis, revision procedures often involve either an extension of fusion for increased fixation, or an additional approach that was not used in the index procedure. It should be noted that radiographically successful revision does not always yield adequate symptomatic relief.[22]

Adjacent Segment Pathology

Much as in other spinal regions, thoracic spine surgery predisposes patients to adjacent segment pathology at levels both proximal and distal to the surgical site. Adjacent segment pathology in the thoracic spine can manifest as a variety of findings ranging from benign spondylosis that is appreciated only on imaging to crippling myelopathy that requires urgent intervention. It should also be noted that there is a lack of precision in the surgical literature with respect to nomenclature as there exist multiple overlapping terms including distal and proximal junctional degeneration, disease, kyphosis, failure, and collapse. While such pathologies exist on a continuum, certain features such as the presence of clinical symptoms or the need for reoperation provide some measure of delineation.

The most benign form of adjacent segment pathology after thoracic spinal fusion is classically described as adjacent segment degeneration that represents radiographic changes in the absence of other clinical findings.[23] This is in contrast to adjacent segment disease, which is typically accompanied by tangible clinical symptoms. Similarly, adjacent segment kyphosis usually refers to radiographic findings of postoperative kyphosis that is increased by at least 10 degrees compared to preoperative imaging in the presence of minimal symptomatology. Proximal junctional failure is considered to be a progression of the same disease process with the presence of symptoms usually necessitating reoperation.[24] We will now explore the details of thoracic adjacent segment pathology in greater detail.

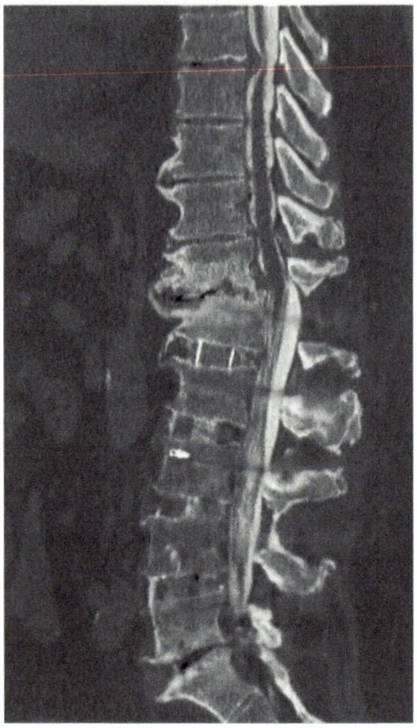

• **Fig. 18.1** Adjacent segment disease at T12-L1 after an L1-L5 fusion. Rates of this complication as well as those of hardware failure and pseudo arthrosis tend to be increased at the cervicothoracic and thoracolumbar junctions.

Proximal Segment Pathology

Proximal segment pathology is widely recognized to be one of the most common indications for reoperation after spinal fusion in all spinal regions and consequently carries a significant cost to the patient and the healthcare system.[24] While proximal segment degeneration is frequently observed after thoracic spinal fusions given adequate follow-up, the presence of proximal junctional kyphosis (PJK) and proximal junctional failure (PJF) is less common. Despite the relative frequency of proximal segment pathology, estimates for its incidence in the thoracic spine still vary significantly from 17% to 61.7%.[25,26] Even though proximal segment pathology is classically considered a long-term postoperative complication, many of the most severe cases are observed within 3 months of surgery.[27]

Multiple patient and surgical factors are acknowledged to increase the probability of proximal segment pathology. Reduced bone mineral density with and without formal diagnoses of osteopenia and osteoporosis has been clearly associated with an increased likelihood of PJK in the thoracic spine.[28,29] A similarly strong association exists between increasing patient age and increasing likelihood of both PJK and PJF in the thoracic spine.[30] However, recent advances in the understanding of age-adjusted alignment parameters may lead to reduced rates of proximal pathology in older patients.[31] Smoking has been identified as an independent risk factor for the development of PJK and PJF after thoracolumbar fusion.[32,33] Despite the known impact of smoking, optimal timing of tobacco cessation and the relevance of nicotine replacement therapy remain unexplored for the prevention of thoracic PJK and PJF.

Surgical factors contributing to increased construct rigidity are generally associated with an increased risk of proximal pathology. Specifically, circumferential fusion has been shown to confer significantly increased risk of PJK in the thoracic spine.[34] Broadly, it appears that larger fusion constructs are associated with higher rates of proximal junctional kyphosis and failure, although this is disputed by some studies.[35] The increase in rigidity resulting from fusion to the sacrum and pelvis has been associated with greater rates of thoracic PJK and PJF[36] as has the utilization of stiffer rod alloys.[37] Constructs terminating at or near the thoracolumbar junction have been classically associated with greater rates of proximal segment pathology (Fig. 18.1). More recently, greater scrutiny has been applied to the extent of deformity correction as a possible predictive factor for subsequent PJK and PJF. Where prior dogma did not consider patient factors when determining postoperative alignment targets, it is now evident that the likelihood of PJK may be reduced by adjusting for patient age.[38]

Extensive ongoing research is currently targeted at the prevention of proximal segment pathology with relatively limited success to date. Various "soft landing zone techniques" have been investigated including flexible rods, transition rods, sublaminar and transverse process hooks, wires, and bands.[25] Prophylactic reinforcement with vertebroplasty of the upper instrumented vertebra (UIV) as well as the UIV +1 and tethering techniques to approximate the surgically disrupted posterior tension band have also been explored.[39] While some of these techniques have shown promise in reducing the rate of thoracic proximal pathology, they also confer potentially increased operative time and complexity. In addition, many of the techniques to mitigate proximal junctional pathology unavoidably reduce construct rigidity and thus increase the risk of pseudoarthrosis. As no clear cost-benefit analysis exists to dictate their utilization, all such techniques remain at the discretion of each individual spine surgeon at present.

Distal Segment Pathology

The nomenclature related to distal junctional pathology matches that used in describing the proximal segment with distal junctional kyphosis (DJK) and distal junctional failure (DJF) representing the most commonly used terms. Compared to proximal segment pathology, distal segment disease in the thoracic spine is both less frequent and more poorly understood. Consequently, many of the risk factors and proposed mitigation techniques for distal segment pathology are inferred from investigations of proximal pathology rather than the result of direct studies.

Nonetheless, some factors have been identified as predisposing patients to distal junctional pathology. Scheuermann's disease and cervical spine deformity are frequently associated with postoperative thoracic DJK/DJF in the literature.[40,41] However, it is notable that these pathologies typically require longer surgical constructs when compared to more routine degenerative conditions that may indirectly explain the association. While longer fusion segments portend greater rates of adjacent segment disease, there is some evidence that longer cervical fusion constructs are associated with more distal segment pathology if they stop short of the cervico-thoracic junction;[42,43] however, these findings are not consistently present in all studies.[44] As with proximal pathology, increased construct rigidity has been demonstrated to increase the likelihood of DJK/DJF,[41] but many studies have struggled to attain sufficient statistical power to demonstrate association with any other factors.[45]

Investigation into the prevention of thoracic distal segment pathology has also been limited to date. Recent studies have indicated that preoperative and postoperative alignment are similarly important considerations with respect to DJF as they are to PJF. Patients with more preoperative deformity and suboptimal alignment postoperatively are more likely to experience DJF after spinal surgery.[41,46] Of note, neither age-adjusted criteria for the prevention of DJK/DJF nor formal targeted surgical techniques for the prevention of DJK/DJF exist at present.

Chronic Sequalae of Acute Complications

Hemothorax and Pneumothorax

The potential space of the thoracic cavity is a well-known consideration for spinal procedures that intentionally or unintentionally violate the pleural lining. While hemothorax and pneumothorax are often identified in the immediate postoperative period, delayed development is a recognized possibility[47] and increased vigilance may be warranted in higher risk procedures. Incidence of both complications appears to be approach-related[48] and is elevated with anterior or combined approaches and reduced with posterior approaches.

In the absence of clear pulmonary or vascular injury, management of a pneumothorax or hemothorax is typically conservative with observation or chest tube placement. Thoracentesis or surgical re-exploration is rarely necessary, with most studies advising protracted maintenance of chest tubes rather than escalation to more aggressive intervention.[49]

The long-term implications of a hemothorax or pneumothorax are poorly studied. Evidence from the trauma literature suggests that patients should be evaluated for pleural decortication in the event of a persistent fluid collection or pain secondary to pleural scarring.[50] If identified, a hemothorax of substantial volume should be evacuated to prevent retention. If retained, a hemothorax has the potential to result in fibrothorax (lung trapping) or pleural empyema,[51] which are both highly morbid conditions. While symptomatic occurrences require action, there is no current evidence that a clinically silent or minimally symptomatic hemothorax or pneumothorax after thoracic spine surgery is associated with long-term sequelae.[49]

Chylothorax

Although a chylothorax can arise spontaneously or as the result of trauma to the thoracic duct, the most frequent cause of this pathology is surgery in the thoracic region.[52] Spine surgery is a relatively rare but acknowledged subset of these procedures;[53] moreover, even posterior-only spinal procedures have been implicated.[54]

While routine conservative or interventional management of chylothorax under the guidance of a thoracic specialist is reportedly successful in up to 90% of cases,[55] surgical intervention can become necessary if the chylothorax does not respond and becomes intractable or chronic. In the most persistent cases, surgical intervention including direct ligation, pleurodesis or pleuroperitoneal shunting may be necessary for definitive control.[52]

Chronic Spinal Cord Injury and Neurological Deficits

Neurologic injuries with spinal surgery are one of the most feared complications for patients and surgeons.[56] High quality evidence suggests that global rates of postoperative neurologic deficit in surgery for degenerative disease are significantly higher in the thoracic spine, 2.67% compared to 0.7% for cervical and 0.52% for lumbar interventions.[57] Sub-analysis based on injury type reveals a predominance of spinal cord injury as compared to individual nerve root or cauda equina injuries. However, it should be noted that even the highest quality studies are limited by the relative rarity of thoracic surgery, which is often more than an order of magnitude less common compared to cervical and lumbar surgeries in most comprehensive studies.

Pathologic ossification of the posterior longitudinal ligament (OPLL) and ligamentum flavum (OLF) are strongly associated with increased rates of neurologic injury in the thoracic spine.[58,59] While formal evidence is sparse, smaller scale studies suggest that the use of a drill may be superior to other methods of decompression in the avoidance of neurologic injury.[60]

Successful long-term recovery from neurologic deficits skews toward nerve root injuries and away from spinal cord injuries, suggesting that the long-term neurologic recovery profile for thoracic surgery is likely to be poorer. Pooled data for iatrogenic cervical, thoracic, and lumbar surgery-related spinal cord injuries reflects a complete recovery rate of 45.7%, suggesting that more than 50% of these injuries become long-term complications.[57] Although specific data do not exist for iatrogenic thoracic injuries, the trauma literature provides clear evidence for poorer rates of recovery for thoracic spinal cord injuries compared to all others.[61]

Global Mitigation of Long-Term Thoracic Complications

Smoking Cessation

While smoking cessation has been broadly associated with reduction of both short- and long-term complications in all spinal regions, relatively little direct evidence exists specifically for long-term complications in the thoracic spine. Multiple studies have specifically investigated the effect of smoking on junctional failure rates with few significant results.[62] Nonetheless, given the strong connection between smoking and increased rates of various complications including surgical site infections and pseudoarthrosis,[63,64] it is likely that preoperative smoking cessation is a worthwhile goal for most elective clinical scenarios.

Bone Mineral Density

Osteoporosis is implicated in many long-term complications following thoracic spine surgery; it is such a pervasive contributing factor that formal guidelines for identification and treatment prior to spine surgery are available.[65] While pharmaceutical interventions to improve spinal bone mineral density are potentially helpful for complication mitigation,[66] it should be noted that the extended timeframes necessary for efficacy are sometime prohibitive.

Weight Loss

Given the greater biomechanical forces associated with elevated BMI, it is not surprising that obesity is a risk factor for various manifestations of long-term mechanical failure after thoracic spinal surgery. The risk of proximal pathologies and pseudoarthrosis have been linked extensively to obesity.[67–70] The recent advent and broad clinical acceptance of injectable agents for weight loss along with legacy surgical and therapeutic methods may represent a significant opportunity for the reduction of complications after thoracic spine surgery. In circumstances where preoperative weight loss is not viable, additional surgical methods such as the utilization of more advanced fusion constructs or biologics may be necessary to reduce the likelihood of long erm complications.

Conclusion

As surgeon experience with the thoracic spine is almost always reduced compared to other spinal regions, extra diligence is required in preoperative planning, patient counseling, and postoperative care to prevent long-term complications for patients undergoing thoracic spine surgery. The increased time required to identify and treat long-term complications further attenuates the feedback loop necessary for optimization of surgical practice and technique. While recent technological developments present an opportunity for improved complication mitigation, they are not a replacement for excellent familiarity with the unique anatomic features and risk profile of the thoracic spine.

References

1. Dekutoski MB, Norvell DC, Dettori JR, fehlings MG, Chapman JR. Surgeon perceptions and reported complications in spine surgery. *Spine (Phila Pa 1976)*. 2010;35(9 Suppl):S9–S21.
2. Aizawa T, Sato T, Ozawa H, et al. Sagittal alignment changes after thoracic laminectomy in adults. *J Neurosurg Spine*. 2008;8(6):510–516.
3. Yasuoka S, Peterson HA, MacCarty CS. Incidence of spinal column deformity after multilevel laminectomy in children and adults. *J Neurosurg*. 1982;57(4):441–445.
4. Hallan D, Mrowczynski OD, McNutt S, Rizk E. Post-laminectomy kyphosis in achondroplasia patients: to concurrently fuse or not. *Cureus*. 2020;12(5).
5. de Jonge T, Slullitel H, Dubousset J, Miladi L, Wicart P, Illés T. Late-onset spinal deformities in children treated by laminectomy and radiation therapy for malignant tumours. *Eur Spine J*. 2005;14:765–771.
6. Kobayashi Y, Kawabata S, Nishiyama Y, et al. Changes in sagittal alignment after surgical excision of thoracic spinal cord tumors in adults. *Spinal Cord*. 2019;57(5):380–387.
7. Millward CP, Bhagawati D, Chan HW, Bestwick J, Brecknell JE. Retrospective observational comparative study of hemilaminectomy versus laminectomy for intraspinal tumour resection; shorter stays, lower analgesic usage and less kyphotic deformity. *Br J Neurosurg*. 2015;29(3):390–395.
8. Amhaz HH, Fox BD, Johnson KK, et al. Postlaminoplasty kyphotic deformity in the thoracic spine: case report and review of the literature. *Pediatr Neurosurg*. 2009;45(2):151–154.
9. Safain MG, Engelberg RB, Riesenburger R, Kryzanski J, Jea A, Hwang SW. Pediatric iatrogenic thoracic kyphosis and tension myelopathy treated with a thoracic pedicle subtraction osteotomy: a case report and review of the literature. *Childs Nerv Syst*. 2014;30:1293–1299.
10. Raizman NM, O'Brien JR, Poehling-Monaghan KL, Yu WD. Pseudarthrosis of the spine. *J Am Acad Orthop Surg*. 2009;17(8):494–503.
11. Yamasaki R, Okuda S, Maeno T, Haku T, Iwasaki M, Oda T. Surgical outcomes of posterior thoracic interbody fusion for thoracic disc herniations. *Eur Spine J*. 2013;22(11):2496–2503.

12. Meredith DS, Kepler CK, Huang RC, Hegde VV. Extreme lateral interbody fusion (XLIF) in the thoracic and thoracolumbar spine: technical report and early outcomes. *HSS J.* 2013;9(1):25–31.
13. Thomsen K, Christensen FB, Eiskjaer SP, Hansen ES, Fruensgaard S, Bünger CE. 1997 Volvo Award winner in clinical studies. The effect of pedicle screw instrumentation on functional outcome and fusion rates in posterolateral fusion: a prospective randomized study. *Spine (Phila Pa 1976).* 1997;22(24):2813–2822.
14. Christensen FB, Hansen ES, Eiskjaer SP, et al. Circumferential lumbar spinal fusion with Brantigan cage versus posterolateral fusion with titanium Cotrel–Dubousset instrumentation: a prospective, randomized clinical study of 146 patients. *Spine (Phila Pa 1976).* 2002;27(23):2674–2683.
15. Sivaganesan A, Chotai S, White-Dzuro G, McGirt MJ, Devin CJ. The effect of NSAIDs on spinal fusion: a cross-disciplinary review of biochemical, animal, and human studies. *Eur Spine J.* 2017;26(11):2719–2728.
16. Brown CW, Orme TJ, Richardson HD. The rate of pseudarthrosis (surgical nonunion) in patients who are smokers and patients who are nonsmokers: a comparison study. *Spine.* 1986;11(9):942–943.
17. Kim YJ, Bridwell KH, Lenke LG, Rhim S, Cheh G. Pseudarthrosis in long adult spinal deformity instrumentation and fusion to the sacrum: prevalence and risk factor analysis of 144 cases. *Spine (Phila Pa 1976).* 2006;31(20):2329–2336.
18. Hofler RC, Swong K, Martin B, Wernhoff M, Jones GA. Risk of pseudoarthrosis after spinal fusion: analysis from the healthcare cost and utilization project. *World Neurosurg.* 2018;120:e194–e202.
19. Streufert BD, Onyedimma C, Yolcu YU, et al. Rheumatoid arthritis in spine surgery: A systematic review and meta-analysis. *Global Spine J.* 2022;12(7):1583–1595.
20. Khanna R, Dlouhy BJ, Smith ZA, Lam SK, Koski TR, Dahdaleh NS. The impact of steroids, methotrexate, and biologics on clinical and radiographic outcomes in patients with rheumatoid arthritis undergoing fusions at the craniovertebral junction. *J Craniovertebr Junction Spine.* 2015;6(2):60–64.
21. Berven S, Kao H, Deviren V, Hu S, Bradford D. Treatment of thoracic pseudarthrosis in the adult: is combined surgery necessary? *Clin Orthop Relat Res.* 2003;411:25–31.
22. Stewart G, Sachs BL. Patient outcomes after reoperation on the lumbar spine. *J Bone Joint Surg Am.* 1996;78(5):706–711.
23. Hilibrand AS, Robbins M. Adjacent segment degeneration and adjacent segment disease: the consequences of spinal fusion? *Spine J.* 2004;4(6 Suppl):S190–S194.
24. Nguyen NLM, Kong CY, Hart RA. Proximal junctional kyphosis and failure—diagnosis, prevention, and treatment. *Current Rev Musculoskelet Med.* 2016;9(3):299–308.
25. Kim HJ, Iyer S. Proximal junctional kyphosis. *J Am Acad Orthop Surg.* 2016;24(5):318–326.
26. Ha Y, Maruo K, Racine L, et al. Proximal junctional kyphosis and clinical outcomes in adult spinal deformity surgery with fusion from the thoracic spine to the sacrum: a comparison of proximal and distal upper instrumented vertebrae. *J Neurosurg Spine.* 2013;19(3):360–369.
27. Hostin R, McCarthy I, O'Brien M, et al. Incidence, mode, and location of acute proximal junctional failures after surgical treatment of adult spinal deformity. *Spine.* 2013;38(12):1008–1015.
28. Yao YC, Elysée J, Lafage R, et al. Preoperative Hounsfield units at the planned upper instrumented vertebrae may predict proximal junctional kyphosis in adult spinal deformity. *Spine.* 2021;46(3):E174–E180.
29. Duan PG, Mummaneni PV, Rivera J, et al. The association between lower Hounsfield units of the upper instrumented vertebra and proximal junctional kyphosis in adult spinal deformity surgery with a minimum 2-year follow-up. *Neurosurg Focus.* 2020;49(2):E7.
30. Liu FY, Wang T, Yang SD, Wang H, Yang DL, Ding WY. Incidence and risk factors for proximal junctional kyphosis: a meta-analysis. *Eur. Spine J.* 2016;25:2376–2383.
31. Passias PG, Passfall L, Williamson T, et al. The clinical impact of failing to achieve ideal proportional realignment in adult spinal deformity patients. *Spine.* 2002;47(14):995–1002.
32. Reames DL, Kasliwal MK, Smith JS, Hamilton DK, Arlet V, Shaffrey CI. Time to development, clinical and radiographic characteristics, and management of proximal junctional kyphosis following adult thoracolumbar instrumented fusion for spinal deformity. *Clin Spine Surg.* 2015;28(2):E106–E114.
33. Maruo K, Ha Y, Inoue S, et al. Predictive factors for proximal junctional kyphosis in long fusions to the sacrum in adult spinal deformity. *Spine (Phila Pa 1976).* 2013;38(23):E1469–E1476.
34. Kim HJ, Yagi M, Nyugen J, Cunningham ME, Boachie-Adjei O. Combined anterior-posterior surgery is the most important risk factor for developing proximal junctional kyphosis in idiopathic scoliosis. *Clin Orthop Relat Res.* 2012;470(6):1633–1639.
35. O'Shaughnessy BA, Bridwell KH, Lenke LG, et al. Does a long-fusion "T3-sacrum" portend a worse outcome than a short-fusion "T10-sacrum" in primary surgery for adult scoliosis? *Spine (Phila Pa 1976).* 2012;37(10):884–890.
36. Smith MW, Annis P, Lawrence BD, Daubs MD, Bridke DS. Acute proximal junctional failure in patients with preoperative sagittal imbalance. *Spine J.* 2015;15(10):2142–2148.
37. Han S, Hyun SJ, Kim KJ, Jahng TA, Lee S, Rhim SC. Rod stiffness as a risk factor of proximal junctional kyphosis after adult spinal deformity surgery: comparative study between cobalt chrome multiple-rod constructs and titanium alloy two-rod constructs. *Spine J.* 2017;17(7):962–968.
38. Lafage R, Schwab F, Glassman S, et al. Age-adjusted alignment goals have the potential to reduce PJK. *Spine (Phila Pa 1976).* 2017;42(17):1275–1282.
39. Bess S, Harris JE, Turner AWL, et al. The effect of posterior polyester tethers on the biomechanics of proximal junctional kyphosis: a finite element analysis. *J Neurosurg Spine.* 2017;26(1):125–133.
40. Denis F, Sun EC, Winter RB. Incidence and risk factors for proximal and distal junctional kyphosis following surgical treatment for Scheuermann kyphosis: minimum five-year follow-up. *Spine (Phila Pa 1976).* 2009;34(20):E729–E734.
41. Passias PG, Vasquez-Montes D, Poorman GW, et al. Predictive model for distal junctional kyphosis after cervical deformity surgery. *Spine J.* 2018;18(12):2187–2194.
42. Cho W, Auerbach JD, Riew KD. Crossing the cervico-thoracic junction in long posterior cervical fusions reduces caudal adjacent segment pathology. *Global Spine J.* 2022;12(8):1636–1639.
43. Schroeder GD, Kepler CK, Kurd MF, et al. Is it necessary to extend a multilevel posterior cervical decompression and fusion to the upper thoracic spine? *Spine J.* 2016;16(10):S115.
44. Truumees E, Singh D, Geck MJ, Stokes JK. Should long-segment cervical fusions be routinely carried into the thoracic spine? A multicenter analysis. *Spine J.* 2018;18(5):782–787.
45. Wang PY, Chen CW, Lee YF, et al. Distal junctional kyphosis after posterior spinal fusion in Lenke 1 and 2 adolescent

idiopathic scoliosis-exploring detailed features of the sagittal stable vertebra concept. *Global Spine J.* 2023;13(4):1112–1119.
46. Passias PG, Krol O, Kummer N, et al. 194. The effect of undercorrection on distal junctional kyphosis in adult cervical deformity patients. *Spine J.* 2021;21(9):S99.
47. Terai H, Toyoda H, Hayashi K, et al. Delayed-onset pneumothorax after posterior spinal fusion for idiopathic scoliosis: Report of two cases. *Indian Spine J.* 2020;3(1):110.
48. Xu R, Garcés-Ambrossi GL, McGirt TF, et al. Thoracic vertebrectomy and spinal reconstruction via anterior, posterior, or combined approaches: clinical outcomes in 91 consecutive patients with metastatic spinal tumors. *J Neurosurg Spine.* 2009;11(3):272–284.
49. Gabel BC, Schnell EC, dettori JR, Jeyamohan S, Oskouian R. Pulmonary complications following thoracic spinal surgery: a systematic review. *Global Spine J.* 2016;6(3):296–303.
50. Yeo TP. Long-term sequelae following blunt thoracic trauma. *Orthop Nurs.* 2001;20(5):35–47.
51. DuBose J, Inaba K, Demetriades D, et al. Management of post-traumatic retained hemothorax: a prospective, observational, multicenter AAST study. *J Trauma Acute Care Surg.* 2012; 72(1):11–22. discussion 22-24; quiz 316.
52. Bender B, Murthy V, Chamberlain RS. The changing management of chylothorax in the modern era. *Eur J Cardio-Thorac Surg.* 2016;49(1):18–24.
53. Doerr CH, Allen MS, Nichols 3rd FC, Ryu JH. Etiology of chylothorax in 203 patients. *Mayo Clin Proc.* 2005;80(7):867–870.
54. Rames RD, Schoenecker PL, Bridwel KHL. Chylothorax after posterior spinal instrumentation and fusion. *Clin. Orthop. Relat. Res.* 1990;261:229–232.
55. Itkin M, Kucharczuk JC, Kwak A, Trerotola SO, Kaiser LR. Nonoperative thoracic duct embolization for traumatic thoracic duct leak: experience in 109 patients. *J Thorac Cardiovasc Surg.* 2010;139(3):584–590.
56. Hart RA, Cabalo A, Bess S, et al. Comparison of patient and surgeon perceptions of adverse events after adult spinal deformity surgery. *Spine (Phila Pa 1976).* 2013;38(9):732–736.
57. Hamilton DK, Smith JS, Sansur CA, et al. Rates of new neurological deficit associated with spine surgery based on 108,419 procedures: a report of the scoliosis research society morbidity and mortality committee. *Spine (Phila Pa 1976).* 2011;36(15):1218–1228.
58. Xu N, Yu M, Liu X, Sun C, Chen Z, Liu Z. A systematic review of complications in thoracic spine surgery for ossification of the posterior longitudinal ligament. *Eur Spine J.* 2017;26(7):1803–1809.
59. Hou X, Chen Z, Sun CG, Zhang G, Wu S, Liu Z. A systematic review of complications in thoracic spine surgery for ossification of ligamentum flavum. *Spinal Cord.* 2018;56(4):301–307.
60. He B, Yan L, Xu Z, Guo H, Liu T, Hao D. Treatment strategies for the surgical complications of thoracic spinal stenosis: a retrospective analysis of two hundred and eighty three cases. *Int Orthop.* 2014;38(1):117–122.
61. Khorasanizadeh M, Yousefifard M, Eskian M, et al. Neurological recovery following traumatic spinal cord injury: a systematic review and meta-analysis. *J Neurosurg Spine.* 2019; 30(5):683–699.
62. Judy BF, Tracz J, Alomari S, Witham TF. Patient optimization for the prevention of proximal junctional kyphosis. *Int J Spine Surg.* 2023;17(3).
63. Kong L, Liu Z, Meng F, Shen Y. Smoking and risk of surgical site infection after spinal surgery: a systematic review and meta-analysis. *Surg Infect (Larchmont).* 2017;18(2):206–214.
64. Berman D, Oren JH, Bendo J, Spivak J. The effect of smoking on spinal fusion. *Int J Spine Surg.* 2017;11(4):29.
65. Sardar ZM, Coury JR, Cerpa M, et al. Best practice guidelines for assessment and management of osteoporosis in adult patients undergoing elective spinal reconstruction. *Spine (Phila Pa 1976).* 2022;47(2):128–135.
66. Wanderman N, Alvi M, Yolcu Y, et al. Is teriparatide beneficial to spinal fusion surgery in the older patient? *Clin Spine Surg.* 2019;32(5):182–190.
67. Park SJ, Lee CS, Chung SS, Lee JY, Kang SS, Park SH. Different risk factors of proximal junctional kyphosis and proximal junctional failure following long instrumented fusion to the sacrum for adult spinal deformity: survivorship analysis of 160 patients. *Neurosurgery.* 2017;80(2):279–286.
68. Wang H, Ma L, Yang D, et al. Incidence and risk factors for the progression of proximal junctional kyphosis in degenerative lumbar scoliosis following long instrumented posterior spinal fusion. *Medicine (Baltimore).* 2016;95(32):e4443.
69. Lazaro BC, Sardi JP, Smith JS, et al. Proximal junctional failure in primary thoracolumbar fusion/fixation to the sacrum/ pelvis for adult symptomatic lumbar scoliosis: long-term follow-up of a prospective multicenter cohort of 160 patients. *J Neurosurg Spine.* 2022;38(3):319–330.
70. Yagi M, Patel R, Boachie-Adjei O. Complications and unfavorable clinical outcomes in obese and overweight patients treated for adult lumbar or thoracolumbar scoliosis with combined anterior/posterior surgery. *J Spinal Disord Tech.* 2015;28(6): E368–E376.

19 When to Operate on the Lumbar Spine

KEVIN C. JACOB, MADHAV R. PATEL, ALEXANDER W. PARSONS, AND KERN SINGH

CHAPTER OUTLINE

Low Back Pain and Lumbar Surgery Indications

Pain due to complications of the lumbar spine is becoming exceedingly prevalent among all age groups. While aging remains a leading risk factor for experiencing low back pain, the increasing prevalence demonstrates the importance of proper diagnostics and treatment plans. The economic burden of low back pain in the United States alone ranges into the billions of dollars when analyzing both direct costs of diagnosis and treatment along with indirect costs of lost wages and employment-related expenses.[1] The burden placed on healthcare systems still fails in comparison to the experience of the patient. Low back pain has been estimated to be the leading cause of years lived with disability since before the turn of the century.[2,3] Common classifications of back pain include axial pain, referred pain, and radicular pain. Pathological causes of low back pain can include neoplastic, infectious, vascular, and musculoskeletal etiologies, among others. Musculoskeletal pain remains the most common cause among these pathologies, with varying causes attributed to acute and/or chronic. Common musculoskeletal etiologies include muscle strain, degenerative diseases, vertebral fractures, intervertebral disk herniation, lumbar radiculopathy, lumbar facet joint syndrome, sacroiliac joint syndrome, lumbar spinal stenosis, and spondylolisthesis.[4–6] Surgical evaluation for progressive weakness, severe pain, or signs or symptoms of cauda equina syndrome warrant an immediate evaluation by a spine surgeon. A significant proportion of patients presenting to the emergency department (ED), urgent care, or primary care will have nonspecific back pain, increasing the difficulty for providers to identify the underlying causes of the pain from the lumbar region. Patients presenting to their primary care health providers often find it difficult to precisely identify the pathological cause of their patients' back pain. This difficult diagnosis can leave the patient with a lack of direction, a dependence on pain medication for management, and an increased susceptibility for mental health concerns. Referral to a spine specialist earlier in the process can help both the patient and primary care provider alike identify and understand the causes and treatment plans to improve well-being for current and future patients.

Obtaining a thorough history with the patient followed by a physical exam and imaging studies, the physician can then approach the patient with a shared decision-making process to gain insight and understanding, integrating their goals for treatment and the best intervention to assist the patient in achieving the desired outcomes. The history should include questions about the onset of symptoms and possible mechanisms of injury, specific location of pain and sensory deficits, characterization of the pain and neurologic symptoms, current treatments or self-remedies, and the effectiveness of initial measures, if there is radicular pain, temporal patterns of the symptoms, and any additional information the patient feels is pertinent. The variable description of low back pain may include throbbing, aching, stabbing, sharp, persistent, and radiating. Additionally, paraesthesias, painful muscle spasms, and difficulty with gait and limb movement can be experienced, leading to significant amounts of disability.[7] Patients presenting with low back pain in the acute setting due to muscle strain may have experienced a history of these injuries, reinforcing the need to review previous symptoms, treatment, and responses to treatment.[4,8] Careful review of the patient's medical history can demonstrate key factors affecting long-term outcomes and additional considerations. Patients with a history of mental health concerns or significant psychological distress can benefit from mental health intervention early in the treatment process and have improved nonsurgical and surgical outcomes.[9] During the history collecting process, key findings may help rule out malignancy or cauda equina syndrome. Specific findings for malignancy include patients in their 50 s with unintentional weight loss and nonspecific symptoms such as fever, insomnia, and generalized fatigue.[10] Cauda equina syndrome can present with low back pain that radiates asymmetrically down the legs, muscle atrophy, late-onset urinary retention, overflow incontinence, bilateral progressive motor deficits, saddle anesthesia, decreased rectal tone or bulbocavernosus reflex, and erectile dysfunction in male patients. Both malignancy and cauda equina syndrome are indications for immediate surgical consultation.[11]

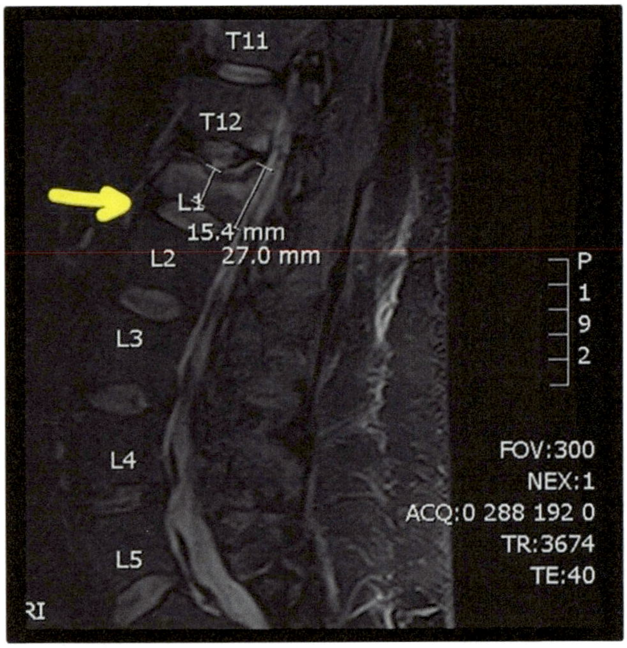

• **Fig. 19.1** Magnetic resonance imaging depicting L1 compression fracture *(arrow)*. From Koda EK. Lumbar compression fracture caused by cardioversion. *Am J Case Rep.* 2020;21:e927064.

Physical exam should include inspection of the skin for visible bruising or deformities, palpation of the entire spine, noting locations of pain and stop-offs, along with the motor and sensory examination of the extremities. In trauma-related injuries, assessment of rectal tone and bulbocavernosus reflexes may be indicated. The variable sensitivity and specificity of physical exam maneuvers, such as the standard straight leg raise test for evaluating low back pain, may lack in comparison to the detailed information gained from imaging. However, the many provocative maneuvers and tests can still provide valuable insight. With patients presenting with pain in the lumbar region where disc herniation is the leading differential, the straight leg raise is often positive. The straight leg raise can help evaluate compression of nerve roots between L4-S1.[4] The femoral nerve stretch test can also help evaluate for nerve compression in the upper lumbar spine. Additional neurological assessments may include sharp/dull sensory tests with decreased sensation in specific regions assisting the examiner to localize to specific regions of the spine. Using physical exam tests and maneuvers can help guide a broad differential but can rarely elicit a specific diagnostic cause. Generally, evaluation for asymmetries, gait, pain pattern, and palpation are starting points.

Radiographic imaging can be an initial attempt to help understand the underlying concern. In traumatic situations, radiographs need to be obtained immediately to assess the injuries' severity. In trauma-related injuries, radiography can be extremely valuable, for instance, in comparing compression fractures and burst fractures (Figs. 19.1 and Fig. 19.2). In compression fractures, the anterior height of the vertebral body is compromised while the posterior height is maintained. Meanwhile, burst fractures where the

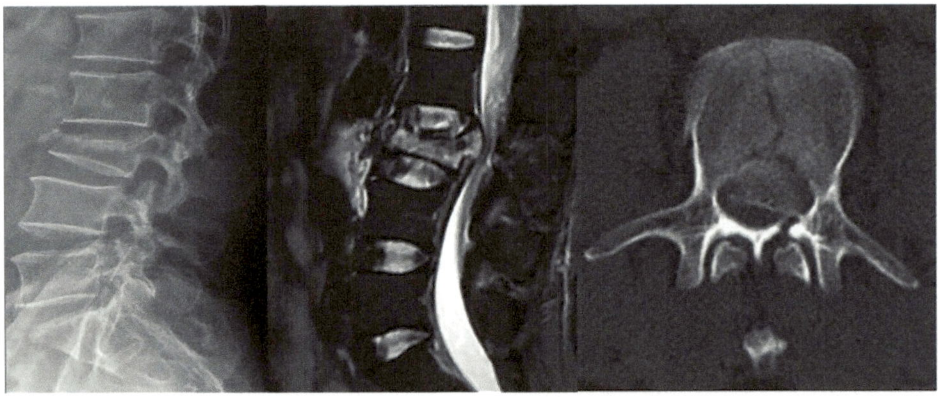

• **Fig. 19.2** X-ray, MRI, and CT examinations revealing L3 lumbar burst fracture with severe spinal cord compression. From Yu S, Zhang H, Chen W, et al. Lessons from a lumbar burst fracture patient infected with SARS-CoV-2. *Aging.* 2020;12:11259–11262.

vertebral body expands anterior-posterior and transversely, leading to reduced height throughout the entire vertebral body with bony fragments in the spinal canal and damage to the posterior longitudinal ligament can occur, and immediate damage surgical consult is required. However, radiographs are generally ineffective at ruling out more severe conditions such as malignancy. Also, radiographic findings often require additional imaging if there is a suspected pathology as the symptomatology of the patient does not always align with the radiographic information.[12] Computed tomography (CT) or magnetic resonance imaging (MRI) evaluation of the spine can be a necessity due to the overlapping presentation of various underlying pathologies. The steps taken early in the diagnostic process to increase patient understanding and education on low back pain will position the patient to understand likely outcomes from the agreed-upon treatment strategy and improve long-term satisfaction. Initially approaching treatment plans in a conservative manner that is safe and effective will help maximize treatments while minimizing overall costs of interventions.[13,14]

Conservative management with a combination of antiinflammatory medications, muscle relaxants, heat, massage therapy, and physical therapy can provide a significant degree of pain relief to most patients, meeting their treatment goals.[4] With conservative management in the acute and subacute phases, generally 2 to 14 weeks, patients can expect to see significant and pronounced improvement within the first month. Pharmacological treatment is started with NSAIDs as the first-line treatment, second-line treatment includes tramadol or duloxetine, and if these measures fail, opioids may be considered.[8] After the first month, patients will likely continue to see steady improvement. Exhausting conservative measures and encouraging adherence to treatment guidelines reduce wasteful healthcare spending, which is often seen in cases where unnecessary imaging or surgical intervention precedes genuinely failed conservative measures. A combination of pharmacological treatment and physical therapy, among other options, increases the potential of conservative measures being successful as a single intervention is less likely to be effective, particularly in patients presenting with chronic or complicated low back pain.[15] If conservative management fails to effectively decrease the symptoms of low back pain, particularly pain lasting longer than 12 weeks, surgical intervention can be warranted. In patients with chronic symptomatology of low back pain, conservative management is likely to prove ineffective for the majority. Discussions between the patient and the spine specialist in an individualized manner will largely determine when to proceed with invasive measures. Guiding patients on when it is the right time to proceed with surgical interventions following exhausting conservative measures is a skill developed through experience, training, and studying of evidence-based principles.

Surgical intervention for chronic lumbar spine pathologies, particularly spinal fusions, has increased in recent years due to increased effectiveness, symptom resolution, improved safety, and shorter downtime in the postoperative period.[16] In addition to the chronicity of the presenting concern, the underlying pathology and presenting symptomatology play a significant role in deciding when to proceed with surgical interventions. Where spinal injuries have occurred, the stability of the surrounding structures needs to be assessed as instability is a crucial indicator for surgical intervention. Additionally, patients who are refractory to conservative management, present with acute neurologic motor deficits, and those who suffer from excruciating pain should be considered for surgery. Furthermore, earlier surgical intervention is advised if a patient's symptoms, exam, and imaging indicate spinal instability (spondylolisthesis is often used as a surrogate for instability). A few of the more common presenting pathologies indicated for lumbar spine surgery include symptomatic degenerative disc disease, symptomatic spondylosis, spondylolisthesis, symptomatic spinal stenosis, and herniated nucleus pulposus.[17–19]

Degenerative Disc Disease

One of the more overused and incorrectly used terms by the general population regarding back pain is the degeneration of the intervertebral discs leading to back pain. The degenerative changes of the spine resulting in the irritation or injury of the adjacent nerve roots and the spinal cord can collectively be termed "spondylosis." While commonly associated with disc herniation, degenerative disc disease is commonly associated with the loss of proteoglycans and the bulk of the intervertebral disc and is impacted by numerous factors, including genetics and chronic mechanical stressors.[20] The loss of disc height (Fig. 19.3A) can then lead to altered structure and increased susceptibility to affect surrounding structures including nerve roots negatively. The intervertebral disc functions as a cushion and shock absorber between the vertebrae, assisting in the dispersion of loading forces on the spine while also improving range of motion and flexibility.[20] Comprised of two distinct layers, the outer annulus fibrosis and inner nucleus pulposus, degeneration of the disc is directly related to increasing age and sex, with men presenting earlier than women.[21] The difficulty in determining when to operate on the lumbar spine for patients with degenerative disc disease depends mainly on the presenting symptoms as a significant majority of patients with degenerative discs are asymptomatic. Furthermore, there is a large degree of ambiguity regarding the definition of degenerative disc disease. Even imaging analysis does not always tell the complete story as current research discusses the increased prevalence of disc degeneration while the patient may be completely asymptomatic. Understanding nomenclature can assist in imaging analysis. As a result of degeneration, a disc bulge occurs when the disc material's displacement extends beyond the disc's outer margins spanning significantly more than 25% of the disc circumference, and can

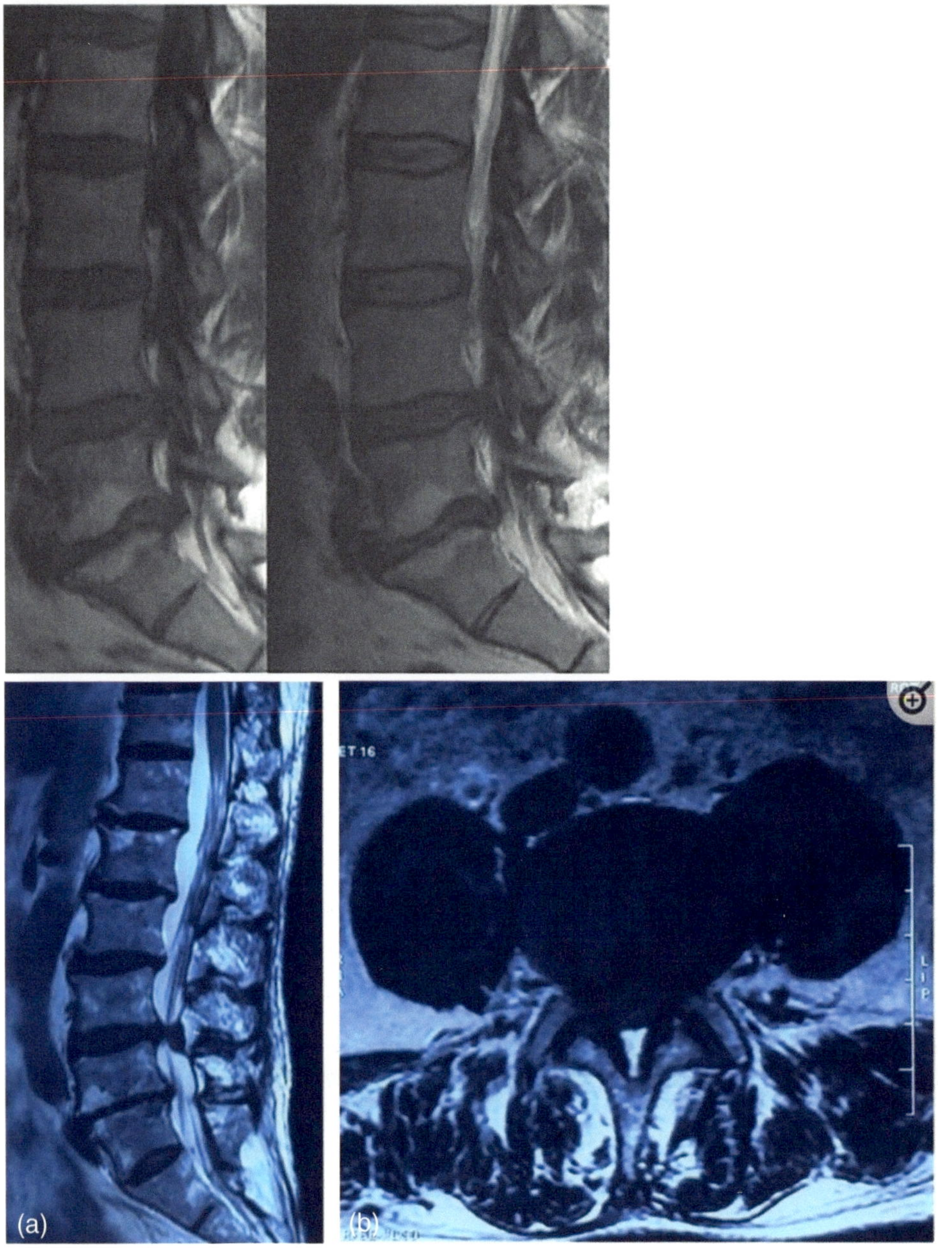

• **Fig. 19.3** Age-related degeneration of disc causing decreased height. (A) Sagittal and axial (B) MRI demonstrating herniated disc at L4-L5. (A) From Kuisma M, Karppinen J, Haapea M, et al. Are the determinants of vertebral endplate changes and severe disc degeneration in the lumbar spine the same? A magnetic resonance imaging study in middle-aged male workers. *BMC Musculoskeletal Disorders*. 2008;9(1). https://doi:10.1186/1471-2474-9-51. (B) Clinical Interventions in Aging 2019:14 2295–2299 - Originally published by and used with permission from Dove Medical Press Ltd.

still be asymptomatic. Research of incidental degenerative disc imaging findings supports the notion that presenting symptoms need to be a significant driver of the treatment strategy. Typically pain is localized to the lumbar spine or buttocks. Generally, extended time in the seated position or increased spine flexion, often when attempting to lift an object, can increase the pain.[22] Additionally, pain relief can be achieved when lying on the side with knees bent towards the chest. Surgical intervention is indicated if the degenerative process leads to symptoms of neurological compromise, limitations of normal activity, decreasing independence, and severe pain.[21]

Herniated Nucleus Pulposus

Along similar lines to degenerative disc disease is the specific pathology of herniated nucleus pulposus causing back pain and other symptoms. Typically seen in a younger population, onset is between 30 and 50 years of age, herniated nucleus pulposus is one of the more common causes of back pain, generally presenting with pain in an L4-S1 nerve root distribution.[23,24] Regarded as one of the more common presenting pathologies underlying a patient's low back pain, herniated nucleus pulposus is a consequence of degeneration of the annulus fibrosus, creating an avenue for the inner nucleus pulposus to bulge or extend beyond the limits of the outer annulus. The extension of the nucleus pulposus beyond the annulus can lead to nerve root compression, causing several problematic symptoms for the patient. In the acute setting, herniation can cause severe pain. Symptoms can be described as shooting or stabbing pain with the pain radiating down the leg in specific patterns.[4,25] In MRI analysis (Fig. 19.3B), herniation is confirmed when the displacement of disc materials spans less than 25% of the circumference. Further imaging classifications of herniations outline two subcategories: protrusions and extrusions. When the base of the herniation is broader than the outward extension, this is protrusion.[13] Alternatively, extrusion is described as herniation where the base is narrower than the outward extension. The specific characterization of the anatomic location of the herniation and the proximity to the nerve root is essential for understanding clinical presentations and symptomatology. Electromyography and nerve conduction velocity (EMG/NCV) tests following an MRI where disk herniation is found may not detect lumbar radiculopathy.[4] In severe cases, spinal cord compression may also occur. Intrusion into the spinal canal in the lumbar region can be associated with cauda equina syndrome, which is an absolute indication for emergent surgical intervention; however, this is a rare complication. Compression of the nerve root can lead to pain associated with a dermatomal distribution, musculoskeletal motor weakness, sensory complications, and radicular pain. Surgical intervention is indicated for symptomatic patients with confirmation CT or MRI of herniation where aggressive pain measures have failed in the subacute and chronic time frames, often when symptoms persist beyond 6 to 8 weeks. Additionally, surgery is indicated for patients suffering from sensory and neurological deficits, including numbness, muscular weakness, and bladder dysfunction, earlier in the evaluation process.[17,23,26]

Spinal Stenosis

Narrowing of the spinal canal leading to the symptomatic presentation of patients to their healthcare provider can be caused by many underlying pathologies, including disc degeneration, ligamentum flavum hypertrophy, and building discs, along with osteophyte formation along various portions of the vertebrae and facet joints.[4,6] Stenosis in the lumbar region (Fig. 19.4) can lead to progressive low back pain and motor and sensory deficits in the lower limbs in nearly a third of all patients.[27] Typically seen in adults over the age of 60 years, pain can occur insidiously and radiate. However, myelopathy is less common in the lumbar region due to the conus medullaris beginning at L1-L2; resulting stenosis below this level can present at neurogenic claudication. Severe spinal stenosis below the terminating point of the spinal cord can produce cauda equina syndrome. Furthermore, physical examination of the patient and a thorough history can provide clues hinting at spinal stenosis. Patients often lack tenderness due to palpation and the straight leg raise may be harmful.[4] Patients describe decreases or increases in pain based on positioning; for example, sitting or leaning forward can create more space in the spinal canal and foramen, which may improve the patient's condition by relieving neurogenic claudication. However, the pain relief from neurogenic claudication can take a few minutes to disappear, which stands in contrast to vascular claudication, which can be relieved in seconds.[4] Conditions that are refractory to treatment or progressively worse are surgical intervention indications.[17] For patients with severe pain, surgery is indicated at an earlier timepoint as long-term management with opioid medications has inherent risks of tolerance and addiction.[4]

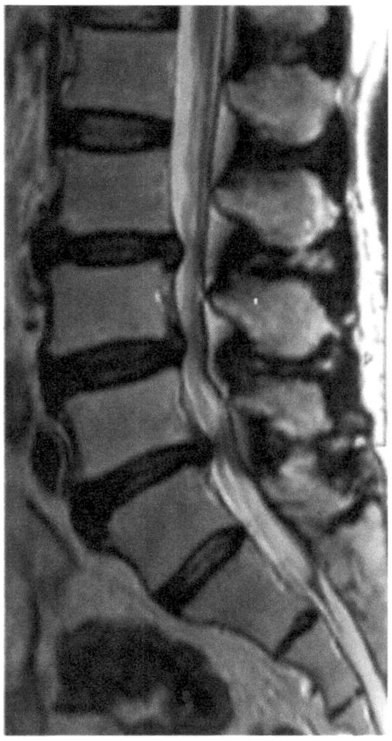

• **Fig. 19.4** T2-weighted midsagittal image showing L3-4 central protrusion, L4-5 central stenosis, and L5-6 central protrusion. From Jin YJ. Quantification of lumbar spinal canal stenosis by quantitative fat-suppressed contrast-enhanced magnetic resonance imaging. *J Clin Med Res*. 2020;9(10). https://doi:10.3390/jcm9103084.

Spondylolisthesis

Spondylolisthesis is a pathological condition of the spine where the vertebral body deviates anteriorly in relation to an adjacent, inferior vertebra. Aging remains a significant risk factor. The etiology of spondylolisthesis can be due to a congenital malformation, an athletic-related injury associated with trauma, or idiopathic. Traumatic causes can occur following high-energy injuries to the lumbar spine, causing fractures and dislocation leading to the anterior slippage of the vertebrae. Spondylolisthesis has two common forms, degenerative and isthmic, primarily seen in the caudal lumbar region. Degenerative spondylolisthesis (Fig. 19.5) results from age-related degeneration changes of the vertebrae, without an associated disruption of the vertebral ring, affecting the posterior ligamentous structures leading to failure of these supportive tissues and anterior slippage. The isthmic subtype is attributed to an abnormality in the pars interarticularis disrupting the vertebral ring. Isthmic spondylolisthesis (Fig. 19.6) most commonly occurs at L5/S1 and is more commonly seen in young athletes where repetitive hyperextension movements are required.

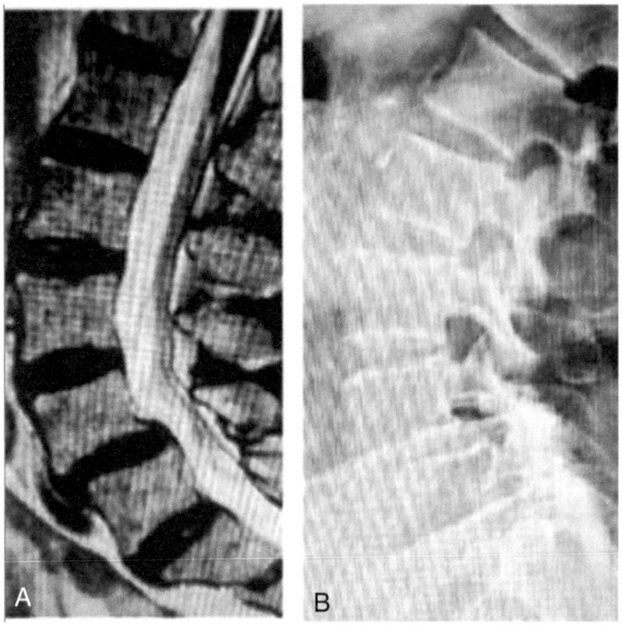

• **Fig. 19.5** Figure (A) and (B) demonstrating degenerative lumbar spondylolisthesis at level L4 with isthmus intact. From Wang PT, Zhang JN, Liu TJ, Yang JS, Hao DJ. Comparison of degenerative lumbar spondylolisthesis and isthmic lumbar spondylolisthesis: effect of pedicle screw placement on proximal facet invasion in surgical treatment. *BMC Musculoskeletal Disorders*. 2022;23(1). https://doi:10.1186/s12891-021-04962-7.

Additionally, spondylolysis, where a fracture of the pars interarticularis occurs, can lead to spondylolisthesis. While often asymptomatic, the instability due to the anterior movement of the vertebrae can cause significant pain in the low back region with or without exertion along with an altered gait, radiating pain, complications related to cauda equina syndrome. A palpable step-off sign can be identified on a physical exam in some instances. When spondylolisthesis is suspected, the diagnosis should be confirmed by imaging. On radiographic analysis of spondylolisthesis at the L5-S1 region, the inverted Napoleon hat sign can be identified in the context of a fracture of the pars interarticularis. An anteroposterior (AP) radiograph will show the anterior border of the transverse process in continuity with the anterior border of the body of the same vertebrae resulting in a projected shadow against the sacrum. Radiographic analysis for spondylolysis (Fig. 19.7) can present with the Scotty dog sign (Fig. 19.8). The outline of a dog can be seen with an oblique view of the lumbar spine, where the transverse process is the nose, pedicle the eyes, pars interarticularis the neck, superior articular facet

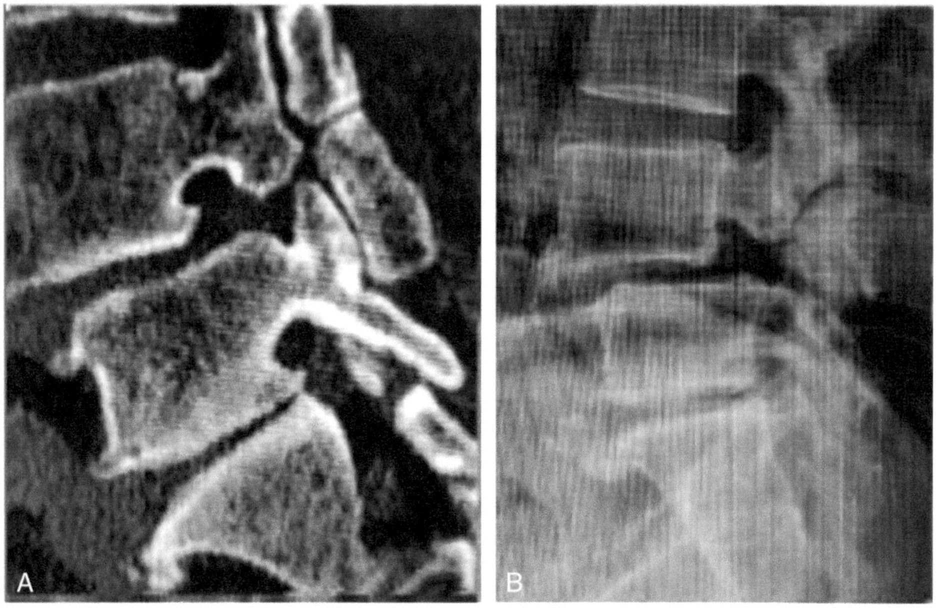

• **Fig. 19.6** (A) and (B) demonstrate that the patient had spondylolisthesis of L4. The isthmus of the bilateral pedicle of the L4 vertebral body is not connected. From Wang PT, Zhang JN, Liu TJ, Yang JS, Hao DJ. Comparison of degenerative lumbar spondylolisthesis and isthmic lumbar spondylolisthesis: effect of pedicle screw placement on proximal facet invasion in surgical treatment. *BMC Musculoskelet Disorders*. 2022;23(1). https://doi:10.1186/s12891-021-04962-7.

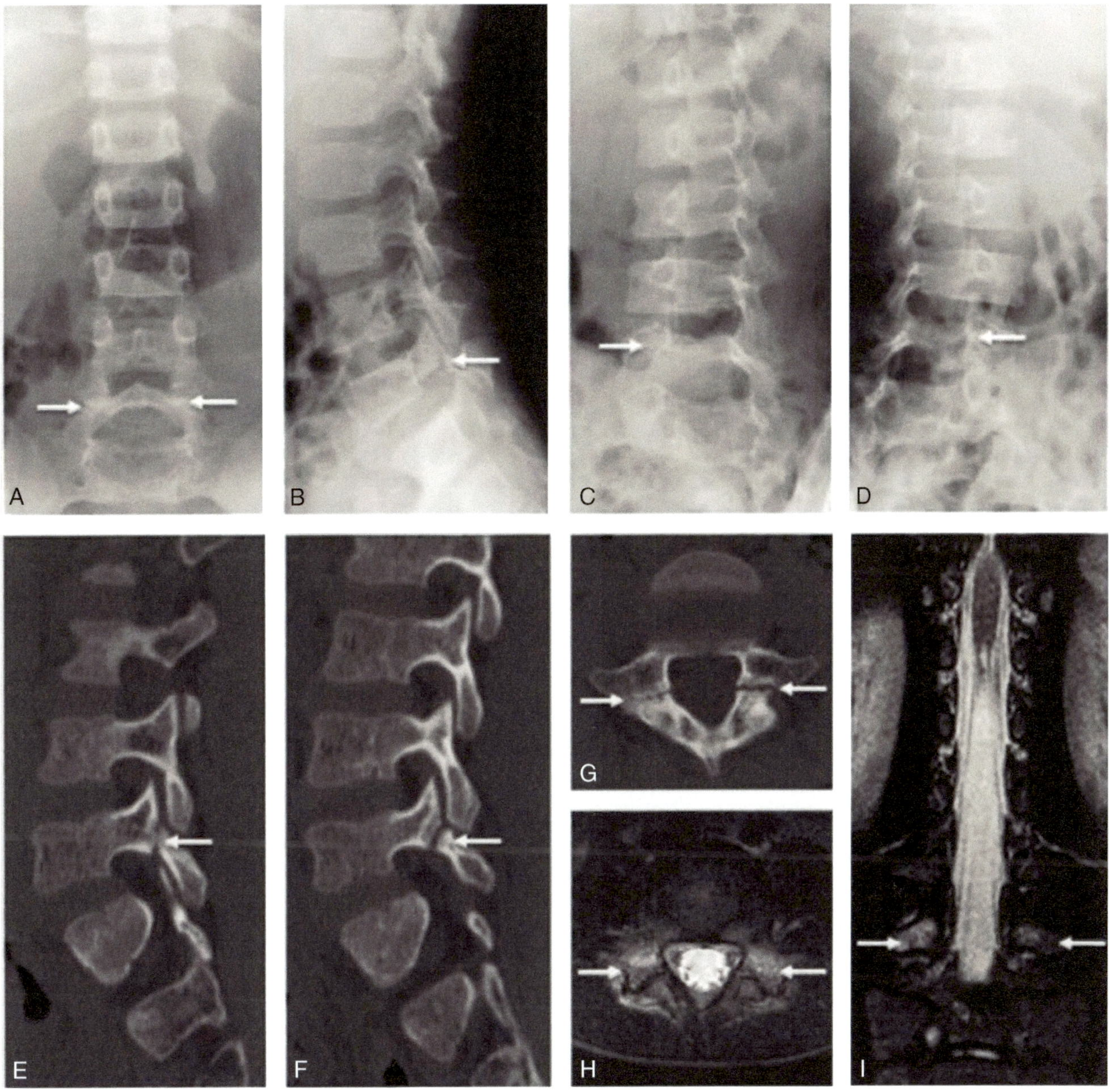

• **Fig. 19.7** Spondylolysis *(white arrows)* is observed at the fifth lumbar vertebra (L5) on posteroanterior (A), lateral (B), 45° right anterior oblique (C), and 45° left anterior oblique (D) radiographs, and right parasagittal (E), left parasagittal (F), and axial CT images parallel to the L5 vertebral arch (G). Axial short tau inversion recovery (STIR)-MRI parallel to the L5 vertebral arch (H) and coronal STIR-MRI (I). Note the signal hyperintensity *(white arrows)* in the pedicle, indicating marrow edema. This is a sign of an early-stage stress fracture of the pars interarticularis. From Kato K, Hakozaki M, Mashiko R, Konno S. Familial development of lumbar spondylolysis: a familial case report of 7- and 4-year-old brothers and their father. *Journal of International Medical Research*. 2021;49(5). https://doi:10.1177/03000605211015559.

the ear, inferior articular facet the front leg. A fracture in the "neck" region, the pars interarticularis, is specific for spondylolysis, leading to spondylolisthesis. Sufficient anterior slippage can lead to compression of the neurological structures in the neighboring region resulting in motor and sensory deficits. If the presenting symptoms are refractory to initial management strategies or symptoms worsen, surgical intervention is indicated and has proven to be safe and effective.[13,26,28]

Deformity

Indications for lumbar spine surgery in spinal deformity are covered in the spine deformity chapter.

Conclusions

The decision for surgical treatment in the lumbar spine is not always an easy one. If surgical treatment is not emergent,

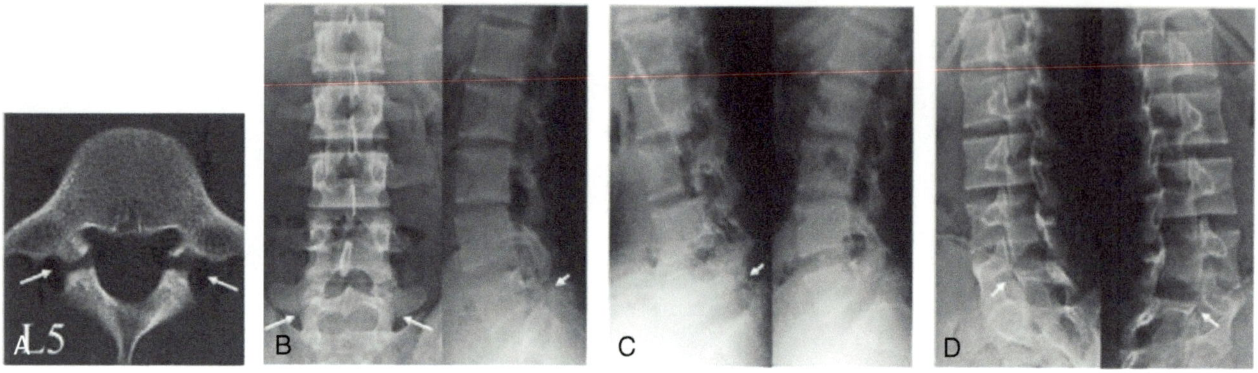

• **Fig. 19.8** A reconstructed CT scan and plain radiographs of a 15-year-old boy with terminal spondylolysis. (A) An oblique-axial CT scan shows pseudoarthrotic changes in the pars interarticularis *(arrow)*. (B–D) Plain radiographs including anteroposterior, lateral (B), dynamic lateral views (C), and oblique views (Scotty dog sign) (D), on which fracture lines are clearly identified *(arrowheads)*. From Morimoto M, Sakai T, Goto T, et al. Is the Scotty dog sign adequate for diagnosis of fractures in pediatric patients with lumbar spondylolysis? *Spine Surg Relat Res*. 2019;3(1):49–53. Licensed under Creative Commons license CC-BY 4.0 International License. http://creativecommons.org/licenses/by/4.0/.

one should look to optimize nonsurgical options first. Then, if the more conservative measures do not provide adequate relief, it is the surgeon's obligation to find and correlate the source of pain to the most appropriate treatment.

References

1. Dieleman JL, Cao J, Chapin A, et al. US health care spending by payer and health condition, 1996-2016. *JAMA*. 2020;323(9): 863–884.
2. Wu A, March L, Zheng X, et al. Global low back pain prevalence and years lived with disability from 1990 to 2017: estimates from the Global Burden of Disease Study 2017. *Ann Transl Med*. 2020; 8(6):299.
3. Fatoye F, Gebrye T, Odeyemi I. Real-world incidence and prevalence of low back pain using routinely collected data. *Rheumatol Int*. 2019;39(4):619–626.
4. Jankovic J, Mazziotta JC, Pomeroy SL, Newman NJ. *Bradley and Daroff's Neurology in Clinical Practice*. Elsevier; 2022.
5. Mekhail NA, Costandi SJ, Armanyous S, et al. The impact of age on the outcomes of minimally invasive lumbar decompression for lumbar spinal stenosis. *Med Devices*. 2020;13:151–161.
6. Lawrence MM, Hayek SM. Minimally invasive lumbar decompression: a treatment for lumbar spinal stenosis. *Curr Opin Anaesthesiol*. 2013;26(5):573–579.
7. Patrick N, Emanski E, Knaub MA. Acute and chronic low back pain. *Med Clin North Am*. 2016;100(1):169–181.
8. Qaseem A, Wilt TJ, McLean RM, Forciea MA, for the Clinical Guidelines Committee of the American College of Physicians. Noninvasive treatments for acute, subacute, and chronic low back pain: A clinical practice guideline from the American College of Physicians. *Annals of Internal Medicine*. 2017;166(7):514. https://doi.org/10.7326/m16-2367.
9. Merrill RK, Zebala LP, Peters C, Qureshi SA, McAnany SJ. Impact of depression on patient-reported outcome measures after lumbar spine decompression. *Spine*. 2018;43(6): 434–439.
10. Goldring S.R. Firestein: Kelley's Textbook of Rheumatology. *Structure and function of Bone, Joints and Connective Tissue*. Published online 2008.
11. Gucalp R, Dutcher JP. Oncologic emergency. *Harrisons Principles of Internal Medicine 19th ed Mc Graw-Hill Education USA*. 2015; 2(19):1787.
12. Cohen SP, Argoff CE, Carragee EJ. Management of low back pain. *BMJ*. 2008;337:a2718.
13. Tehranzadeh J. *Basic Musculoskeletal Imaging. Second Edition*. McGraw-Hill Education; 2021.
14. Azar FM, Terry Canale S, Beaty JH. *Campbell's Operative Orthopaedics, E-Book*. Elsevier Health Sciences; 2020.
15. Airaksinen O, Brox JI, Cedraschi C, et al. Chapter 4 European guidelines for the management of chronic nonspecific low back pain. *European Spine Journal*. 2006;15(S2):s192–s300. https://doi.org/10.1007/s00586-006-1072-1.
16. Weinstein JN, Lurie JD, Olson PR, Bronner KK, Fisher ES. United States' trends and regional variations in lumbar spine surgery: 1992-2003. *Spine*. 2006;31(23):2707–2714.
17. Ebraheim NA, Thomas BJ, Fu FH, et al. Orthopedic surgery. *Schwartz's Principles of Surgery*. 11th ed. New York: McGraw-Hill Education. Published online 2019. https://onlinelibrary.wiley.com/page/journal/17577861/homepage/free_review_articles.htm.
18. Doherty GM. *Current Diagnosis and Treatment Surgery*. 14th ed. McGraw-Hill Education/Medical; 2014.Accessed March 11, 2022. http://www.kubalibri.cz/files/127---Current-Diagnosis-and-Treatment-Surgery.pdf.
19. Parks E. *Practical Office Orthopedics*. McGraw Hill Professional; 2018.
20. Bogduk N. Degenerative joint disease of the spine. *Radiol Clin North Am*. 2012;50(4):613–628.
21. Donnally III CJ, Hanna A, Varacallo M. *Lumbar degenerative disk disease. StatPearls*. StatPearls Publishing; 2021.
22. Karppinen J, Shen FH, Luk KDK, Andersson GBJ, Cheung KMC, Samartzis D. Management of degenerative disk disease and chronic low back pain. *Orthop Clin North Am*. 2011; 42(4):513–528, viii.

23. De Cicco FL, Camino Willhuber GO. *Nucleus pulposus herniation*. StatPearls Publishing; 2021.
24. Dydyk AM, Ngnitewe Massa R, Mesfin FB. *Disc herniation. StatPearls*. StatPearls Publishing; 2022.
25. Dydyk AM, Khan MZ, Das JM. *Radicular back pain*. StatPearls Publishing; 2021.
26. Hines RL, Jones SB. *Stoelting's anesthesia and co-existing disease e-book*. Elsevier Health Sciences; 2021.
27. Raja A, Hoang S, Patel P, Mesfin FB. *Spinal stenosis. StatPearls*. StatPearls Publishing; 2021.
28. Shamrock AG, Donnally III CJ, Varacallo M. *Lumbar spondylolysis and spondylolisthesis. StatPearls*. StatPearls Publishing; 2021.

20

General Complication in Lumbar Spine Surgery

SRIKANTH N. DIVI, KAMIL OKROJ, AND ALPESH A. PATEL

CHAPTER OUTLINE

Introduction

Lumbar spine surgery has seen significant advances over the last century for the treatment of degenerative disease, metastatic tumors, infection, and traumatic injuries. Many of these disease processes cause malalignment, instability, and neurologic compression in the lumbar spine resulting in symptomatic back and leg pain for patients. Today, lumbar surgery is performed through three major approaches—anterior (transperitoneal or retroperitoneal), lateral retroperitoneal, and posterior. Each approach possesses a different complication profile, unique to its relevant surgical anatomy. In general, these complications can be divided into five groups: 1) neurovascular injuries, 2) postoperative superficial or deep surgical site infections, 3) cerebrospinal fluid (CSF) leaks, 4) pseudarthrosis, and 5) medical complications.

Neurovascular Injuries

Among all of the complications encountered in spine surgery, neurovascular injuries can be the most devastating due to their associated morbidity and mortality. Given that the spinal cord usually terminates at the level of the L1 vertebral body in the average adult, the main risk of neurologic injury in lumbar procedures is at the level of each individual nerve root. Vascular injuries in the lumbar spine can involve both the aorta and vena cava and their associated iliac branches, which lie directly anterior to the spine. Also at risk for injury are the segmental arteries that run along the anterolateral aspect of the spine at each vertebral segment. Treatment of neurovascular injuries may range from observation (e.g., neuropraxia) to immediate repair in consultation with other surgeons for direct repair (e.g., catastrophic intraoperative vascular injuries).

Neurologic Injury

Injuries to nerve roots present as radicular symptoms, which can include pain, numbness, and/or weakness in a nerve-specific distribution. Severity and duration of these symptoms vary widely and are entirely dependent on the nature and severity of the injury as well as the patient's physiology. However, the majority of these injuries are mild and result in neuropraxia, which is defined as focal demyelination without axonal injury—resulting in transient weakness and/or paresthesias.

Nerve injuries generally occur with direct trauma; such as an inadvertent tearing injury from a Kerrison rongeur, laceration injury from an osteotome, or stretch-related injury from excessive intraoperative traction. Extra care must be taken during direct spinal decompression to identify the exiting and traversing nerve roots in order to prevent iatrogenic injury. Neurologic injury can also occur during instrumentation with the placement of pedicle screws or interbody implants. Surgical cases with implants have twice the rate of new neurologic deficits compared to cases without implants.[1] The main culprit for these injuries is inaccurate placement of pedicle screws with a medial or inferior breach (Fig. 20.1). The use of CT navigation and robotic surgery can potentially reduce the risk of pedicle wall breaches during lumbar spine surgery.[2] Furthermore, the use of stimulated electromyography can help detect pedicle breaches intraoperatively. Although much less common, neurologic injury can also happen indirectly through intraoperative reduction maneuvers. Reduction can cause excessive tension on the nerve roots or their vascular supply, leading to a neurologic deficit. Common examples include reduction

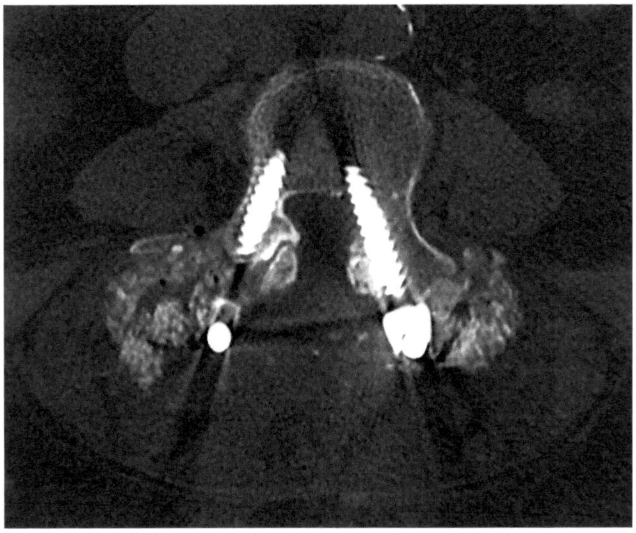

• **Fig. 20.1** Scan showing medial breach of pedicle screw.

of a high-grade spondylolisthesis or compression/distraction maneuvers in combination with osteotomies to correct deformities. Delayed neurologic decline after lumbar spine surgery can occur in the setting of a compressive postoperative hematoma, with an incidence reported around 0.1% to 0.24%.[3] Patients can present up to 1 month after surgery with a wide spectrum of symptoms ranging from radicular pain to significant bilateral weakness and/or cauda equina syndrome.

Each approach to the lumbar spine introduces its own separate risk profile. The lateral transpsoas approach uniquely places the lumbar plexus at risk, which is located within the confines of the psoas muscle. It is not uncommon for patients undergoing lateral lumbar fusions to experience transient radiculitis and postoperative weakness with rates reported as high as 24%.[4] However, Ahmadian et al. found that a majority of these symptoms resolve after the first 6 months after surgery.[5] Also, utilizing both stimulated and continuous EMG monitoring and decreasing retraction time can both help prevent neurologic injury to the lumbar plexus.

The anterior lumbar approach poses less risk to the nerve roots but risks injury to the genitofemoral nerve and hypogastric plexus. Injury to the hypogastric plexus can result in retrograde ejaculation, which is reported in up to 5.9% of males having undergone an anterior lumbar interbody fusion.[6] Injury to the genitofemoral nerve is much less common, but can result in pain and paresthesias along the groin and medial thigh.

Postoperative neurologic injuries are treated differently depending on the type of symptoms and their severity. New postoperative numbness without pain or weakness is most often temporary and can be observed. In the setting of acute postoperative weakness or severe radicular pain, an immediate CT scan and MRI with and without contrast should be obtained to evaluate for implant positioning or any compressive etiology (e.g., hematoma, bone fragment, etc). If an epidural hematoma is identified, emergent evacuation of the hematoma is warranted. Likewise, if spinal implants such as pedicle screws or interbody grafts have compromised neural structures, they should be immediately revised. In general, it is believed that outcomes after a neurologic injury are related to the severity of the deficit and the time elapsed until the intervention. However, in the absence of any identifiable source for the pain or weakness, patients should be treated symptomatically with steroids, neuromodulators (gabapentin, pregabalin, etc.) and observed.

Vascular Injury

Vascular injuries around the lumbar spine occur most commonly during anterior procedures given its proximity to the major vessels. The incidence of major vascular injury during an open approach to the anterior lumbar spine has been reported to be between 1.4% and 15.6%.[7] Risk factors for injury include smoking, a history of vascular disease, and previous abdominal surgery. The most frequently injured vessel is the left common iliac vein (0.7% incidence).[8] The iliolumbar vein is a branch of the common iliac vein that is located anterior to the L5 level, putting it at high risk for injury during retraction or surgery at the L5 level.

In addition to direct injury of these vessels, there is the added risk of thrombosis from extended retraction of these vessels. This can result in limb ischemia and/or deep venous thrombosis and pulmonary embolism. Brau et al. reported 6 episodes of thrombosis in 1315 patients undergoing anterior lumbar interbody fusion (incidence = 0.45%). Of these patients, four required thrombectomy, two required a bypass type procedure, and two developed a compartment syndrome.[9]

Vascular injuries from the lateral approach generally involve the segmental arteries, which lie just along the anterolateral aspect of the spine at the mid-vertebral body. The incidence of vascular injuries via the lateral approach have been reported from 0.056% to 2.6%.[10] Placement of shims along the anterior aspect of the disc space can result in damage to the segmental artery at that level. Damage to the segmental artery can also occur during a release of the contralateral annulus, which leads to a psoas hematoma and can also result in a neurologic deficit.[11] There have been reports of injuries to the major vessels (aorta, vena cava) during lateral lumbar surgery; however, these are quite uncommon. Injuries to the segmental vessels should be identified during surgery and subsequently isolated and ligated with bipolar cautery or vessel clips. If identified postoperatively, embolization can be considered. Injuries to the major vessels are more concerning and require emergent vascular consultation.

Major vascular injuries are exceedingly rare during posterior lumbar surgery. During exposure of the transverse processes, surgeons should take extra care not to violate the transverse membrane as this can put the segmental arteries at risk. Pedicle screw instrumentation in the lumbar spine poses minimal risk for vessel injury. Lonstein et al. reported that 2.8% of 4790 pedicle screws were found to have penetrated the anterior cortex of the vertebral body but that none of these injuries resulted in major complications.[12] Discectomies and interbody fusions from the posterior or transforaminal approach pose a slightly higher risk to the major anterior vessels. Great care should be taken to avoid anterior penetration of the annulus in such surgery. Osteotomies also pose a higher risk to the anterior vasculature and segmental vessels both from direct injury and from indirect manipulation of the vessels in the deformity correction. The incidence of vascular injuries from these posterior approaches ranges from 1.6 to 17 in 10,000.[13] They may be hard to detect intraoperatively and can be devastating, with mortality rates reported to range from 15% to 61%.[14,15] If there is any suspicion for a vascular injury postoperatively, an emergent angiogram should be obtained followed by vascular surgery consultation.

Although major vascular injuries via posterior lumbar surgery are rare, there is still potential for large amounts of total blood loss over the full duration of a case. Common sources of bleeding during the posterior lumbar exposure involve terminal branches of the segmental arteries located at the lateral aspect of the facets and pars. Any excessive bleeding identified intraoperatively should be controlled with electrocautery in order to limit total blood loss and prevent postoperative hematomas. Furthermore, almost all multilevel open posterior lumbar decompressions and/or fusions should have a drain placed at the end of the case to prevent hematoma formation.

Infection

Among the most frequent postoperative complications in lumbar spine surgery are postoperative surgical site infections. Despite vast advances in the technology of spinal surgery and emergence of minimally invasive surgical techniques, there has been little improvement in infection rates over the last decade. The latest National Nosocomial Infections Surveillance report from the federal Centers for Disease Control and Prevention (CDC) over a 12-year period reported an infection rate of 2.1% following spinal fusion and 1.25% after laminectomy.

Postoperative infections can range from superficial infections to deep (subfascial and epidural) abscesses with sepsis. Furthermore, they can develop at any stage after surgery: early (<4 weeks), subacute (>4 weeks to 3 months), or late (>3 months), especially with the presence of spinal implants. Major patient risk factors for postoperative infections include obesity, smoking, diabetes, alcohol abuse, and malnutrition (albumin <3.5 g/dL). Surgical risk factors include length of surgery, blood loss, surgeries for tumor/trauma, posterior approach, and use of steroids postoperatively.[16]

Superficial infections are usually diagnosed early in the postoperative period since they generally present with an erythematous, draining, or nonhealing wound. Late infections are more difficult to diagnose since they usually do not present with wound complications. Instead, patients can present with nonspecific symptoms such as fevers/chills, weight loss, or worsening back or radicular symptoms after an initial period of improvement postoperatively. These patients require further workup, which should include labs (CBC with differential, erythrocyte sedimentation rate [ESR], C-reactive protein [CRP]) and imaging (XR, CT, MRI). Plain radiographs can show subtle changes in spinal alignment to obvious hardware failure. CT scans can more accurately assess implant position and adequate ongoing fusion. Conversely, subtle signs such as lucency around screws or implants may be indicative of hardware loosening. An MRI with and without contrast may help differentiate a normal postoperative fluid collection from an infection. For example, a peripherally enhancing fluid collection in the epidural space may be indicative of a deep surgical site infection (Fig. 20.2). If there is still uncertainty in a clinical diagnosis of postoperative infection in the setting

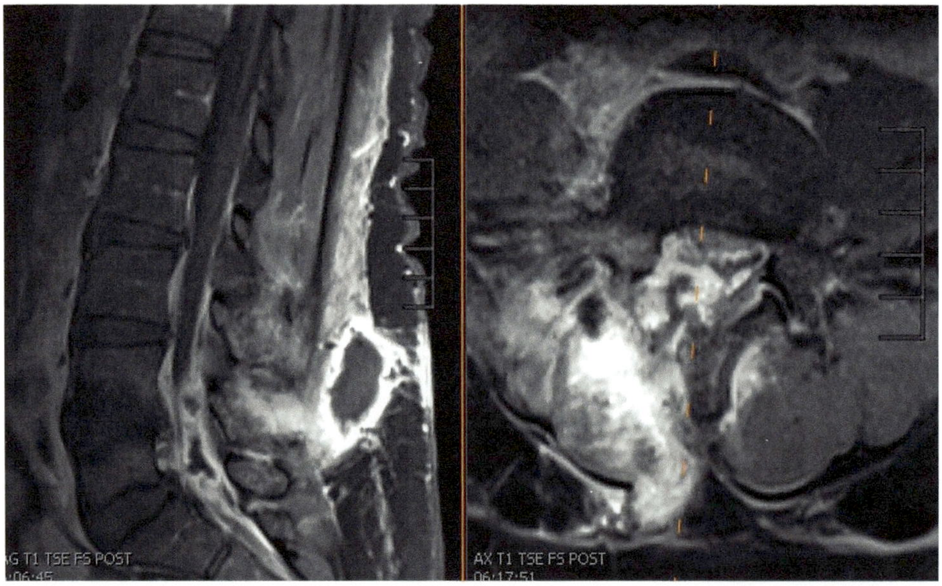

• **Fig. 20.2** T1 postconstrast MRI showing rim-enhancing postoperative epidural collection.

of a postoperative fluid collection, an interventional radiology (IR) aspiration may help discern a postoperative seroma/hematoma from an infection. However, caution should be warranted with this approach if there is any concern for a CSF leak, since an aspiration increases the risk of further neurologic injury, subdural hematoma, or brainstem herniation.

Treatment of postoperative lumbar infections generally requires irrigation and debridement and treatment with a course of antibiotics. Deep infections may at times necessitate removal of implants and/or revision fixation due to pseudarthrosis followed by a period of IV antibiotics. Implants are usually retained in early infections to preserve spinal stability.[17] On the other hand, superficial infections, regardless of acuity, do not require removal or revision of hardware and can often be treated with a period of oral antibiotics following a thorough irrigation and debridement. Closed suction drains after irrigation and debridement are helpful in decreasing functional dead space for bacteria to accumulate. Overall, patients can still achieve good results after receiving treatment for a postop lumbar spine infection. Petilon et al. demonstrated that Oswestry Disability Index (ODI) and SF-36 scores improved from baseline after resolution of infection, albeit to a lesser extent than the control group without infection.[18]

Although prevention of postoperative infections remains a challenge, the use of appropriately dosed perioperative antibiotics is crucial. In addition, the use of vancomycin powder in surgical wounds has demonstrated a significant decrease in postop spine infections, both deep and superficial.[19] Finally, several studies have shown that optimization of modifiable risk factors prior to surgery (obesity, serum glucose, smoking, and stopping immunocompromising medications) can decrease infection rates.[20]

Spinal Fluid Leaks

CSF has a critical role in the maintenance and function of the spinal cord, brain, and nerve roots. CSF is contained within the thecal sac, which is made up of three layers of meninges: the pia, arachnoid membrane, and dura mater.[21] A common complication in lumbar spine surgery involves inadvertent violation of the dura intraoperatively. This can happen with routine exposure of the dura during many lumbar procedures, as well as placement of pedicle screws around the thecal sac and nerve roots. Ultimately, the occurrence of CSF leaks both increase a patient's length of stay and overall medical costs, so extra vigilance and good surgical technique should be utilized to prevent these complications.[22]

If both the dura mater and arachnoid membrane are violated, there will be extravasation of clear CSF and, occasionally, nerve roots, from the dura. CSF leaks may be more difficult to identify intraoperatively if they are out of the surgeon's direct line of sight (i.e., due to a medial breach from a pedicle screw). Clues like decreased thecal sac turgor can suggest to the surgeon that there may be a dural tear. Occasionally, CSF leaks may happen in a more delayed fashion due to lacerations from residual sharp bony edges after a lumbar decompression procedure.

Patients with persistent CSF leaks most commonly present with postural headaches sometimes associated with nausea, vomiting, dizziness, photophobia, and tinnitus. These symptoms are related to a decrease in intraspinal pressure, which subsequently decreases intracranial pressure. Although uncommon, this caudally directed pressure can lead to a subdural hematoma due to rupture of fragile bridging veins in more elderly individuals.[23]

A persistent CSF leak can result in a pseudomeningocele or CSF fistula. Pseudomeningoceles are defined as a contained extradural CSF collection (Fig. 20.3), whereas CSF fistulas are not contained and continue to drain through the surgical wound. Nerve roots may become entrapped in pseudomeningoceles, which can cause radiculopathy and impede healing of the dura. CSF fistulas can lead to meningitis, arachnoiditis, or even an epidural abscess.[24] Although minimally invasive surgery (MIS) approaches have equivalent to slightly higher rates of dural laceration than traditional open approaches, they have been shown to have lower rates of CSF fistula or pseudomeningocele development.[25]

Upon identification of a CSF leak, efforts should be made to expose the laceration and repair it in a watertight manner with a combination of suture and various dural sealants. A Valsalva maneuver should then be performed intraoperatively to confirm the quality of the dural repair. Bovine-derived collagen or autologous fat, muscle, or fascial patch grafts can also be used to help augment repairs if there is a persistent leak.[26] One example of a commercially available dural sealant is DuraSeal Exact, which is an absorbable hydrogel that can be used as an adjunct for dural closure and is the only product specifically approved by the FDA for use as a dural sealant in spinal surgeries. Compared to sutures alone, a sutured closure supplemented with DuraSeal (Integra, Princeton, NJ) had higher rates of intraoperative

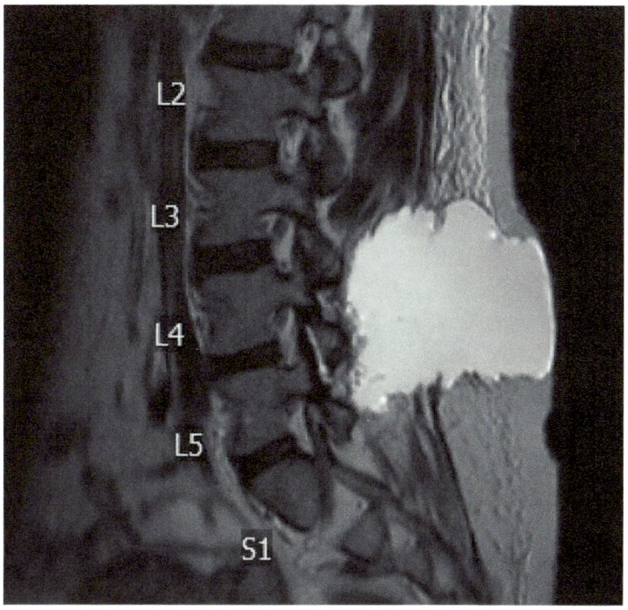

• **Fig. 20.3** MRI showing pseudomeningocele.

sealing (100%, hydrogel vs 79%, control), lower rates of postoperative CSF leakage (6.8% vs 12.5%), and a similar complication profile.[27]

Postoperatively, a period of flat bedrest decreases hydrostatic pressure in the lumbar spine and can theoretically help facilitate healing of the dura. However, the use of bedrest in the management of incidental durotomies continues to evolve and varies greatly among surgeons. In a study by Gautschi et al. surveying 175 neurosurgeons and orthopedic spine surgeons, 14.9% of surgeons never use bedrest, 35% use a 24-hour period, 28% use a 48-hour period of bedrest, and only 6.3% use a bedrest period of 72 hours.[28] Literature has shown that there is no advantage to prolonged bedrest as long as a watertight repair is achieved.[26] Therefore, the surgeon's perceived quality of dural repair often dictates how aggressive they are in mobilizing patients postoperatively.

Pseudarthrosis

Since the introduction of spinal fusion surgery in the early 1900s, pseudarthrosis—or the failure to achieve solid fusion—has been a major issue. Successful spinal fusion depends on the presence of appropriate biologic and mechanical factors. Although advances in posterior instrumentation techniques and osteobiologics over the last century have significantly improved fusion rates, it still remains a prevalent complication with rates reported between 5% and 35%.[29] However, the true incidence of pseudarthrosis is hard to determine since a large percentage of these patients are asymptomatic.

Patients with symptomatic pseudarthrosis generally present with persistent pain after surgery, new onset of pain after a pain free postoperative period, or progressive deformity. When suspecting a possible pseudarthrosis, it is important to first rule out other causes of pain and progressive deformity including adjacent segment degeneration, proximal junctional kyphosis, and infection. The diagnosis cannot be made until at least 1 year postoperatively and should involve multiple imaging modalities including AP, lateral, and dynamic plain radiographs as well as high-resolution CT scans with contiguous 1-mm-thick axial cuts. The FDA set radiographic guidelines for successful fusion to be less than 3 mm translational motion and less than 5 degrees of angular motion for the lumbar spine. However, in the absence of obvious implant failure or progressive deformity, plain radiographs have a relatively low sensitivity for the diagnosis of pseudarthrosis.[30] CT scans provide a more accurate assessment of bridging trabecular bone and can also identify haloing around pedicle screws (Fig. 20.4), which is suggestive of implant loosening.

There are multiple risk factors for pseudarthrosis after lumbar spinal fusion surgery that can be divided into biologic and mechanical factors. Significant systemic factors that have been shown to decrease fusion rates include smoking, diabetes, infection, malnutrition, peripheral vascular disease, and autoimmune disease. It has also been shown that patients >55 years old have higher pseudarthrosis rates

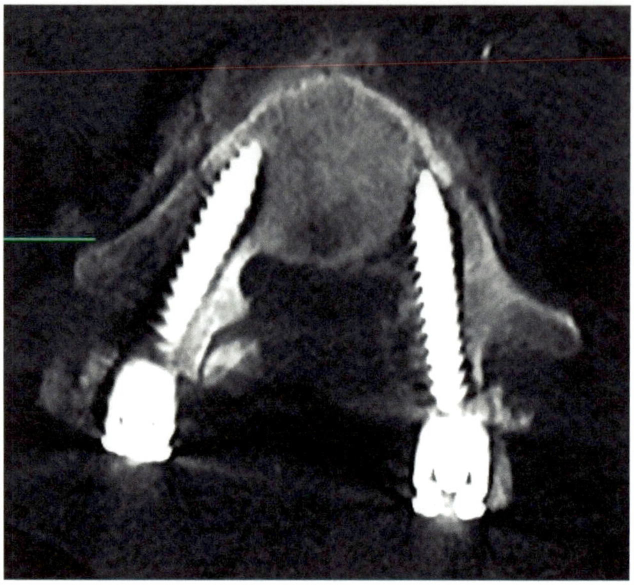

• **Fig. 20.4** CT scan of pseudarthrosis showing haloing around screws.

than younger patients.[31] Surgeon technique also plays a significant role in creating a favorable fusion environment. This involves adequate disc preparation in lumbar interbody fusions, exposure and decortication of the transverse processes, and bone grafting. In the absence of adequate amounts of autograft, or in patients at high risk for pseudarthrosis, additional autograft can be harvested from the patient's iliac crest. However, with the increasing off-label use of recombinant human bone morphogenetic protein 2 (rhBMP-2) in lumbar spinal fusions, harvesting iliac crest autograft has become much less common. Recent studies have shown higher fusion rates in long spinal deformity surgery when rhBMP-2 was used.[32] Additional sources of bone grafting material can include: allograft bone, bone marrow aspirate, and bone graft substitutes (demineralized bone matrix, calcium phosphate, etc).[33]

The mechanical risk factors associated with increased pseudarthrosis rates include excessive motion or shear forces at the fusion site, inadequate load sharing, and poor fixation. Failure of fusion in the lumbar spine occurs most commonly at the lumbosacral junction due to high biomechanical demands and poor bone quality in the sacrum. Factors independently associated with increased pseudarthrosis at L5-S1 include global sagittal imbalance >5 cm, longer fusion constructs, and significant hip arthritis. All of these factors increase biomechanical stress across the lumbosacral junction. Bone health also plays a significant role in mechanical stability of a construct and can significantly impact the rate of hardware failure prior to achieving a solid fusion. In patients with significant osteoporosis, cement augmentation can be added to the more cranial and caudal fixation segments to prevent loosening.

The mainstay of treatment for symptomatic pseudarthrosis is revision fusion surgery. However, prior to proceeding with revision surgery, the surgeon must work with the patient to minimize biologic risk factors that might have contributed to the pseudarthrosis in the first place. This may include interventions such as smoking cessation, improving glucose control, nutritional optimization, and improving bone density.[34]

Although revision techniques vary greatly depending on patient-specific parameters and surgeon preference, the basic principles are the same—maximize biology and mechanical stability to promote fusion. This usually involves replacing loose or failed hardware, adding additional load sharing and mechanical stability with interbody fusions and/or pelvic fixation, and providing extra osteoconductive and osteoinductive grafts to the fusion bed. In instances with significant global sagittal imbalance, a pedicle subtraction osteotomy (PSO) may be warranted to provide sagittal correction and decrease shear forces across the lumbosacral junction. Cultures should be sent during revision cases when concomitant infection is suspected.

Medical Complications

Although a lot of a surgeon's attention is centered around preventing intraoperative complications and perioperative complications related to surgical technique, postoperative medical complications can be equally, if not more, devastating. Common medical complications after lumbar spine surgery include (but are not limited to): urinary tract infections (UTI), ileus, acute kidney injury (AKI), deep vein thrombosis (DVT)/pulmonary embolus (PE), and myocardial infarction (MI).[35]

Urinary tract infections are perhaps the most commonly seen medical complication after lumbar spine surgery, reported to be as high as 20%.[36] These UTIs are attributed to the use of Foley catheters during lumbar fusion surgeries, which can introduce bacteria into the urethra and bladder; thus, Foley use should be minimized when possible and, when used, removed as soon as possible. In these cases of UTI, prompt antibiotic treatment should be initiated with either a third-generation cephalosporin or quinolone.

Postoperative ileus occurs in 5% to 12% of all patients undergoing lumbar spine surgery and is more common in patients undergoing anterior lumbar surgery or deformity correction.[36] Manipulation or retraction of bowel during anterior lumbar surgery causes a decrease in gastrointestinal motility postoperatively, which significantly contributes to the increase in ileus rates. Additional risk factors include narcotic use, electrolyte abnormalities, and dehydration. Treatment is typically conservative and involves limiting solid food intake, an aggressive bowel regimen, adequate intravenous hydration, and correcting electrolyte abnormalities.

Thromboembolism related to DVT is another known complication of lumbar spine surgery. DVT prophylactic measures, both mechanical and chemical, should be considered for all inpatient cases and the benefits must be weighed against the risk of hematoma formation and wound drainage. Prophylactic preoperative inferior vena cava (IVC) filter placement may be considered in high-risk patients and subsequently removed 2 to 3 weeks postoperatively. Treatment options after a DVT/PE is identified include therapeutic anticoagulation, IVC filter placement, or thrombolysis.

Myocardial infarction (MI) following any surgery is a very serious complication with a reported mortality rate as high as 70%.[37] Daubs et al. found a 1.8% rate of postoperative chest pain associated with ECG changes and a 0.6% rate of arrhythmia in 169 patients undergoing spinal fusion.[36] Preprocedure medical consultation and testing for elective procedures is helpful to identify patients with cardiac risk factors. If a patient is diagnosed with an MI postoperatively, they should be transferred immediately to a closely monitored unit and receive a cardiac consultation.

Conclusion

Complications in lumbar surgery have the ability to cause significant morbidity and mortality in patients, but also stress for surgeons. Therefore, it is imperative to know how to prevent these complications or, if they do arise, how to manage them in order to prevent poor outcomes. Although the trend in lumbar spine surgery is moving towards more minimally invasive techniques and approaches, these carry with them their own subset of complications and appropriate patient selection is crucial in order to minimize complications.

References

1. Hamilton DK, Smith JS, Sansur CA, et al. Rates of new neurological deficit associated with spine surgery based on 108,419 procedures: A report of the scoliosis research society morbidity and mortality committee. *Spine (Phila Pa 1976)*. 2011;36(15):1218–1228. https://doi.org/10.1097/BRS.0b013e3181ec5fd9.
2. Shin BJ, James AR, Njoku IU, Härtl R. Pedicle screw navigation: A systematic review and meta-analysis of perforation risk for computer-navigated versus freehand insertion - A review. *J Neurosurg Spine*. 2012;17(2):113–122. https://doi.org/10.3171/2012.5.SPINE11399.
3. Yi S, Yoon DH, Kim KN, Kim SH, Shin HC. Postoperative spinal epidural hematoma: risk factor and clinical outcome. *Yonsei Med J*. 2006;47(3):326–332.
4. Epstein N. More nerve root injuries occur with minimally invasive lumbar surgery: Let's tell someone. *Surg Neurol Int*. 2016;7:S96–S101. https://doi.org/10.4103/2152-7806.174896.
5. Ahmadian A, Deukmedjian AR, Abel N, Dakwar E, Uribe JS. Analysis of lumbar plexopathies and nerve injury after lateral retroperitoneal transpsoas approach: Diagnostic standardization. *J Neurosurg Spine*. 2013;18(3):289–297. https://doi.org/10.3171/2012.11.SPINE12755.
6. Sasso RC, Burkus JK, Lehuec JC. Retrograde ejaculation after anterior lumbar interbody fusion transperitoneal versus retroperitoneal exposure. *Spine (Phila Pa 1976)*. 2003;28(10):1023–1026. https://doi.org/10.1097/01.BRS.0000062965.47779.EB.
7. Baker JK, Reardon PR, Reardon MJ, Heggeness MH. Vascular injury in anterior lumbar surgery. *Spine (Phila Pa 1976)*. 1993;18(15):2227–2230.

8. Kulkarni SS, Lowery GL, Ross RE, Sankar KR, Lykomitros V. Arterial complications following anterior lumbar interbody fusion: Report of eight cases. *Eur Spine J.* 2003;12(1):48–54. https://doi.org/10.1007/s00586-002-0460-4.
9. Brau SA, Delamarter RB, Schiffman ML, Williams LA, Watkins RG. Vascular injury during anterior lumbar surgery. *Spine J.* 2004; 4(4):409–412. https://doi.org/10.1016/j.spinee.2003.12.003.
10. Kueper J, Fantini GA, Walker BR, Aichmair A, Hughes AP. Incidence of vascular complications during lateral lumbar interbody fusion: an examination of the mini-open access technique. *Eur Spine Jl.* 2015;24(4):800–809. https://doi.org/10.1007/s00586-015-3796-2.
11. Beckman JM, Vincent B, Park MS, et al. Contralateral psoas hematoma after minimally invasive, lateral retroperitoneal transpsoas lumbar interbody fusion: A multicenter review of 3950 lumbar levels. *J Neurosurg Spine.* 2017;26(1):50–54. https://doi.org/10.3171/2016.4.SPINE151040.
12. Lonstein JE, Denis F, Perra JH, Pinto MR, Smith MD, Winter RB Complications associated with pedicle screws. *J Bone Joint Surg Am.* 1999;81(11):1519–1528. https://doi.org/10.2106/00004623-199911000-00003.
13. Inamasu J, Guiot BH. Vascular injury and complication in neurosurgical spine surgery. *Acta Neurochir (Wien).* 2006;148(4): 375–386. https://doi.org/10.1007/s00701-005-0669-1.
14. Harbison SP. Major vascular complications of intervertebral disc surgery. *Ann Surg.* 1954;140(3):342–348. https://doi.org/10.1097/00000658-195409000-00010.
15. Bingol H, Cingoz F, Turan Yilmaz A, Yasar M, Harun Tatar A. Vascular complications related to lumbar disc surgery. *J Neurosurg.* 2004;100(3 Suppl Spine):249-253. https://doi.org/10.3171/spi.2004.100.3.0249.
16. Olsen MA, Mayfield J, Lauryssen C, et al. Risk factors for surgical site infection in spinal surgery. *J Neurosurg.* 2003;98(2 Suppl): 149–155.
17. Ahmed R, Greenlee JDW, Traynelis VC. Preservation of spinal instrumentation after development of postoperative bacterial infections in patients undergoing spinal arthrodesis. *J Spinal Disord Tech.* 2012;25(6):299–302.
18. Petilon JM, Glassman SD, Dimar JR, Carreon LY, Clinical outcomes after lumbar fusion complicated by deep wound infection: a case-control study. *Spine (Phila PA 1976).* 2012;37(16):1370–1374. https://doi.org/10.1097/BRS.0b013e31824a4d93.
19. Sweet FA, Roh M, Sliva C. Intrawound application of vancomycin for prophylaxis in instrumented thoracolumbar fusions: Efficacy, drug levels, and patient outcomes. *Spine (Phila Pa 1976).* 2011;36(24):2084–2088. https://doi.org/10.1097/BRS.0b013e3181ff2cb1.
20. Kanayama M, Hashimoto T, Shigenobu K, Oha F, Togawa D. Effective prevention of surgical site infection using a Centers for Disease Control and Prevention guideline-based antimicrobial prophylaxis in lumbar spine surgery. *J Neurosurg Spine.* 2007; 6(4):327–329.
21. Sakka L, Coll G, Chazal J. Anatomy and physiology of cerebrospinal fluid. *Eur Ann Otorhinolaryngol Head Neck Dis.* 2011;128(6): 309–316. https://doi.org/10.1016/j.anorl.2011.03.002.
22. Cammisa FP, Girardi FP, Sangani PK, Parvataneni HK, Cadag S, Sandhu HS. Incidental durotomy in spine surgery. Spine (Phila Pa 1976). 2000;25(20):2663–2667. https://doi.org/10.1097/00007632-200010150-00019.
23. Lu C, Ho S, Kong S. Intracranial subdural hematoma after unintended durotomy during spine surgery. *Can J Anesth.* 2002; 49:100–102.
24. Hawk MW, Kim KD. Review of spinal pseudomeningoceles and cerebrospinal fluid fistulas. *Neurosurg Focus.* 2000;9(1):e5.
25. Klingler JH, Volz F, Krüger MT, et al. Accidental durotomy in minimally invasive transforaminal lumbar interbody fusion: Frequency, risk factors, and management. *Sci World J.* 2015; 2015:532628. https://doi.org/10.1155/2015/532628.
26. Bosacco SJ, Gardner MJ, Guille JT. Evaluation and treatment of dural tears in lumbar spine surgery: a review. *Clin Orthop Relat Res.* 2001(389):238–247.
27. Wright NM, Park J, Tew JM, et al. Spinal sealant system provides better intraoperative watertight closure than standard of care during spinal surgery: A prospective, multicenter, randomized controlled study. *Spine (Phila Pa 1976).* 2015;40(8): 505–513. https://doi.org/10.1097/BRS.0000000000000810.
28. Gautschi OP, Stienen MN, Smoll NR, Corniola MV, Tessitore E, Schaller K. Incidental durotomy in lumbar spine surgery - A three-nation survey to evaluate its management. *Acta Neurochir (Wien).* 2014;156(9):1813–1820. https://doi.org/10.1007/s00701-014-2177-7.
29. Kim YJ, Bridwell KH, Lenke LG, Rhim S, Cheh G. Pseudarthrosis in long adult spinal deformity instrumentation and fusion to the sacrum: prevalence and risk factor analysis of 144 cases. *Spine (Phila Pa 1976).* 2006;31(20):2329–2336. https://doi.org/10.1097/01.brs.0000238968.82799.d9.
30. Blumenthal SL, Gill K. Can lumbar spine radiographs accurately determine fusion in postoperative patients? Correlation of routine radiographs with a second surgical look at lumbar fusions. *Spine (Phila Pa 1976).* 1993;18(9):1186–1189. https://doi.org/10.1097/00007632-199307000-00010.
31. Dickson DD, Lenke LG, Bridwell KH, Koester LA. Risk factors for and assessment of symptomatic pseudarthrosis after lumbar pedicle subtraction osteotomy in adult spinal deformity. *Spine (Phila Pa 1976).* 2014;39(15):1190–1195. https://doi.org/10.1097/BRS.0000000000000380.
32. Kim HJ, Buchowski JM, Zebala LP, Dickson DD, Koester L, Bridwell KH. RhBMP-2 Is superior to iliac crest bone graft for long fusions to the sacrum in adult spinal deformity. *Spine (Phila Pa 1976).* 2013;38(14):1209–1215. https://doi.org/10.1097/BRS.0b013e31828b656d.
33. Kannan A, Dodwad SNM, Hsu WK Biologics in spine arthrodesis. *J Spinal Disord Tech.* 2015;28(5):163–170.
34. Albert TJ, Pinto M, Denis F. Management of symptomatic lumbar pseudarthrosis with anteroposterior fusion. A functional and radiographic outcome study. Spine *(Phila Pa 1976).* 2000;25(1):123–129; discussion 130. https://doi.org/10.1097/00007632-200001010-00021.
35. Nasser R, Yadla S, Maltenfort MG, et al. Complications in spine surgery a review. *J Neurosurg Spine.* 2010;13(2):141–143. https://doi.org/10.3171/2010.3.SPINE09369.
36. Daubs MD, Lenke LG, Cheh G, Stobbs G, Bridwell KH. Adult spinal deformity surgery complications and outcomes in patients over age 60. *Spine (Phila Pa 1976).* 2007;32(20):2238–2244. https://doi.org/10.1097/BRS.0b013e31814cf24a.
37. Adams JE 3rd, Sicard GA, Allen BT, et al. Diagnosis of perioperative myocardial infarction with measurement of cardiac troponin I. *N Engl J Med.* 1994;330(10):670–674. https://doi.org/10.1056/NEJM199403103301003.

21 Avoiding Complications Associated With Anterior Lumbar Surgery

AARON W. STEVENSON AND CHRISTOPHER MARDEN JOHN CAIN

CHAPTER OUTLINE

Introduction

Anterior lumbar surgical techniques were initially developed in the management of spinal infection.[1,2] The approach was subsequently adopted in the management of degenerative conditions.[3–6] Burns[3] and Mercer[4] reported a direct transperitoneal approach whilst Ito[2] described a retroperitoneal approach. Hodgson[7,8] later expanded the technique and reported the use of anterior and lateral approaches to the lumbar spine, including their application in the management of spinal tumors, trauma, spondylolisthesis, and degenerative disc disease.

The oblique muscle splitting approach to the retroperitoneal space was reported by Fraser[9] in 1992, which was further modified by Mayer[10] and Brau.[11] A direct midline anterior or paramedian approach is preferred today that has reduced the morbidity of the approach.

Prior to the introduction of stable segmental pedicle screw instrumentation systems,[12–14] fusion rates and the clinical outcomes of anterior spinal surgery were considered superior to those of posterior spinal surgery. Improved fusion rates with these systems led to a fairly rapid move away from anterior fusion techniques in the mid-1990s. As a result of this, surgeons trained during this era were not regularly exposed or trained to utilize this approach.

It was not until the introduction of the lumbar disc replacement[15,16] and the development of "stand-alone" anterior fusion cages[17] that the merits of anterior spinal surgery were again realized. Improved restoration of segmental lordosis and foraminal height, along with improved fusion rates,[18,19] have led to a resurgence in the use of anterior lumbar spinal surgery techniques.

Due to greater sub-specialization of surgical practice and changes in surgical training programs, the majority of these anterior spinal procedures are now performed with a vascular or general co-surgeon employed to facilitate safe access to the anterior lumbar spine.

Today, anterior access to the lumbar spine is generally performed via a retroperitoneal approach. Whilst this description is somewhat all encompassing, including the lateral trans psoas and oblique anterior to psoas approach, this chapter will focus upon the direct anterior retroperitoneal approach performed in the supine position through a midline or paramedian incision.

This direct anterior approach, medial to the rectus, can be performed through either a horizontal or vertical incision. The anterior rectus sheath is divided just lateral to the linea alba and the rectus is elevated and retracted laterally. The inferior epigastric vessels will be encountered in the lateral aspect of the sheath, and tributaries of these vessels should be coagulated and divided to avoid their avulsion. The arcuate line is identified in the iliac fossa and the peritoneum mobilized from the sheath using blunt dissection. The posterior sheath is then divided laterally over sufficient distance to gain access to the operative levels. Once the retroperitoneal space is accessed and vessel retraction completed, direct anterior visualization of the spine is afforded for disc clearance and instrumentation with balanced abdominal wall tissue on both sides of the incision.

Preoperative Factors

Identification of potential challenges and risks prior to surgery, and assessing your ability to overcome these challenges, is the single most important way to minimize complications.

Careful patient selection is paramount to success and this includes factors related to the patient, their anatomy, and their pathology.

Body habitus: Obesity is associated with an increased risk of complications in spine surgery,[20] but when looking specifically at anterior lumbar surgery while there is generally a need for longer incisions and an expectation of longer operating times, the incidence of major complications may not be increased.[21] A critical factor is being able to achieve and maintain adequate exposure with available retraction systems. Examination of the abdomen with the patient supine and the hips and knees slightly flexed allows assessment of the likely depth and tension of the abdomen.

An access surgeon may be unable to review the patient preoperatively prior to meeting them on the day of surgery; in this situation, the depth of the exposure may be gauged by the scout view of a recent lumbar CT or MRI (Fig. 21.1A,B). The maximum standard depth of many retraction systems is 18 or 20 cm, which becomes a limiting factor when performing anterior lumbar surgery. Retraction of abdominal contents in larger patients may be overcome using handheld retractors; however, assistant fatigue may limit the quality of exposure. An alternative is demonstrated in Fig. 21.1C where guarded Steinmann pins are used in combination with the SynFrame (DePuy Synthes, Raynham, MA) to maintain exposure.

Patients should ideally lose weight prior to surgery. When this is not possible or practical, utilize strategies to reduce the volume and tension of intraperitoneal contents. These strategies include having the patient complete a bowel preparation prior to admission. The placement of a nasogastric or orogastric tube after intubation will also reduce gaseous distension of the gut during surgery.

Obesity may also lead to wound healing issues due to both abdominal tension and the depth of adipose tissue. Planning to utilize abdominal binders, drains, and vacuum-assisted closure devices can reduce tension and the risk of fat necrosis and wound dehiscence.

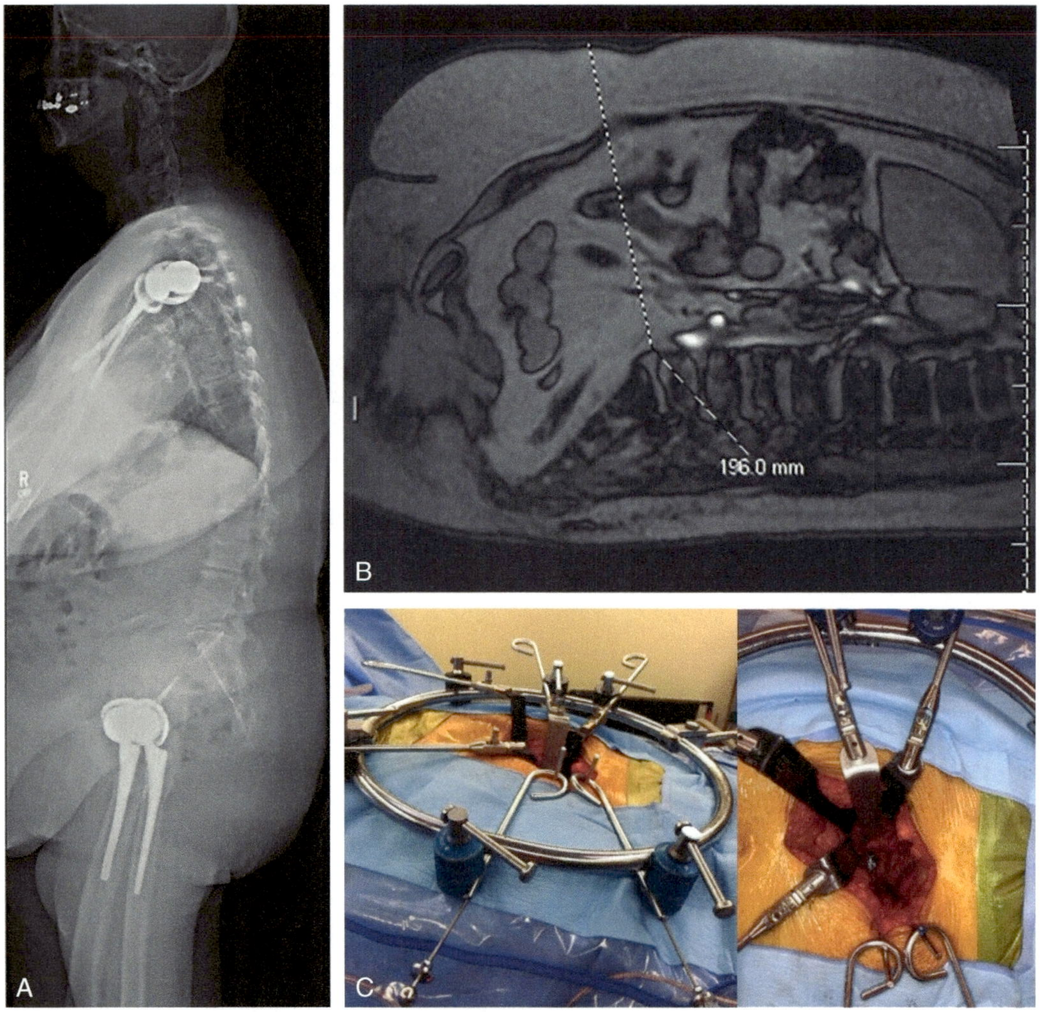

• **Fig. 21.1** (A) Standing lateral radiograph of obese woman scheduled for anterior lumbar surgery. (B) Scout view of supine MRI of the woman in Fig. 21.1(A) showing the depth of the abdomen to be expected when performing an anterior exposure. (C) Adaptation of the SynFrame retractor (DePuy Synthes, Raynham, MA) utilizing a combination of long retractor blades and guarded Steinmann pins to maintain anterior exposure.

Previous Surgery

Previous abdominal procedures, particularly those that utilized the retroperitoneal space, can result in challenges exposing the anterior lumbar spine.

Previous major **vascular surgery** involving the distal aorta and common iliac vessels represent a contraindication to this approach.

Renal surgery may violate the retroperitoneal space, but this surgery is usually undertaken from a more lateral approach above L3. In this case, access to the lower lumbar spine is generally not compromised. While access to the anterior spine may be possible in patients who have undergone pelvic placement of a transplanted kidney, access obtained from the contralateral side may disrupt the arterial supply or venous outflow of the transplanted kidney. Should anterior surgery be considered the best option in this situation, great care must be taken to minimize vessel displacement in the region of the transplant.

Previous anterior spinal exposure, either at the same level, or from the same side to an adjacent level, is a relative contraindication for repeat exposure. Expect retroperitoneal scarring to tether the vasculature to the anterior aspect of the spine, not only at the previously instrumented level but also the adjacent levels. Scarring will make mobilization of the vessels difficult, if not impossible, and identification of the margins of the vasculature, particularly the inferior vena cava and common iliac vein, may also be challenging, significantly increasing the risk of vessel injury.

However, there are cases where revision exposure is both indicated and feasible. The vascular anatomy, extent, and nature of the previous surgery and the patient's pathology will determine this. Review of the initial preoperative imaging allows assessment of the original vascular anatomy and the potential window for access. If the anterior vasculature is not well visualized on standard preoperative imaging, CT angiography may be considered. Where possible, review the previous operation record to identify whether difficulties or a vascular injury were encountered. Do not be fooled into thinking the use of vessel guards or membranes will make a revision exposure easier. These products have not proven to be effective in preserving tissue planes.

Revision exposure at L5-S1 can generally be performed from the contralateral side to the initial exposure, provided the vascular anatomy is favorable. The risks inherent to a revision exposure at L4-5 are such that it should not be attempted. In a situation such as implant failure or infection where repeat exposure is desirable, the use of a lateral or anterolateral approach is recommended to minimize the need for mobilization of the vessels.

The ureter is also at risk of injury during revision exposures as it is often obscured by or adherent to scar tissue. The placement of a ureteric stent prior to surgery allows identification and protection of this structure.

Inguinal hernia repair with mesh, particularly when performed via a laparoscopic approach, is not uncommon and represents a challenge gaining access to the L5-S1 level. The peritoneum is usually adherent to the inferior abdominal wall, tethering the vas deferens and testicular vessels or round ligament distally, which makes medial and distal mobilization of these structures more difficult. In this situation, it is recommended to dissect between the mesh and the abdominal wall as the plane develops with greater ease than trying to mobilize the mesh from the peritoneum. Where possible, approach the L5-S1 level from the contralateral side to the hernia repair. Access to L4-5 and above is generally not compromised, but initial access to the retroperitoneal space distally may take a little more time.

Caesarian section and **abdominal hysterectomy** surgery seldom causes an issue once the retroperitoneal space has been identified. Adhesion of the rectus muscle within its sheath distally is likely to be encountered, but this can usually be released relatively easily with minimal additional risk of complications.

Midline laparotomies to address intraperitoneal pathology may lead to adhesion of the medial margin of the rectus, but once these adhesions are mobilized the exposure is generally not compromised. In patients having undergone an **abdominoplasty** it may be difficult to identify the anterior rectus sheath during superficial dissection. Once the sheath has been divided the deeper structures should be free of adhesions.

Laparoscopic portals encountered following a variety of abdominal surgeries cause little more than small regions of scar when developing access planes. These areas generally pose no obstruction to achieving safe access.

The presence of an **umbilical hernia** or **rectus diastasis** does not preclude anterior retroperitoneal access; however, care must be taken to avoid inadvertent injury to the peritoneum. Consideration should also be given to the reconstruction or repair of these defects at the time of surgery. A slightly more lateral incision and division of the anterior rectus sheath may be beneficial in patients having undergone an **umbilical hernia repair** if exposure above L4-5 is being performed.

Vessel Anatomy

Critical to achieving safe access to the anterior spine is the mobilization and retraction of the anterior vasculature. Careful review of preoperative MRI imaging enables identification of potential challenges.

Lumbosacral (L5-S1) exposures in the bifurcation of the vessels are generally considered straightforward.[22] Fig. 21.2 demonstrates variations in the lumbosacral "window" that may be encountered at this level. Fig. 21.2A is an example of a wide window between the iliac vessels and Fig. 21.2B the MRI of a patient with a very low bifurcation where both the L4-5 and L5-S1 discs were approached from the left. The presence of a high bifurcation (Fig. 21.3) usually indicates relatively easy access to L5-S1, but greater challenges should be anticipated when gaining access to the L4-5 level. Finding the level of the crotch or apex of the bifurcation on

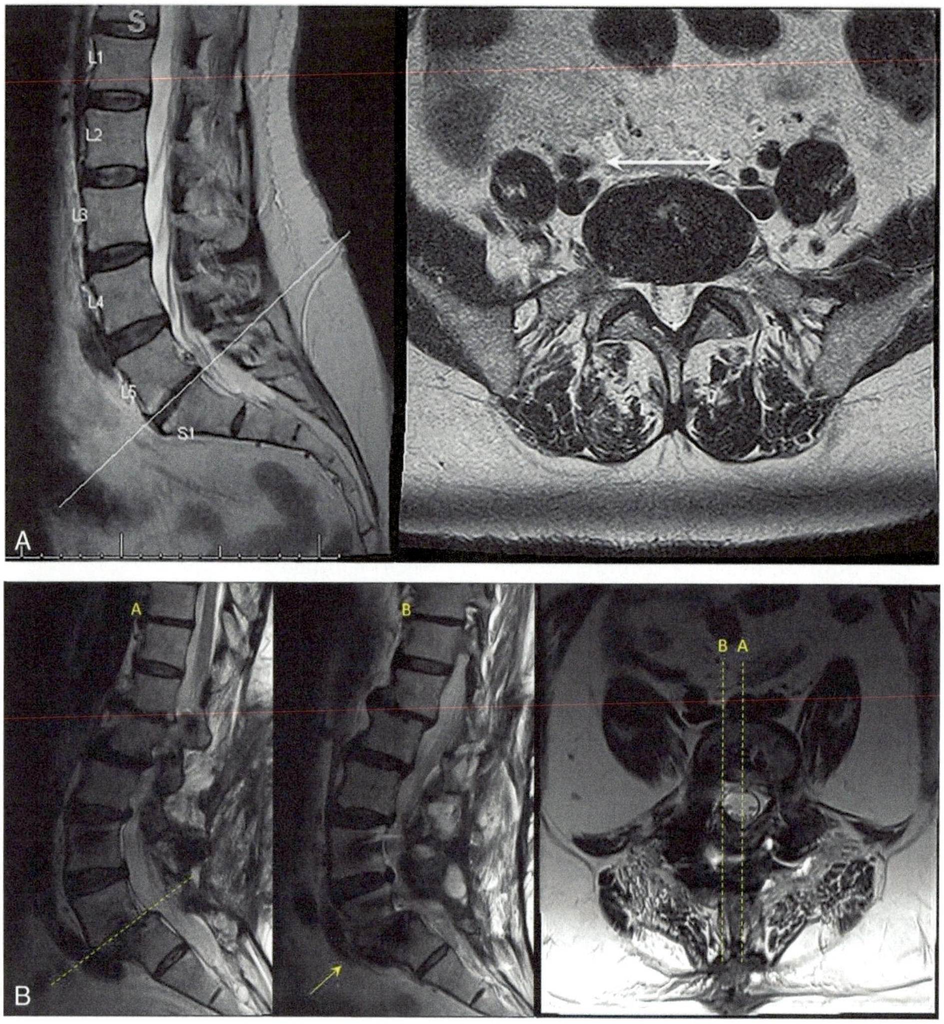

• **Fig. 21.2** (A) Midline sagittal T2-weighted MRI and disc axial at L5-S1 demonstrating a wide opening between the iliac vessels **(arrow)**. (B) Midline sagittal (left) and paramedian sagittal (middle) T2-weighted MRI and disc axial at L5-S1 (right) demonstrating a low bifurcation. The **arrow** indicates the level of the crotch or apex of the bifurcation

the sagittal MRI helps to assess the likelihood of being able to access L4-5 in the bifurcation (Fig. 21.2B).

Exposure of the L4-5 level generally presents the most challenging exposure. The left common iliac vein will become evident as the distal aorta and common iliac artery is mobilized medially and distally. At this point, an effort should be made to identify whether an iliolumbar vein is likely to limit mobilization of the vessel. The presence of an iliolumbar vein does not mandate its ligation, but continued observation is required to identify when the limits of retraction are being reached.

Many surgeons utilize vascular clips to ligate vessels whilst some still prefer silk ties. Regardless of the method used, ensure good and stable exposure of the vessel prior to its ligation. Have sufficient length exposed such that the vessel may be divided without the clip or tie slipping off. If using clips, ensure an appropriate size is used to avoid ongoing bleeding or dislodgement. The use of a silk tie takes a little more time but is less likely to be displaced as vessels are mobilized. An appreciation of the tolerance of the vessels to manipulation, mobilization, and retraction comes with experience.

Exposure of the L3/4 and L2/3 levels are usually less challenging with respect to vascular mobilization. However, isolated exposure of the more proximal levels can lead to more difficulty gaining access to the retroperitoneal space if the arcuate line of the posterior rectus sheath cannot be identified. In such cases, the posterior rectus sheath can be carefully divided laterally using a scalpel, without penetration of the peritoneum. The peritoneum can then be mobilized from the lateral abdominal wall using blunt dissection and the posterior rectus sheath divided over sufficient distance to complete the desired exposure.

Segmental vessels are to be expected in the middle third of each vertebra and should be coagulated, tied off, or clipped if they limit mobilization of the vessels. Be sure to check the presence of segmental vessels at the proximal end of the exposure, as their avulsion during medial retraction of the vessels can be very difficult to control.

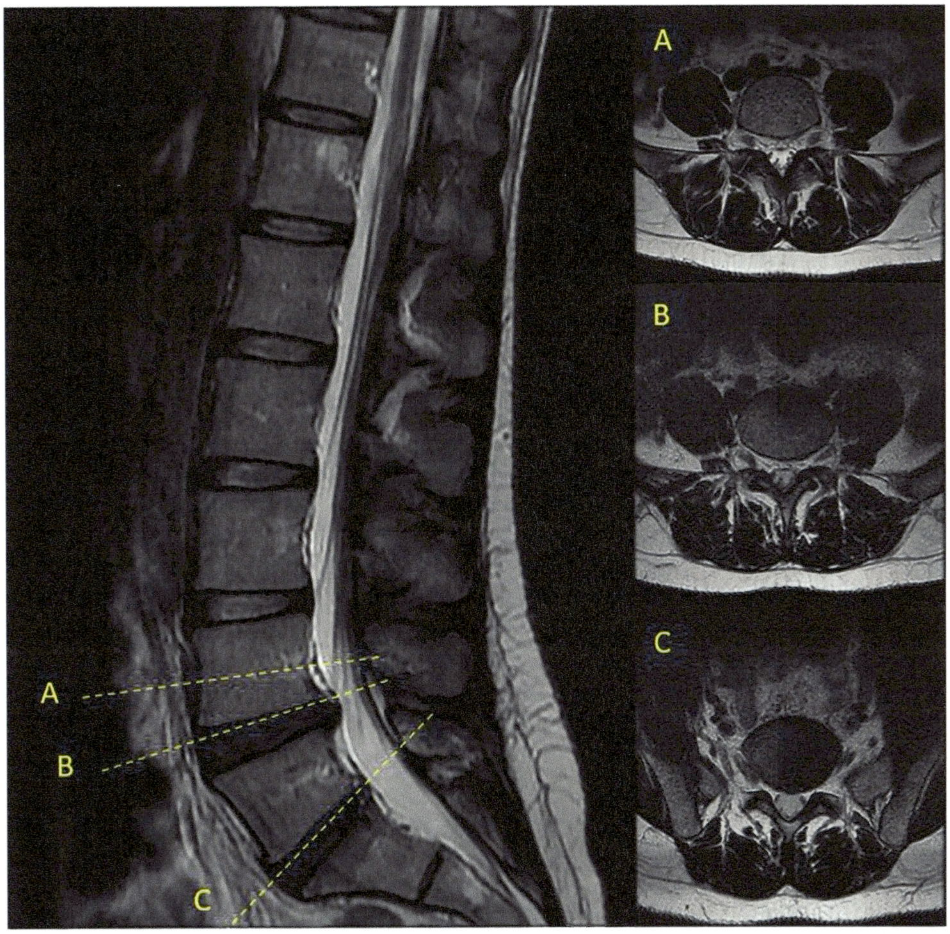

• **Fig. 21.3** Midline sagittal and axial T2 weighted MRIs in the middle of the L4 vertebra (A), the inferior endplate of L4 (B), and the inferior endplate of L5 (C) demonstrating a high bifurcation where both the L4-5 and L5-S1 discs were approached and instrumented in the bifurcation.

A pulse oximeter should be placed on the left, and in some cases also the right, great toe to monitor distal perfusion as retraction of the vessels may lead to loss of perfusion to the lower limb or limbs. Should this occur, the time should be noted. Release of the retraction and restoration of normal vascular flow should be considered after 30 minutes, and definitely performed after 60 minutes. Loss of perfusion for more than 90 minutes risks lower limb ischemic injury.

The renal vessels limit the proximal extent that an anterior exposure can safely be performed. These vessels seldom branch from the aorta and inferior vena cava (IVC) below L2. However, variations occur and Fig. 21.4A,B shows an example of a patient with only one kidney where an L2 to S1 exposure was planned but the presence of an aberrant left renal vein at the level of the L3 vertebra limited the exposure to L3-4.

Other vascular anomalies are not uncommon, and careful examination of preoperative imaging will usually reveal these variations. While CT angiography is effective in identifying the vascular anatomy,[23] the routine use of this technique is not associated with a reduction in intraoperative or overall complications.[24]

Atherosclerosis: Atrial calcification demonstrated on plane radiographs or an abdominal CT scan denotes significant underlying atherosclerosis. Circumferential atheromatous plaques indicate a nonpliable vessel, and if this extends from the distal aorta into the common iliac vessels, adequate mobilization of the vessels is challenging and associated with greater risk of distal emboli. This situation represents a contraindication for this approach. Localized plaques may also be associated with the risk of plaque dislodgment and distal ischemia. In this situation, assess how much mobilization of the vessels will be required to adequately expose the anterior aspect of the spine and if this can be done safely. It is important to ensure atheromatous vessels are not kinked, and this may be achieved by performing a wider exposure that allows more gradual vascular retraction. Atheroma may also be associated with reduced compliance in segmental vessels that are less receptive to electrocautery. In this situation, clips or ties should may be required to ligate these vessels. In patients with significant atheroma, it is prudent to use pulse oximetry on both lower limbs, and urgent vascular evaluation and intervention should be sought upon detection of a persistent ischemic limb. Consideration should also be given to lower limb compartment fasciotomy should ischemia persist for more than 180 minutes.[25]

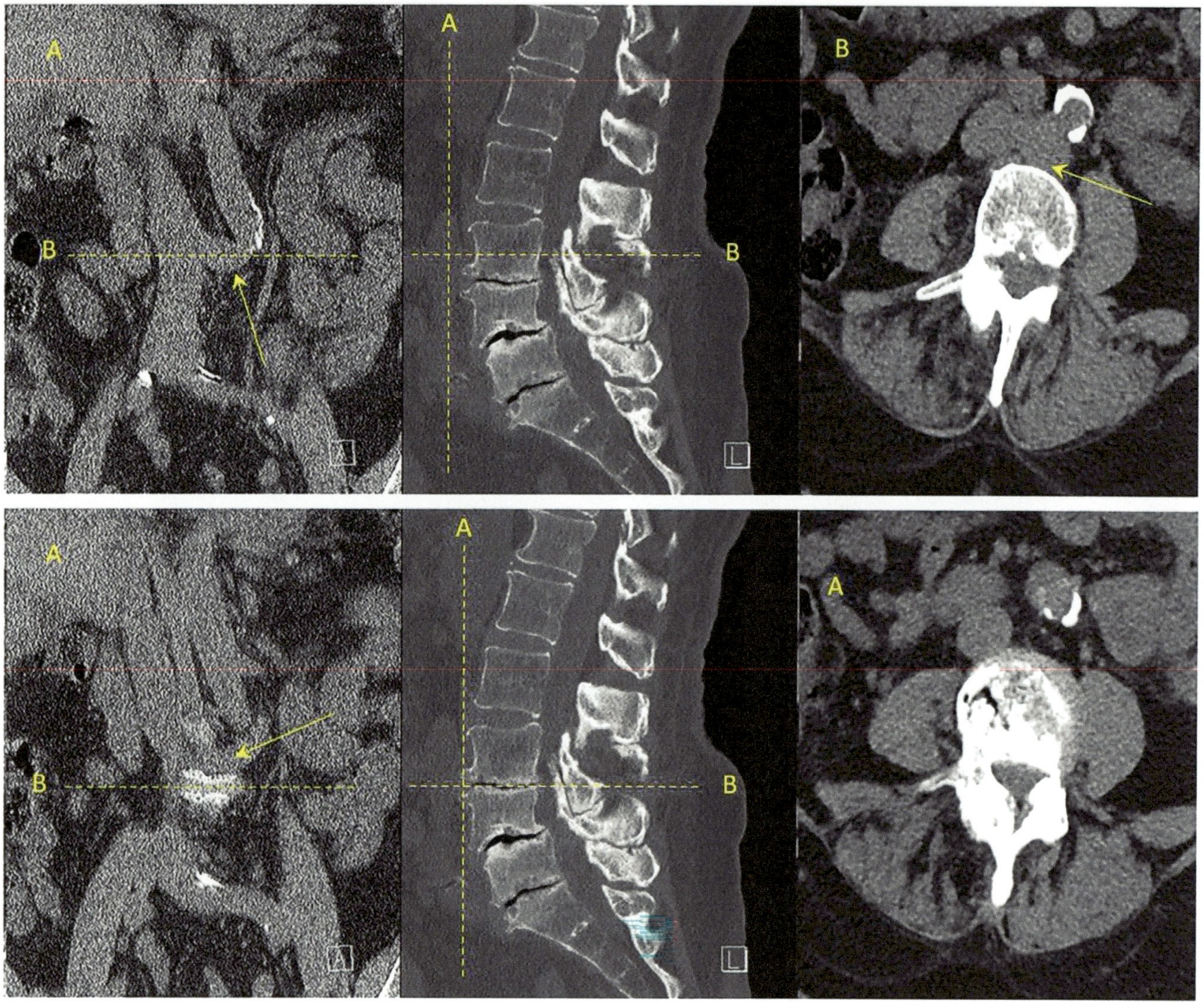

• **Fig. 21.4** The **top** row of images represents coronal, sagittal, and axial image at the midpoint of the L3 vertebra of a woman with only one kidney. The **arrow** indicates the origin of a large renal vein passing to the left and behind the aorta. The **bottom** row of images represents coronal, sagittal, and axial images at the level of the L3-4 disc of the same woman. The location of this vein and the fact she had only one kidney limited exposure to the L3-4 interspace.

Scoliosis: In cases of significant scoliosis, the vessels often become tortuous due to shortening of the trunk and tethering by segmental vessels. In the absence of significant atheroma, the vessels will usually realign as the deformity is corrected. Consider this when performing the initial access, as when distal levels are instrumented and distracted, the proximal exposure may become limited. In cases where a long anterior fusion is being performed in the presence of a scoliosis, it may pay to instrument the proximal level(s) before completing the distal instrumentation.

Lumbar lordosis and listhesis: A steep sacral slope, often in association with an L5-S1 spondylolisthesis and transitional anatomy, may not pose a barrier to anterior exposure, but may create challenges in relation to disc clearance and instrumentation. It is the pubis that limits access to the disc in this situation and it is not always evident on a standard lateral lumbar radiograph. If suspected, a standing EOS or similar image or the scout view of a lumbar CT scan may show this relationship. Alternatively, obtain a supine lateral radiograph showing the position of the pubis relative to a line drawn along the superior surface of the sacrum (Fig. 21.5A,B). This will identify any challenges that might be encountered during disc clearance and instrumentation, which may in turn lead to a change in the surgical plan.

Limitations may also be encountered proximally due to the sternum and costal margin when exposing the upper lumbar spine.

Infection: Osteomyelitis and discitis requiring anterior spinal surgery represents one of the most challenging and risky situations for anterior exposure of the lumbar spine. In this setting, tissue planes and landmarks may be grossly

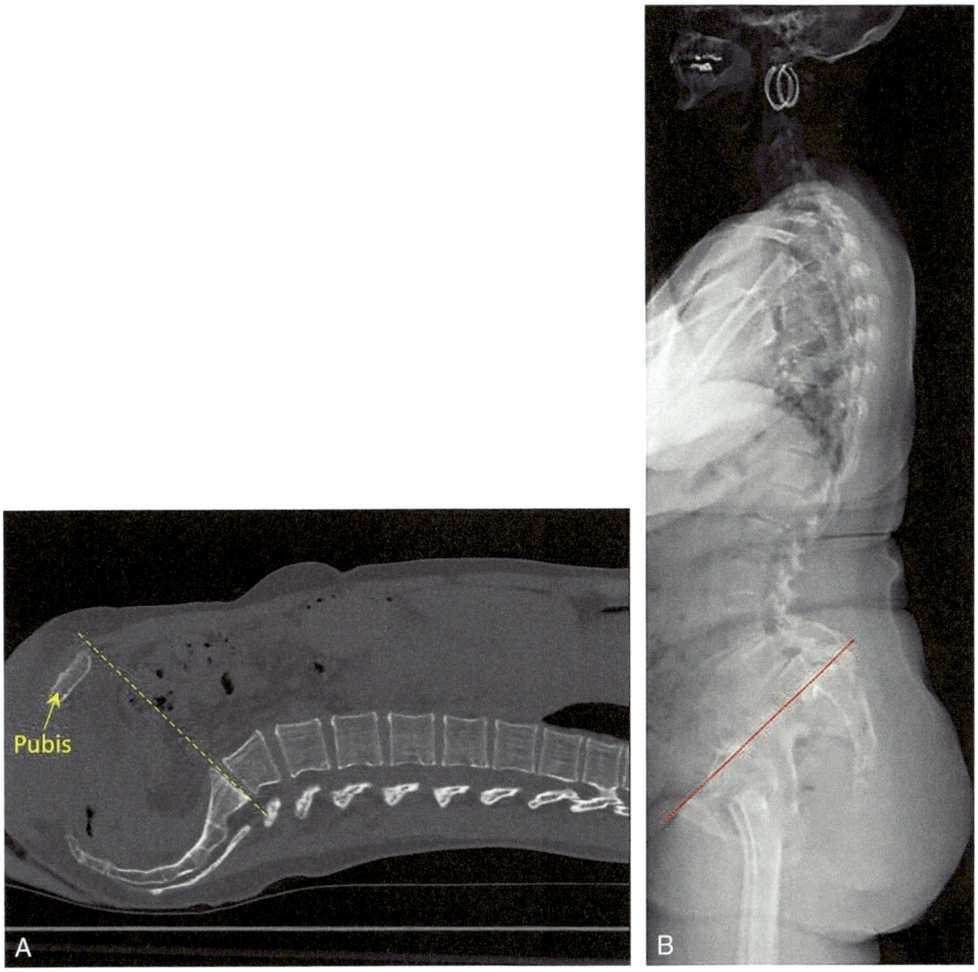

• **Fig. 21.5** (A) Scout view of a young woman with a steep sacral slope showing access to the L5-S1 disc just above the pubis. (B) Standing EOS view of a middle-aged women with degenerative spondylolisthesis at L3-4, L4-5, and L5-S1 with increased lumbar lordosis and a steep sacral slope such that direct access to the L5-S1 disc should not be expected. In this case, posterior instrumentation, distraction, and realignment was done prior to the anterior instrumentation.

distorted or lost. Tissue integrity is often compromised, either by scar or granulation tissue if the infection is chronic, or by increased fragility due to active inflammation. This is of most concern in relation to the vasculature, as repair of a friable vessel is very difficult and the use of grafts, patches, and stents is problematic in the presence of infection. The ureter is also at risk as it becomes encased in scar and inflammatory tissue, and in this situation the preoperative placement of a stent is advisable.

In situations where anatomy and tissue planes are distorted, it is advisable to perform a wider exposure and start in areas of more normal anatomy before working towards the focus of infection or scaring.

Malignancy and previous radiotherapy: Unlike infection, most primary and secondary malignant lesions in the lumbar spine do not compromise adjacent vascular structures. Patients who have undergone previous radiation treatment to the lumbar spine, however, are likely to have adherent tissues, but the friability encountered with infection is seldom experienced.

Osteoporosis: Poor bone quality does not add significantly to the risks of the exposure but certainly leads to additional challenges in relation to disc clearance, instrument failure, and avoiding subsidence through endplate failure. In this situation, care should be taken during disc clearance to preserve the integrity of the endplate. Appropriately sized and anatomical implant designs should be utilized to prevent point loading of the endplate, which leads to endplate failure, and supplemental posterior fixation should be utilized.

Intraoperative Complications

Intraoperative complications during anterior spinal access surgery are rare but can be devastating.

Vascular injury avoidance is a better strategy than being skilled at vessel repair, which is probably a factor in relation to the finding that vessel injuries are more common when an access surgeon is utilized.[26] Vascular surgeons are comfortable handling and repairing these structures and will often approach the vessels directly and then move them out of the way to expose the spine. The approach of many spine surgeons still performing their own access is more focused on the spine, just mobilizing the vessels sufficiently to complete the required procedure. Jarrett et al.[26] reported a 7% incidence of a vessel injury when an access surgeon was utilized compared to a 2% incidence when the spine surgeon performed their own access. Bateman et al.[24] reported from their meta-analysis of complications related to anterior lumbar surgery, somewhat surprisingly, lower rates of reoperation, prosthesis-related complications, and neurologic injury but significantly higher rates of venous thrombosis when an access surgeon was utilized. The rates of venous thrombosis may be attributed to increased vessel manipulation and longer operation times.

While the incidence of vessel injuries overall is relatively low, at around 3%,[24] the consequence can be life-threatening. As such, developing and maintaining the exposure should be undertaken in such a way that if a vessel injury occurs it can be readily controlled and addressed. To this end, surgeons should not be performing this sort of surgery unless they have the skills to deal with complications as they arise, or have appropriate backup readily available should they need it.

Maintaining good exposure is paramount, and several table-mounted retraction systems exist to facilitate this. Become familiar with what is available in your hospital and if needed request the system that is most appropriate to your needs.

Being prepared also means having blood products available and/or cell saver systems for collection, filtration, and re-infusion of any blood lost. Direct repair of any vessel injury is ideal, but for minor vessel injuries simple packing and the use of clotting agents and patches may suffice. Having ties, vascular clips, sutures, and thrombotic agents readily available in the operating room or close by is also advisable. As you gain experience, items not needed often can be left off the operative field but should still be available in or close to the operating room.

As soon as a vessel injury is identified, immediate control is the priority. Once controlled, communicate with the anesthesiology team and operating room personnel to ensure everything that may be required is readily available. It may also pay to call for an extra pair of hands for suction or retraction to ensure the surgeon has two hands free to address the vessel injury.

Vessel injuries will usually occur during the exposure or placement of the implant and while it is preferable to address the injury as soon as possible, in some cases doing so may limit the ability to complete the planned procedure. Subject to the stability of the patient and control of the bleeding, packing or application of pressure on the bleeding site may allow completion of the disc clearance or resection and instrumentation prior to repairing the vessel defect. Vessel patches like TachoSil (Baxter, Deerfield, IL), a collagen sponge with human coagulation factors fibrinogen and thrombin, do not respond well to manipulation once secured so this sort of patch should be applied once the instrumentation is complete and the vessel is allowed to sit back in place without requiring further manipulation.

Rarely a vessel injury will be encountered where the procedure should be abandoned once the vessel has been repaired or patched, and this is a decision to be made by the surgical and anesthesiology teams together to ensure the safety of the patient.

Today there is also a range of endovascular tools available to control and address vessel injuries that most spine surgeons will not be familiar with or be able to utilize. For this reason, it is a good idea for any spine surgeon performing their own access to have a good working relationship with the vascular team in their hospital to provide assistance if required. For cases where difficulty is expected, asking a vascular or general surgeon to assist is also a good way to minimize the risk of complications.

Uretic or bladder injury is rare[24]; however, should a ureteric injury be identified, immediate direct repair and stent placement is best completed by a surgeon with expertise in this area. More commonly, ureteric complications result from ischemic injury due to dissection of the ureter from the investing retroperitoneal fat during the exposure, which compromises the supporting vasculature. Injury of this type is generally not apparent immediately but can lead to ureteric dilatation, an ischemic stricture formation, or rarely segmental ureteric necrosis. The ureter may also be caught beneath a retractor blade and compressed for the duration of the procedure. To avoid this, identify this structure early on in the exposure and pay attention to its location throughout the procedure.

Bladder injury is very rare and generally mitigated by the placement of an indwelling catheter preoperatively to decompress this structure and remove it from the operative field.

Bowel injury is more common during a transperitoneal approach, but can still occur when peritoneal defects are created and loops of bowel herniate into the operative field. In this situation, bowel may be caught beneath retractors leading to direct trauma or ischemia. When bowel herniates into the wound through a peritoneal defect, it is usually possible to repair the defect, but if this is not possible the use of a moist lap sponge over the bowel can protect the bowel and help preserve the operative field during completion of the procedure. If loops of bowel become dilated, placement of an orogastric or nasogastric tube will help decompress the bowel and make retraction easier. Small peritoneal defects are more likely to lead to problems due to bowel herniation than larger defects, so if a small defect cannot be repaired, small defects should be made larger. A bowel injury due to direct trauma or ischemia may not be evident immediately, so have a high index of suspicion following the development of abdominal complications in patients having undergone this approach.

Brau[11] reported **sympathetic dysfunction** as indicated by a warm ipsilateral lower limb in 8.8% of 686 anterior access cases performed over 3 years at all levels. However, a large number of these exposures were confined to L5-S1, and the incidence is closer to 25% for procedures undertaken at L4-5 and above.

It is good practice to identify the location of the sympathetic trunk in the gutter between the spine and the psoas muscle. This can usually be done by palpation prior to mobilizing the vessels. If the sympathetic trunk is not palpable, commence dissection close to the aorta and left common iliac artery and retract the vessels medially and the retroperitoneal fat in this area laterally. As tissues are mobilized, the sympathetic trunk will generally be evident laterally.

In the vast majority of cases, symptoms related to sympathetic irritation resolve over 2 to 3 months. The incidence of long-term sympathetic dysfunction, as indicated by vasodilatation, increased warmth, and **anhidrosis** of the affect limb, is very rare. Patients with a history of chronic regional pain syndrome or reflex sympathetic dystrophy may also experience exacerbations of these symptoms following anterior procedures to this region.

Lymphatic injury may not be recognized as a problem intraoperatively but can lead to a postoperative retroperitoneal seroma. Lymphatic channels typically lie along the common iliac artery and distal aorta and can be differentiated from vessels by their thin and translucent walls and clear contents. Lymph nodes may be evident along their path, and coagulation of these vessels will often suffice, but their walls can be friable and larger lymphatic vessels will not be occluded in this way. Use of ties or clips will certainly control the escape of lymphatic fluid but their use is rarely indicated. A simple way to avoid seroma formation is to create a peritoneal defect in the dorsal aspect of the peritoneal sack at the completion of the procedure to allow absorption of the lymphatic fluid through the peritoneum.

Vas deferens and round ligament are at risk during initial stages of the approach in the iliac fossa, usually when identifying and dividing the arcuate line of the posterior rectus sheath. By rolling the distal margin of posterior rectus sheath between your fingertips you can identify if a cord-like structure is evident. This indicates the presence of either of these structures and the need to gain access to the retroperitoneal space more proximally. While exposure of L5-S1 may be possible distal to these structures, their presence proximally will limit the proximal extent of the exposure as these structures should not be divided. Should injury to the vas deferens occur, repair should be undertaken in those wanting to preserve their fertility. In those of non-childbearing age, it may be sufficient to tie off this structure but seek advice from a urological colleague regarding how best to manage this situation should it occur.

Other intraoperative complications such as a **dural tear** when performing the anterior disc clearance may occur and require use of a nonsuturable dural patch, use of sealants such as DuraSeal (Integra, Princeton, NJ) the placement of a decompressive epidural catheter, and bedrest if direct repair is not feasible.

With a direct anterior approach, injury to the **lumbar plexus** in the psoas is unlikely, but the use of retractor systems placed around the lateral margin of the vertebra may cause injury or irritation to these structures. While the routine use of neural monitoring for anterior access cases is not recommended, it is important to be aware of these structures and take care when placing and manipulating retractors.

Retrograde ejaculation is caused by irritation or injury to the superior hypogastric plexus that lies just beneath the peritoneum and is closely related to the distal aorta and common iliac vessels. This plexus controls bladder sphincter control during ejaculation and injury results in ejaculate passing into the bladder rather than out the penis. While it does not render a male with this condition sterile, it does reduce fertility and has been a major concern for males of reproductive age when considering anterior surgery in the past. The risk of this complication is greatest with anterior exposure of the L5-S1 disc, and the incidence is 10-fold higher with a transperitoneal compared to a retroperitoneal approach. The incidence is accepted as being 2% to 3%,[24] and in at least 50% of cases resolution is expected after several months. The risk is reduced by careful mobilization of the peritoneum over the vessels and disc, staying close to the vessels and sweeping the peritoneum to the opposite side to expose the L5-S1 disc and median sacral vessels. It also pays to dissect vertically rather than transversely, and to avoid use of unipolar diathermy.

Carragee[27] suggested the rate of retrograde ejaculation was considerably increased when rhBMP-2 was used in the disc space, but this has failed to be supported by other reviews.[28,29]

Implant-related complications can occur and modern anterior cage and implant designs incorporate a myriad of surface technologies that enhance the stability and biologic features of these implants. Some have spikes or keels, others rough and abrasive surfaces that may catch and damage viscera as they are being manipulated into place. They may also catch and tether tissue, swabs, or lap sponges as the implant is positioned and secured. The retraction system chosen can help preserve an adequate window of exposure but remain vigilant as implants are being placed to avoid these issues. It is also advantageous if the access surgeon is familiar with the implants to be placed as there are different access requirements for many of the different implants utilized.

Postoperative Complications

Postoperative **ileus** is common and more prevalent with protracted anterior surgery, proximal lumbar exposure, and where large peritoneal defects have been created. This typically resolves within 12 to 24 hours but can rarely persist for several days. Management includes avoidance of oral intake and maintenance of hydration with IV fluids until audible bowel sounds or passage of flatus is confirmed.

A **superficial hematoma** may develop if the superficial epigastric vein or artery is injured during the initial exposure, closure, or placement of drains. If apparent, intraoperative bleeding should be controlled prior to closure. If these vessels are damaged by the placement or removal of a drain or bleeding develops as a result of anticoagulation, open drainage may be required, but placement of a percutaneous drain by interventional radiology will usually address the situation.

Deep **retroperitoneal hematomas** should be rare if all bleeding is controlled prior to closure. Where persistent bleeding is encountered, drain placement is recommended so as to track the progress of any bleed. Bleeding may also be initiated following commencement of anticoagulant therapy or increased venous pressure postoperatively and displacement of clips or ties. If bleeding persists or is problematic, re-exploration to evacuate the hematoma to address any ongoing bleeding may be indicated.

Seroma formation is usually the result of lymphatic injury, which has been discussed above. If not identified intraoperatively and if the collection is significant and persistent, the laparoscopic creation of a peritoneal defect will generally address this issue.

Superficial infection is seen in approximately 1% and **deep infection** in <0.1% of cases.[24] Superficial infections can be treated with appropriate wound care and antibiotics. Dehiscence is uncommon and usually only seen in patients with an obese and tense abdomen. **Reoperation** is required in this situation and the use of abdominal binders or mesh reinforcement may be indicated. Deep infection may not become evident for some time and when it occurs, depending on the organism and status of the patient, may be controlled medially. Where this is not the case, considerable challenges, which have been outlined previously, may be encountered during **reoperation.**

Incisional hernia formation was more common with approaches undertaken lateral to the rectus where failure of the fascial repair resulted in a direct route for peritoneal herniation through the defect. This complication is rare when utilizing an approach through the anterior rectus sheath medially and the posteriorly sheath laterally where the rectus muscle provides a barrier to peritoneal herniation.

Implant and **technique-related complications** can be encountered, and with any surgical procedure it is important to consider all risks associated with the procedure and balance them against the potential benefits. This includes considering revision strategies to address implant-related complications such as cage or implant displacement, subsidence, implant breakage, and nonunion. What are the risk of these complications, and can they be managed without having to perform a revision anterior exposure? Take into consideration the bone quality and the patient's age and comorbidities. Optimizing bone mineral density, careful endplate preparation, and implant sizing will help to avoid early endplate fracture of subsidence, but procedures like lumbar disc replacement is contraindicated, and "stand-alone" anterior fusion should be avoided in patients with poor bone quality. Supplemental posterior fusion should be considered if stability or bone quality is considered an issue.

Conclusion

Anterior spinal surgery offers an incredibly powerful means to address spinal pathology. Safe anterior spinal access and instrumentation is, however, reliant upon both the spinal surgeon and anterior access surgeon recognizing the limitations of the approach. Patient selection is probably the most important factor to ensure successful anterior spinal access. Having the necessary training and insight regarding your limitations is also important. A team approach, whereby the spinal and access surgeon understand the requirements and limitations of the approach, the nature of the patients' pathology and the surgical goals, and being prepared for any possible challenges will ensure safe anterior lumbar spinal surgery is performed.

References

1. Matur AV, Mejia-Munne JC, Plummer ZJ, Cheng JS, Prestigiacomo CJ. The history of anterior and lateral approaches to the lumbar spine. *World Neurosurg.* 2020;144:213–221.
2. Ito H, Tsuchiya J, Asami G. A new radical operation for Pott's disease: A report of ten cases. *JBJS.* 1934;16(3):499–515.
3. Burns BH. An operation for spondylolisthesis. *The Lancet.* 1933;1 (5728):1233.
4. Mercer W. Spondylolisthesis: With a description of a new method of operative treatment and notes of ten cases. *Edinb Med J.* 1936;43:545–572.
5. Southwick WO, Robinson RA. Surgical approaches to the vertebral bodies in the cervical and lumbar regions. *J Bone Joint Surg Am.* 1957;39-A:631–644.
6. Harmon PH. Anterior extraperitoneal lumbar disc excision and vertebral body fusion. *Clin Orthop Relat Res.* 1960;18: 169–198.
7. Hodgson AR, Stock FE, Fang HS, Ong GB. Anterior spinal fusion. The operative approach and pathological findings in 412 patients with Pott's disease of the spine. *Br J Surg.* 1960;48: 172–178.
8. Hodgson AR, Wong SK. A description of a technic and evaluation of results in anterior spinal fusion for deranged intervertebral disc and spondylolisthesis. *Clin Orthop Relat Res.* 1968;56: 133–162.
9. Fraser RD, Gogan WJ. A modified muscle-splitting approach to the lumbosacral spine. *Spine.* 1992;17:943–948.
10. Mayer HM. A new microsurgical technique for minimally invasive anterior lumbar interbody fusion. *Spine.* 1997;22:691–700.
11. Brau SA. Mini-open approach to the spine for anterior lumbar interbody fusion: Description of the procedure, results and complications. *Spine J.* 2002;2(3):216–223.
12. Roy-Camille R, Saillant G, Mazel C. Internal fixation of the lumbar spine with pedicle screw plating. *Clin Orthop Relat Res.* 1986;203:7–17.
13. Steffee RD, Biscup RS, Sitkowski DJ. Segmental spine plates with pedicle screw fixation: A new internal fixation device for disorders of the lumbar and thoracolumbar spine. *Clin Orthop Relat Res.* 1986;203:45–53.
14. Cotrel Y, Dubousset J, Guillaumat M. New universal instrumentation in spinal surgery. *Clin Orthop Relat Res.* 1988;227:10–23.

15. Buttner-Janz K, Schellnack K, Zippel H. Biomechanics of the SB Charite lumbar intervertebral disc prosthesis. *Int Orthop.* 1989;13:173–176.
16. Tropiano P, Huang R, Girardi FP, Marnay T. Lumbar disc replacement: Preliminary results with ProDisc II after a minimum follow-up period of 1 year. *J Spinal Disord Tech.* 2003; 16(4):362–368.
17. Cain CMJ, Schleicher P, Gerlach R, Pflugmacher R, Scholz M, Kandziora F. A new stand-alone anterior lumbar interbody fusion device: Biomechanical comparison with established fixation techniques. *Spine.* 2005;30(23):2631–2636.
18. Bassani R, Morselli C, Querenghi AM, Nuara A, Sconfienza LM, Peretti GM. Functional and radiological outcome of anterior retroperitoneal versus posterior transforaminal interbody fusion in the management of single-level lumbar degenerative disease. *Neurosurg Focus.* 2020;49(3):E2.
19. Bozzio AE, Johnson CR, Fattor JA, Kleck CJ, Patel VV, Burger EL, Noshchenko A, Cain CMJ. Stand-alone anterior lumbar interbody, transforaminal lumbar interbody, and anterior/posterior fusion: Analysis of fusion outcomes and costs. *Orthopedics.* 2018;41(5):e655–e662.
20. Patel N, Bagan B, Vadera S, Maltenfort MG, Deutsch H, Vaccaro A, Harrop J, Sharan A, Ratliff J. Obesity and spine surgery: relation to perioperative complications. *J Neurosurg Spine.* 2007;6(4):291–297.
21. Peng CW, Bendo JA, Goldstein JA, Nalbandian MM. Perioperative outcomes of anterior lumbar sugery in obese versus non-obese patients. *Spine J.* 2009;9(9):715–720.
22. Ng JP, Scott-Young M, Chan DN, Oh JY. The feasibility of anterior spinal access: The vascular corridor at the L5-S1 level for anterior lumbar interbody fusion. *Spine (Phila Pa 1976).* 2021; 46(15):983–989.
23. Barrey C, Ene B, Louis-Tisserand G, Montagna P, Perrin G, Simon E. Vascular anatomy in the lumbar spine investigated by three-dimensional computed tomography angiography: the concept of vascular window. *World Neurosurg.* 2013;79(5-6): 784–791.
24. Bateman DK, Millhouse PW, Shahi N, Kadam AB, Maltenfort MG, Koerner JD, Vaccaro AR. Anterior lumbar spine surgery: A systemic review and meta-analysis of associated complications. *Spine J.* 2015;15:1118–1132.
25. Labbe R, Lindsay T, Walker PM. The extent and distribution of skeletal muscle necrosis after graded periods of complete ischemia. *J Vasc Surg.* 1987;6(2):152–157.
26. Jarrett CD, Heller JG, Tsai L. Anterior exposure of the lumbar spine with and without an "access surgeon": morbidity analysis of 265 consecutive cases. *J Spinal Disord Tech.* 2009;22(8): 559–564.
27. Carragee EJ, Hurwitz EL, Weiner BK. A critical review of recombinant human bone morphogenic protein-2 trials in spinal surgery: emerging safety concerns and lessons learned. *Spine J.* 2011;11:471–491.
28. Lindley EM, McBeth ZL, Henry SE, et al. Retrograde ejaculation after anterior lumbar spine surgery. *Spine.* 2012;37:1785–1789.
29. Tepper G, Rabbani R, Yousefzadeh M, Prince D. Quantitative assessment of retrograde ejaculation using semen analysis, comparison with a standardized quantitative questionnaire, and investigating the impact of rhBMP-2. *Spine.* 2013;38(10): 841–845.

22

Lateral Approach Related Complications

SHANE BURCH AND JENNIFER MARIE O'DONNELL

CHAPTER OUTLINE

Lateral approaches to the spine have been described since the late 1990s and have provided novel and more muscle-sparing approaches to the spine. With these new methods, they bring new potential complications and challenges. These include complications related to the muscles: the abdominal wall muscles that have to be split and the psoas that has to be split or retracted; the nerves: the nerves on the surface of the psoas, the lumbar plexus that runs through the psoas, and the exiting nerve roots in the foramina; and the vessels: the segmental arteries and veins, and the great vessels. While there are many dangers associated with this approach, careful planning and meticulous technique can help avoid all of them.

Background

Lateral approaches to the spine can be divided into either a transpsoas or antepsoas approach. Each carry potential complications as well as advantages. The transpsoas approach has been utilized since 1998 and first described by Pimenta in 2001[1] and was then published by Bergey et al. in 2004.[2] The extreme lateral interbody fusion approach, or XLIF, the technique as it is performed currently with approach specific retractors, was described by Ozgur in 2006.[3]

The antepsoas approach was first described by Mayer as the anterior oblique lateral interbody fusion in 1997[4] as a modification on the direct anterior approach. Both transpsoas and antepsoas lateral approaches have become increasingly utilized, and the goal is to place a cage from lateral in the desired anterior-posterior plane of the vertebral body. Typically, the transpsoas approach relies on palpation and neuromonitoring to avoid neural structures with limited direct visualization. In contrast the antepsoas approach relies on direct visualization and may be utilized without neuromonitoring. The transpsoas approach splits the psoas muscle to access the disc while the antepsoas approach docks a retractor anterior to the psoas and reflects the psoas posteriorly. Both approaches advocate for placement of the cages in a direct lateral trajectory.

It is important to be aware of the structures at risk during these approaches and therefore the possible complications. The approach utilizes a muscle splitting approach dissecting through the external oblique, internal oblique, and transversus abdominus (Fig. 22.1). When developing the plane between the internal and external oblique muscles, the ilioinguinal and iliohypogastric nerves can be identified. These peripheral nerves also travel within the retroperitoneal space and can on occasion be palpated. Once in the retroperitoneal space the genitofemoral nerve can be identified upon the psoas muscle. The lateral femoral cutaneous nerve (LFCN) is also traveling across the surgical field in these approaches. The psoas muscle itself is of course at risk for damage and trauma, more commonly when using the transpsoas approach that directly violates the muscle. The ureters lie on the undersurface of the transversalis fascia and cross the posterior one-third of the upper lumbar vertebrae, as described in the cadaveric study by Voin et al.[5] Usually, the ureter is reflected anteriorly during an antepsoas approach, similar to an anterior retroperitoneal approach.

The sympathetic chain lies on the anterior lateral aspect of the vertebral body and can also be visualized anterior to the psoas. The aorta and inferior vena cava run along the anterior aspect of the spine and can be visualized with careful dissection. Segmental arteries lying along the vertebrae can also be visualized with careful dissection. The iliolumbar vein can also be a sizeable vessel and is often interdigitated with lumbar nerve roots; it can be encountered in both ante- and transpsoas approaches.[6]

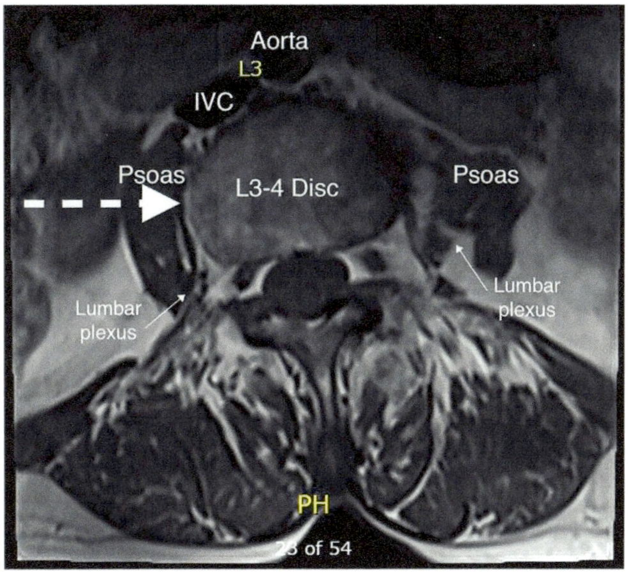

• **Fig. 22.1** An axial image of L3-4 disc showing the lateral transpsoas approach and relevant anatomy.

Anatomic studies have demonstrated the proximity of the plexus in relation to the vertebral body and psoas.[7,8] The lumbar plexus is comprised of nerve roots from L1-L4, with some contribution from T12 as well. The ilioinguinal nerve branches from the anterior ramus of L1 and innervates the scrotum and base of the penis or the labia majora and mons pubis and the upper medial thigh. The iliohypogastric nerve is also a branch of L1 and provides sensation over the lateral gluteal skin. Both the ilioinguinal and iliohypogastric nerves contribute motor function to the internal oblique and transversalis abdominus muscles. Abdominal pseudohernia ("abdominal pooching") may occur if these nerves are injured during the approach. This leads to asymmetry of the abdominal wall. A case of incisional hernia was described by Galan et al.[9] They advised that careful repair of tranversalis fascia avoids this.

Davis et al. described the changes in position of the lumbar plexus at different levels based off of their study of cadavers.[8] Specifically, as one moves distal the lumbar plexus is more anterior. This makes the safe window narrower until it is no longer possible to place an interbody cage through the psoas at the L4-5 level. At the L4-5 level, the femoral nerve was encountered in most specimens. Additionally, the impact of retractor blades and retractor time on the plexus may contribute to a neuropraxia or other injury. Caution must be taken at the more distal levels.

The genitofemoral nerve has genital and femoral branches. It originates from L1 and L2 off the lumbar plexus and supplies sensation of the upper thigh and the mons pubis or scrotum. Injury to these nerves can lead to pain or numbness in the penis, scrotum, or vagina. Finally, the LFCN arises from the lumbar plexus from the L2 and L3 nerve roots and supplies sensation over the anterior and lateral proximal thigh. The LFCN supplies no motor function. The use of neuromonitoring is crucial in understanding the proximity and safety of any nerves in the transpsoas approach.[10] Triggered electromyography (EMG) can provide real-time direct threshold responses to the surgeon, allowing them to safely place retractors. Additional techniques include motor-evoked potentials (MEPs) and somatosensory-evoked potentials (SSEPs) of the saphenous nerve.[11]

In the lateral approach, anterior releases must be performed carefully as well. An anterior annulotomy can be performed sharply, and one must be cautious of penetrating across to the contralateral psoas muscle.[12] Complications from this including psoas seromas, hematomas, and motor deficits have been described.[13,14] The proximity of the great vessels increases the risk to vascular injuries as well. It is important to fully release the annulus and anterior longitudinal ligament as needed, to allow for an interbody cage that spans the full width.

In addition to complications specific to the lateral approach, there are the generalizable complications of spinal fusion, including pseudoarthrosis, implant subsidence, wound complications, and adjacent segment disease. Complications associated with these approaches can be exacerbated by patient body habitus.[15]

Overall complication rates of the transpsoas and antepsoas approaches vary widely in the literature, as many do not include certain side effects such as psoas irritation as complications. This is a substantial limitation to the literature and to determining the actual rates of these complications. With the transpsoas approach, Rodgers et al. reports a complication rate of 6.2%, while others have reports as high as 52% when including transient nerve symptoms.[16–18] With the antepsoas lateral approach, intraoperative complication rates have been reported as 1.5% and postoperatively as 9.9%.[19,20] Again, these may be even higher when including known side effects such as transient psoas irritation or nerve symptoms.

General Complications

Complications of interbody fusions include cage subsidence, adjacent segment disease, pseudoarthrosis or nonunion, and lack of relief from the indirect decompression provided. Additional surgical complications such as need for blood transfusion, infection, or damage to nearby structures are seen as well, with any approach.

With all interbody fusions, there is concern for subsidence of the cages into the endplates. Careful endplate preparation without violating subchondral bone can help to avoid this. Pimenta first cautioned of subsidence with lateral approaches in 2011, and the first prospective randomized study of transpsoas versus transforaminal lumbar interbody fusion, in 2009 by Isaacs et al., found that subsidence rates were significantly lower than a transforaminal (TLIF) approach.[21] A recent systematic review found a rate of cage subsidence of 10.3%.[22,23] The same study found reoperation rate for subsidence was 2.7%.[22]

Other reasons for reoperation noted include adjacent segment disease, pseudoarthrosis, and inadequate relief from indirect decompression. These results are common to all approaches, but it is important to examine whether the lateral approach is associated with increased rates of occurrence. For the lateral transpsoas approach, Walker et al. found in a 2019 meta-analysis a rate of 7.5% for pseudarthrosis.[24] Rates of pseudarthrosis have been shown to be 3.6% for the lumbar antepsoas approach, with only half of these patients being symptomatic, and a 0.9% reoperation rate for pseudarthrosis in one study.[25] Higher rates of pseudarthrosis were seen with smokers and it was most common at the L5-S1 level.

Lateral Transpsoas Complications

The most common complications associated with the lateral transpsoas technique are neurological deficits, with the majority of these being transient. The rates are as high at 30% to 40% but range in the literature from 0% to 75% prevalence.[26] Postoperative thigh symptoms, ranging from paresthesia to hypoesthesia, pain, numbness, and weakness can come from multiple sources. The iliopsoas muscle itself is irritated during surgery, and thus weakness can be present. This is most common when operating on the L4-5 level due to the position of the plexus in relation to the middle of the disc. Paresthesia in the thigh is most common when working at the L1-2 level. Overall, sensory deficits are more common than motor weakness.

Between the antepsoas and transpsoas approaches, there are higher rates of hip flexor weakness and temporary sensory deficits with the transpsoas approach, as studied by Walker et al. in 2019.[24]

The sensory nerves discussed, including LFCN, genitofemoral, ilioinguinal, and iliohypogastric nerves, can also be irritated or develop a postoperative neuropraxia. Retractor placement can contribute to neuropraxia; retractor time and dimensions have both been associated with symptomatic neuropraxia.[27] Prevention of frank nerve injury can be achieved with intraoperative monitoring, using less than 5 milliamps as a level, which indicates direct contact of the dilators with a nerve. Between 5 and 10 indicates close proximity.[3] Rates of sensory nerve symptoms range from 0% and 75%, with permanent symptoms in 62%.[28] The LFCN is symptomatic and results in meralgia paresthetica in 12.5% to 25% of patients.[28]

Lateral Antepsoas Complications

When approaching the spine anterior to the psoas, the sympathetic chain lies in the anterior one-third of the vertebral body and is vulnerable with this approach. Kim et al.[29] reported a prevalence of sympathetic chain injury of 13.4% for antepsoas approaches at L4-5, but this is likely underestimated as findings are subtle and diagnosis can be missed.

In total, Tannoury et al. showed the complication rate associated with antepsoas approach as 8.2%.[30] The most common complications from their study included anterior thigh pain (1.3%) and persistent paresthesias (2.6%). Complications were associated with smokers, age greater than 65 years, and more than three levels fused.[30]

Major Complications

Beyond the most common complications, one must be aware of the complications that are the most dangerous and problematic. The lateral approaches can place the surgeon in a difficult situation, as any serious complication is difficult to treat while in a lateral position. Awareness and quick recognition will allow the surgeon to manage these more readily.

In the transpsoas approach, a dreaded complication is visceral injury, such as perforation of the small bowel.[31] The rate of this was reported as 0.08% in a study of nearly 13,000 cases.[32] The rate has ranged from 0.03% to as high as 12.5% (1 in a series of n = 8).[16,33] Bowel injury can present insidiously, for example as postop nausea or vomiting. In a case series of bowel injuries secondary to lateral approaches, laparotomies were necessary for 6 of these 11 patients.[31] While the rate of this complication is small, the consequences can be quite significant. Transitional anatomy with a high bifurcation of the iliac vessels should be considered when choosing the appropriate approach to access the anterior aspect of the spine. Not considering these anatomical variants may lead to injury of vascular structures.

Another serious but rare complication is vascular injury. The rate of these has been reported as ranging from 0% to 0.4%.[24,33,34] Fatal complication with vascular injury from XLIF was first described by Assina et al.[35] Case reports have described superior mesenteric or celiac artery compression syndromes.[36] The common iliac vein can be injured as well, typically requiring stenting or direct repair.[37] Vascular injuries reported in the literature can be fatal, highly morbid resulting in hemorrhagic shock, and many can be treated with vascular interventions.[28,35] These vascular complications are rare but must be recognized and treated urgently. Careful review of preoperative imaging must be performed to minimize the risk.[38]

Wound infections are much less prevalent with the lateral approaches, as these incisions tend to be much smaller than standard posterior approaches. The rate of deep and superficial wound infection has been 0.14% and 0.27%, respectively, as shown by Uribe et al. amongst 13,000 patients.[32]

The ureters are at risk in these approaches as well. Anatomic studies have shown the ureters to be more at risk in women and at the lower lumbar levels.[39,40] Rates of ureteral injury have been reported from 0.1% to 0.3%.[33] This injury can be subtle and can even go unnoticed intraoperatively, as described in some case reports.[39] Additional rare complications have been reported as case studies. Chang et al. reported the incidence of a ventral dural tear.[41]

In addition to the use of intraoperative neuromonitoring, complication rates in the lateral approach can be minimized with navigation.[42] Navigation can increase imaging accuracy and reduce radiation exposure.[43]

Conclusions

The lateral approaches to the spine, both transpsoas and antepsoas, allow for a minimally invasive interbody fusion. This can yield better results, with faster recovery and less blood loss.[44] The transpsoas approach relies on intraoperative neuromonitoring, either with triggered EMG, MEPs, or SSEPs to safely place retractors without direct injury to the nearby nerves including the lumbar plexus. The antepsoas approach relies on direct visualization to safely place retractors. Transpsoas can allow for large interbody cages to be placed, but antepsoas has less psoas muscle irritation and lumbar plexus injuries. Both lateral approaches can have rare but serious complications such as visceral or vascular injuries, and understanding of the anatomy is paramount to avoiding these. Further development of the equipment and technologies such as navigation assistance and neuromonitoring can continue to improve the ease, safety, and accuracy of these approaches for spine surgery.

References

1. Pimenta L, ed. Lateral endoscopic transpsoas retroperitoneal approach for lumbar spine surgery. VIII Brazilian Spine Society Meeting; 2001: Belo Horizonte, Minas Gerais Brazil.
2. Bergey DL, Villavicencio AT, Goldstein T, Regan JJ. Endoscopic lateral transpsoas approach to the lumbar spine. *Spine*. 2004;29 (15):1681–168.
3. Ozgur BM, Aryan HE, Pimenta L, Taylor WR. Extreme lateral interbody fusion (XLIF): a novel surgical technique for anterior lumbar interbody fusion. *Spine J*. 2006;6(4):435–443.
4. Mayer MH. A new microsurgical technique for minimally invasive anterior lumbar interbody fusion. *Spine*. 1997;22(6):691–699.
5. Voin V, Kirkpatrick C, Alonso F, Rustagi T, Sanders FH, Drazin D, et al. Lateral transpsoas approach to the lumbar spine and relationship of the ureter: anatomic study with application to minimizing complications. *World Neurosurg*. 2017;104: 674–678.
6. Davis M, Jenkins S, Bordes S, Iwanaga J, Loukas M, Uribe J, et al. Iliolumbar vein: Anatomy and surgical importance during lateral transpsoas and oblique approaches to lumbar spine. *World Neurosurg*. 2019;128:e768–e772.
7. Uribe JS, Arredondo N, Dakwar E, Vale FL. Defining the safe working zones using the minimally invasive lateral retroperitoneal transpsoas approach: an anatomical study. *J Neurosurg Spine*. 2010;13(2):260–266.
8. Davis TT, Bae HW, Mok MJM, Rasouli A, Delamarter RB. Lumbar plexus anatomy within the psoas muscle: implications for the transpsoas lateral approach to the L4-L5 disc. *J Bone Joint Surg Am*. 2011;93(16):1482–1487.
9. Galan TV, Mohan V, Klineberg EO, Gupta MC, Roberto RF, Ellwitz JP. Case report: incisional hernia as a complication of extreme lateral interbody fusion. *Spine J*. 2012;12(4):e1–e6.
10. Cheng I, Acosta F, Chang K, Pham M. Point-counterpoint: The use of neuromonitoring in lateral transpsoas surgery. *Spine (Phila Pa 1976)*. 2016;41(Suppl 8):S145–S151.
11. Alluri R, Mok JK, Vaishnav A, Shelby T, Sivaganesan A, Hah R, et al. Intraoperative neuromonitoring during lateral lumbar interbody fusion. *Neurospine*. 2021;18(3):430–436.
12. Kwon B, Kim DH. Lateral lumbar interbody fusion: Indications, outcomes, and complications. *J Am Acad Orthop Surg*. 2016; 24(2):96–105.
13. Taher F, Hughes AP, Lebl DR, Sama AA, Pumberger M, Aichmair A, et al. Contralateral motor deficits after lateral lumbar interbody fusion. *Spine (Phila Pa 1976)*. 2013;38(22):1959–1963.
14. Taher F, Lebl DR, Hughes AP, Girardi FP. Contralateral psoas seroma after transpsoas lumbar interbody fusion with bone morphogenetic protein-2 implantation. *Spine J*. 2013;13(2):e1–e5.
15. Xi Z, Burch S, Mummaneni PV, Mayer RR, Eichler C, Chou D. The effect of obesity on perioperative morbidity in oblique lumbar interbody fusion. *J Neurosurg Spine*. 2020:1–8.
16. Tormenti MJ, Maserati MB, Bonfield CM, Okonkwo DO, Kanter AS. Complications and radiographic correction in adult scoliosis following combined transpsoas extreme lateral interbody fusion and posterior pedicle screw instrumentation. *Neurosurg Focus*. 2010;28(3):E7.
17. Rodgers WB, Gerber EJ, Patterson J. Intraoperative and early postoperative complications in extreme lateral interbody fusion: an analysis of 600 cases. *Spine*. 2011;36(1):26–32.
18. Regev GJ, Kim CW. Safety and the anatomy of the retroperitoneal lateral corridor with respect to the minimally invasive lateral lumbar intervertebral fusion approach. *Neurosurg Clin N Am*. 2014;25(2):211–218.
19. Li JXJ, Phan K, Mobbs R. Oblique lumbar interbody fusion: technical aspects, operative outcomes, and complications. *World Neurosurg*. 2017;98:113–123.
20. Silvestre C, Mac-Thiong J-M, Hilmi R, Roussouly P. Complications and morbidities of mini-open anterior retroperitoneal lumbar interbody fusion: oblique lumbar interbody fusion in 179 patients. *Asian Spine J*. 2012;6(2):89.
21. Isaacs RE, Sembrano JN, Tohmeh AG. Two-year comparative outcomes of MIS lateral and MIS transforaminal interbody fusion in the treatment of degenerative spondylolisthesis. *Spine*. 2016;41(1):S133–S144.
22. Macki M, Anand SK, Surapaneni A, Park P, Chang V. Subsidence rates after lateral lumbar interbody fusion: a systematic review. *World Neurosurg*. 2019;122:599–606.
23. Pimenta L, Marchi L, Coutinho E, Oliveira L, editors. A comparative study on cage subsidence following standalone lateral interbody fusion. Proceedings of the 4th Annual SOLAS Research Meeting; 2011.
24. Walker CT, Farber SH, Cole TS, Xu DS, Godzik J, Whiting AC, et al. Complications for minimally invasive lateral interbody arthrodesis: a systematic review and meta-analysis comparing prepsoas and transpsoas approaches. *J Neurosurg Spine*. 2019;30(4):446–460.
25. Tannoury C, Bhale R, Vora M, Saade A, Kortbawi R, Orlando G, et al. Pseudarthrosis following lumbar and lumbosacral fusion using the antepsoas technique. *Spine*. 2021;46(24):1690–1695.
26. Epstein NE. Review of risks and complications of extreme lateral interbody fusion (XLIF). *Surg Neurol Int*. 2019;10:237.
27. Uribe JS, Isaacs RE, Youssef JA, Khajavi K, Balzer JR, Kanter AS, et al. Can triggered electromyography monitoring throughout retraction predict postoperative symptomatic neuropraxia after XLIF? Results from a prospective multicenter trial. *Eur Spine J*. 2015;24(Suppl 3):378–385.
28. Epstein NE. Extreme lateral lumbar interbody fusion: Do the cons outweigh the pros? *Surg Neurol Int*. 2016;7(Suppl 25): S692–S700.
29. Kim J-S, Choi WG, Lee S-H. Minimally invasive anterior lumbar interbody fusion followed by percutaneous pedicle screw

fixation for isthmic spondylolisthesis: minimum 5-year follow-up. *Spine J.* 2010;10(5):404–409.
30. Tannoury T, Kempegowda H, Haddadi K, Tannoury C. Complications associated with minimally invasive anterior to the psoas (ATP) fusion of the lumbosacral spine. *Spine.* 2019;44 (19):E1122–E1129.
31. Balsano M, Carlucci S, Ose M, Boriani L. A case report of a rare complication of bowel perforation in extreme lateral interbody fusion. *Eur Spine J.* 2015;24(3):405–408.
32. Uribe JS, Deukmedjian AR. Visceral, vascular, and wound complications following over 13,000 lateral interbody fusions: a survey study and literature review. *Eur Spine J.* 2015;24(3):386–396.
33. Fujibayashi S, Kawakami N, Asazuma T, Ito M, Mizutani J, Nagashima H, et al. Complications associated with lateral interbody fusion: nationwide survey of 2998 cases during the first 2 years of its use in Japan. *Spine.* 2017;42(19):1478–1484.
34. Epstein NE. Incidence of major vascular injuries with extreme lateral interbody fusion (XLIF). *Surg Neurol Int.* 2020;11:70.
35. Assina R, Majmundar NJ, Herschman Y, Heary RF. First report of major vascular injury due to lateral transpsoas approach leading to fatality: case report. *J Neurosurg Spine.* 2014;21(5):794–798.
36. Kotani T, Sakuma T, Iijima Y, et al. Acute celiac artery compression syndrome with superior mesenteric artery stenosis and aortic stenosis: A rare but life-threatening complication after adult spinal deformity surgery. *J Orthop Sci.* 2023;28(2):490–493.
37. Buric J, Bombardieri D. Direct lesion and repair of a common iliac vein during XLIF approach. *Eur Spine J.* 2016;25(1): 89–93.
38. Sakai T, Tezuka F, Wada K, et al. Risk management for avoidance of major vascular injury due to lateral transpsoas approach. *Spine.* 2016;41(5):450–453.
39. Lee H-J, Kim J-S, Ryu K-S, Park CK. Ureter injury as a complication of oblique lumbar interbody fusion. *World Neurosurg.* 2017;102693e7-e14.
40. Kagami Y, Nakashima H, Satake K, Ito K, Tanaka S, Segi N, et al. Assessment of ureters at dangerous locations in lateral lumbar interbody fusion. *Spine Surg Relat Res.* 2022;6(1): 38–44.
41. Chang J, Kim J-S, Jo H. Ventral dural injury after oblique lumbar interbody fusion. *World Neurosurg.* 2017;98:881 e1–e4.
42. Xi Z, Chou D, Mummaneni PV, Burch S. The navigated oblique lumbar interbody fusion: accuracy rate, effect on surgical time, and complications. *Neurospine.* 2020;17(1):260–267.
43. Sembrano JN, Yson SC, Theismann JJ. Computer navigation in minimally invasive spine surgery. *Curr Rev Musculoskeletal Med.* 2019;12(4):415–424.
44. Xi Z, Chou D, Mummaneni PV, et al. Anterior lumbar compared to oblique lumbar interbody approaches for multilevel fusions to the sacrum in adults with spinal deformity and degeneration. *J Neurosurg Spine.* 2020:1–10.

23

Posterior Approach Related Complications

GASTON CAMINO-WILLHUBER, JUSTIN P. CHAN, SOHAIB HASHMI, YU-PO LEE, AND NITIN BHATIA

CHAPTER OUTLINE

Introduction

Despite the increasing popularity of lateral and anterior approaches to the lumbar spine, the posterior approach remains the gold standard for many conditions. Posterior approach related complications range from wound complications such as incision dehiscence and surgical site infections to deeper fluid accumulations including seromas and epidural hematomas. Patient risk factors such as nutritional status, smoking, and other medical comorbidities are major contributors to the overall complication risk, but surgical technique including hemostasis and operative time also plays a role.

Surgical Site Infections

Postoperative surgical site infections (SSI) are relatively common complications that all spine surgeons will encounter, making effective diagnosis and treatment paramount.

Despite a focused effort to improve infection control including preoperative patient optimization, antibiotic prophylaxis, aseptic technique, and the advent of minimally invasive spine surgery, postoperative infections still represent a significant cause of morbidity, readmission, prolonged hospital stay, and health costs in spine surgery.[1–4] They also remain one of the leading causes of hospital-acquired infections along with urinary tract infection and pneumonia.[4] Moreover, postoperative spinal infections have been associated with a threefold increase in hospital length of stay after elective spine surgery,[3] as well as increased pseudarthrosis rates after lumbar fusion surgery.[5] Less frequently, infections following spine surgery can also lead to devastating consequences including neurological compromise, sepsis, and even death.

Classification

The Centers for Disease Control and Prevention (CDC) classifies SSIs into three categories: superficial, deep, and organ space.[6] Superficial SSIs involve skin and subcutaneous tissues above the thoracolumbar fascia and are commonly accompanied by purulent drainage, positive drain cultures, or signs of skin infection such as redness, swelling, or pain. Deep SSIs affect fascial and subfascial muscle layers and are associated with purulent drainage, abscess formation, and positive drain cultures (Fig. 23.1). Organ space SSIs occur deep to the muscle and fascia but share the same criteria as deep infections. SSIs usually occur within 30 days of the index surgery; however, in cases of spinal instrumentation the window of time may be up to 1 year.[3]

Risk Factors

Numerous risk factors have been reported in the development of postoperative wound infection. These can be classified as patient-related factors such as poor nutritional status, smoking, and obesity. In particular, albumin levels have been shown to be a good predictor of nutritional status

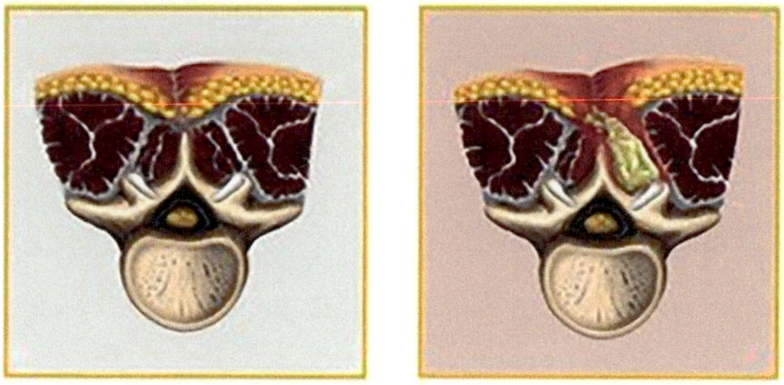

• **Fig. 23.1** Illustration of the most common surgical site infections. Superficial infections do not compromise the fascial layer and usually can be treated with antibiotics; deep infections account below the fascia and are usually treated by irrigation and debridement.

and hypoalbuminemia has been associated with higher rates of infection and dehiscence due to the delayed wound healing process.[7] Other factors can also be classified as surgery-related factors such as surgery duration, blood loss, use of instrumentation, and surgeon experience.

Posterior Approach

Compared with anterior approaches in spine surgery, the posterior approach has been shown to have increased rates of surgical site infections. Wimmer et al. observed significantly higher rates of SSI after posterior approaches among 850 patients treated with instrumented fusion.[8] In a recent systematic review, Zhou et al. found that incidence of SSI after posterior approaches was more than twice that of anterior approaches (5% vs 2.3%).[9]

Diagnosis

As there is no universally accepted diagnostic criteria for SSI, a combination of clinical, laboratory, and radiological parameters are required. Persistent wound drainage is one of the most common clinical signs, whereas the most reliable laboratory marker is the elevated C-reactive protein. Persistent elevations in other parameters such as white blood cell count and erythrocyte sedimentation rate (ESR) can also be suspicious for infection. Imaging studies can be helpful for identifying an abscess, but are difficult to interpret during the early postoperative period due to postsurgical changes. Clinical evaluation remains the most important diagnostic tool and is supplemented by laboratory markers.

Treatment

Standard treatment for surgical site infections consists of deep wound cultures with open irrigation and debridement followed by broad-spectrum antibiotic therapy that can later be fine-tuned according to culture results. A recent systematic review performed by Khan et al.[10] found that for infections after fusion procedures, most surgeons employ early wound irrigation and debridement with or without negative pressure wound therapy and retain implants except in refractory cases where implant removal is necessary to eradicate infection. The most common antibiotic treatment plan includes 6 weeks of culture-directed intravenous antibiotics. In a prospective study with 85 patients, Fernandez-Gerlinger et al.[11] demonstrated good outcomes in 91% of infections treated with 6 weeks of intravenous antibiotics, and noted that in most cases of treatment failure, the infection was caused by anaerobic bacteria.

Wound Dehiscence

Wound dehiscence represents another significant cause of reoperation and readmission after posterior spine surgery. Albumin is considered to play a critical role in the normal wound healing process, and hypoalbuminemia has been shown to increase the rate of postoperative complications, unplanned readmission, and hospital stay.[12–15] This is likely due to poor nutritional status and inflammation impairing the wound healing process.[16] He et al.[17] has also demonstrated a significant association between low albumin levels and wound dehiscence in 554 patients that underwent single-level posterior lumbar fusion surgery.

Some studies have shown decreased rates of wound dehiscence after fusion surgery when negative pressure wound therapy (NPWT) is used routinely.[18] One retrospective study by Akhter et al. found decreased rates of superficial wound dehiscence, infection, and revision rates when NPWT was used instead of standard dressings.[19] NPWT has long been used to treat soft tissue defects and open wounds but has increasingly been used over closed wounds to decrease the risk of seroma formation and wound infection.[20] NPWT works by increasing local blood flow and angiogenesis, as well as causing accumulation of beneficial growth factors and removing excess interstitial fluid. Additionally, the closed sealing effect provides a barrier to bacterial growth and physically helps maintain wound edge approximation.[21,22] Despite proven benefits in the trauma, orthopaedic, and vascular surgery literature,[23–25] indications for the use of NPWT in spine surgery still have not been clearly defined.

Treatment

Large wound dehiscence can present a significant risk for infection and should be treated with surgical exploration and wound closure under sterile conditions in the operating room. Smaller, superficial wound dehiscence may be amenable to a trial of nonoperative management and healing by second-intention healing in the reliable patient that can be closely monitored. There are no clear evidence-based guidelines on the size or depth of wound dehiscence that need to be treated operatively versus nonoperatively.

Symptomatic Postoperative Epidural Hematoma

Postoperative epidural hematomas are rare complications but can cause significant morbidity with devastating consequences if not properly treated. First described by Jackson in 1969,[26] a spinal epidural hematoma is an accumulation of blood in the epidural space that can cause mechanical compression of the spinal cord or cauda equina (Fig. 23.2). A recent study using the American College of Surgeons National Surgical Quality Improvement Program (NSQIP) database found the incidence of epidural hematomas after elective cervical spine surgery to be 0.48%.[27] They also found that male gender, revision surgery, dural tear, prolonged operative time, perioperative transfusion, bleeding disorders, and American Society of Anesthesiologists (ASA) physical status classification 3–5 were significant risk factors.[27] In the lumbar spine, Knusel et al.[28] found an incidence of 0.27% after posterior elective lumbar surgery in 75,878 patients. In half of the cases, symptoms associated with the epidural hematoma presented within the first 5 days postoperatively. The authors also found that increased age, obesity, multilevel surgery, perioperative transfusion, and dural tear repair were risk factors. Although symptomatic epidural hematomas are rare, the resultant cord compression can cause bowel and bladder dysfunction, saddle anesthesia, motor weakness, and increased pain.

Physical exam remains the most important way to quickly detect neurologic changes, but MRI is the gold standard for diagnosis of spinal cord compression and can differentiate between recurrent disc herniation, epidural abscesses or hematomas, and cerebrospinal fluid (CSF) leakage. The MRI features of an epidural hematoma change over time due to hemoglobin oxidation. They are typically hypointense on both T1- and T2-weighted images during the first 24 hours. During days 1 to 3, they can then become isointense in T1 and hypointense in T2-weighted images as deoxyhemoglobin is converted to methemoglobin, increasing the T1 intensity. After 2 weeks, the presence of ferritin and hemosiderin causes them to become T1 and T2 hypointense once again.[29]

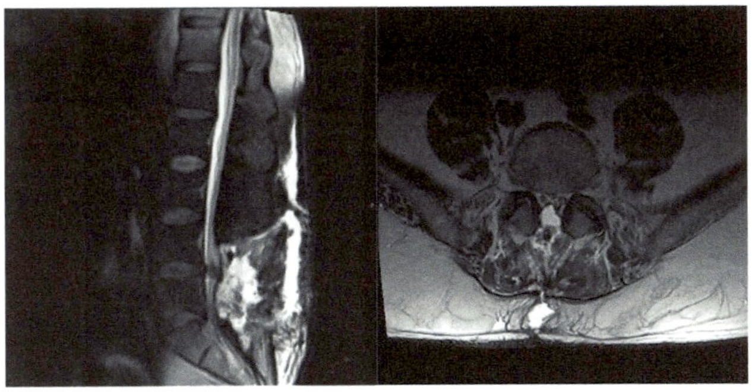

• **Fig. 23.2** Lumbar MRI 24 hours after decompressive laminectomy showing an epidural hematoma. Patient developed cauda equina–like symptoms and required emergent hematoma drainage.

Symptomatic epidural hematomas causing cord compression or cauda equina symptoms should be treated with urgent surgical evacuation in order to prevent irreversible neurologic damage. The literature has shown higher recovery rates when surgery was performed within 12 hours after symptoms onset,[30] and some authors even recommend surgery within 6 hours for the best outcome.[31]

Some surgeons routinely place surgical drains during surgery to decrease the risk of epidural hematoma; however, their efficacy in this regard has not been proven.[32] The authors of this chapter still recommend its use routinely in fusion surgery and after laminectomies. The drain can typically be maintained until there is less than 30 mL of output during a 24-hour period. Although the communication between the surgical site and the outside environment created by the drain carries a theoretical increased risk of infection, recent studies have found no association between drain placement and the risk of infection in spine surgery.[33,34]

Muscle Flap Reconstruction In Complex Spine Surgery

In high-risk patients, such as those with diabetes, poor nutritional status, and obesity, elective surgery should be avoided if possible. In many cases, however, surgery is necessary, and surgeons may need to take extra steps to proactively minimize the risk of wound complications. One viable option after multilevel spine surgery is the use of local musculocutaneous flaps to provide more robust soft tissue coverage over the surgical site.[35] Flap coverage promotes wound healing by increasing blood flow, obliterating dead spaces, and reducing the tension of wound edges. Most cases reported in the literature employ local flaps in high-risk patients with a history of radiation, neoplasms, exposed hardware, and multiple revision surgeries.[36–39] Recent studies have also shown a decreased risk of wound complications when prophylactic local flap coverage is used in multilevel spine surgery done for degenerative spine disease.[40] Inglesby et al. reported a significant decrease in wound complications among 58 complex spine wound patients treated with paraspinal muscle flaps.[41]

Prevention

Prevention of complications is always preferable to treating their consequences. It also reduces the need for revision surgery and decreases hospital costs associated with prolonged hospital stays and readmissions.[3,4] Modifiable risk factors for SSI have included contamination from surgical scrub technique, surgical gowns, C-arm misplacement, poor light manipulation, excessive operating room traffic, and lapses in implant sterilization techniques.[42] Gruenberg et al.[43] analyzed the role of vertical laminar flow in the operating room and demonstrated a significant reduction in infection rates compared with conventional flow method, although more recent studies have replicated this benefit.[44]

Prophylactic antibiotics are also commonly used in spinal surgery to prevent infections. The North American Spine Society (NASS) evidence-based guidelines suggest a single preoperative dose of antibiotics to decrease the risk of infection and/or discitis in uncomplicated lumbar laminectomy or discectomy. In patients with comorbidities or for those undergoing more complex spine procedures, consideration of intraoperative antibiotics redosing, addition of gram-negative coverage, and locally placed antibiotic powder are suggested to decrease the rate of infection.[45] The use of antibiotic powder directly applied into the wound during the closure phase has been shown to result in a significant reduction of staphylococcal infections, particularly in trauma, cervical procedures, and complex spine surgery.[46–48] Some authors also recommend redosing after 4 hours of surgery. Although there is not robust evidence supporting this recommendation in spine surgery,[49] some authors have shown a decrease in SSI when antibiotics are redosed intraoperatively.[50]

For the prevention of wound seromas and hematomas, preoperative optimization including screening for coagulation disorders and poorly managed hypertension are important. Following this, intraoperative placement of deep surgical drains can be used to minimize risk of fluid accumulation.[51,52] Criteria for deep drain placement in spine surgery still have not yet been defined, however, and surgeon discretion based on the quality of hemostasis, as well as the duration and complexity of the procedure, is required. Interestingly, some studies have shown no benefit of drain placement in preventing hematoma formation and subsequent neurological compromise.[51,53] The use of drains also creates an open communication with the external environment, theoretically increasing the risk of wound contamination, especially when kept for long periods of time.[54] A study by Buser et al. found no increased risk of infection when drains were used, however, regardless of the levels involved or duration of surgery.[33]

We recommend the routine use of drains except after microdiscectomy, or for one- or two-level laminectomies in patients without bleeding disorders.

Finally, prophylactic negative pressure wound therapy (PNPWT) is increasingly being used to prevent wound complications in fusion surgery. A recent meta-analysis showed that PNPWT significantly reduced the risk of surgical site infection with no significant effect on wound dehiscence, readmission and reoperation.[55] To our knowledge, this prophylactic therapy could be useful in selected cases in which the risk of wound complications is higher, such as obese, diabetic, poor nutritional status, and prolonged complex spine surgery.

Conclusion

Despite the advances in technology and minimally invasive techniques, posterior approach related complications are not uncommon. The most common complications are wound dehiscence and postoperative wound infection, whereas the most serious complication is epidural hematoma. Proper identification of risk factors for these complications is important. Early recognition and treatment are associated with better outcomes.

References

1. Petilon JM, Glassman SD, Dimar JR, Carreon LY. Clinical outcomes after lumbar fusion complicated by deep wound infection: a case-control study. *Spine (Phila Pa 1976)*. 2012;37(16): 1370–1374.
2. Bernatz JT, Anderson PA. Thirty-day readmission rates in spine surgery: systematic review and meta-analysis. *Neurosurg Focus*. 2015;39(4):E7.
3. Camino-Willhuber G, Guiroy A, Servidio M, et al. Unplanned readmission following early postoperative complications after fusion surgery in adult spine deformity: A multicentric study. *Global Spine J*. 2023;13(1):74–80.
4. Camino Willhuber G, Elizondo C, Slullitel P. Analysis of postoperative complications in spinal surgery, hospital length of stay, and unplanned readmission: Application of Dindo-Clavien classification to spine surgery. *Global Spine J*. 2019;9(3):279–286.
5. Boishardy A, Bouyer B, Boissière L, et al. Surgical site infection a major risk factor of pseudarthrosis in adult spinal deformity surgery. *Spine J*. 2022;22(12):2059–2065.
6. Edwards JR, Peterson KD, Mu Y, et al. National Healthcare Safety Network (NHSN) report: data summary for 2006 through 2008, issued December 2009. *Am J Infect Control*. 2009; 37:783–805.
7. Camino-Willhuber G, Oyadomari S, Ochoa J, et al. The impact of stratified hypoalbuminemia and dialysis on morbidity/mortality after posterior spinal fusion surgery: An ACS-NSQIP study. *Surg Neurol Int*. 2022;13:359.
8. Wimmer C, Gluch H, Franzreb M, Ogon M. Predisposing factors for infection in spine surgery: a survey of 850 spinal procedures. *J Spinal Disord*. 1998;11(2):124–128.
9. Zhou J, Wang R, Huo X, Xiong W, Kang L, Xue Y. Incidence of surgical site infection after spine surgery: A systematic review and meta-analysis. *Spine (Phila Pa 1976)*. 2020;45(3):208–216.
10. Khan SA, Choudry U, Salim A, Nathani KR, Enam SA, Shehzad N. Current management trends for surgical site infection after posterior lumbar spinal instrumentation: A systematic review. *World Neurosurg*. 2022;164:374–380.
11. Fernandez-Gerlinger MP, Arvieu R, Lebeaux D, et al. Successful 6-week antibiotic treatment for early surgical-site infections in spinal surgery. *Clin Infect Dis*. 2019;68(11):1856–1861.
12. Yoshida B, Nguyen A, Formanek B, Alam M, Wang JC, Buser Z. Hypoalbuminemia and elevated CRP are risk factors fordeep infections and urinary tract infections after lumbar spine surgery in a large retrospective patient population. *Global Spine J*. 2023;13(1):33–44.
13. Yamamoto Y, Shigematsu H, Iwata E, et al. Hypoalbuminemia increased the length of stayin the treatment of postoperative acute surgical site infec-tion in spinal surgery. *Spine (Phila Pa 1976)*. 2020;45:E1564–1571.
14. Bohl DD, Shen MR, Mayo BC, et al. Malnutrition predicts infectious and woundcomplications following posterior lumbar spinal fusion. *Spine (Phila Pa 1976)*. 2016;41:1693–1699.
15. Camino-Willhuber G, Franklin A, Rosecrance K, et al. Preoperative hypoalbuminemia and dialysis increase morbidity/mortality after spine surgery for primary pyogenic spinal infections (ACS-NSQIP Study). *Surg Neurol Int*. 2022;13:193.

16. Russell L. The importance of patients' nutritional status in wound healing. *Br J Nurs*. 2001;10(Suppl):S429.
17. He Z, Zhou K, Tang K, Quan Z, Liu S, Su B. Perioperativehypoalbuminemia is a risk factor for wound complications following posterior lumbar interbody fusion. *J Orthop Surg Res*. 2020;15:538.
18. Adogwa O, Fatemi P, Perez E, et al. Negative pressure wound therapy reduces incidence of postoperative wound infection and dehiscence after long-segment thoracolumbar spinal fusion: a single institutional experience. *Spine J*. 2014;14(12):2911–2917.
19. Akhter AS, McGahan BG, Close L, et al. Negative pressure wound therapy in spinal fusion patients. *Int Wound J*. 2021; 18(2):158–163.
20. Dyck BA, Bailey CS, Steyn C, et al. Use of incisional vacuum assisted closure in the prevention of postoperative infection in high-risk patients who underwent spine surgery: a proof-of concept study. *J Neurosurg Spine*. 2019;31:1–10.
21. Shah A, Sumpio BJ, Tsay C, et al. Incisional negative pressure wound therapy augments perfusion and improves wound healing in a swine model pilot study. *Ann Plast Surg*. 2019;82 (4S Suppl 3):S222–s227.
22. Orgill DP, Manders EK, Sumpio BE, et al. The mechanisms of action of vacuum assisted closure: more to learn. *Dermatol Surg*. 2009;146(1):40–51.
23. Stevens P. Vacuum-assisted closure of laparostomy wounds: a critical review of the literature. *Int Wound J*. 2009;6(4):259–266.
24. Stannard JP, Volgas DA, Stewart R, McGwin G Jr, Alonso JE. Negative pressure wound therapy after severe open fractures: a prospective randomized study. *J Orthop Trauma*. 2009;23(8): 552–557.
25. Hasselmann J, Bjork J, Svensson-Bjork R, Acosta S. Inguinal vascular surgical wound protection by incisional negative pressure wound therapy: a randomized controlled trial-INVIPS trial. *Ann Surg*. 2019;271(1):48–53.
26. Jackson R. Case of spinal apoplexy. *Lancet*. 1869;2:5–6.
27. Abola MV, Du JY, Lin CC, Schreiber-Stainthorp W, Passias PG. Symptomatic epidural hematoma after elective cervical spine surgery: Incidence, timing, risk factors, and associated complications. *Oper Neurosurg (Hagerstown)*. 2021;21(6):452–460.
28. Knusel K, Du JY, Ren B, Kim CY, Ahn UM, Ahn NU. Symptomatic epidural hematoma after elective posterior lumbar decompression: Incidence, timing, risk factors, and associated complications. *HSS J*. 2020;16(Suppl 2):230–237.
29. Braun P, Kazmi K, Nogues-Melendez P, Mas-Estelles F, Aparici-Robles F. MRI findings in spinal subdural and epidural hematomas. *Eur J Radiol*. 2007;64(1):119–125.
30. Lawton MT, Porter RW, Heiserman JE, Jacobowitz R, Sonntag VK, Dickman CA. Surgical management of spinal epidural hematoma: relationship between surgical timing and neurological outcome. *J Neurosurg*. 1995;83(1):117.
31. Kebaish KM, Awad JN. Spinal epidural hematoma causing acute cauda equina syndrome. *Neurosurg Focus*. 2004;16(6):e1. pii 160601.
32. Muthu S, Ramakrishnan E, Natarajan KK, Chellamuthu G. Risk-benefit analysis of wound drain usage in spine surgery: a systematic review and meta-analysis with evidence summary. *Eur Spine J*. 2020;29(9):2111–2128.
33. Buser Z, Chang KE, Kall R, et al. Lumbar surgical drains do not increase the risk of infections in patients undergoing spine surgery [published online ahead of print, 2022 Feb 11]. *Eur Spine J*. 2022. https://doi.org/10.1007/s00586-022-07130-0.
34. Adogwa O, Elsamadicy AA, Sergesketter AR, et al. Postoperative drain use in patients undergoing decompression and fusion: incidence of complications and symptomatic hematoma. *J Spine Surg*. 2018;4(2):220–226.
35. Cohen LE, Fullerton N, Mundy LR, et al. Optimizing successful outcomes in complex spine reconstruction using local muscle flaps. *Plast Reconstr Surg*. 2016;137:295–301.
36. Mericli AF, Tarola NA, Moore JH Jr, et al. Paraspinous muscle ap reconstruction of com- plex midline back wounds: Risk factors and postreconstruction complications. *Ann Plast Surg*. 2010;65:219–224.
37. Hultman CS, Jones GE, Losken A, et al. Salvage of infected spinal hardware with paraspinous muscle flaps: anatomic considerations with clinical correlation. *Ann Plast Surg*. 2006;57: 521–528.
38. Garvey PB, Rhines LD, Dong W, et al. Immediate soft tissue reconstruction for complex defects of the spine following surgery for spinal neoplasms. *Plast Reconstr Surg*. 2010;125: 1460–1466.
39. Dumanian GA, Ondra SL, Liu J, et al. Muscle flap salvage of spine wounds with soft tissue defects or infection. *Spine (Phila Pa 1976)*. 2003;28:1203–1211.
40. Adapa N, Jain N, Capek A, et al. Prophylactic muscle flap reconstruction after complex spine surgery for degenerative disease: case series and institutional protocol. *J Spine Surg*. 2018;4(3): 560–567.
41. Inglesby DC, Young ZT, Alshareef M, et al. Paraspinous muscle flaps for the treatment of complex spinal wounds. *Spine (Phila Pa 1976)*. 2020;45(9):599–604.
42. Weber DJ, Anderson D, Rutala WA. The role of the surface environment in healthcare-associated infections. *Curr Opin Infect Dis*. 2013;26(4):338–344.
43. Gruenberg MF, Campaner GL, Sola CA, Ortolan EG. Ultraclean air for prevention of postoperative infection after posterior spinal fusion with instrumentation: a comparison between surgeries performed with and without a vertical exponential filtered airflow system. *Spine*. 2004;29(20):2330–2334.
44. Brandt C, Hott U, Sohr D, Daschner F, Gastmeier P, Rüden H. Operating room ventilation with laminar airflow shows no protective effect on the surgical site infection rate in orthopedic and abdominal surgery. *Ann Surg*. 2008;248(5):695–700.
45. Shaffer WO, Baisden JL, Fernand R, Matz PG. North American Spine Society. An evidence-based clinical guideline for antibiotic prophylaxis in spine surgery. *Spine J*. 2013;13(10):1387–1392.
46. O'Neill KR, Smith JG, Abtahi AM, Archer KR, Spengler DM, McGirt MJ, Devin CJ. Reduced surgical site infections in patients undergoing posterior spinal stabilization of traumatic injuries using vancomycin powder. *Spine J*. 2011;11(7): 641–646.
47. Caroom C, Tullar JM, Benton EG Jr, Jones JR, Chaput CD. Intrawound vancomycin powder reduces surgical site infections in posterior cervical fusion. *Spine*. 2013;38(14):1183–1187.
48. Lemans JVC, Öner FC, Wijdicks SPJ, Ekkelenkamp MB, Vogely HC, Kruyt MC. The efficacy of intrawound vancomycin powder and povidone-iodine irrigation to prevent surgical site infections in complex instrumented spine surgery. *Spine J*. 2019;19(10):1648–1656.
49. Dodson V, Majmundar N, Swantic V, Assina R. The effect of prophylactic vancomycin powder on infections following spinal surgeries: a systematic review. *Neurosurg Focus*. 2019;46(1):E11.

50. Glotzbecker M, Troy M, Miller P, et al. Implementing a multidisciplinary clinical pathway can reduce the deep surgical site infection rate after posterior spinal fusion in high-risk patients. *Spine Deform.* 2019;7(1):33–39.
51. Kou J, Fischgrund J, Biddinger A, et al. Risk factors for spinal epidural hematoma after spinal surgery. *Spine.* 2002;27(15): 1670–1673.
52. Walid MS, Abbara M, Tolaymat A, et al. The role of drains in lumbar spine fusion. *World Neurosurg.* 2012;77(3-4):564–568.
53. Awad JN, Kebaish KM, Donigan J, et al. Analysis of the risk factors for the development of post-operative spinal epidural haematoma. *J Bone Joint Surg Br.* 2005;87(9):1248–1252.
54. Pennington Z, Lubelski D, Molina C, et al. Prolonged post-surgical drain retention increases risk for deep wound infection after spine surgery. *World Neurosurg.* 2012;130:e846–e853.
55. Chen Z, Sun J, Yao Z, Song C, Liu W. Can prophylactic negative pressure wound therapy improve clinical outcomes in spinal fusion surgery? A meta-analysis. *Eur Spine J.* 2022;31(6):1546–1552.

24 Long-Term Complications of Lumbar Spine Surgery

JESSE SHEN AND JEAN-CHRISTOPHE LEVEQUE

CHAPTER OUTLINE

Introduction

Lumbar spine surgery is amongst the most common interventions performed in orthopedic surgery. A variety of surgeries can be performed ranging from simple decompressive procedures to stabilization procedures involving fusions with instrumentation. Despite many of these interventions being beneficial to patients, they are not without risk of both short- and long-term complications that can worsen postoperative quality of life.

This chapter will focus on describing the long-term complications from lumbar spine surgery, specifically focusing primarily on those complications arising from fusion surgery. We will review and cover complications such as pseudarthrosis, adjacent level disease, and failed back surgery syndrome. The complication rates, diagnosis, strategies for avoidance, and the management of these complications will be reviewed.

Pseudarthrosis

Pseudarthrosis is the failure to achieve bony fusion after surgery. It is one of the most common long-term complications with reported incidence ranging from 5% to 35%.[1] The practicing spine surgeon must be aware of the risk factors, diagnosis, avoidance strategies, and management of this complication.

Risk Factors

Successful fusion needs both adequate biology and sufficient mechanical stability to promote bone growth. The spine surgeon usually controls the latter through the use of fixation devices such as pedicle screws, hooks, and other segmental fixation. Optimal patient biology is often outside of a surgeon's direct control, and therefore requires diligence to adequately screen for risk factors, optimize medical conditions, and ultimately select the proper patient for surgery.

Tobacco smoking is one of the most important modifiable risk factors for pseudarthrosis.[2–5] Glassman et al.[2] evaluated posterolateral lumbar fusions in smokers compared to nonsmokers and found that smokers had significantly higher pseudarthrosis rates than nonsmokers (26.5% vs 14.2%). Smokers who had stopped for 6 months after surgery had a trend towards similar rates of pseudarthrosis as nonsmokers (17.1%). Furthermore, a recent study by Bydon et al.[3] has shown that for two-level posterolateral fusion the rates of pseudarthrosis were two times greater in smokers than nonsmokers (29.17% vs 10.92%). Hermann et al.[6] reported higher pseudarthrosis rates and a greater rate of surgery in patients who smoked as compared to nonsmokers. Brown et al.[4] showed a similar trend of increased pseudarthrosis rates in smokers compared to nonsmokers (40% vs 8%), although their study did not involve any instrumentation, making it perhaps less applicable to fusion surgery as typically performed nowadays. The literature evidence supports smoking as a modifiable risk factor for pseudarthrosis, and patients should be counseled to undergo smoking cessation prior to lumbar fusion surgery.

Metabolic disorders are also risk factors for pseudarthrosis. Osteoporosis, vitamin D deficiency, diabetes, and hypothyroidism have all been described as potential risk factors.[7] In a study by Hills et al.,[7] 82% of the patients undergoing revision surgery for pseudarthrosis had a preexisting metabolic condition. Their prevalence in this often-older patient population should not be underestimated. Stoker et al.[8] demonstrated in their analysis of adult patients undergoing fusion that there is a high prevalence of vitamin D deficiency. These metabolic disorders may also play a role in the development of surgical site infection (SSI), which has independently been described as a risk factor for pseudarthrosis. Weiss et al.[9] reported a more than 30% risk of pseudarthrosis after surgical site infection while Hollern et al.[10] have shown that higher BMI and increased number of fusion levels are independent risk factors of pseudarthrosis in patients who have developed a postoperative SSI. Given that the adult fusion population is often older and therefore may have an increased prevalence of metabolic disorders that may contribute directly to pseudarthrosis or SSI, it is of critical importance that these disorders be screened and managed preoperatively

As previously mentioned, mechanical stability also influences the rate of pseudarthrosis. Fischgrund et al.[11] compared the fusion rates in patients with and without pedicle screw instrumentation for lumbar laminectomy and fusion. Their results demonstrate higher pseudarthrosis rates for patients without instrumentation (55% vs 18%). The Spine Patient Outcomes Research Trial also noted a higher fusion rate for patients with posterolateral fusions with instrumentation compared to noninstrumented fusions.[12] Controversy remains on whether circumferential fusion using interbody devices improves outcomes and fusion rates. Christensen et al.[13] demonstrated excellent fusion rates, decreased reoperation rates, and improved lordosis alignment in patients undergoing circumferential fusion. However, the Spine Outcomes Research Trial did not differentiate between posterolateral fusion and circumferential fusions.[12] We can gather that stability with instrumentation can provide improved fusion rates and that noninstrumented fusions are a risk factor for pseudarthrosis.

Diagnosis of Pseudarthrosis

Radiographic pseudarthrosis can be present in either symptomatic or asymptomatic patients. Pseudarthrosis should be in the differential diagnosis for any patient with postoperative pain or new neurologic symptoms, yet the rates of asymptomatic pseudarthrosis can be as high as 50%.[11,14] A detailed history, physical exam, and judicious usage of imaging for all of these patients will allow the clinician to obtain an accurate diagnosis. Although physical examination may not be abnormal in cases of pseudarthrosis, ensuring that the proper wound healing is essential, as infection can be a risk factor for nonunion. Gross instability and deformity can also be noted on the physical exam, which may reflect pseudarthrosis of the spine.[1] While symptomatic patients will often require further treatment, a purely radiographic but asymptomatic pseudarthrosis can be a challenging situation and requires a thorough history and discussion with the patient about the clinical situation. Detailing the patient's pain to pinpoint a mechanical etiology may help guide the clinician as to whether the nonunion is symptomatic or not. Furthermore, screening for risk factors of pseudarthrosis can also aid in the diagnosis.

Imaging is an important noninvasive test to help diagnose pseudarthrosis. Implant failure, new radiolucency, loss of fixation, or new deformity suggest pseudarthrosis and can be noticed on simple x-rays. Flexion and extension x-rays may help detect pseudarthrosis not easily identified on static films,[15] although an absence of motion on flexion and extension x-rays cannot be assumed to be due to solid fusion.[16] CT scan is the most accurate modality for diagnosing pseudarthrosis.[17,18] Although the exact postoperative time point that can define pseudarthrosis remains under debate, Kanemura et al.[19] suggest that the final determination of nonunion should be 3 years after surgery since some patients may go on to fuse after 2 years postop, although many surgeons would consider reoperation for a symptomatic pseudarthrosis much earlier, especially in the setting of implant failure or a new neurologic deficit.

Complication Avoidance

Preoperative patient optimization is vital to avoid pseudarthrosis in lumbar spine surgery. Modifiable patient risk factors such as smoking or BMI need to be addressed before elective surgery. Optimization of comorbid conditions such as diabetes and osteoporosis are also critical for patient management before surgery. The rationale for a multidisciplinary team to optimize these patients preoperatively is thus essential and has been shown to decrease complications.[20]

The surgeon and surgical technique also play an important role in avoiding pseudarthrosis. Meticulous attention to surgical detail with proper preparation of the fusion bed by removal of all soft tissue and decortication of all bony surfaces is imperative. The choice of bone graft may also influence the rate of fusion. The usage of local autograft or demineralized bone matrices may offer an 89% fusion rate.[21] Recent meta-analyses have suggested that demineralized bone matrices combined with autograft may have greater fusion rates but these are not statistically significant when compared to autograft alone.[22] Bone morphogenic protein has shown high fusion rates over 94%[21,22] but has its own specific complications that may limit its use in all cases.

As previously discussed, the use of instrumentation during surgery may increase the rates of fusion and therefore consideration of a circumferential fusion at the index surgery is warranted.[13] These preoperative and intraoperative strategies both can help decrease the rate of pseudarthrosis.

Management

The asymptomatic patient with radiographic findings alone may not require any surgical intervention. Pseudarthrosis may not significantly impact the patient, especially in the short-term,[11,14] and some patients with pseudarthrosis may have excellent clinical outcomes, making surgery unnecessary.[1] Hassanzadeh et al. suggested in their small case series that patients with rod fractures may not necessarily reflect a true bony pseudarthrosis and therefore may not need any intervention,[23] although this result was demonstrated in patients undergoing long posterior spinal fusion for spinal deformity and may not be representative of the population as a whole. Although immediate surgical intervention may not be required, long-term follow-up of these patients to ensure good clinical outcomes is suggested.

The symptomatic patient with pseudarthrosis often requires treatment, as this pseudarthrosis is a potential source of disability and pain. Once diagnosed, the cause of and factors contributing to pseudarthrosis need to be evaluated and managed. Smoking cessation, diabetes control, and optimization of other risk factors will all play an essential role in ensuring successful treatment of pseudarthrosis. Surgical management may be offered for these symptomatic patients, as recent evidence has shown that surgical management may provide benefit.[24,25] Circumferential fusion has been advocated as a strategy to treat these patients.[26–28] High satisfaction and fusion rates of over 90% were noted in patients treated with circumferential fusion while revision surgery with posterolateral fusion and instrumentation had inferior fusion rates of 49%,[29] although patients need to be appropriately counseled that solid fusion may not always correlate with improved outcomes for revision procedures.[30]

Adjacent Segment Disease

Adjacent segment disease (ASD) refers to the clinical symptoms associated with radiographic degeneration at an adjacent segment to a fusion construct, while the radiographic manifestation without relevant clinical symptoms is usually referred to as adjacent segment degeneration.[31] This section will discuss the diagnosis, avoidance, and management of adjacent segment disease.

Natural History, Risk Factors, and Diagnosis

The natural history of adjacent segment degeneration and disease is subject to debate. Radcliff et al.[32] suggested that although surgical intervention is associated with degeneration it is unclear that it accelerates the process. Furthermore, Mannion et al.[33] demonstrated that adjacent segment degeneration but not adjacent segment disease is associated with surgical intervention. Moreover, this degeneration does not impact patient outcomes. Park et al.[34] described similar findings with radiographic degeneration not influencing functional outcomes in their review. Hence, there is a rationale for nonoperative management for these asymptomatic patients.

Although the natural history remains unclear, the biomechanical contribution of fusion seems intuitive. Increased disc pressure, increased mobility at the adjacent segment, and increased facet joint loading have been described as biomechanical factors contributing to ASD.[34] Furthermore, Kumar et al.[35] have shown that sagittal parameters alter the biomechanical environment around the fusion construct and influence ASD. Multiple patient-specific risk factors such as female gender, age, and osteoporosis have also been associated with the development of ASD.[34] It is essential that the spine surgeon be aware of these risk factors and utilize perioperative management to minimize the occurrence of ASD. The overall incidence has been reported as 9% for patients with lumbar spine fusion on an average follow-up period of 4.7 years.[36] Sears et al.[37] further stratified the risk of ASD based on the number of levels fused, with 1-level, 2-level, and 3-4 level fusions leading to a mean annual incidence of 1.7%, 3.6%, and 5%, respectively. It is apparent that the incidence is greater with longer fusion constructs, and therefore the addition of fusion levels carries a risk that extends beyond the immediate perioperative time period.

Several radiological criteria have been described for adjacent segment degeneration. Anteroposterior translation of more than 3 mm, >10° of segmental kyphosis, and loss of 50% of height at the adjacent segment.[38] The diagnosis of ASD requires both imaging changes of degeneration at an adjacent segment and clinical symptoms related to these changes. Typical examples include radicular symptoms related to spinal stenosis at an adjacent segment to fusion or degenerative changes in the facets or disc adjacent to a fusion leading to a symptomatic spondylolisthesis or spondylosis. Malalignment both preoperatively and postoperatively may predispose to ASD, especially mismatches between pelvic incidence and lumbar lordosis as well as sagittal balance.[39]

Avoidance and Management of ASD

Surgical treatment of ASD can be complex, as revision surgery often involves extending the fusion construct and decompression within an area of potentially significant scarring. The risk of complications is thus greater than primary surgeries, again emphasizing the importance of recognizing and mitigating the preoperative risk factors. Judicious selection of fusion length and meticulous surgical technique to preserve adjacent soft tissues and avoid violation of adjacent facet joints are elements within the surgeon's control that may reduce the risk of ASD.[40–42] The restoration or maintenance of proper spinal alignment is also critical in reducing the development of ASD.[39] Osteoporosis is a modifiable patient risk factor, and patients affected by this condition should be preoperatively optimized.[43] Although T scores may aid in the determination of bone health, Hounsfield units (HU) lower than 110 within the instrumented vertebral body on lumbar CT scan may also be indicative of osteoporosis and an increased risk of ASD, so treatment strategies should take this radiographic data into account.[44,45] Recent evidence has suggested that in patients with osteoporosis who may be at higher risk of failure, cement augmentation may help prevent radiological failure while providing similar outcomes to solid pedicle patients.[46] Ghobrial et al.[47] have described cementing the upper instrumented vertebra and the vertebra proximal to it to avoid adjacent failure in an adult deformity population, and this strategy should be considered in degenerative cases at higher risk of failure.[48,49]

Minimally invasive techniques may be an option conceptually to avoid adjacent segment disease. These techniques involve less soft tissue dissection and, in theory, may help preserve adjacent segments. However, current evidence does not seem to suggest a difference in the development of adjacent segment disease between open versus minimally invasive techniques, and in fact percutaneous pedicle screw fixation has a higher incidence of superior facet joint violation, which may help to explain its lack of benefit in the reduction of ASD.[50,51] Dynamic stabilization techniques and junctional tethers are newer technologies that have garnered some interest but there is currently limited evidence in their prevention of adjacent segment disease.[52] Some evidence exists in the adult spinal deformity literature that proximal tether placement may help decrease the incidence of adjacent segment disease,[53] but this benefit remains to be proven for shorter-segment-fusion lumbar spine pathology and so spine surgeons should be careful when incorporating these new technologies with the goal of preventing ASD.

Managing adjacent segment disease is tailored based on the clinical symptoms as well as the correlating radiological abnormalities. Instability is typically treated with fusion techniques, while stenosis of neurologic structures requires decompression, although adjacent level decompression and fusion have been described as treatment for stenosis above a previously fused segment.[34] Minimally invasive techniques can also be utilized to treat ASD and avoid the morbidity of open procedures, especially in areas with previous scarring. Lateral interbody fusion is a minimally invasive technique that uses a lateral corridor to the spine and can provide indirect decompression for central and foraminal stenosis. This technique can also be used as a standalone method of treatment for ASD.[54] However, we recommend that if there are signs of instability at the adjacent segment, posterior or lateral instrumentation at the adjacent level should accompany the lateral interbody technique.[55]

Failed Back Surgery Syndrome

Failed back surgery syndrome (FBSS) is a vague term that describes a patient's clinical scenario with either dissatisfaction from surgery or residual symptoms after spine surgery.[56–58] Despite this umbrella term being likely outdated, it warrants discussion as many patients may be referred for this problem. In an Internet survey, Inoue et al.[59] found a prevalence of 20.6% of failed back surgery syndrome in 1842 lumbar surgery patients surveyed. A 40% prevalence has also been reported for FBSS.[60] This prevalence is even more alarming given that the economic burden of this syndrome is comparable to chronic medical conditions such as heart failure.[61] The prevalence and economic burden support the rationale that these patients need to be carefully assessed and managed, which may be made more difficult by the negative stigma around this label that may be a barrier for clinicians to delineate a cause and subsequent appropriate treatment.

Risk Factors, Etiology, and Diagnosis

Baber et al.[62] have described both preoperative and postoperative factors contributing to FBSS. Preoperatively, patient-centered factors such as obesity, smoking, and worker's compensation status need to be identified by the clinician for optimization or patient counseling on expected outcomes. Psychological conditions are also an important risk factor that should be assessed preoperatively and treated.[63] Postoperatively, a multitude of factors may contribute to FBSS. Progression of degenerative changes can explain persistent or new-onset symptoms that are not necessarily related to the initial surgical site. Altered biomechanics of surrounding soft tissues, atrophy, spasm, and stiffness have been described as potential contributors to postoperatively persistent symptoms.[62]

The underlying etiology of FBSS therefore requires a wide differential diagnosis. The three most common diagnoses underlying FBSS are foraminal stenosis (29%), recurrent painful disc (17%), and pseudarthrosis (14%).[56] In patients having undergone fusion with instrumentation, a diagnosis such as pseudarthrosis, hardware-related issues, adjacent segment disease, and unaddressed malalignment are all potential causes that require assessment. Surgeons also need to scrutinize the rationale that led to the patient having undergone surgery as errors in diagnosis or wrong surgical site can be an etiology of FBSS.[64] The history, physical exam, imaging, operative notes, and indications need to be reviewed. A careful clinical exam and patient history need to be performed to orient the diagnostic investigation. Simple plain radiographs are often the first diagnostic modality employed and can immediately orient the surgeon to potential diagnoses such as instability, pseudarthrosis, or persistent deformity. CT scans and MRI can provide further information if initial investigations are negative and can reveal potential problems such as misplaced hardware or adjacent level stenosis. The surgeon needs to be aware of all potential problems and diagnoses relative to the index surgery to have an appropriate differential diagnosis for a patient presenting with FBSS.

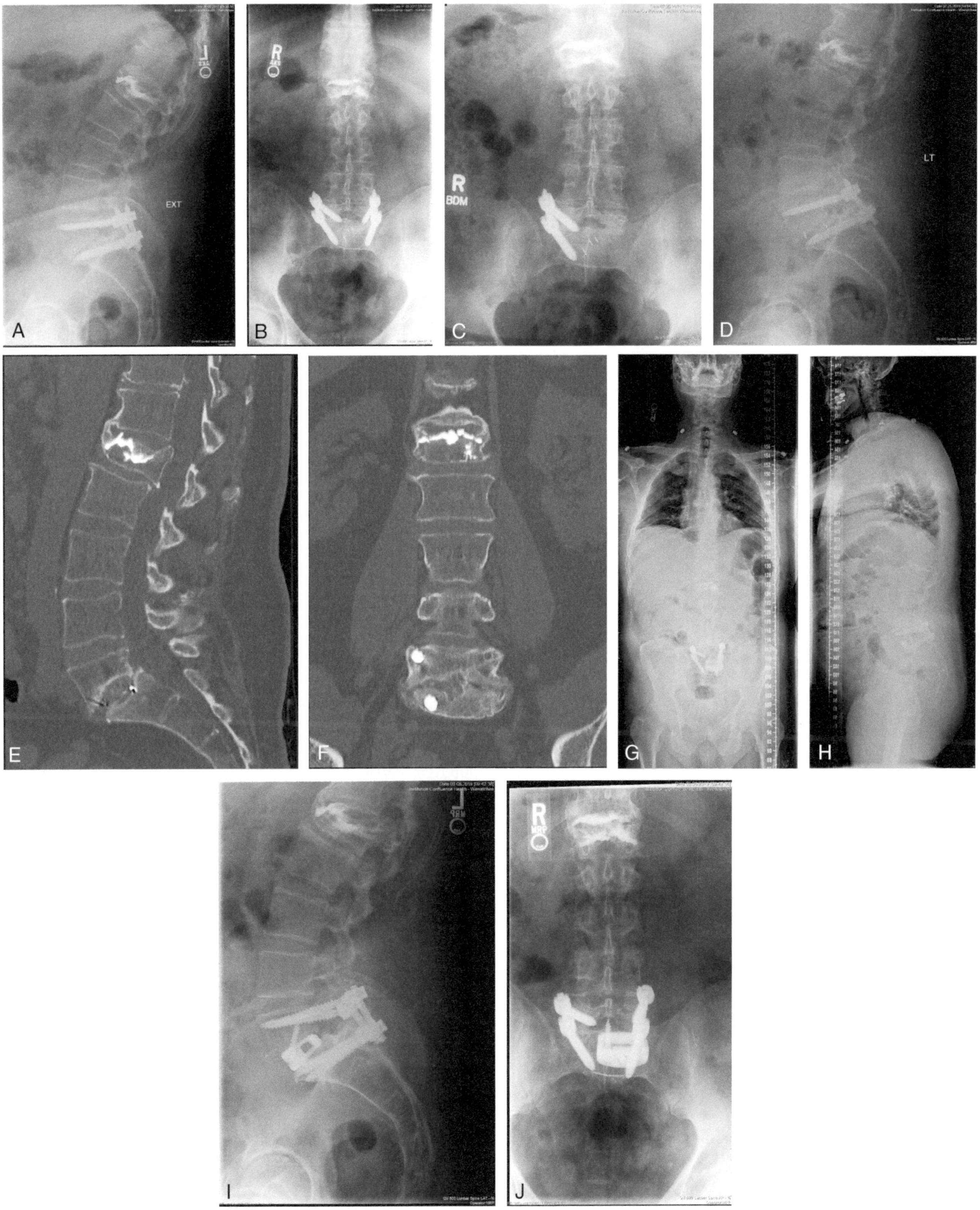

• **Fig. 24.1** Case example of a patient with pseudarthrosis after lumbar spine surgery. (A–F) show a patient suffering from symptomatic pseudarthrosis following an initial L5-S1 transforaminal lumbar interbody fusion (TLIF). (G–J) show the subsequent revision surgery.

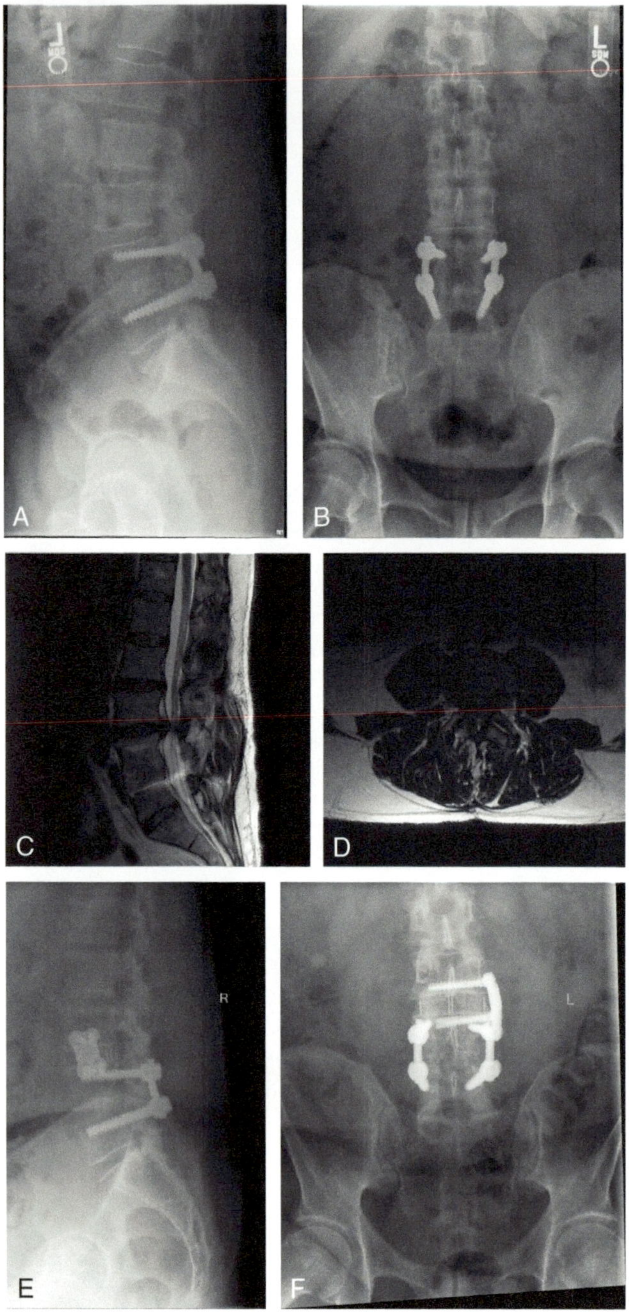

• **Fig. 24.2** Case example of an adjacent segment disease following L4-5 lumbar spine fusion. (A–D) show the initial imaging. The subsequent surgical management is shown in (E) and (F).

Management

The management of FBSS is highly dependent on the established diagnosis. Patients should have exhausted all options of nonsurgical care before consideration of surgery. Surgical management will be tailored based on the clinical and radiological findings.

Revision surgery should be offered in patients who have residual symptoms and have a surgically manageable problem. Wrong-level surgical cases should be offered revision surgery as the initial symptoms were not treated with the index surgery. Long-term complications of the index surgery, such as adjacent segment disease or pseudarthrosis, should be managed as described previously within this chapter. Patients who do not have a clear diagnosis or imaging abnormalities that do not correlate with the patient's symptoms should not be offered revision surgery. The surgeon should be wary of offering surgery without a precise diagnosis of the underlying problem causing FBSS. These patients should be referred to physical medicine and rehabilitation services to explore all nonoperative modalities in managing their symptoms, including the use of spinal cord stimulation for postoperative pain management.[58,65,66]

Case example of a pseudarthrosis following lumbar spine surgery (Fig. 24.1). This is a patient that initially had an L5-S1 transforaminal lumbar interbody fusion (TLIF) with posterior spinal fusion and instrumentation (A and B). This patient had persistent symptoms postoperatively and had the left-sided instrumentation removed for a presumed diagnosis of symptomatic hardware (C and D). He was referred for persistent symptoms despite the two surgical interventions. A CT-scan demonstrated a pseudarthrosis at L5-S1 (E and F). This was then treated with a revision anterior lumbar interbody fusion (ALIF) and revision of the posterior spinal instrumentation and fusion (G to J). His postop evolution was favorable.

Case example of adjacent segment disease following lumbar spine fusion at L4-L5 (Fig. 24.2). This patient was referred for neurogenic claudication after L4-5 lumbar spine. Of note, his initial x-rays showed that he had successfully fused, but fused relatively flat at the L4-L5 level. A lumbar lordosis to pelvic incidence mismatch was perhaps iatrogenically induced by the first surgery. This could have predisposed this patient to ASD. A to D show this patient's preoperative x-rays and MRI. His MRI shows degeneration at the adjacent L3-L4 level with important central stenosis and collapse. A revision lateral interbody fusion with plate construct was performed (E and F).

References

1. Chun DS, Baker KC, Hsu WK. Lumbar pseudarthrosis: a review of current diagnosis and treatment. *Neurosurg Focus.* 2015; 39(4):E10.
2. Glassman SD, Anagnost SC, Parker A, et al. The effect of cigarette smoking and smoking cessation on spinal fusion. *Spine (Phila Pa 1976).* 2000;25(20):2608–2615.
3. Bydon M, De la Garza-Ramos R, Abt NB, et al. Impact of smoking on complication and pseudarthrosis rates after single- and 2-level posterolateral fusion of the lumbar spine. *Spine (Phila Pa 1976).* 2014;39(21):1765–1770.
4. Brown C, Orme T, Richardson H. The rate of pseudarthrosis (surgical nonunion) in patients who are smokers and patients who are nonsmokers: a comparison study. *Spine (Phila Pa 1976).* 1986;11:942–943.
5. Berman D, Oren JH, Bendo J, Spivak J. The effect of smoking on spinal fusion. *Int J Spine Surg.* 2017;11(4):29.
6. Hermann PC, Webler M, Bornemann R, et al. Influence of smoking on spinal fusion after spondylodesis surgery: A comparative clinical study. *Technol Health Care.* 2016;24(5):737–744.

7. Hills JM, Khan I, Archer KR, et al. Metabolic and endocrine disorders in pseudarthrosis. *Clin Spine Surg.* 2019;32(5): E252–E257.
8. Stoker GE, Buchowski JM, Bridwell KH, Lenke LG, Riew KD, Zebala LP. Preoperative vitamin D status of adults undergoing surgical spinal fusion. *Spine (Phila Pa 1976).* 2013;38(6): 507–515.
9. Weiss LE, Vaccaro AR, Scuderi G, McGuire M, Garfin SR. Pseudarthrosis after postoperative wound infection in the lumbar spine. *J Spinal Disord.* 1997;10(6):482–487.
10. Hollern DA, Woods BI, Shah NV, et al. Risk factors for pseudarthrosis after surgical site infection of the spine. *Int J Spine Surg.* 2019;13(6):507–514.
11. Fischgrund JS, Mackay M, Herkowitz HN, Brower R, Montgomery DM, Kurz LT. Volvo Award winner in clinical studies. Degenerative lumbar spondylolisthesis with spinal stenosis: a prospective, randomized study comparing decompressive laminectomy and arthrodesis with and without spinal instrumentation. *Spine (Phila Pa 1976).* 1997;22(24): 2807–2812.
12. Abdu WA, Lurie JD, Spratt KF, et al. Degenerative spondylolisthesis: does fusion method influence outcome? Four-year results of the spine patient outcomes research trial. *Spine (Phila Pa 1976).* 2009;34(21):2351–2360.
13. Christensen FB, Hansen ES, Eiskjaer SP, et al. Circumferential lumbar spinal fusion with Brantigan cage versus posterolateral fusion with titanium Cotrel-Dubousset instrumentation: a prospective, randomized clinical study of 146 patients. *Spine (Phila Pa 1976).* 2002;27(23):2674–2683.
14. Gruskay JA, Webb ML, Grauer JN. Methods of evaluating lumbar and cervical fusion. *Spine J.* 2014;14(3):531–539.
15. Shen FH, Samartzis D. Assessment of lumbar fusion: importance of dynamic plain standing x-rays. *J Am Coll Surg.* 2008; 207(6):955–956.
16. Choudhri TF, Mummaneni PV, Dhall SS, et al. Guideline update for the performance of fusion procedures for degenerative disease of the lumbar spine. Part 4: radiographic assessment of fusion status. *J Neurosurg Spine.* 2014;21(1):23–30.
17. Peters MJM, Bastiaenen CHG, Brans BT, Weijers RE, Willems PC. The diagnostic accuracy of imaging modalities to detect pseudarthrosis after spinal fusion-a systematic review and meta-analysis of the literature. *Skeletal Radiol.* 2019;48(10): 1499–1510.
18. Carreon LY, Djurasovic M, Glassman SD, Sailer P. Diagnostic accuracy and reliability of fine-cut CT scans with reconstructions to determine the status of an instrumented posterolateral fusion with surgical exploration as reference standard. *Spine (Phila Pa 1976).* 2007;32(8):892–895.
19. Kanemura T, Matsumoto A, Ishikawa Y, et al. Radiographic changes in patients with pseudarthrosis after posterior lumbar interbody arthrodesis using carbon interbody cages: a prospective five-year study. *J Bone Joint Surg Am.* 2014;96(10):e82.
20. Sethi R, Buchlak QD, Yanamadala V, et al. A systematic multidisciplinary initiative for reducing the risk of complications in adult scoliosis surgery. *J Neurosurg Spine.* 2017;26(6): 744–750.
21. Hsu WK, Nickoli MS, Wang JC, et al. Improving the clinical evidence of bone graft substitute technology in lumbar spine surgery. *Global Spine J.* 2012;2(4):239–248.
22. Han S, Park B, Lim J-W, et al. Comparison of fusion rate between demineralized bone matrix versus autograft in lumbar fusion: Meta-analysis. *J Korean Neurosurg Soc.* 2020;63(6):673–680.
23. Hassanzadeh H, Dafrawy MH, Kim TJ, et al. Is rod fracture always a sign of pseudoarthrosis in patients with a long posterior spinal fusion (PSF)? *Spine J.* 2012;12(9 Suppl):S160.
24. Adogwa O, Carr RK, Kudyba K, et al. Revision lumbar surgery in elderly patients with symptomatic pseudarthrosis, adjacent-segment disease, or same-level recurrent stenosis. Part 1. Two-year outcomes and clinical efficacy: Clinical article. *J Neurosurg Spine.* 2013;18(2):139–146.
25. Glassman SD, Carreon LY, Djurasovic M, et al. Lumbar fusion outcomes stratified by specific diagnostic indication. *Spine J.* 2009; 9(1):13–21.
26. Albert TJ, Pinto M, Denis F. Management of symptomatic lumbar pseudarthrosis with anteroposterior fusion. A functional and radiographic outcome study. *Spine (Phila Pa 1976).* 2000;25(1):123–129; discussion 130.
27. Gertzbein SD, Hollopeter MR, Hall S. Pseudarthrosis of the lumbar spine. Outcome after circumferential fusion. *Spine (Phila Pa 1976).* 1998;23(21):2352–2356; discussion 2356–2357.
28. Slosar PJ, Reynolds JB, Schofferman J, Goldthwaite N, White AH, Keaney D. Patient satisfaction after circumferential lumbar fusion. *Spine (Phila Pa 1976).* 2000;25(6):722–726.
29. Lauerman WC, Bradford DS, Ogilvie JW, Transfeldt EE. Results of lumbar pseudarthrosis repair. *J Spinal Disord.* 1992; 5(2):149–157.
30. Dede O, Thuillier D, Pekmezci M, et al. Revision surgery for lumbar pseudarthrosis. *Spine J.* 2015;15(5):977–982.
31. Hilibrand AS, Carlson GD, Palumbo MA, Jones PK, Bohlman HH. Radiculopathy and myelopathy at segments adjacent to the site of a previous anterior cervical arthrodesis. *J Bone Joint Surg Am.* 1999;81(4):519–528.
32. Radcliff KE, Kepler CK, Jakoi A, et al. Adjacent segment disease in the lumbar spine following different treatment interventions. *Spine J.* 2013;13(10):1339–1349.
33. Mannion AF, Leivseth G, Brox J-I, Fritzell P, Hägg O, Fairbank JCT. ISSLS Prize winner: Long-term follow-up suggests spinal fusion is associated with increased adjacent segment disc degeneration but without influence on clinical outcome: results of a combined follow-up from 4 randomized controlled trials. *Spine (Phila Pa 1976).* 2014;39(17):1373–1383.
34. Park P, Garton HJ, Gala VC, Hoff JT, McGillicuddy JE. Adjacent segment disease after lumbar or lumbosacral fusion: review of the literature. *Spine (Phila Pa 1976).* 2004;29(17):1938–1944.
35. Kumar MN, Baklanov A, Chopin D. Correlation between sagittal plane changes and adjacent segment degeneration following lumbar spine fusion. *Eur Spine J.* 2001;10(4):314–319.
36. Okuda S, Yamashita T, Matsumoto T, et al. Adjacent segment disease after posterior lumbar interbody fusion: A case series of 1000 patients. *Global Spine J.* 2018;8(7):722–727.
37. Sears WR, Sergides IG, Kazemi N, et al. Incidence and prevalence of surgery at segments adjacent to a previous posterior lumbar arthrodesis. *Spine J.* 2011;11(1):11–20.
38. Moreau P-E, Ferrero E, Riouallon G, Lenoir T, Guigui P. Radiologic adjacent segment degeneration 2 years after lumbar fusion for degenerative spondylolisthesis. *Orthop Traumatol Surg Res.* 2016;102(6):759–763.
39. Matsumoto T, Okuda S, Maeno T, et al. Spinopelvic sagittal imbalance as a risk factor for adjacent-segment disease after single-segment posterior lumbar interbody fusion. *J Neurosurg Spine.* 2017;26(4):435–440.
40. Levin JM, Alentado VJ, Healy AT, Steinmetz MP, Benzel EC, Mroz TE. Superior segment facet joint violation during instrumented lumbar fusion is associated with higher reoperation rates

and diminished improvement in wuality of life. *Clin Spine Surg.* 2018;31(1):E36–e41.
41. Wang H, Ma L, Yang D, et al. Incidence and risk factors of adjacent segment disease following posterior decompression and instrumented fusion for degenerative lumbar disorders. *Medicine (Baltimore).* 2017;96(5):e6032.
42. Oh HS, Seo HY. The relationship between adjacent segment pathology and facet joint violation by pedicle screw after posterior lumbar instrumentation surgery. *J Clin Med.* 2021;10(13):2911.
43. Dimar J, Bisson EF, Dhall S, et al. Congress of Neurological Surgeons systematic review and evidence-based guidelines for perioperative spine: Preoperative osteoporosis assessment. *Neurosurgery.* 2021;89(Suppl 1):S19–S25.
44. Demir Ö, Öksüz E, Deniz FE, Demir O. Assessing the effects of lumbar posterior stabilization and fusion to vertebral bone density in stabilized and adjacent segments by using Hounsfield unit. *J Spine Surg.* 2017;3(4):548–553.
45. Zaidi Q, Danisa OA, Cheng W. Measurement techniques and utility of Hounsfield unit values for assessment of bone quality prior to spinal instrumentation: A review of current literature. *Spine (Phila Pa 1976).* 2019;44(4):E239–e244.
46. Son HJ, Choi SH, Heo DR, et al. Outcomes of the use of cement-augmented cannulated pedicle screws in lumbar spinal fusion. *Spine J.* 2021;21(11):1857–1865.
47. Ghobrial GM, Eichberg DG, Kolcun JPG, et al. Prophylactic vertebral cement augmentation at the uppermost instrumented vertebra and rostral adjacent vertebra for the prevention of proximal junctional kyphosis and failure following long-segment fusion for adult spinal deformity. *Spine J.* 2017;17(10): 1499–1505.
48. Kim KH, Lee S-H, Lee DY, Shi CS, Maeng DH. Anterior bone cement augmentation in anterior lumbar interbody fusion and percutaneous pedicle screw fixation in patients with osteoporosis. *J Neurosurg Spine.* 2010;12(5):525–532.
49. McCoy S, Tundo F, Chidambaram S, Baaj AA. Clinical considerations for spinal surgery in the osteoporotic patient: A comprehensive review. *Clin Neurol Neurosurg.* 2019;180:40–47.
50. Radcliff KE, Kepler CK, Maaieh M, et al. What is the rate of lumbar adjacent segment disease after percutaneous versus open fusion? *Orthop Surg.* 2014;6(2):118–120.
51. Yee TJ, Terman SW, L Marca F, Park P. Comparison of adjacent segment disease after minimally invasive or open transforaminal lumbar interbody fusion. *J Clin Neurosci.* 2014;21 (10):1796–1801.
52. Fu L, France A, Xie Y, Fang K, Gan Y, Zhang P. Functional and radiological outcomes of semi-rigid dynamic lumbar stabilization adjacent to single-level fusion after 2 years. *Arch Orthop Trauma Surg.* 2014;134(5):605–610.
53. Buell TJ, Chen C-J, Quinn JC, et al. Alignment risk factors for proximal junctional kyphosis and the effect of lower thoracic junctional tethers for adult spinal deformity. *World Neurosurg.* 2019;121:e96–e103.
54. Wang MY, Vasudevan R, Mindea SA. Minimally invasive lateral interbody fusion for the treatment of rostral adjacent-segment lumbar degenerative stenosis without supplemental pedicle screw fixation. *J Neurosurg Spine.* 2014;21(6):861–866.
55. Louie PK, Varthi AG, Narain AS, et al. Stand-alone lateral lumbar interbody fusion for the treatment of symptomatic adjacent segment degeneration following previous lumbar fusion. *Spine J.* 2018;18(11):2025–2032.
56. Waguespack A, Schofferman J, Slosar P, Reynolds J. Etiology of long-term failures of lumbar spine surgery. *Pain Med.* 2002; 3(1):18–22.
57. Weigel R, Capelle HH, Al-Afif S, Krauss JK. The dimensions of "failed back surgery syndrome": what is behind a label? *Acta Neurochir (Wien).* 2021;163(1):245–250.
58. North RB, Campbell JN, James CS, et al. Failed back surgery syndrome: 5-year follow-up in 102 patients undergoing repeated operation. *Neurosurgery.* 1991;28(5):685–690; discussion 690–691.
59. Inoue S, Kamiya M, Nishihara M, et al. Prevalence, characteristics, and burden of failed back surgery syndrome: the influence of various residual symptoms on patient satisfaction and quality of life as assessed by a nationwide Internet survey in Japan. *J Pain Res.* 2017;10:811–823.
60. Thomson S. Failed back surgery syndrome - definition, epidemiology and demographics. *Br J Pain.* 2013;7(1):56–59.
61. Taylor RS, Taylor RJ. The economic impact of failed back surgery syndrome. *Br J Pain.* 2012;6(4):174–181.
62. Baber Z, Erdek MA. Failed back surgery syndrome: current perspectives. *J Pain Res.* 2016;9:979–987.
63. Sikora M, Nemani VM, Winnett RL, et al. Helping spine surgeons detect pre-surgical psychological distress in complex spine patients: an observational pilot study. *Spine Deform.* 2020; 8(3):413–420.
64. Guyer RD, Patterson M, Ohnmeiss DD. Failed back surgery syndrome: diagnostic evaluation. *J Am Acad Orthop Surg.* 2006;14(9):534–543.
65. Turner JA, Loeser JD, Deyo RA, Sanders SB. Spinal cord stimulation for patients with failed back surgery syndrome or complex regional pain syndrome: a systematic review of effectiveness and complications. *Pain.* 2004;108(1-2):137–147.
66. Leveque JC, Villavicencio AT, Bulsara KR, Rubin L, Gorecki JP. Spinal cord stimulation for failed back surgery syndrome. *Neuromodulation.* 2001;4(1):1–9.

25

Complications of Minimally Invasive Surgery of the Lumbar Spine

ANDREW S. CHUNG AND NEEL ANAND

CHAPTER OUTLINE

Introduction

The number of minimally invasive spine surgical (MISS) techniques that are now available to spine surgeons has increased significantly in the last decade. As a result of notable technological advancements in implant science and instrumentation, there is increasing evidence to show that MISS decreases blood loss, shortens hospital lengths of stay, mitigates complications, decreases perioperative pain, and enables quicker return to function when compared to equivalent open surgical techniques.[1–7] Concomitant advancements in perioperative pain management protocols have led to further improvements in outcomes as many MISS procedures are now able to be safely performed in an outpatient setting. Further, by maximally preserving normal anatomy, MISS techniques may theoretically mitigate the risks of iatrogenic instability and adjacent segment degeneration in the long term, further decreasing the overall incidence of negative sequelae following surgical intervention. In this chapter, we will discuss the complications related to MISS techniques for the treatment of lumbar pathology.

MISS Decompression and Discectomy

MISS decompressions were first introduced for the treatment of disc herniations in 1997 by Foley and Smith, who utilized tubular retractors and an endoscope to visualize pertinent pathology. Both Fessler and Palmer translated this MISS approach to the decompression of lumbar spinal stenosis in 2002.[8,9] Traditional open treatment of lumbar stenosis involves a wide laminectomy via a midline posterior approach that results in extensive damage to the posterior musculoligamentous complex—which both helps to maintain spinal stability and secondarily contains important proprioceptors.[10] On the contrary, MISS techniques minimize damage to these crucial structures without compromising patient outcomes. The types of complications encountered are similar in MISS decompression compared to open decompressions, but rates of complications appear to be less in MISS decompression (MISS: 1.6%–7.9% vs open: up to 16.1%).[11,12] Specifically, surgical site infections appear to be less common (Relative Risk 0.23, 95% Confidence Interval 0.07 to 0.079),[13] and while rates of dural tears have been reported at up to 6.4% with use of MISS, in general these latter complications seem to be less common in MISS than in open surgery (15.9%; $P < 0.05$).[14]

Lateral Interbody Fusion

First described in 2006, the lateral lumbar interbody fusion (LLIF) utilizes a retroperitoneal transpsoas corridor to allow direct access to the interbody space. It intrinsically circumvents the need for manipulation of the posterior neural elements. In comparison to posterior approaches, it offers improved visualization of the interbody space allowing a more thorough discectomy and consequent insertion of a larger interbody device,[15] which may mitigate rates of subsidence.[16] This may facilitate more powerful restoration of disc and foraminal height and correction of sagittal and coronal contours.[17,18] The most worrisome limitation of the

LLIF is the risk of direct injury to the lumbar plexus while it traverses the psoas muscle.[19–21]

Similar to other MISS approaches, LLIF may result in improved short-term postoperative outcomes in regards to estimated blood loss (EBL), length of stay, and mobility when compared to equivalent open approaches.[16,20,22] Furthermore, LLIF may enable more powerful correction of radiographic spinopelvic parameters including lumbar lordosis when compared to comparable posterior interbody approaches, as it enables the placement of a larger interbody implant.[23] Subsidence is not uncommon but may be mitigated with use of posterior fixation and maximizing the footprint of the selected implant.[24]

A meta-analysis comparing a total of 1874 patients who received an oblique lumbar interbody fusion (OLIF) to 4607 patients who received a LLIF found the rates of transient hip weakness and sensory deficits to be much higher with LLIF (19.7% and 21.7%, respectively) when compared to those associated with OLIF (5.7% and 8.7%, respectively). These differences were statistically significant.[20] Furthermore, persistent neurologic injury may be higher with LLIF when compared to OLIF (2.8% vs 1.0%; $P = 0.005$).[20] Permanent sensory deficits appear to be more common that motor deficits.[21] On the contrary, risk of vascular injury and injury to the sympathetic nerve plexus appear to be less likely with LLIF.[20] Other possible complications of LLIF include pseudohernia, due to injury of the motor innervation to the abdominal musculature (1.8%). Visceral injuries, vertebral fractures, and wound complications have all been reported but are much less common.[24]

Oblique Lumbar Interbody Fusion

By exploiting the interval between the great vessels and the psoas, the psoas-sparing OLIF circumvents the weaknesses of the transpsoas approach (LLIF) and the morbidity associated with the open anterior lumbar interbody fusion (ALIF). Furthermore, it enables more reliable access to the L4-5 disc space that is less accessible via LLIF due to the intervening bony anatomy of the pelvis. Furthermore, the OLIF corridor may enable more optimal visualization of the disc space. Consequently, a more thorough discectomy can be performed allowing for a larger interbody cage to be placed, potentially mitigating risk of subsidence.[25] Existing clinical data are promising, demonstrating excellent fusion rates[26,27] and significant improvements in patient-reported outcome measures in patients undergoing OLIF.[26,28] Consequently, for some surgeons, the OLIF procedure has significant appeal.

As might be expected given the surgical corridor utilized, complications of OLIF may include any of the following: incisional pain, injury to the sympathetic chain, injury to the lumbar plexus, postop ileus, vascular injury, abdominal visceral injury, and peritoneal injury. These rates are relatively low, and as discussed previously, the rates of neurologic injury are substantially less in OLIF when compared to LLIF.[20]

Minimally Invasive Transforaminal Lumbar Interbody Fusion

The transforaminal lumbar interbody fusion (TLIF) is a posterior-based approach to the disc space that minimizes the need for neural retraction by taking advantage of the foraminal corridor. Conventionally, a complete facetectomy allows easy access to the lateral disk space via Kambin's triangle, facilitating discectomy and interbody insertion. The minimally invasive transforaminal lumbar interbody fusion (MIS-TLIF) offers further benefits via a less-invasive Wiltse-type approach. A major criticism of TLIF, however, particularly when comparing it to other more anterior-based interbody approaches, is that it fails to adequately re-establish lumbar lordosis.[23,29,30] However, more recent studies have suggested that anterior placement of curvilinear or hyperlordotic interbody devices in combination with posterior column shortening osteotomies may allow for more optimal lordotic corrections.[23] It has also been suggested that use of an expandable cage may potentially improve correction; however, this remains to be definitively proven.[31] Nonetheless, numerous studies have demonstrated excellent improvements in patient-reported outcome measures with MIS-TLIF that are comparable to that of open approaches. Further, it appears that decreased iatrogenic musculoligamentous and osseous damage mitigates postoperative pain, perioperative blood loss, and shortens operative times compared to traditional open approaches.[32,33] Similar to other less invasive approaches to the spine, the risk of iatrogenic segmental destabilization and resultant adjacent segment degeneration and disease may theoretically be minimized in the long term.

In general, it appears that the complication profile is at least similar (if not better) to that of open techniques. In a large series of patients undergoing MIS-TLIF rates of complications were as follows: durotomy (5.1%), hardware failure (2.3%), neurologic deficit (0.8%), and wound hematoma (0.8%). Of the 11 hardware failures in this series, 5 patients had cage migration and 6 patients had an intraoperative fracture of the K-wire used for pedicle screw placement.[34]

Spinal Endoscopy

Spinal endoscopy is becoming an increasingly acceptable option for the treatment of disc herniations and spinal stenosis[35–37] and may represent the most minimally invasive surgical technique currently available to surgeons. Surgical indications have expanded to include spinal instrumentation and even the management of tumors and infection.[38,39]

Several randomized-controlled trials and meta-analyses to date have demonstrated equivalent outcomes in patients undergoing spinal endoscopy for the treatment of lumbar stenosis,[40] lumbar disc herniations,[41–43] when compared to the use of more conventional MISS techniques.

It is important to note, that while in experienced hands, complication rates may be comparable to MISS, the risk of complications during the initial learning phase may be notably higher. This learning curve appears to be procedure specific,[44,45] with more complex cases necessitating a minimum 70 or more cases to achieve surgical competency.[46] Durotomies, neural injury, iatrogenic facet damage, and postoperative diskitis are all described complications with overall rates of complications reported in the literature varying from 0.14% to up to 21%.[47,48] There fortunately appears to be an inverse relationship between surgeon experience and the rate of related complications, that is, in experienced hands, the risk of complications and rates of treatment failures approach that of similar MISS procedures.[48,49]

Minimally Invasive Deformity Correction

Adult spinal deformity correction, while potentially effective, comes with a high risk of patient morbidity with rates of all cause complications reported at up to 86%[50–52] with correction of the most severe deformities.[53] Rod fractures alone have an incidence of 18.4% in this surgical setting[54] with even higher rates noted in patients undergoing more significant deformity correction. In this context, rates of revision surgery in open deformity correction have been reported between 24% and 33%.[53–55] Furthermore, rates of mortality have been reported at 0.5%.[56]

In contrast, with use of circumferential minimally invasive deformity correction, rates of complications have been reported at 9.4%[57] with no surgery-related mortalities.[58,59] Furthermore, the rate of hardware failure requiring revision surgery with use of minimally invasive techniques is 3.9% with a low prevalence of rod fracture at 1.8%.

Proximal junctional kyphosis (PJK) and proximal junctional failure (PJF) are common complications following adult spinal deformity correction with a high prevalence of PJK (up to 61%)[60,61] and PJF (up to 35%)[62,63] reported in the open deformity literature. With use of minimally invasive techniques, however, the prevalence of PJK and PJF appears to be much lower. In a series of 184 patients undergoing adult spinal deformity surgery (mean follow-up of 85.2 months), the combined rate of PJK or PJF was 10.8% (21 patients). Only 10 of these patients (4.9%) met criteria for PJF (symptomatic PJK) with no catastrophic PJFs identified in this series.[64] Therefore, the majority of PJFs in this series occurred after at least 1 year following the index surgery and were the result of progressively increasing proximal junctional angles secondary to pelvic decompensation and a gradual loss of sagittal alignment.

Conclusion

Over the last decade, there has been a rapid expansion in the number of minimally invasive techniques that have become available for the management of lumbar spinal conditions. It appears that MISS techniques are associated with less blood loss, shorter hospital lengths of stay, decreased perioperative pain and postoperative narcotics usage, and enable faster return to daily activities. Complication profiles are at least equal to if not better when compared to equivalent open techniques. Furthermore, preservation of native anatomy may mitigate negative sequelae following surgical intervention including iatrogenic instability, proximal junctional issues, and adjacent segment disease.

However, it is imperative that surgeons understand that the adoption of MISS techniques is associated with a significant learning curve during which complications may be more prevalent. Therefore, adoption of MISS techniques should be slow and gradual, exercising strict patient selection to minimize these latter risks and, to maximize the chance of an optimal perioperative outcome.

While higher quality evidence is necessary to support the safety and efficacy of the latest minimally invasive techniques, more established MISS techniques for the management of lumbar spinal conditions may be associated with superior perioperative outcomes and a lesser complication profile when compared to more conventional open surgical approaches.

References

1. Allen RT, Garfin SR. The economics of minimally invasive spine surgery. *Spine*. 2010;35(26 Suppl):S375–382.
2. Avila MJ, Walter CM, Baaj AA. Outcomes and complications of minimally invasive surgery of the lumbar spine in the elderly. *Cureus*. 2016;8(3):e519. https://doi.org/10.7759/cureus.519.
3. Alimi M, Hofstetter CP, Pyo SY, Paulo D, Härtl R. Minimally invasive laminectomy for lumbar spinal stenosis in patients with and without preoperative spondylolisthesis: clinical outcome and reoperation rates. *J Neurosurg Spine*. 2015;22(4):339–352. https://doi.org/10.3171/2014.11.SPINE13597.
4. Al-Khouja LT, Baron EM, Johnson JP, Kim TT, Drazin D. Cost-effectiveness analysis in minimally invasive spine surgery. *Neurosurg Focus*. 2014;36(6):E4. https://doi.org/10.3171/2014.4.FOCUS1449.
5. Parker SL, Adogwa O, Witham TF, Aaronson OS, Cheng J, McGirt MJ. Post-operative infection after minimally invasive versus open transforaminal lumbar interbody fusion (TLIF): Literature review and cost analysis. *Minim Invasive Neurosurg*. 2011;54(1):33–37. https://doi.org/10.1055/s-0030-1269904.
6. Phan K, Hogan JA, Mobbs RJ. Cost–utility of minimally invasive versus open transforaminal lumbar interbody fusion: systematic review and economic evaluation. *Eur Spine J*. 2015;24(11):2503–2513. https://doi.org/10.1007/s00586-015-4126-4.
7. Swamy G, Lopatina E, Thomas KC, Marshall DA, Johal HS. The cost effectiveness of minimally invasive spine surgery in the treatment of adult degenerative scoliosis: a comparison of transpsoas and open techniques. *Spine J Off J North Am Spine Soc*. 2019;19(2):339–348. https://doi.org/10.1016/j.spinee.2018.05.040.
8. Guiot BH, Khoo LT, Fessler RG. A minimally invasive technique for decompression of the lumbar spine. *Spine*. 2002;27(4):432–438. https://doi.org/10.1097/00007632-200202150-00021.
9. Khoo LT, Fessler RG. Microendoscopic decompressive laminotomy for the treatment of lumbar stenosis. *Neurosurgery*. 2002;51(5 Suppl):S146–154.

10. Arai Y, Hirai T, Yoshii T, et al. A prospective comparative study of 2 minimally invasive decompression procedures for lumbar spinal canal stenosis: unilateral laminotomy for bilateral decompression (ULBD) versus muscle-preserving interlaminar decompression (MILD). *Spine.* 2014;39(4):332–340. https://doi.org/10.1097/BRS.0000000000000136.
11. Montano N, Stifano V, Papacci F, Mazzucchi E, Fernandez E. Minimally invasive decompression in patients with degenerative spondylolisthesis associated with lumbar spinal stenosis. Report of a surgical series and review of the literature. *Neurol Neurochir Pol.* 2018;52(4):448–458. https://doi.org/10.1016/j.pjnns.2018.06.004.
12. Rahman M, Summers LE, Richter B, Mimran RI, Jacob RP. Comparison of techniques for decompressive lumbar laminectomy: the minimally invasive versus the "classic" open approach. *Minim Invasive Neurosurg MIN.* 2008;51(2):100–105. https://doi.org/10.1055/s-2007-1022542.
13. Rasouli MR, Rahimi-Movaghar V, Shokraneh F, Moradi-Lakeh M, Chou R. Minimally invasive discectomy versus microdiscectomy/open discectomy for symptomatic lumbar disc herniation. *Cochrane Database Syst Rev.* 2014;9:CD010328. https://doi.org/10.1002/14651858.CD010328.pub2.
14. Sharma A, Shakya A, Singh V, et al. Incidence of dural tears in open versus minimally invasive spine surgery: A single-center prospective study. *Asian Spine J.* 2022;16(4):463–470. https://doi.org/10.31616/asj.2021.0140.
15. Tatsumi R, Lee YP, Khajavi K, Taylor W, Chen F, Bae H. In vitro comparison of endplate preparation between four mini-open interbody fusion approaches. *Eur Spine J.* 2015;24(Suppl 3):372–377. https://doi.org/10.1007/s00586-014-3708-x.
16. Marchi L, Abdala N, Oliveira L, Amaral R, Coutinho E, Pimenta L. Radiographic and clinical evaluation of cage subsidence after stand-alone lateral interbody fusion. *J Neurosurg Spine.* 2013;19(1):110–118. https://doi.org/10.3171/2013.4.SPINE12319.
17. Phillips FM, Isaacs RE, Rodgers WB, et al. Adult degenerative scoliosis treated with XLIF: clinical and radiographical results of a prospective multicenter study with 24-month follow-up. *Spine.* 2013;38(21):1853–1861. https://doi.org/10.1097/BRS.0b013e3182a43f0b.
18. Nakashima H, Kanemura T, Satake K, et al. Changes in sagittal alignment following short-level lumbar interbody fusion: Comparison between posterior and lateral lumbar interbody fusions. *Asian Spine J.* 2019;13(6):904–912. https://doi.org/10.31616/asj.2019.0011.
19. Davis TT, Bae HW, Mok JM, Rasouli A, Delamarter RB. Lumbar plexus anatomy within the psoas muscle: implications for the transpsoas lateral approach to the L4-L5 disc. *J Bone Joint Surg Am.* 2011;93(16):1482–1487. https://doi.org/10.2106/JBJS.J.00962.
20. Walker CT, Farber SH, Cole TS, et al. Complications for minimally invasive lateral interbody arthrodesis: a systematic review and meta-analysis comparing prepsoas and transpsoas approaches. *J Neurosurg Spine.* 2019:1–15. https://doi.org/10.3171/2018.9.SPINE18800.
21. Lykissas MG, Aichmair A, Hughes AP, et al. Nerve injury after lateral lumbar interbody fusion: a review of 919 treated levels with identification of risk factors. *Spine J.* 2014;14(5):749–758. https://doi.org/10.1016/j.spinee.2013.06.066.
22. Katz AD, Singh H, Greenwood M, Cote M, Moss IL. Clinical and radiographic evaluation of multilevel lateral lumbar interbody fusion in adult degenerative scoliosis. *Clin Spine Surg.* 2019;32(8):E386–E396. https://doi.org/10.1097/BSD.0000000000000812.
23. Ahlquist S, Park HY, Gatto J, Shamie AN, Park DY. Does approach matter? A comparative radiographic analysis of spinopelvic parameters in single-level lumbar fusion. *Spine J.* 2018;18(11):1999–2008. https://doi.org/10.1016/j.spinee.2018.03.014.
24. Salzmann SN, Shue J, Hughes AP. Lateral lumbar interbody fusion-outcomes and complications. *Curr Rev Musculoskelet Med.* 2017;10(4):539–546. https://doi.org/10.1007/s12178-017-9444-1.
25. Peck JH, Kavlock KD, Showalter BL, Ferrell BM, Peck DG, Dmitriev AE. Mechanical performance of lumbar intervertebral body fusion devices: An analysis of data submitted to the Food and Drug Administration. *J Biomech.* 2018;78:87–93. https://doi.org/10.1016/j.jbiomech.2018.07.022.
26. Abbasi A, Khaghany K, Orandi V, Abbasi H. Clinical and radiological outcomes of oblique lateral lumbar interbody fusion. *Cureus.* 2019;11(2):e4029. https://doi.org/10.7759/cureus.4029.
27. Woods KRM, Billys JB, Hynes RA. Technical description of oblique lateral interbody fusion at L1-L5 (OLIF25) and at L5-S1 (OLIF51) and evaluation of complication and fusion rates. *Spine J.* 2017;17(4):545–553. https://doi.org/10.1016/j.spinee.2016.10.026.
28. Li HM, Zhang RJ, Shen CL. Radiographic and clinical outcomes of oblique lateral interbody fusion versus minimally invasive transforaminal lumbar interbody fusion for degenerative lumbar disease. *World Neurosurg.* 2019;122:e627–e638. https://doi.org/10.1016/j.wneu.2018.10.115.
29. Champagne PO, Walsh C, Diabira J, et al. Sagittal balance correction following lumbar interbody fusion: A comparison of the three approaches. *Asian Spine J.* 2019;13(3):450–458. https://doi.org/10.31616/asj.2018.0128.
30. Saadeh YS, Joseph JR, Smith BW, Kirsch MJ, Sabbagh AM, Park P. Comparison of segmental lordosis and global spinopelvic alignment after single-level lateral lumbar interbody fusion or transforaminal lumbar interbody fusion. *World Neurosurg.* 2019;126:e1374–e1378. https://doi.org/10.1016/j.wneu.2019.03.106.
31. Alvi MA, Kurian SJ, Wahood W, Goyal A, Elder BD, Bydon M. Assessing the difference in clinical and radiologic outcomes between expandable cage and nonexpandable cage among patients undergoing minimally invasive transforaminal interbody fusion: A systematic review and meta-analysis. *World Neurosurg.* 2019;127:596–606. https://doi.org/10.1016/j.wneu.2019.03.284.e1.
32. Miller LE, Bhattacharyya S, Pracyk J. Minimally invasive versus open transforaminal lumbar interbody fusion for single-level degenerative disease: Systematic review and meta-analysis of randomized controlled trials. *World Neurosurg.* 2020;133:358–365. https://doi.org/10.1016/j.wneu.2019.08.162.e4.
33. Goldstein CL, Phillips FM, Rampersaud YR. Comparative effectiveness and economic evaluations of open versus minimally invasive posterior or transforaminal lumbar interbody fusion: A systematic review. *Spine.* 2016;41(Suppl 8):S74–89. https://doi.org/10.1097/BRS.0000000000001462.
34. Wong AP, Smith ZA, Nixon AT, et al. Intraoperative and perioperative complications in minimally invasive transforaminal lumbar interbody fusion: a review of 513 patients. *J Neurosurg Spine.* 2015;22(5):487–495. https://doi.org/10.3171/2014.10.SPINE14129.
35. Gibson JNA, Subramanian AS, Scott CEH. A randomised controlled trial of transforaminal endoscopic discectomy vs microdiscectomy. *Eur Spine.* 2017;26(3):847–856. https://doi.org/10.1007/s00586-016-4885-6.

36. Komp M, Hahn P, Oezdemir S, et al. Bilateral spinal decompression of lumbar central stenosis with the full-endoscopic interlaminar versus microsurgical laminotomy technique: a prospective, randomized, controlled study. *Pain Physician*. 2015;18(1):61–70.
37. Nomura K, Yoshida M. Assessment of the learning curve for microendoscopic decompression surgery for lumbar spinal canal stenosis through an analysis of 480 cases involving a single surgeon. *Glob Spine J*. 2017;7(1):54–58. https://doi.org/10.1055/s-0036-1583943.
38. Telfeian AE, Veeravagu A, Oyelese AA, Gokaslan ZL. A brief history of endoscopic spine surgery. *Neurosurg Focus*. 2016;40(2):E2. https://doi.org/10.3171/2015.11.FOCUS15429.
39. Mayer HM. A history of endoscopic lumbar spine surgery: What have we learnt? *BioMed Res Int*. 2019;2019:4583943. https://doi.org/10.1155/2019/4583943.
40. Ruetten S, Komp M, Merk H, Godolias G. Surgical treatment for lumbar lateral recess stenosis with the full-endoscopic interlaminar approach versus conventional microsurgical technique: a prospective, randomized, controlled study. *J Neurosurg Spine*. 2009;10(5):476–485. https://doi.org/10.3171/2008.7.17634.
41. Ruetten S, Komp M, Merk H, Godolias G. Full-endoscopic interlaminar and transforaminal lumbar discectomy versus conventional microsurgical technique: a prospective, randomized, controlled study. *Spine*. 2008;33(9):931–939. https://doi.org/10.1097/BRS.0b013e31816c8af7.
42. Ruetten S, Komp M, Merk H, Godolias G. Recurrent lumbar disc herniation after conventional discectomy: a prospective, randomized study comparing full-endoscopic interlaminar and transforaminal versus microsurgical revision. *J Spinal Disord Tech*. 2009;22(2):122–129. https://doi.org/10.1097/BSD.0b013e318175ddb4.
43. Qin R, Liu B, Hao J, et al. Percutaneous endoscopic lumbar discectomy versus posterior open lumbar microdiscectomy for the treatment of symptomatic lumbar disc herniation: A systemic review and meta-analysis. *World Neurosurg*. 2018;120:352–362. https://doi.org/10.1016/j.wneu.2018.08.236.
44. Hsu HT, Chang SJ, Yang SS, Chai CL. Learning curve of full-endoscopic lumbar discectomy. *Eur Spine J*. 2013;22(4):727–733. https://doi.org/10.1007/s00586-012-2540-4.
45. Xu H, Liu X, Liu G, Zhao J, Fu Q, Xu B. Learning curve of full-endoscopic technique through interlaminar approach for L5/S1 disk herniations. *Cell Biochem Biophys*. 2014;70(2):1069–1074. https://doi.org/10.1007/s12013-014-0024-3.
46. Morgenstern R, Morgenstern C, Yeung AT. The learning curve in foraminal endoscopic discectomy: experience needed to achieve a 90% success rate. *SAS J*. 2007;1(3):100–107. https://doi.org/10.1016/SASJ-2007-0005-RR.
47. Anichini G, Landi A, Caporlingua F, et al. Lumbar endoscopic microdiscectomy: Where are we now? An updated literature review focused on clinical outcome, complications, and rate of recurrence. *BioMed Res Int*. 2015;2015:417801. https://doi.org/10.1155/2015/417801.
48. Lewandrowski KU. Incidence, management, and cost of complications after transforaminal endoscopic decompression surgery for lumbar foraminal and lateral recess stenosis: A value proposition for outpatient ambulatory surgery. *Int J Spine Surg*. 2019;13(1):53–67. https://doi.org/10.14444/6008.
49. Yeung A, Roberts A, Zhu L, Qi L, Zhang J, Lewandrowski KU. Treatment of soft tissue and bony spinal stenosis by a visualized endoscopic transforaminal technique under local anesthesia. *Neurospine*. 2019;16(1):52–62. https://doi.org/10.14245/ns.1938038.019.
50. Sciubba DM, Yurter A, Smith JS, et al. A comprehensive review of complication rates after surgery for adult deformity: A reference for informed consent. *Spine Deform*. 2015;3(6):575–594. https://doi.org/10.1016/j.jspd.2015.04.005.
51. Yeramaneni S, Robinson C, Hostin R. Impact of spine surgery complications on costs associated with management of adult spinal deformity. *Curr Rev Musculoskelet Med*. 2016;9(3):327–332. https://doi.org/10.1007/s12178-016-9352-9.
52. Smith JS, Shaffrey CI, Klineberg E, et al. Complication rates associated with 3-column osteotomy in 82 adult spinal deformity patients: retrospective review of a prospectively collected multicenter consecutive series with 2-year follow-up. *J Neurosurg Spine*. 2017;27(4):444–457. https://doi.org/10.3171/2016.10.SPINE16849.
53. Lertudomphonwanit T, Kelly MP, Bridwell KH, et al. Rod fracture in adult spinal deformity surgery fused to the sacrum: prevalence, risk factors, and impact on health-related quality of life in 526 patients. *Spine J*. 2018;18(9):1612–1624. https://doi.org/10.1016/j.spinee.2018.02.008.
54. Smith JS, Klineberg E, Lafage V, et al. Prospective multicenter assessment of perioperative and minimum 2-year postoperative complication rates associated with adult spinal deformity surgery. *J Neurosurg Spine*. 2016;25(1):1–14. https://doi.org/10.3171/2015.11.SPINE151036.
55. Crawford CH, Glassman SD, Carreon LY, et al. Prevalence and indications for unplanned reoperations following index surgery in the adult symptomatic lumbar scoliosis NIH-sponsored clinical trial. *Spine Deform*. 2018;6(6):741–744. https://doi.org/10.1016/j.jspd.2018.04.006.
56. Lee NJ, Kothari P, Kim JS, et al. Early complications and outcomes in adult spinal deformity surgery: An NSQIP study based on 5803 patients. *Glob Spine J*. 2017;7(5):432–440. https://doi.org/10.1177/2192568217699384.
57. Anand N, Cohen JE, Cohen RB, Khandehroo B, Kahwaty S, Baron E. Comparison of a newer versus older protocol for circumferential minimally invasive surgical (CMIS) correction of adult spinal deformity (ASD)-evolution over a 10-year experience. *Spine Deform*. 2017;5(3):213–223. https://doi.org/10.1016/j.jspd.2016.12.005.
58. Anand N, Sardar ZM, Simmonds A, Khandehroo B, Kahwaty S, Baron EM. Thirty-day reoperation and readmission rates after correction of adult spinal deformity via circumferential minimally invasive surgery-analysis of a 7-year experience. *Spine Deform*. 2016;4(1):78–83. https://doi.org/10.1016/j.jspd.2015.08.002.
59. Smith JS, Shaffrey CI, Kelly MP, et al. Effect of serious adverse events on health-related quality of life measures following surgery for adult symptomatic lumbar scoliosis. *Spine*. 2019;44(17):1211–1219. https://doi.org/10.1097/BRS.0000000000003036.
60. Maruo K, Ha Y, Inoue S, et al. Predictive factors for proximal junctional kyphosis in long fusions to the sacrum in adult spinal deformity. *Spine*. 2013;38(23):E1469–1476. https://doi.org/10.1097/BRS.0b013e3182a51d43.
61. Lee JH, Kim JU, Jang JS, Lee SH. Analysis of the incidence and risk factors for the progression of proximal junctional kyphosis following surgical treatment for lumbar degenerative kyphosis: minimum 2-year follow-up. *Br J Neurosurg*. 2014;28(2):252–258. https://doi.org/10.3109/02688697.2013.835369.
62. Hostin R, McCarthy I, O'Brien M, et al. Incidence, mode, and location of acute proximal junctional failures after surgical treatment of adult spinal deformity. *Spine*. 2013;38(12):1008–1015. https://doi.org/10.1097/BRS.0b013e318271319c.

63. Smith MW, Annis P, Lawrence BD, Daubs MD, Brodke DS. Acute proximal junctional failure in patients with preoperative sagittal imbalance. *Spine J*. 2015;15(10):2142–2148. https://doi.org/10.1016/j.spinee.2015.05.028.
64. Anand N, Agrawal A, Ravinsky R, Khanderhoo B, Kahwaty S, Chung A. The prevalence of proximal junctional kyphosis (PJK) and proximal junctional failure (PJF) in patients undergoing circumferential minimally invasive surgical (cMIS) correction for adult spinal deformity: long-term 2- to 13-year follow-up. *Spine Deform*. 2021;9(5):1433–1441. https://doi.org/10.1007/s43390-021-00319-1.

26 When to Operate on Pediatric Spine Deformity

TYLER A. TETREAULT AND MICHAEL J. HEFFERNAN

CHAPTER OUTLINE

When to Operate on Early Onset Scoliosis

Natural History

Early onset scoliosis (EOS) is defined as the presence of spinal deformity with a major Cobb angle greater than 10 degrees before 10 years of age. The etiology for EOS is broad, and causes may be idiopathic, neuromuscular, congenital, or syndromic (as seen with neurofibromatosis). The primary concern with EOS is the potential for patients to develop restrictive lung disease. Patients with thoracic cage deformity due to EOS can have small lung volumes, diminished chest wall compliance, and respiratory muscle dysfunction.[1,2] Due to the significant growth potential in young children, these curves can have a high risk for progression and the development of thoracic insufficiency syndrome (TIS), defined as an inability for the thorax to support normal lung growth. TIS, first described in cases of congenital scoliosis with fused ribs, is highlighted by the presence of respiratory insufficiency, reduced chest wall compliance, worsening spinal deformity on radiographs, and a decline in pulmonary function tests.[3]

Indications for Surgery

The goals of treatment in this age group are to prevent curve progression while allowing continued spinal growth, as early fusion and short thoracic height results in poor pulmonary function.[4] However, there is a high complication rate associated with growth-friendly instrumentation (GFI) and therefore initiation of surgical treatment should be delayed as long as possible.[5,6] The initial treatment in the youngest children is often serial elongation, flexion, and derotation (EDF) casting. For some, casting is curative. Of 136 children prospectively studied by Mehta,[7] 94 children had resolution of their scoliosis with EDF casting. The primary determinant of success from casting was early initiation of treatment once there was evidence of progression, a rib vertebral angle difference greater than 20 degrees, or a phase 2 rib head (where the rib head overlaps the vertebral body) on PA spine radiographs.[7] Even for patients whose curvatures do not resolve, EDF casting is beneficial in delaying the need for growth friendly instrumentation and thus the time available for complications to arise. In patients with syndromic, congenital, or neuromuscular early onset scoliosis, Fletcher et al. showed that serial casting can delay growing spine instrumentation for 3 years on average and allowed for the avoidance of growing rods in 72% of patients in this cohort.[8] However, casting is contraindicated in patients with frail pulmonary status, fragile medical condition, sharp and rigid congenital scoliosis, and cervical spine instability.

For young patients who fail casting/bracing (either due to poor tolerance or continued curve progression while in a cast or brace), GFI such as traditional growing rods (TGR)

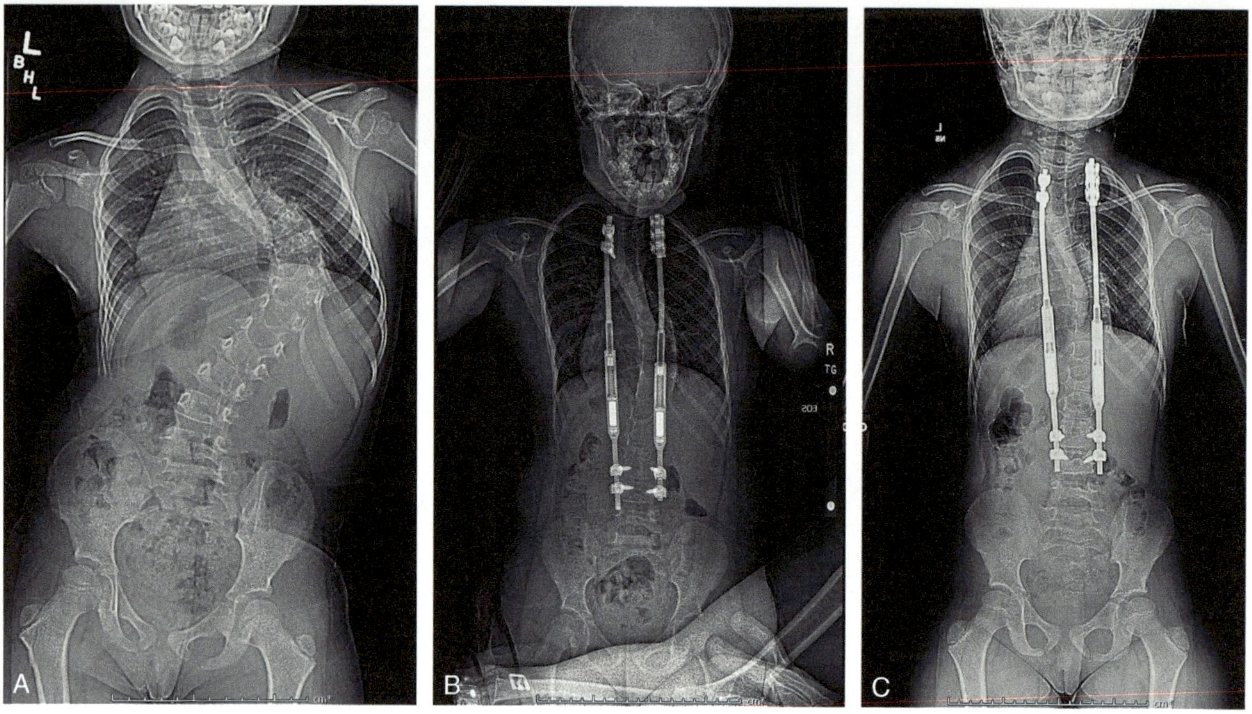

• **Fig. 26.1** (A) Five-year-old female with early onset scoliosis (EOS) prior to magnetically controlled growing rods (MCGR) instrumentation. (B) At 7 years old rods had been fully lengthened, though curve remained well controlled. (C) The patient underwent MCGR reimplantation to allow for continued lengthening.

or magnetically controlled growing rods (MCGR) is indicated. Because EOS encompasses such a heterogeneous population, there is not a well-defined curve magnitude for when GFI should be implemented. Rather, the surgeon must consider additional factors such as rate of progression, apex of deformity, global alignment, and curve flexibility when deciding when to proceed with GFI (Fig. 26.1). There are high complication rates with GFI that tend to increase with time, and numerous studies have shown that auto fusion of the spine occurs around 5 years after instrumentation.[5,6,9,10] Ideally, patients are at least 5 years old prior to instrumentation so that when spine auto fusion occurs around age 10 they will have adequate spinal height for conversion to definitive fusion.

There are a few factors to consider when choosing between MCGR and TGR implants. In a case-matched study, MCGR and TGR achieved similar deformity correction, similar spinal growth, and had similar numbers of *unplanned* surgeries, though TGR had three times greater total surgeries due to the need for surgical lengthening every 6 months.[11] Although patients with MCGR undergo fewer total surgeries, quality-of-life metrics remain the same.[12] MCGR are contraindicated in patients who require serial spinal MRI, as in cases of neurofibromatosis, tumor, spinal cord syrinx, or tethered cord. While MCGR are safe to undergo MRI, the imaging around the rods is nondiagnostic.[13] Obesity, stiff/rigid curves, and hyperkyphosis are additional contraindications to MCGR.[14] In these cases, or when MCGR are unavailable, traditional growing rods are an excellent option.

Vertical expandable prosthetic titanium rib (VEPTR) implants were first FDA approved in 2004 for the treatment of Jeune thoracic dystrophy, Jarcho-Levin syndrome, and congenital scoliosis with fused ribs. This was then expanded to include progressive EOS. While effective in the treatment of EOS, high complication rates have been documented, and for this reason VEPTR has fallen out of favor for EOS.[15,16] VEPTR remains a good surgical option for thoracic dystrophy patients.

While we know that early posterior spinal fusion (PSF) results in poor pulmonary outcomes for young patients with EOS, there is growing evidence to support spinal fusion in the older "tweener" aged EOS patient who is 8 to 10 years old. When comparing primary PSF to GFI followed by conversion to PSF in this age group, patients with GFI had a mean of 2 cm greater thoracic height gain, but at a cost of higher complication rates (14%–28% of primary PSF patients vs 61%–80% of GFI patients), higher need for additional surgery, and less deformity correction than patients undergoing primary PSF.[17,18] The patient's stature, medical frailty, ability to undergo multiple surgical events, and family expectations are other factors to consider when formulating a plan for patients in this transitional age group.

When to Operate on Congenital Scoliosis

Natural History

Congenital scoliosis is a unique type of EOS caused by a failure of vertebral segmentation or formation during embryonic development. This leads to spinal anomalies due to a failure of formation (i.e., wedged or hemivertebra) or from a failure of segmentation (i.e., vertebral bar or block vertebra). More complex deformities with a mixture of anomalies and congenitally fused or absent ribs can also occur. The mere presence of a congenital anomaly does not require intervention, rather the presence and rate of deformity progression dictates treatment. The risk of progression depends on anomaly type. A block vertebra has the most benign course with an average progression of <2 degrees per year during growth, while a hemivertebra with a contralateral bar behaves the most aggressively with an average progression of 5 to 10 degrees per year.[19] The course of progression for an isolated hemivertebra is variable and depends on the presence (or absence) of the adjacent discs. An incarcerated hemivertebra, with thin, underdeveloped discs or synostoses to the adjacent vertebrae, will likely progress <1 degree per year. In contrast, a fully segmented hemivertebra with healthy discs above and below is likely to progress and require surgical intervention, especially if located in the upper thoracic or thoracolumbar region.[20] The wide variability in vertebral anomalies means that no two curves behave alike and treatment decisions must be made on a case-by-case basis.

Indications for Surgery

Deformities with demonstrated rapid progression, those with high risk for rapid progression based on anomaly type, and patients with decompensated spinal balance are indicated for surgical intervention. In contrast to other types of EOS, early surgical intervention is often warranted in congenital scoliosis. The goal of treatment is to prevent further deformity progression while preserving as much motion and normal spine growth as possible. The focal nature of many congenital scoliosis anomalies allows for more limited surgical approach involving only a few spinal levels. Addressing the deformity at an earlier age, before further spinal decompensation occurs, can limit the morbidity of the procedure. Klemme et al. showed that in a patient with progressive congenital scoliosis, young age is not a contraindication to surgical intervention.[21]

Correction Techniques

The spectrum of unique treatment options for congenital scoliosis includes limited in situ fusion, convex hemiepiphysiodesis, and hemivertebra excision. The magnitude of deformity, number, location, and type of vertebral anomalies and overall spinal alignment are key factors to assess on both radiographs and clinical appearance when formulating a surgical plan.

Limited in situ fusion is an excellent option for short-segment progressive congenital scoliosis without substantial spinal deformity. While safe in young patients, crankshaft phenomenon can develop and consideration of a combined anterior and posterior fusion is warranted, though in theory this is less of a concern with modern all pedicle screw constructs.[22]

Convex hemiepiphysiodesis is indicated for an isolated hemivertebra with substantial spinal curvature where in situ fusion would yield an unacceptable spinal balance. In theory, this allows for continued growth on the concave side of the curve while arresting growth along the convexity. Early techniques described uninstrumented fusion following decortication of the hemivertebra and excision of the convex disc and apophyses via a dual anterior/posterior approach, or a posterior-only transpedicular approach.[23,24] Modern techniques now describe posterior-only convex pedicle screw instrumentation to achieve three-column fixation.[25] The correction from convex hemiepiphysiodesis is variable and somewhat unpredictable, though efficacy appears to be greatest in younger patients <5 years old and for lumbar level hemivertebrae that cause more substantial spinal decompensation.[26–28]

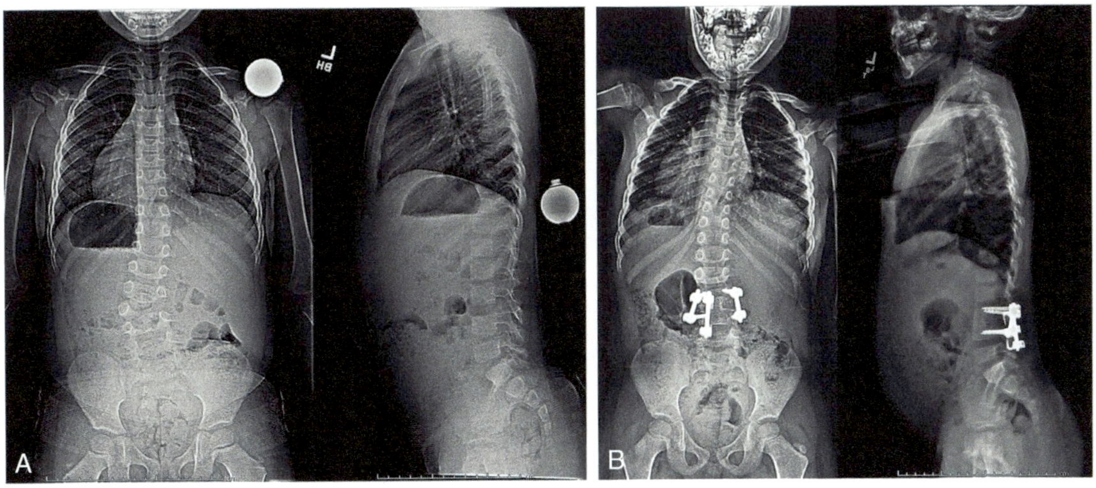

• **Fig. 26.2** (A) Posteroanterior (PA) and lateral x-rays of a 3-year-old male with an isolated lumbar hemivertebra, prior to excision. (B) X-rays at 4 years old demonstrated good correction of spinal deformity. A third rod with sublaminar hooks was used to reduce the deformity once the hemivertebra was excised.

For an isolated hemivertebra causing significant trunk imbalance, typically those at a lower lumbar or lumbosacral level, correction with hemivertebra excision allows for an acute correction and can restore spinal balance when convex epiphysiodesis is unlikely to provide sufficient correction (Fig. 26.2). While surgery at a very young age has been shown to be safe and effective, it is our preference to wait until a child is 3 years of age, or when they are large enough for spinal instrumentation.[21]

When to Operate on Adolescent Idiopathic Scoliosis

Natural History

Adolescent idiopathic scoliosis (AIS) is a condition of asymmetric spinal growth that results in a three-dimensional spinal deformity. A diagnosis of AIS is made when a patient 10 years or older develops a spinal curvature with a major Cobb angle of greater than 10 degrees and has no underlying medical conditions to explain their spinal curvature. With a prevalence of 1.5% to 3% of adolescents, AIS is the most common pediatric spine deformity.

Prior to skeletal maturity, three major factors influence the risk of curve progression: gender, curve magnitude, and remaining growth. Females are at greater risk for curve progression compared to males.[29,30] As curve magnitude increases, so does the risk for progression. Curves less than 20 degrees are at low risk for progression, while those greater than 25 degrees are at a higher risk for curve progression, though skeletal age and relationship to peak height velocity also play an important role in predicting curve behavior.[31,32] The Sanders skeletal maturity scoring system provides the best predictor of future curve progression based on curve magnitude and Sanders stage. This has supplanted the Tanner-Whitehouse-III staging system and is often used in conjunction with the Risser staging system and menarchal status for predicting curve behavior.[33]

After skeletal maturity, there is a risk of continued curve progression for curves over 40 to 50 degrees. On average, these curves progress at a rate of 1 degree per year.[34–37] This can lead to substantial spinal deformity decades later. Weinstein's prospective 50-year natural history study on patients with untreated idiopathic scoliosis showed that while in general these patients have minimal physical impairment, there is an increased rate of chronic back pain and more body dissatisfaction compared to a matched cohort.[38] In addition, patients with thoracic curves greater than 50 degrees at skeletal maturity are at greater risk for pulmonary dysfunction, and patients in this group reported increased shortness of breath with activity.[38]

Indications for Surgery

The foundational goals for surgical treatment of idiopathic scoliosis are to prevent deformity progression and achieve a solid fusion with good spinal balance. The ideal results of surgery also include deformity correction and improved clinical appearance. The surgical indications are relatively well defined due to long-term natural history studies. Thoracic curves greater than 50 degrees, and thoracolumbar or lumbar curves greater than 40 to 45 degrees, are indicated for posterior spinal fusion surgery, as these are the curves that are expected to progress after skeletal maturity.[36]

Correction Techniques

Posterior spinal fusion aims to achieve the above goals while involving the minimum numbers of spinal levels so that spinal motion is preserved as much as possible. The Lenke classification helps identify which curves are structural and which are compensatory, or nonstructural. In general, all structural curves should be included in the fusion.[39] Compared to historic techniques such as uninstrumented fusions, Harrington rods, and sublaminar bands and hooks, modern pedicle screw constructs allow for greatly improved spinal deformity correction. Pedicle screws give three-column segmental control of the spine to achieve coronal plane correction, derotation of the vertebral bodies, and restoration of thoracic kyphosis (Fig. 26.3). Implant factors to consider during surgical planning include screw density and rod stiffness. Higher density screw constructs are often used in younger patients to prevent crankshaft deformity, or when more points of fixation are needed to share the load during reduction maneuvers. Stiffer rods put a greater force on the spine and can help with correction, though this must be balanced with the risk of screw pullout, which can occur in patients with decreased bone density. Reduction maneuvers include differential rod bending, en bloc or segmental derotation, in situ rod bending, and compression or distraction across vertebral levels. The selection of and sequence in which these techniques are employed is surgeon dependent.

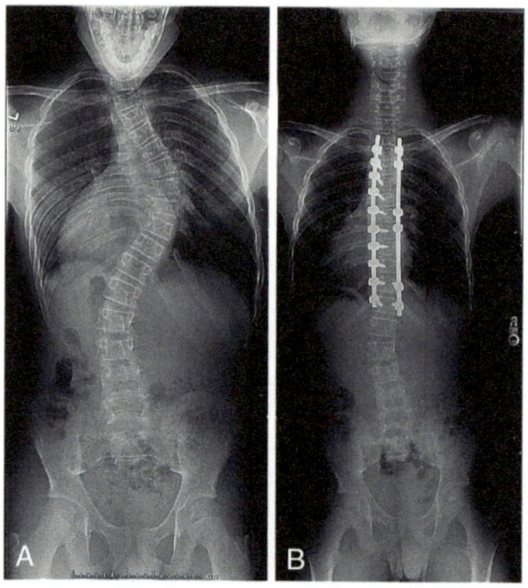

• **Fig. 26.3** PA x-rays of a 13-year-old male with adolescent idiopathic scoliosis (AIS) (A) before and (B) after T3-T12 posterior spinal fusion (PSF). Note that postoperatively the patient's shoulders are level and there is excellent coronal balance. The lumbar curve was nonstructural and not included in the spinal fusion.

In addition to the above correction maneuvers, adjunctive techniques such as posterior column osteotomies, anterior release, and thoracoplasty can further mobilize the spine and improve overall correction, though at the cost of increased surgical risk. Preoperative factors such as patient age, curve magnitude, and curve flexibility help guide the decision making for when to use these techniques.

Posterior column osteotomies (PCOs) increase spinal mobility by resecting the articular facets and soft tissue attachments (namely, the ligamentum flavum and facet capsule) at the involved level. There is significant variability in surgeon technique for performing posterior column osteotomies, which has led to some controversy regarding their efficacy in mobilizing the spine.[40–42] Generally, PCOs are performed through the apex of deformity, where the curve is the most rotated and most rigid. PCOs are performed at the surgeon's discretion, weighing the risks of increased surgical time, potential for increased blood loss, and exposing the spinal canal with the benefit of improved curve flexibility.

Anterior release is a spinal mobilization technique that entails an anterior resection of the discoligamentous complex, performed via a thoracotomy or thoracoscopic approach. This allows for increased flexibility of the spine and shortening of the anterior column, which can help with restoration of kyphosis. Once a frequently used tool for spinal deformity correction, anterior release has been widely replaced by posterior mobilization techniques and all pedicle screw instrumentation, as many studies have shown equivalent deformity correction with posterior-only approaches.[43–46] For severe rigid curves, there is still an indication for anterior release in the trained surgeon's hands.

Thoracoplasty involves partial resection of the three to six ribs at the apex of deformity to improve the rib hump prominence. Previously, thoracoplasty was relatively indicated for patients with greater than 10 degrees of rib prominence, curves greater than 60 degrees, or less than 20% curve flexibility.[47] Now, with improved three-dimensional correction due to pedicle screw instrumentation, posterior column releases, and derotation maneuvers, the rib hump deformity is almost always adequately addressed without need for thoracoplasty. For petite patients with a sharp rib hump deformity that persists after spinal correction, thoracoplasty remains a viable option.

A desire to achieve a fusionless solution for spinal deformity correction, allowing for continued spinal growth and spinal motion, led to a series of translational work in the early 2000s. These studies demonstrated an ability to modulate spinal growth in animal models by applying compression across the vertebral physis with a flexible tether system.[48–50] Early clinical trials then led to an FDA Humanitarian Device Exemption in 2019, which indicated anterior vertebral body tethering (AVBT) for skeletally immature patients with a major Cobb angle of 30 to 65 degrees who had failed a trial of bracing. Continued experience has narrowed these indications to patients with a hypokyphotic curve of 45 to 65 degrees, skeletal maturity of Risser 0-1, and Sanders stage 3-4.[51] Early outcomes are now emerging, and the results are mixed. As indications for AVBT narrow, clinical success (defined as a curve of <30 degrees at skeletal maturity) rates appear to be improving, with some multicenter studies reporting up to 77% success.[52–54] However, complications such as overcorrection and tether breakage are common. Reoperation rates remain unacceptably high, reported at 14% to 41%.[52–55] Thus, even among experts there remains a lack of consensus on when to proceed with AVBT versus PSF.[56] Further research and experience will help further narrow indications for AVBT.

When to Operate on Neuromuscular Scoliosis

Natural History

Neuromuscular scoliosis is a form of scoliosis that results from disorders of the nervous or muscular systems, such as cerebral palsy, spina bifida, spinal muscular atrophy, or muscular dystrophy. It is postulated that spinal deformity develops from asymmetric forces across the spine during growth that can cause a large, sweeping C-shaped curvature with marked pelvic obliquity. The etiology of the condition plays a significant role in the expected natural history. Here, we will focus on neuromuscular scoliosis in patients with cerebral palsy, which is one of the most frequently encountered subtypes. Long-term studies of institutionalized adults with cerebral palsy suggest that curves greater than 40 to 50 degrees at skeletal maturity are likely to continue to progress in adulthood, at a rate of 1.4 to 4.4 degrees per year.[57–59] Although this natural history is worrisome, the impact of progressive deformity on nursing care and general medical status remains unclear, with no differences found in incidence of decubitus ulcers, physical function, pulmonary status, or time required for daily care between those with severe untreated scoliosis and those without significant spinal deformity.[60,61] While there are no longitudinal studies evaluating quality-of-life scores in nonoperatively treated patients with neuromuscular scoliosis, in a small retrospective study Sewell et al. demonstrated that health-related quality of life, as measured with the Caregiver Priorities and Health Child Index of Life with Disabilities (CPCHILD) questionnaire, slightly decreased in the observed cohort, and this decrease was primarily due to changes in pain.[62]

Indications for Surgery

Regardless of etiology, the goals for posterior spinal fusion in the neuromuscular population are the same: prevent further curve progression and achieve good seating balance. In general, progressive curves greater than 50 degrees are indicated for surgery (Fig. 26.4). However, a thorough discussion assessing the family's goals, the patient's comfort and seating tolerance, and ability to perform nursing care, is imperative. While scores on the CP CHILD increase after surgery, and many families report high satisfaction rates postoperatively regarding the patient's appearance, quality

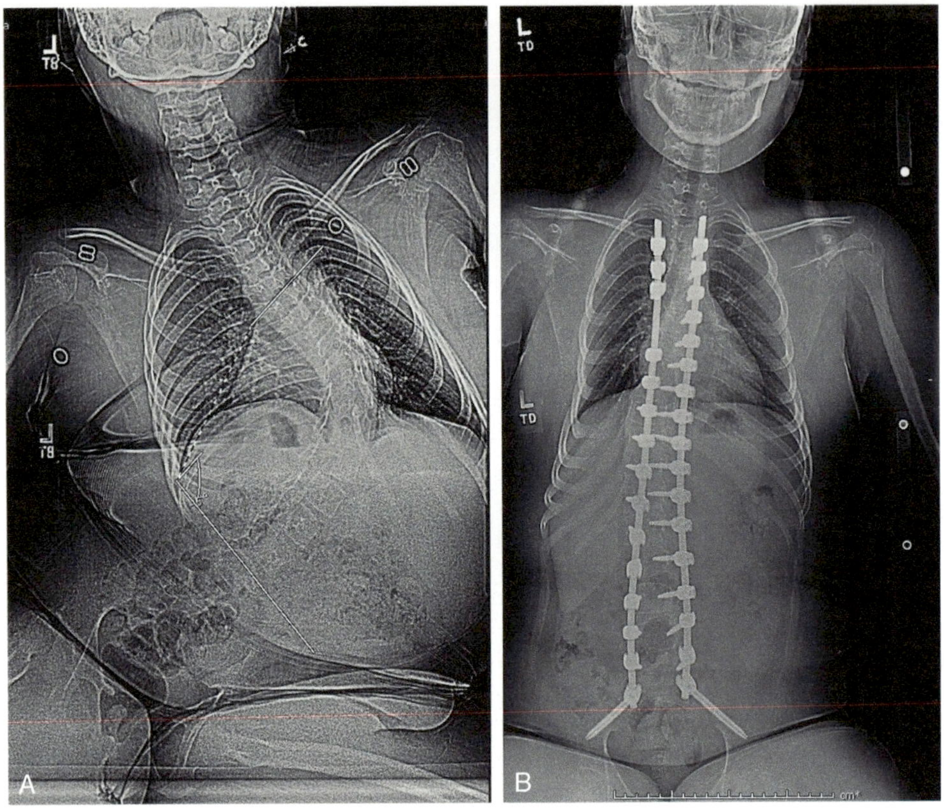

• **Fig. 26.4** (A) Sitting PA x-rays of an 11-year-old female with cerebral palsy and neuromuscular scoliosis demonstrate the typical sweeping C-shaped curvature seen in this population with marked pelvic obliquity. (B) After T3-pelvis PSF with a high screw density construct there is significant improvement in the patient's pelvic obliquity and coronal balance.

of life, improved comfort, and ease of care, the decision to proceed with posterior spinal fusion should be made on a case-by-case basis, with a shared decision-making process that also addresses the high rate of complications in neuromuscular spine surgery.[62–66]

Because patients with neuromuscular scoliosis often have underlying comorbidities, surgery is only indicated in those that can endure surgery with an acceptable risk profile. Comorbidities common in patients with neuromuscular scoliosis include decreased pulmonary function, poor nutritional status, decreased cognitive function, and seizure disorders. Involvement of a patient's pulmonary and nutrition teams, as well as a cardiac evaluation, are necessary to optimize their condition for surgery. At some institutions, this is performed through a high-risk scoliosis multidisciplinary pathway, which has been shown to minimize intensive care and hospital length of stay and decrease perioperative complications.[67] After a global health assessment is performed, a meeting with the family and consulting teams can allow the family to make a fully informed decision prior to proceeding with surgery.

Correction Techniques

Correction of deformity in neuromuscular patients can pose a challenge. Often, bone quality is quite poor due to the patient's nonambulatory status and suboptimal nutrition. As such, indirect correction techniques that do not rely on the bone-pedicle screw interface are helpful to prevent loss of screw fixation. Halo femoral traction, which can be placed prior to the initiation of surgery, allowed for improved correction of the scoliosis and pelvic obliquity in a case-matched group, and Bane et al. achieved 53% coronal plane correction and 65% correction of pelvic obliquity with this method.[68,69] Traction is applied to the head after Mayfield tong application, and rather than placing a femoral traction pin, we elect to place skin traction on the buttock of the elevated hemipelvis. We have found this to both be more efficient and minimize the morbidity associated with placement of a femoral traction pin.

When to Operate on Scheuermann's Kyphosis

Natural History

Scheuermann's kyphosis (SK) is a fixed deformity of the thoracic spine with anterior vertebral body wedging of at least 5 degrees at three or more levels and irregular vertebral apophyses.[70,71] The natural history regarding this condition is poorly understood. Few long-term studies have assessed rates of back pain and associated disability in adults with SK. Patients with SK tended to select less strenuous occupations

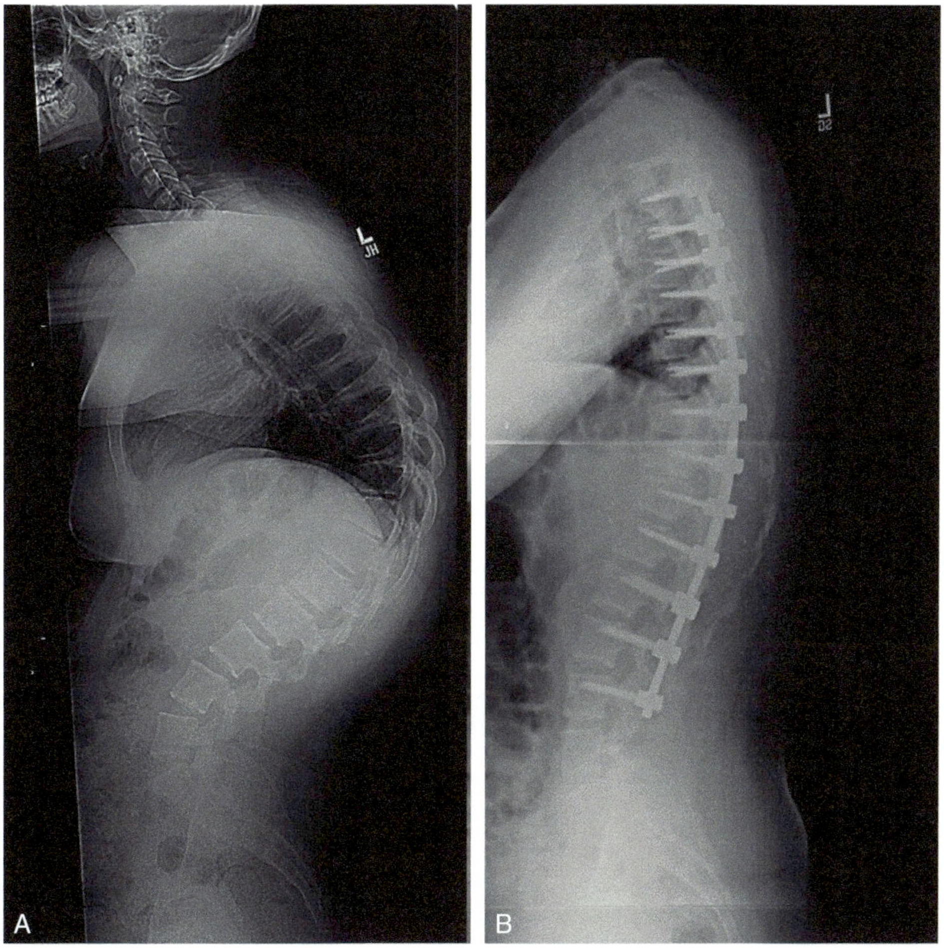

• **Fig. 26.5** (A) Lateral x-ray of a 13-year-old female with Scheuermann's kyphosis. Note the endplate changes and anterior vertebral body wedging through the apex of the deformity. (B) The patient underwent T2-L3 PSF.

and demonstrated diminished thoracic motion compared to controls but reported good physical function and no significant difference in pulmonary function was noted unless the kyphosis was greater than 100 degrees.[72,73] The deformity appears to be relatively stable over time, with only a mild increase in mean thoracic kyphosis over a 46-year period from mean of 46 degrees (range 25–78 degrees) at onset to 60 degrees (range 34–82 degrees) at final follow-up.[72] However, this study includes SK patients with normal kyphosis and does not fully address the natural history of those with hyperkyphosis over time and our understanding of the natural history of those with severe SK is lacking.

Indications for Surgery

The goals of PSF for SK are to improve deformity and decrease thoracic kyphosis. Surgery is reserved for patients with pain, rigid deformity, and/or an unacceptable cosmetic appearance (Fig. 26.5). There is no well-defined threshold for when to surgically treat SK, though 75 degrees of kyphosis is often cited.[74,75] A multicenter study of the Spine Deformity Study Group showed significant variability in surgical indications, and no significant difference in thoracic kyphosis between those treated with and without surgery, though those treated with surgery had a greater mean BMI and worse pretreatment SRS-22 and Spinal Assessment Questionnaire Scores.[76] In addition, numerous studies evaluating surgical outcomes have shown a significant improvement in back pain and SRS-22 compared to non-surgically managed patients.[77–79] These findings suggest that the patient's symptoms and global well-being are equally as important as their radiographic measurements when formulating a treatment plan, and that surgery can improve pain and function in the appropriately selected patient.

Conclusion

The decision to operate on the pediatric spine must account for the etiology of the condition, magnitude of deformity, evidence of progression, and remaining growth. In early onset scoliosis, we employ delay tactics such as casting or bracing to delay or forego growth-friendly instrumentation. Congenital early onset scoliosis is an exception to this strategy as early surgical intervention can prevent the development of a large spinal deformity that would require a more extensive surgical procedure at an older age.

Natural history studies on adolescent idiopathic scoliosis have led to well-defined surgical indications for curves greater than 50 degrees in the thoracic spine or 40 to 45 degrees in the thoracolumbar or lumbar spine. Different surgical maneuvers can be employed to improve spine flexibility and achieve a well-balanced spine with good cosmetic results. The indications for anterior vertebral body tethering continue to evolve.

Patients with neuromuscular scoliosis often have progressive, sweeping deformities with pelvic obliquity that can make seating balance difficult. The decision to proceed with surgery needs to be made with a heavy consideration for the family's goals of care and the patient's overall medical status.

The natural history of Scheuermann's kyphosis is poorly understood but some patients can experience pain and disability. The presence of pain and unacceptable physical appearance are important factors in the decision to proceed with surgery.

References

1. Whittaker AL. Are ethnic differences in lung function explained by chest size? *Arch Dis Child - Fetal Neonatal Ed.* 2005;90(5): F423–F428. https://doi.org/10.1136/adc.2004.062497.
2. Emans JB, Ciarlo M, Callahan M, Zurakowski D. Prediction of thoracic dimensions and spine length based on individual pelvic dimensions in children and adolescents: An age-independent, individualized standard for evaluation of outcome in early onset spinal deformity. *Spine.* 2005;30(24):2824–2829. https://doi.org/10.1097/01.brs.0000190865.47673.6a.
3. Campbell RM, Smith MD, Mayes TC, et al. The characteristics of thoracic insufficiency syndrome associated with fused ribs and congenital scoliosis. *J Bone Jt Surg-Am Vol.* 2003;85(3):399–408. https://doi.org/10.2106/00004623-200303000-00001.
4. Karol LA, Johnston C, Mladenov K, Schochet P, Walters P, Browne RH. Pulmonary function following early thoracic fusion in non-neuromuscular scoliosis. *J Bone Jt Surg.* 2008;90(6): 1272–1281. https://doi.org/10.2106/JBJS.G.00184.
5. Bess S, Akbarnia BA, Thompson GH, et al. Complications of growing-rod treatment for early-onset scoliosis: Analysis of one hundred and forty patients. *J Bone Jt Surg-Am Vol.* 2010; 92(15):2533–2543. https://doi.org/10.2106/JBJS.I.01471.
6. Upasani VV, Parvaresh KC, Pawelek JB, et al. Age at initiation and deformity magnitude influence complication rates of surgical treatment with traditional growing rods in early-onset scoliosis. *Spine Deform.* 2016;4(5):344–350. https://doi.org/10.1016/j.jspd.2016.04.002.
7. Mehta MH. Growth as a corrective force in the early treatment of progressive infantile scoliosis. *J Bone Joint Surg Br.* 2005;87-B(9): 1237–1247. https://doi.org/10.1302/0301-620X.87B9.16124.
8. Fletcher ND, McClung A, Rathjen KE, Denning JR, Browne R, Johnston CE. Serial casting as a delay tactic in the treatment of moderate-to-severe early-onset scoliosis. *J Pediatr Orthop.* 2012; 32(7):664–671. https://doi.org/10.1097/BPO.0b013e31824bdb55.
9. Sankar WN, Skaggs DL, Yazici M, et al. Lengthening of dual growing rods and the law of diminishing reeturns. *Spine.* 2011; 36(10):806–809. https://doi.org/10.1097/BRS.0b013e318214d78f.
10. Noordeen HM, Shah SA, Elsebaie HB, Garrido E, Farooq N, Al Mukhtar M. In vivo distraction force and length measurements of growing rods: Which factors influence the ability to lengthen? *Spine.* 2011;36(26):2299–2303. https://doi.org/10.1097/BRS.0b013e31821b8e16.
11. Akbarnia BA, Pawelek JB, Cheung KMC, et al. Traditional growing rods versus magnetically controlled growing rods for the surgical treatment of rarly-onset scoliosis: A case-matched 2-year study. *Spine Deform.* 2014;2(6):493–497. https://doi.org/10.1016/j.jspd.2014.09.050.
12. Aslan C, Olgun ZD, Ayik G, et al. Does decreased surgical stress really improve the psychosocial health of early-onset scoliosis patients?: A comparison of traditional growing rods and magnetically-controlled growing rods patients reveals disappointing results. *Spine.* 2019;44(11):E656–E663. https://doi.org/10.1097/BRS.0000000000002938.
13. Woon RP, Andras LM, Noordeen H, et al. Surgeon survey shows no adverse events with MRI in patients with magnetically controlled growing rods (MCGRs. *Spine Deform.* 2018;6(3): 299–302. https://doi.org/10.1016/j.jspd.2017.10.004.
14. Seidel CP, Gilday SE, Jain VV, Sturm PF. How much does depth matter? Magnetically controlled growing rod distraction directly influenced by rod tissue depth. *Spine Deform.* 2022;10(1): 177–182. https://doi.org/10.1007/s43390-021-00399-z.
15. El-Hawary R, Kadhim M, Vitale M, Smith J, Samdani A, Flynn JM. VEPTR implantation to treat children with early-onset scoliosis without rib abnormalities: Early results from a prospective multicenter study. *J Pediatr Orthop.* 2017;37(8):e599–e605. https://doi.org/10.1097/BPO.0000000000000943.
16. Lucas G, Bollini G, Jouve JL, et al. Complications in pediatric spine surgery using the vertical expandable prosthetic titanium rib: The French experience. *Spine.* 2013;38(25):E1589–E1599. https://doi.org/10.1097/BRS.0000000000000014.
17. Mackey C, Hanstein R, Lo Y, et al. Magnetically controlled growing rods (MCGR) versus single posterior spinal fusion (PSF) versus vertebral body tether (VBT) in older early onset scoliosis (EOS) patients: How do early outcomes compare. *Spine.* 2022;47(4): 295–302. https://doi.org/10.1097/BRS.0000000000004245.
18. Keil LG, Nash AB, Stürmer T, et al. When is a growth-friendly strategy warranted? A matched comparison of growing rods versus primary posterior spinal fusion in juveniles with early-onset scoliosis. *J Pediatr Orthop.* 2021;41(10):e859–e864. https://doi.org/10.1097/BPO.0000000000001926.
19. McMaster M, Ohtsuka K. The natural history of congenital scoliosis. A study of two hundred and fifty-one patients. *J Bone Jt Surg Am.* 1982;64(8):1128–1147.
20. McMaster M, David C. Hemivertebra as a cause of scoliosis. A study of 104 patients. *J Bone Jt Surg Br.* 1968;68(4):588–595.
21. Klemme WR, Polly DW, Orchowski JR. Hemivertebral excision for congenital scoliosis in very young children. *J Pediatr Orthop.* 2001;21(6):761–764. https://doi.org/10.1097/01241398-200111000-00011.
22. Terek R, Wehner J, Lubick J. Crankshaft phenomenon in congenital scoliosis: a preliminary report. *J Pediatr Orthop.* 1991; 11(4):527–532.
23. Andrew T, Piggott H. Growth arrest for progressive scoliosis. Combined anterior and posterior fusion of the convexity. *J Bone Jt Surg Br.* 1985;67(2):193–197.
24. Keller P, Lindseth R, DeRosa G. Progressive congenital scoliosis treatment using a transpedicular anterior and posterior convex

hemiepiphysiodesis and hemiarthrodesis. A preliminary report. *Spine*. 1994;19:1933–1939.

25. Demirkiran G, Yilmaz G, Kaymaz B, et al. Safety and efficacy of instrumented convex growth arrest in treatment of congenital scoliosis. *J Pediatr Orthop*. 2014;34(3):275–281. https://doi.org/10.1097/BPO.0000000000000090.
26. Thompson A, Marks D, Sayampanathan S, Piggott H. Long-term results of combined anterior and posterior convex epiphysiodesis for congenital scoliosis due to hemivertebrae. *Spine*. 1995;20(12):1380–1385.
27. Ginsburg G, Mulconrey DS, Browdy J. Transpedicular hemiepiphysiodesis and posterior instrumentation as a treatment for congenital scoliosis. *J Pediatr Orthop*. 2007;27(4):387–391. https://doi.org/10.1097/01.bpb.0000271312.95621.b0.
28. Uzumcugil A, Cil A, Yazici M, et al. Convex growth srrest in the treatment of congenital spinal deformities, Revisited. *J Pediatr Orthop*. 2004;24(6):9.
29. Rogala E, Drummond D, Gurr J. Scoliosis: incidence and natural history. A prospective epidemiological study. *J Bone Jt Surg Am*. 1978;60(2):173–176.
30. Asher M, Green P, Orrick J. A six-year report: spinal deformity screening in Kansas school children. *J Kans Med Soc*. 1980;81(12):568–571.
31. Lonstein JE, Carlson J. The prediction of curve progression in untreated idiopathic scoliosis during growth. *J Bone Jt Surg Am*. 1984;66(7):1061–1071.
32. Nachemson AL, Peterson LE. Effectiveness of treatment with a brace in girls who have adolescent idiopathic scoliosis. A prospective, controlled study based on data from the brace study of the Scoliosis Research Society. *J Bone Jt Surg Am*. 1995;70(6):815–822.
33. Sanders JO, Khoury JG, Kishan S, et al. Predicting scoliosis progression from skeletal maturity: A simplified classification during adolescence. *J Bone Jt Surg-Am Vol*. 2008;90(3):540–553. https://doi.org/10.2106/JBJS.G.00004.
34. Asher MA, Burton DC. Adolescent idiopathic scoliosis: natural history and long term treatment effects. *Scoliosis*. 2006;1(2):1–10. https://doi.org/10.1186/1748-7161-1-2.
35. Danielsson AJ. Natural history of adolescent idiopathic scoliosis: A tool for guidance in decision of surgery of curves above 50°. *J Child Orthop*. 2013;7(1):37–41. https://doi.org/10.1007/s11832-012-0462-7.
36. Weinstein SL, Ponseti I. Curve progression in idiopathic scoliosis. *J Bone Jt Surg Am*. 1983;65(4):447–455.
37. Weinstein SL. The natural history of adolescent idiopathic scoliosis. *J Pediatr Orthop*. 2019;39(Supplement 1):S44–S46. https://doi.org/10.1097/BPO.0000000000001350.
38. Weinstein SL, Dolan LA, Spratt KF. Health and function of patients with untreated idiopathic scoliosis: A 50-year natural history study. *JAMA*. 2003;289(5):559–567.
39. Lenke LG, Betz RR, Harms J, et al. Adolescent idiopathic scoliosis: a new classification to determine extent of spinal arthrodesis. *J Bone Jt Surg Am*. 2001;83(8):1169–1181.
40. Halanski MA, Cassidy JA. Do multilevel Ponte osteotomies in thoracic idiopathic scoliosis surgery improve curve correction and restore thoracic kyphosis? *J Spinal Disord Tech*. 2013;26(5):252–255. https://doi.org/10.1097/BSD.0b013e318241e3cf.
41. Samdani AF, Bennett JT, Singla AR, et al. Do Ponte osteotomies enhance correction in adolescent idiopathic scoliosis? An analysis of 191 Lenke 1A and 1B curves. *Spine Deform*. 2015;3(5):483–488. https://doi.org/10.1016/j.jspd.2015.03.002.
42. Ponte A, Orlando G, Siccardi GL. The true Ponte osteotomy: By the one who developed it. *Spine Deform*. 2018;6(1):2–11. https://doi.org/10.1016/j.jspd.2017.06.006.
43. Ferrero E, Pesenti S, Blondel B, Jouve JL, Mazda K, Ilharreborde B. Role of thoracoscopy for the sagittal correction of hypokyphotic adolescent idiopathic scoliosis patients. *Eur Spine J*. 2014;23(12):2635–2642. https://doi.org/10.1007/s00586-014-3566-6.
44. Shi Z, Chen J, Wang C, et al. Comparison of thoracoscopic anterior release combined with posterior spinal fusion versus posterior-only approach with an all-pedicle screw construct in the treatment of rigid thoracic adolescent idiopathic scoliosis. *J Spinal Disord Tech*. 2015;28(8):E454–E459. https://doi.org/10.1097/BSD.0b013e3182a2658a.
45. Theologis AA, Sing DC, Chekeni F, Diab M. National trends in the surgical management of adolescent idiopathic scoliosis: Analysis of a national estimate of 60,108 children from the national inpatient sample over a 13-year time period in the United States. *Spine Deform*. 2017;5(1):56–65. https://doi.org/10.1016/j.jspd.2016.09.001.
46. Li M, Ni J, Fang X, et al. Comparison of selective anterior versus posterior screw instrumentation in Lenke5C adolescent idiopathic scoliosis. *Spine*. 2009;34(11):1162–1166. https://doi.org/10.1097/BRS.0b013e31819e2b16.
47. Harvey CJ, Betz RR, Clements D, Huss G, Clancy M. Are there indications for partial rib resection in patients with adolescent idiopathic scoliosis treated with Cotrl-Dubousset instrumentation? *Spine*. 1993;18(12):1593–1598.
48. Chay E, Patel A, Ungar B, et al. Impact of unilateral corrective tethering on the histology of the growth plate in an established porcine model for thoracic scoliosis. *Spine*. 2012;37(15):E883–E889. https://doi.org/10.1097/BRS.0b013e31824d973c.
49. Newton PO, Farnsworth CL, Faro FD, et al. Spinal growth modulation with an anterolateral flexible tether in an immature bovine model: Disc health and motion preservation. *Spine*. 2008;33(7):724–733. https://doi.org/10.1097/BRS.0b013e31816950a0.
50. Newton PO, Upasani VV, Farnsworth CL, et al. Spinal growth modulation with use of a tether in an immature porcine model. *J Bone Jt Surg-Am Vol*. 2008;90(12):2695–2706. https://doi.org/10.2106/JBJS.G.01424.
51. Newton PO. Spinal growth tethering: indications and limits. *Ann Transl Med*. 2020;8(2):27. https://doi.org/10.21037/atm.2019.12.159.
52. Newton PO, Kluck DG, Saito W, Yaszay B, Bartley CE, Bastrom TP. Anterior spinal growth tethering for skeletally immature patients with scoliosis: A retrospective look two to four years postoperatively. *J Bone Jt Surg*. 2018;100(19):1691–1697. https://doi.org/10.2106/JBJS.18.00287.
53. Baker CE, Kiebzak GM, Neal KM. Anterior vertebral body tethering shows mixed results at 2-year follow-up. *Spine Deform*. 2021;9(2):481–489. https://doi.org/10.1007/s43390-020-00226-x.
54. Miyanji F, Pawelek J, Nasto LA, Rushton P, Simmonds A, Parent S. Safety and efficacy of anterior vertebral body tethering in the treatment of idiopathic scoliosis: a multicentre review of 57 consecutive patients. *Bone Jt J*. 2020;102-B(12):1703–1708. https://doi.org/10.1302/0301-620X.102B12.BJJ-2020-0426.R1.
55. Shin M, Arguelles GR, Cahill PJ, Flynn JM, Baldwin KD, Anari JB. Complications, reoperations, and mid-term outcomes following anterior vertebral body tethering versus posterior

spinal fusion: A meta-analysis. *JBJS Open Access.* 2021;6(2): https://doi.org/10.2106/JBJS.OA.21.00002.e21.00002.

56. Shaw KA, Welborn MC, Matsumoto H, et al. To tether or fuse? Significant equipoise remains in treatment recommendations for idiopathic scoliosis. *Spine Deform.* 2022;10(4):763–773. https://doi.org/10.1007/s43390-022-00497-6.
57. Majd M, Muldowny D, Holt R. Natural history of scoliosis in the institutionalized adult cerebral palsy population. *Spine.* 1997;22(13):1461–1466.
58. Thometz J, Simon S. Progression of scoliosis after skeletal maturity in institutionalized adults who have cerebral palsy. *J Bone Jt Surg Am.* 1988;70(9):1290–1296.
59. Saito N, Ebara S, Ohotsuka K, Kumeta H, Takaoka K. Natural history of scoliosis in spastic cerebral palsy. *The Lancet.* 1998;351(9117):1687–1692. https://doi.org/10.1016/S0140-6736(98)01302-6.
60. Kalen V, Conklin M, Sherman F. Untreated scoliosis in severe cerebral palsy. *J Pediatr Orthop.* 1992;12(3):337–340.
61. Cassidy C, Craig C, Perry A, Karlin L, Goldberg M. A reassessment of spinal stabilization in severe cerebral palsy. *J Pediatr Orthop.* 1994;14(6):731–739.
62. Sewell MD, Malagelada F, Wallace C, et al. A preliminary study to assess whether spinal fusion for scoliosis improves carer-assessed quality of life for children with GMFCS Level IV or V cerebral palsy. *J Pediatr Orthop.* 2016;36(3):299–304. https://doi.org/10.1097/BPO.0000000000000447.
63. Miyanji F, Nasto LA, Sponseller PD, et al. Assessing the risk-benefit ratio of scoliosis surgery in cerebral palsy: Surgery is worth it. *J Bone Jt Surg.* 2018;100(7):556–563. https://doi.org/10.2106/JBJS.17.00621.
64. Bohtz C, Meyer-Heim A, Min K. Changes in health-related quality of life after spinal fusion and scoliosis correction in patients with cerebral palsy. *J Pediatr Orthop.* 2011;31(6): 668–673. https://doi.org/10.1097/BPO.0b013e318221093c.
65. Tsirikos AI, Chang WN, Dabney KW, Miller F. Comparison of parents' and caregivers' satisfaction after spinal fusion in children with cerebral palsy. *J Pediatr Orthop.* 2004;24(1):54–58.
66. DiFazio RL, Miller PE, Vessey JA, Snyder BD. Health-related quality of life and care giver burden following spinal fusion in children with cerebral palsy. *Spine.* 2017;42(12):E733–E739. https://doi.org/10.1097/BRS.0000000000001940.
67. Miller NH, Benefield E, Hasting L, Carry P, Pan Z, Erickson MA. Evaluation of high-risk patients undergoing spinal surgery: A matched case series. *J Pediatr Orthop.* 2010;30(5):496–502. https://doi.org/10.1097/BPO.0b013e3181df16ac.
68. Takeshita K, Lenke LG, Bridwell KH, Kim YJ, Sides B, Hensley M. Analysis of patients with nonambulatory neuromuscular scoliosis surgically treated to the pelvis with intraoperative halo-femoral traction. *Spine.* 2006;31(20):2381–2385. https://doi.org/10.1097/01.brs.0000238964.73390.b6.
69. Bane T, Luhmann SJ. Predicting the impact of intraoperative halo-femoral traction from preoperative imaging in neuromuscular scoliosis. *Spine Deform.* 2022;10(3):679–687. https://doi.org/10.1007/s43390-021-00461-w.
70. Scheuermann H. Deforming osteochondritis of the spine. *Ugeskr Laeger.* 1920;82:385.
71. Sorenson K. *Scheuermann's juvenile kyphosis: clinical appearances, radiography, aetiology, and prognosis.* [Thesis Dissertation]. Denmark, Copenhagen: Aarhus Universitet; 1964.
72. Ristolainen L, Kettunen JA, Heliövaara M, Kujala UM, Heinonen A, Schlenzka D. Untreated Scheuermann's disease: a 37-year follow-up study. *Eur Spine J.* 2012;21(5):819–824. https://doi.org/10.1007/s00586-011-2075-0.
73. Murray PM, Weinstein SL, Spratt KF. The natural history and long-term follow-up of Scheuermann kyphosis. *J Bone Jt Surg.* 1993;75(2):236–248. https://doi.org/10.2106/0000 4623-199302000-00011.
74. Arlet V, Schlenzka D. Scheuermann's kyphosis: surgical management. *Eur Spine J.* 2005;14(9):817–827. https://doi.org/10.1007/s00586-004-0750-0.
75. Geck MJ, Macagno A, Ponte A, Shufflebarger HL. The Ponte procedure: Posterior only treatment of Scheuermann's kyphosis using segmental posterior shortening and pedicle screw instrumentation. *J Spinal Disord Tech.* 2007;20(8):586–593. https://doi.org/10.1097/BSD.0b013e31803d3b16.
76. Polly DW, Ledonio CGT, Diamond B, et al. What are the indications for spinal fusion surgery in Scheuermann kyphosis? *J Pediatr Orthop.* 2019;39(5):217–221. https://doi.org/10.1097/BPO.0000000000000931.
77. Suominen EN, Saarinen AJ, Syvänen J, et al. Health-related quality of life outcomes in adolescent Scheuermann's kyphosis patients treated with posterior spinal fusion: A comparison with age- and sex-matched controls. *J Child Orthop.* 2022;16(4): 290–296. https://doi.org/10.1177/18632521221106384.
78. Audat ZA, Kheirallah KA, Ababneh BF, et al. Assessment of quality of life for Scheuermann's kyphosis patients with Cobb's angle 50°–65° treated conservatively or surgically in North Jordan: A prospective comparative study. *Clin Orthop Surg.* 2022;14(2):244. https://doi.org/10.4055/cios20219.
79. Green C, Brown K, Caine H, Dieckmann RJ, Rathjen KE. Prospective comparison of patient-selected operative versus nonoperative treatment of Scheuermann kyphosis. *J Pediatr Orthop.* 2020;40(8):e716–e719. https://doi.org/10.1097/BPO.0000000000001576.

27

General Complications in Pediatric Spinal Deformity

GABRIEL S. MAKAR, AND MEAGAN DELBAGGIO FERNANDEZ

CHAPTER OUTLINE

Introduction

Posterior spinal fusion is a common technique for pediatric adolescent idiopathic scoliosis (AIS) as well as other pediatric spinal deformities and traumatic injuries. Although a reliable procedure with good outcomes, performing a posterior spinal fusion does not come without complications, both intraoperative as well as postoperative. Intraoperative complications include neurologic injury to the spinal cord or peripheral nerve injury, dural tears, and hemorrhage or significant blood loss among other complications. Similarly, hemorrhage and thromboembolic events may present in the postoperative period along with surgical site infections, pseudoarthrosis, proximal junctional kyphosis, and implant-associated complications.

Complications in spinal fusion range from 3.6% to as high as 20%.[1–5] Fusions are predominantly done through a posterior-only approach; however, many times complex spines require the surgeon to include an anterior approach for further correction. Combined anterior and posterior instrumentation and fusion has an approximate complication rate of over 10%, double that of posterior spinal fusion alone.[2] Although much of our discussion and the literature refers to complications during the posterior approach, it is important to note that the addition of an anterior approach doubles the complication rate. It is unclear whether the complications are secondary to the complex nature of the spines, requiring the additional approach or the approach itself, but the discussion with patients and families regarding these findings is essential. As previously mentioned, complications in corrective scoliotic surgery are largely variable. The most common complications include surgical site infections, thromboembolism, gastrointestinal complications, blood loss requiring transfusions, and nerve injury.[6]

A number of pediatric patients undergoing spinal fusion are medically complex and carry an array of comorbid conditions that further complicate their care.[7] One study reviewed over 7000 patients undergoing spinal fusion and found the most common cohorts requiring fusion were those with cerebral palsy, brain malformations, and chromosomal syndromes. In their study, the majority of patients had more than four chronic medical comorbidities, the most common of which were epilepsy, gastroesophageal reflux disease, asthma, and dysphagia. They also noted that 42% percent of patients required the assistance of additional medical devices, the most common being an enterostomy (27.9%) followed by neurological and respiratory-related devices such as CSF shunts and tracheostomies, respectively.[7] These patients, especially those with neuromuscular scoliosis, tend to have significant spinal deformities requiring operative correction. However, given their medical complexity they often are at higher risk for complications both intraoperatively as well as postoperatively.[1] Therefore, it is important to understand the double hit phenomena that many of these patients encounter, namely increased spinal deformity and complex medical conditions.

Neurologic Injury in Posterior Spinal Fusion

Neurologic injury is a common complication among patients undergoing posterior spinal fusion. Injury can range from permanent spinal cord damage or cauda equina injury to temporary peripheral neurapraxia. Rates of neurologic injury span from 0.17% to 4%.[8,9] Rates of nerve injury are also higher in patients undergoing revision surgery compared to their index procedures.[10] Given the broad range of injury, treatment options vary identically as well.

Treatment options for neurologic injury can include lessening correction and removal of instrumentation to close observation. A large percentage of nerve injuries likely results from peripheral neuropraxias and are not reported. However, more critical complications such as cord injury may also go underreported secondary to the consequences that occur after such a complication.

Peripheral nerve injury after posterior spinal fusion can be transient or permanent, depending on the cause of nerve injury. Given the numerous factors that play a role in the pre-, peri-, and postoperative management of patients undergoing corrective surgery, the majority of cases of peripheral neuropathy are not well understood.[11,12] An additional analysis by the American Society of Anesthesiologists reviewing closed claims in patients with peripheral nerve injuries was not able to locate singular events in the instances of each claim, suggesting a singular event is not the cause of most nerve injuries.[12]

In general, transient nerve injuries are due to stretch of the nerve secondary to correction, compression from surrounding structures, or instrumentation. One study of 1136 patients undergoing posterior spinal fusion found a low rate of nerve injury (0.17%). The study reviewed 15 studies spanning posterior spinal fusion with either Harrington rods, Cotrel-Dubousset construct, or all-pedicle screw fixation. They found two patients with peripheral nerve injury, both of which underwent fixation with a Cotrel-Dubousset constructs. No neurologic injury was reported in the studies that included Harrington rods or all-pedicle screw fixation. The two patients sustained transient lower extremity paralysis in the immediate postoperative period. Both had complete recovery within a few months; however, one was noted to have persistent hyperreflexia.[8]

Prevention and early detection of nerve injury is essential to optimize outcomes and decrease risk for future nerve injury. A thorough neurological exam should be documented at each patient visit as the patients' curve progresses. Serial radiographs should be reviewed and measured for Cobb angles to document the ultimate degree of curvature as well as the rate of progression. Although many patients may elect to have their curves monitored nonoperatively and followed up at their interval clinic visit, they should be counseled on the risk of nerve injury with increasing curvature. As patients' curves increase, they may develop neurologic symptoms prior to undergoing their spinal fusion, and they additionally are at increased risk of nerve injury intraoperatively with the greater scoliotic curve. These discussions are essential in the office so that if a complication were to arise, the patient and family have been primed on the increased risk with prolonged monitoring of progressive curves.

Simple and periodically overlooked procedures such as proper patient positioning can help eliminate postoperative transient neuropraxias. Neurological monitoring, monitoring with both somatosensory evoked potentials (SSEPs) and motor evoked potentials (MEPs), has also largely become standard of care. Although neuromonitoring has become standard across many operating rooms across the nation, studies discuss that there is no true Level 1 evidence on neuromonitoring. For this reason, it should be used in a multimodal approach to prevent complications.[13] When the primary neurophysiologist is establishing the leads for the case, it's important for everyone on the team to keep the place of the leads in mind from time of positioning throughout the length of the case. If not closely considered, leads can easily become loosened from a patient and will be both difficult to replace intraoperatively as well as resulting in possible faults in monitoring throughout the case.

There are some concerns regarding the use of anesthetics and their effect on intraoperative neuromonitoring. Neuromuscular blocking agents have largely been found to not affect SSEPs while affecting other thermoregulatory mechanisms such as body temperature and blood pressure.[14,15] Propofol has not been found to have significant amplitude effects on SSEPs and MEPs and is a popular anesthetic for spinal deformity cases. Ketamine has been found to increase SSEPs and MEPs and may be used cautiously.[16] Anesthetic technique is important to discuss preoperatively with the team, so that proper anesthetic agents are used if neuromonitoring will be used.

If there are changes found during intraoperative neuromonitoring, each institution should have a checklist or protocol to decipher the cause for those changes. Various articles discuss not only their own checklists but techniques in developing one's own at their respective institution.[17–19] These checklists, as described by Vitale et al., should include a range of modalities such as gaining control of the room, anesthetic and systemic concerns, technical or neurophysiological status, and possible surgical causes such as malplaced hardware, significant curve correction, etc.[19] Furthermore, once the cause for the neuromonitoring change is recognized one should regularly revisit the checklist to prevent further changes as deficits can become additive and have a more significant effect on the cord.

Proper patient position may be commonly ignored but is critical in reducing the additive effect of all the variables that can cause patient's complications. It is also crucial to understand that many surrounding staff assist in the positioning of the patient, but ultimately it is the responsibility of the attending surgeon to ensure proper positioning. At our institution, it is paramount that the attending surgeon is present and directing the patient's positioning. A collaborative environment including all perioperative personnel aides in this process. Additionally, patient position should be maintained from the initial setup throughout the procedure and should be frequently checked. It is easy to lose sight of the patient's position given the extensive draping and the addition of technologies such as robotics, but one must keep in mind that altering the patient's position at any time increases the patient's risk of complications. Likewise, appropriate positioning aids in optimal operative site exposure, which will additionally decrease the risk for iatrogenic nerve injury.

Iatrogenic nerve injury in positioning commonly relates to compression of the lateral femoral cutaneous nerve (LFCN). The injury typically occurs below the anterosuperior iliac spine (ASIS) secondary to the positioning.[20] The injury is commonly seen in patients positioned on a Relton-Hall frame, but can occur with any frame or prone positioning that stabilizes the pelvis anteriorly.[21] The injury was found to occur in approximately 20% of patients undergoing spine surgery, of which 90% recovered by 3 months. It is appropriate to educate patients regarding transient neuropraxia to the LFCN and its benign nature as they might confuse the meralgia paresthetica for a more serious concern.

There are additionally various optic complications that may occur secondary to not only positioning but also intra- and postoperative measures.[22] Prone positioning significantly increases patients' cranial pressures and with various other measures, such as hypoperfusion and a low mean arterial pressure (MAP), optical complications increase significantly. Studies have found that pediatric patients undergoing posterior spinal surgery in the prone position may benefit from cervical traction to decrease facial contact pressure. One study suggested a combination of upward vectored 45 degree traction angle with 15 lbs of weight statistically significantly decreased facial contact pressure.[23] Less commonly, patients can experience orbital compartment syndrome secondary to prone positioning, but this is largely found in case reports and few case series. The rate of orbital compartment syndrome is remarkably low, but clinically patients may present with facial swelling, edema, proptosis, and no light perception.[24] Diagnosis is made with increased intraorbital tension. Being aware of the clinical signs and symptoms for orbital compartment syndrome can help early recognition and treatment.[25]

Ischemic optic neuropathy (ION) and central retinal artery occlusion (CRAO) are other optical complications in patients undergoing posterior spinal corrective surgery. Posterior ION is more common than anterior secondary to the blood supply to the optic nerve. The nature of the posterior blood supply creates a watershed area that is predominantly susceptible to vascular compromise and ischemia.[26,27] CRAO is less commonly found in the pediatric population compared to adults undergoing posterior spine surgery. CRAO is likely due to similar causes of ION; however, it also can be due to emboli, which are not commonly seen in the pediatric population. The relatively pathognomonic cherry-red spot on the fovea can be found in approximately 90% of patients.[28] Additional findings such as retinal opacity in the posterior pole and retinal artery attenuation were less commonly reported.

Prolonged operative times resulting in extended time in the prone position, significant blood loss, and intra- as well as postoperative hypotension are risk factors for orbital complications. As previously mentioned, this highlights the importance of having a well-rounded and educated team in the positioning of a patient. It is critically important that anesthesia is aware of the possible optical complications and attentive to the eye protection necessary to help prevent such instances.

Spinal Cord Injury in Posterior Spinal Fusion

Spinal cord injury during corrective scoliotic curves is also remarkably rare. Reports discuss rates lower than those for peripheral nerve injury, but nonetheless, these devastating complications occur for a multitude of reasons.

Cervical cord injury has been reported in a few case reports. Most recently, a report discussed the cervical injury in a patient with a 50-degree curve and Risser III.[29] This patient underwent instrumented fusion from T2-L1 with Ponte osteotomies at T5-T6 and T9-T10. MAPs were maintained above 80 mmHg. The case reported a loss of 1200 mL of blood and no changes to the SSEPs or MEPs during the case. Postoperatively the patient had weakness and an inability to move their right lower extremity. This returned once the MAPs were raised from 70 to approximately 90 mmHg. The patient was unable to move their right arm and this weakness persisted overnight. The patient obtained both a CT, which showed the hardware in appropriate position, as well as an magnetic resonance imaging (MRI), which appeared to show increased signal at the C5-C6 levels, suggestive of cord edema. The authors suggested that the likely cause of the edema was related to intraoperative hypotension, positioning, and preoperative cervical stenosis. Another reported case of cervical cord injury occurred in a female patient undergoing correction for her 55 degree right thoracic curve with 45 degree left lumbar curve. She underwent posterior spinal fusion without intraoperative correction but was noted to lose 1200 mL of blood. SSEPs were at baseline throughout the case. On the second postoperative morning the patient was noted to have neck pain and subsequently no motor function in the lower extremities bilaterally. The patient was then taken to the operating room where neuromonitoring showed loss of SSEPs below C7. Implants were removed but did not result in any improvement in the SSEPs. The suspected cause for the patient's findings was venous congestion secondary to arteriovenous shunting in the T4 vertebral body with engorgement of the epidural venous plexus at the lower cervical spine.[30] A second alternative considered was an unrecognized syrinx that was appreciated on the 6 month postoperative MRI. Overall, studies have shown that preoperative MRIs are not indicated in typical scoliotic curves, and therefore an MRI would not have been indicated in this patient.[31] This case illustrates that cord injury may occur secondarily to vascular anomalies as well as undetected syrinx. Although these malformations might have been detected by a preoperative MRI, studies do not largely support obtaining a preop MRI of the cervical spine for idiopathic thoracic and thoracolumbar curves.

A third study identified two cases of incomplete cervical spinal cord injury after posterior spinal fusion.[32] The first patient underwent T5-T11 PSF without any acute intraoperative complications, and neuromonitoring did not reveal any changes. Total blood loss was 600 mL and the patient required 1 unit of pRBCs with the lowest recorded hemoglobin of 6./7 g/dL. MAPs intraoperatively reached as low as approximately 40 mmHg at the start of the case and fluctuated between the 40 s and 50 s throughout the case. Postoperatively, the patient reported gradual onset of bilateral upper extremity paresthesia and later the next day endorsed bilateral motor and sensory deficits in the lower extremities. MRI was obtained and revealed a hyperintense lesion in the C4-C6 region of the cord. The patient was taken back for removal of hardware that did not improve SSEPs, but was placed on bedrest postop for 2 weeks, during which the clinical exam progressively improved. This patient was later taken to the operating room for repeat fixation that was uneventful. Overall, the likely cause in the first case was secondary to cord ischemia. Briefly, the second case mentioned is in a neuromuscular patient undergoing T11-L4 Ponte osteotomies and T3-L4 posterior spinal fusion. During the procedure the patient lost motor signals in both lower extremities and required a wake-up test. The patient was able to move the left extremities but not the right. They repeated inserting the rods; however, motor and sensory function was lost in all four extremities. A repeat wake-up test revealed similar results. The rods were finally inserted to a lesser curvature with motor signals present in the lower extremities but absent in the upper extremities. Postoperatively, the patient was found to have left hand weakness and difficulty with fine motor movement. MRI revealed edema in the cervical spinal cord from C3-T1.[32] The cord ischemia in the latter case may likely have been exacerbated by the correction. The additive effect of anatomic irregularities, low MAPs, tension on the cord, and vascular system and positioning could each have had a small hand in the resulting cord ischemia for both cases. Although a singular event may not cause cord ischemia, the additive measure of each factor plays a vital role in ensuring the proper safety for each patient.

Maintaining appropriate MAPs can be vital as seen in some of the cases mentioned above. MAPs play an important role in both the prevention of spinal cord injury as well as the recovery of any injury. Additionally, studies have shown that it is critical to maintain an appropriate MAP postoperatively, especially in patients that have sustained spinal cord injury. Research suggests maintaining MAPs greater than 85 mmHg in patients who have a spinal cord injury recover at a faster rate.[33] The study reviewed average MAPs for 100 patients and found that a large proportion of measurements were below the recommended measurement of 85 mmHg. Close observation must be made regarding patients' MAPs as periods of low pressure can not only negatively affect healing but also cause further damage with limited blood flow to the already damaged cord.

General Nonneurologic Postoperative Complications

Rates of postoperative complications range from 4% to 25% for patients with general AIS and higher rates up to 35% for patients with neuromuscular scoliosis including bleeding, infection, hardware failure, and pseudoarthrosis, of which many occur both perioperatively as well as postoperatively.[34] Significant deformity surgery can results in massive intraoperative blood loss that may require transfusion. Risk of excessive bleeding is found to be lower than 1% of overall nonneurologic complications in spinal deformity correction.[4] Appropriate hemostasis if not managed appropriately intraoperatively can lead to postoperative hemorrhage as well as hematoma formation, subsequently increasing risk of wound complications. Multiple agents such as tranexamic acid (TXA), bovine and bipolar electrocautery, as well as intraoperative local hemostatic agents have brought down risks of excessive hemorrhage and therefore subsequent complications.[35] Additional measures can be taken to decrease infection along with hemostatic control including intraoperative use of povidone-iodine irrigation solution as well as topical local vancomycin powder.[36] Minimally invasive techniques have also become more commonplace with reported smaller incisions, less intraoperative bleeding, and infection.[37] Other complications including pseudarthrosis additionally occur at an infrequent rate of approximately less than 1% of all patients undergoing deformity correction. Studies have investigated various grafting options to help increase fusion rates including local bone grafts, allograft, iliac crest bone graft, and other bone substitutes.[38,39] Hardware failure including proximal junction kyphosis (PJK) from adjacent segment disease may occur in as many as 39% of patients.[40] Numerous risks present increased rates of PJK such as construct length and preoperative thoracic kyphosis and lumbar lordosis; however, the vast majority of patients are largely asymptomatic, not requiring revision surgery.[41] Although deformity correction for adolescent idiopathic scoliosis is a largely successful procedure, it is not without its own risks, most commonly including infection, pseudarthrosis, hardware failure, and bleeding.

Complications must be fought head on in patients undergoing large deformity corrections. Without properly appreciating the risks of surgery and the modalities available to decrease risks of complications, surgeons will be faced with dire complications that can have lasting effects on patients. From neurologic complications such as spinal cord injuries, dural tears, and root injuries to nonneurologic complications of hemorrhage, infection, proximal junctional kyphosis, and hardware failure, patients must be well informed of the risks of surgery and their potential consequences. Prevention and early detection through well-developed preestablished protocols will aid surgeons and their teams on providing patients with the best care available.

Conflict of Interest Statement

The authors declare that there is no conflict of interest regarding the publication of this paper.

References

1. Reames DL, Smith JS, Fu KMG, et al. Complications in the surgical treatment of 19,360 cases of pediatric scoliosis: a review of the Scoliosis Research Society Morbidity and Mortality database. *Spine*. 2011;36(18):1484–1491.
2. Coe JD, Arlet V, Donaldson W, et al. Complications in spinal fusion for adolescent idiopathic scoliosis in the new millennium. A report of the Scoliosis Research Society Morbidity and Mortality Committee. *Spine*. 2006;31(3):345–349.
3. Abu-Bonsrah N, Goodwin CR, Ortega G, et al. Risk factors associated with short-term complications and mortality after pediatric spinal arthrodesis. *Neurosurg Focus*. 2017;43(4):E7.
4. Carreon LY, Puno RM, Lenke LG, et al. Non-neurologic complications following surgery for adolescent idiopathic scoliosis. *J Bone Joint Surg Am*. 2007;89(11):2427–2432.
5. Vigneswaran HT, Grabel ZJ, Eberson CP, Palumbo MA, Daniels AH. Surgical treatment of adolescent idiopathic scoliosis in the United States from 1997 to 2012: an analysis of 20,346 patients. *J Neurosurg Pediatr*. 2015;16(3):322–328.
6. Murphy RF, Mooney JF. Complications following spine fusion for adolescent idiopathic scoliosis. *Curr Rev Musculoskelet Med*. 2016; 9(4):462–469.
7. Berry JG, Glotzbecker M, Rodean J, Leahy I, Hall M, Ferrari L. Comorbidities and Complications of Spinal Fusion for Scoliosis. *Pediatrics*. 2017;139(3):e20162574.
8. Lykissas MG, Jain VV, Nathan ST, et al. Mid- to long-term outcomes in adolescent idiopathic scoliosis after instrumented posterior spinal fusion: A meta-analysis. *Spine*. 2013;38(2):E113.
9. Wilber RG, Thompson GH, Shaffer JW, Brown RH, Nash CL. Postoperative neurological deficits in segmental spinal instrumentation. A study using spinal cord monitoring. *J Bone Joint Surg Am*. 1984;66(8):1178–1187.
10. Hamilton DK, Smith JS, Sansur CA, et al. Rates of new neurological deficit associated with spine surgery based on 108,419 procedures: a report of the scoliosis research society morbidity and mortality committee. *Spine*. 2011;36(15):1218–1228.
11. Caplan RA. Will we ever understand perioperative neuropathy? A fresh approach offers hope and insight. *Anesthesiology*. 1999; 91(2):335–336.
12. Cheney FW, Domino KB, Caplan RA, Posner KL. Nerve injury associated with anesthesia: a closed claims analysis. *Anesthesiology*. 1999;90(4):1062–1069.
13. Howick J, Cohen BA, McCulloch P, Thompson M, Skinner SA. Foundations for evidence-based intraoperative neurophysiological monitoring. *Clin Neurophysiol*. 2016;127(1):81–90.
14. Banoub M, Tetzlaff JE, Schubert A. Pharmacologic and physiologic influences affecting sensory evoked potentials: implications for perioperative monitoring. *Anesthesiology*. 2003;99(3): 716–737.
15. Sloan TB, Heyer EJ. Anesthesia for intraoperative neurophysiologic monitoring of the spinal cord. *J Clin Neurophysiol*. 2002;19 (5):430–443.
16. Frei FJ, Ryhult SE, Duitmann E, Hasler CC, Luetschg J, Erb TO. Intraoperative monitoring of motor-evoked potentials in children undergoing spinal surgery. *Spine*. 2007;32(8):911–917.
17. Ziewacz JE, Berven SH, Mummaneni VP, et al. The design, development, and implementation of a checklist for intraoperative neuromonitoring changes. *Neurosurg Focus*. 2012;33(5):E11.
18. Lall RR, Lall RR, Hauptman JS, et al. Intraoperative neurophysiological monitoring in spine surgery: indications, efficacy, and role of the preoperative checklist. *Neurosurg Focus*. 2012;33(5):E10.
19. Vitale MG, Skaggs DL, Pace GI, et al. Best practices in intraoperative neuromonitoring in spine deformity surgery: Development of an intraoperative checklist to optimize response. *Spine Deform*. 2014;2(5):333–339.
20. Schonauer C, Bocchetti A, Barbagallo G, Albanese V, Moraci A. Positioning on surgical table. *Eur Spine J*. 2004;13(Suppl 1): S50–S55.
21. Mirovsky Y, Neuwirth M. Injuries to the lateral femoral cutaneous nerve during spine surgery. *Spine*. 2000;25(10):1266–1269.
22. Kwee MM, Ho YH, Rozen WM. The prone position during surgery and its complications: A systematic review and evidence-based guidelines. *Int Surg*. 2015;100(2):292–303.
23. Koreckij J, Price N, Schwend RM. Vectored cranial-cervical traction limits facial contact pressure from prone positioning during posterior spinal deformity surgery. *Spine*. 2011;36(15): E993–997.
24. Leibovitch I, Casson R, Laforest C, Selva D. Ischemic orbital compartment syndrome as a complication of spinal surgery in the prone position. *Ophthalmology*. 2006;113(1):105–108.
25. McCallum E, Keren S, Lapira M, Norris JH. Orbital compartment syndrome: An update with review of the literature. *Clin Ophthalmol Auckl NZ*. 2019;13:2189–2194.
26. Hayreh SS. The blood supply of the optic nerve head and the evaluation of it - myth and reality. *Prog Retin Eye Res*. 2001;20(5): 563–593.
27. Hayreh SS. In vivo choroidal circulation and its watershed zones. *Eye Lond Engl*. 1990;4(Pt 2):273–289.
28. Hayreh SS, Zimmerman MB. Fundus changes in central retinal artery occlusion. *Retina Phila Pa*. 2007;27(3):276–289.
29. Kristobak A, Helgeson MD, Jex J. Cervical cord injury following posterior spinal fusion in a patient with adolescent idiopathic scoliosis: A case report. *JBJS Case Connect*. 2019;9(3):e0331.
30. Dapunt UA, Mok JM, Sharkey MS, Davis AA, Foster-Barber A, Diab M. Delayed presentation of tetraparesis following posterior thoracolumbar spinal fusion and instrumentation for adolescent idiopathic scoliosis. *Spine*. 2009;34(25):E936–941.
31. Winter RB, Lonstein JE, Heithoff KB, Kirkham JA. Magnetic resonance imaging evaluation of the adolescent patient with idiopathic scoliosis before spinal instrumentation and fusion. A prospective, double-blinded study of 140 patients. *Spine*. 1997;22 (8):855–858.
32. Youlo ST, Merrick MT, Cassidy JA, Halanski MA. Cervical spinal cord injury after thoracic spinal instrumentation: a case series. *Spine*. 2013;38(26):E1704–1708.
33. Hawryluk G, Whetstone W, Saigal R, et al. Mean arterial blood pressure correlates with neurological recovery after human spinal cord injury: Analysis of high frequency physiologic data. *J Neurotrauma*. 2015;32(24):1958–1967.
34. Bartley CE, Yaszay B, Bastrom TP, et al. Perioperative and delayed major complications following surgical treatment of adolescent idiopathic scoliosis. *J Bone Joint Surg Am*. 2017;99(14): 1206–1212.
35. Grant JA, Howard J, Luntley J, Harder J, Aleissa S, Parsons D. Perioperative blood transfusion requirements in pediatric

scoliosis surgery: The efficacy of tranexamic acid. *J Pediatr Orthop.* 2009;29(3):300.
36. Mallet C, Meissburger V, Caseris M, et al. Does the use of intra-wound povidone-iodine irrigation and local vancomycin powder impact surgical site infection rate in adolescent idiopathic scoliosis surgery? *Eur Spine J.* 2022;31(11):3020–3028.
37. Park SC, Son SW, Yang JH, et al. Novel surgical technique for adolescent idiopathic scoliosis: Minimally invasive scoliosis surgery. *J Clin Med.* 2022;11(19):5847.
38. Betz RR, Lavelle WF, Samdani AF. Bone grafting options in children. *Spine.* 2010;35(17):1648–1654.
39. Yataganbaba A, Gahukamble A, Antoniou G, Freeman BJC, Cundy PJ. Local bone grafting is sufficient for instrumented adolescent idiopathic scoliosis surgery: A preliminary study. *J Pediatr Orthop.* 2021;41(8):e641–e645.
40. Al-Mohrej OA, Aldakhil SS, Al-Rabiah MA, Al-Rabiah AM. Surgical treatment of adolescent idiopathic scoliosis: Complications. *Ann Med Surg.* 2020;52:19–23.
41. Erkilinc M, Baldwin KD, Pasha S, Mistovich RJ. Proximal junctional kyphosis in pediatric spinal deformity surgery: a systematic review and critical analysis. *Spine Deform.* 2022;10(2): 257–266.

28

Complications Associated with Congenital and Neuromuscular Scoliosis

SUMEET GARG AND BRENNAN ROPER

CHAPTER OUTLINE

Congenital Scoliosis

Congenital scoliosis is caused by failures of formation, segmentation, or both prior to birth.[1] Adjacent rib abnormalities (fusions or absence of ribs) may also contribute to the overall deformity. Congenital scoliosis is often associated with other abnormalities, including neural axis abnormalities in 21% to 37% of patients.[2] Roughly 60% patients with congenital scoliosis have associated abnormalities of other body systems, with cardiac and genitourinary being most common.[3,4] Progression of deformity is variable and often dependent upon the type and severity of the malformation(s) present. Commonly, compensatory curves develop in response to the congenital deformity, especially in those with congenital curves with apex at T5, T6, or T7.[2] Bracing and other nonoperative treatment modalities are usually unsuccessful at preventing curve progression; however, they may be used as temporizing methods to delay surgical intervention in very young patients.[5] Surgical treatment for congenital scoliosis typically is with spinal fusion, with severe angular deformities often requiring three column osteotomies.

The progression of congenital spinal deformities is dependent upon the type and severity of the abnormality; patients with balanced congenital abnormalities are less likely to progress than those with unbalanced abnormalities. Overall, 25% curves do not significantly progress, 25% progress slowly, and 50% progress rapidly.[6] In the most severe scenario, a thoracolumbar unilateral unsegmented bar with contralateral hemivertebra may worsen by an average of 7 degrees per year before 10 years of age and 14 degrees per year during the adolescent growth spurt.[2] This progression is often accompanied by progression of compensatory curves. Early spinal fusion was often performed in the past involving both anterior and posterior approaches; however, progressive deformity requiring repeat surgery was common.[7] There have also been reports demonstrating the adverse impact of early spinal fusion on pulmonary function.[8] Currently, serial casting as a temporizing modality to allow for further maturation of the patient has demonstrated some success.[9,10] Progressive congenital scoliosis, however, will generally require surgical treatment to restore spinal balance and prevent progression. Depending on the curve characteristics and age this may include nonfusion or fusion techniques.

Neuromuscular Scoliosis

Neuromuscular scoliosis results from a wide variety of neuropathic and/or myopathic conditions (Table 28.1).[11] Depending upon the diagnosis, progressive scoliosis may be present in 25% to 100% of patients (Table 28.2). Studies evaluating the natural history of neuromuscular scoliosis suggest that most progress, especially those in patients with more severe underlying disease, patients with more severe curves at initial presentation, and those presenting at an earlier age.[12–15] Similar to congenital scoliosis, nonoperative

TABLE 28.1 Scoliosis Research Society classification of neuromuscular spinal deformity.

Primary neuropathies
Upper motor neuron pathologies
Cerebral palsy
Spinocerebellar degeneration
Friedreich's ataxia
Charcot-Marie-Tooth disease
Roussy-Levy disease
Syringomyelia
Spinal cord tumor
Spinal cord trauma
Lower motor neuron pathologies
Poliomyelitis
Other viral myelitides
Traumatic
Spinal muscular atrophy
Werdnig-Hoffmann disease
Kugelberg-Welander disease
Dysautonomia
Riley-Day syndrome
Combined upper and lower pathologies
Myelomeningocele
Primary myopathies
Muscular dystrophy
Duchenne muscular dystrophy
Limb-girdle dystrophy
Facioscapulohumeral dystrophy
Arthrogryposis
Fiber-type disproportion
Congenital hypotonia
Myotonia dystrophica

TABLE 28.2 Incidence of scoliosis with various neuromuscular conditions.

Diagnosis	Incidence of Scoliosis
Cerebral palsy (2 limbs involved)	25%
Myelodysplasia (lower lumbar)	60%
Spinal muscle atrophy	67%
Friedreich's ataxia	80%
Cerebral palsy (4 limbs involved)	80%
Duchenne muscular dystrophy	90%
Myelodysplasia (thoracic level)	100%
Traumatic paralysis (<10years)	100%

treatment of neuromuscular scoliosis is usually ineffective at preventing curve progression. Surgery is often undertaken in patients with neuromuscular scoliosis to improve sitting position and overall spinal balance but carries high rates of medical and surgical complications. Limited case series demonstrate improvement in health-related quality of life with surgery, independent of degree of curvature correction,[16] as has parental satisfaction.[17] Current treatment algorithms rely on growth-friendly surgical modalities used as a temporizing therapy until the patient reaches approximately 8 to 10 years of age, at which definitive fusion is more appropriate and better tolerated long term.

Complications in the Treatment of Congenital and Neuromuscular Scoliosis

Both congenital and neuromuscular scoliosis patients have increased risk of medical and surgical complications when compared to patients with idiopathic scoliosis. In a review of over 19,000 pediatric patients undergoing surgical correction, those with congenital scoliosis were found to have a complication rate of 10.6%, while those with neuromuscular scoliosis were found to have a complication rate of 17.9%.[18] Severely involved patients with cerebral palsy (Gross Motor Function Classification System [GMFCS] 4/5) are reported to have complication rates approaching 50%.[19] Knowledge of these complications and utilizing techniques to reduce or prevent these complications is essential to the safety and ultimate outcome for these patients.

Systemic Complications

Positioning Complications

Surgery for congenital and neuromuscular scoliosis commonly is performed via a posterior approach with patients in the prone position. Potential complications from prone positioning include perioperative visual loss (POVL), brachial plexus injuries, and pressure sores. POVL, while rare in patients <12 years of age, is devasting when it does occur; recommendations to prevent this complication include avoiding direct pressure to the eyes, keeping the neck in a neutral position, keeping the head above the heart, frequent evaluation during surgery, and avoiding severe hypotension.[20] Brachial plexopathies have been observed to occur in 3.6% to 15% of patients undergoing scoliosis correction in a prone position.[21,22] Plexopathy is more common in the prone position and when arms are abducted to greater than 90 degrees, extended, and externally rotated.[23] Use of somatosensory evoked potential signals of the ulnar nerve can reliably identify changes as they occur and alert the team to the need for repositioning; immediate improvement is usually achieved once addressed.[24] If using rib-based fixation, take care to not place implants higher than the second rib to prevent brachial plexus injury.[25] Patients with neuromuscular scoliosis often have significant soft tissue and joint contractures that makes prone positioning challenging. Diligent attention to padding of all bony prominences, feeding access points (e.g., G tube), and implanted devices (e.g., baclofen pumps) is recommended to decrease risk of pressure sores.[26]

Intraoperative Blood Loss and Need for Transfusion

Blood loss can be substantial during spinal deformity surgery in patients with congenital and neuromuscular scoliosis. Patients with neuromuscular disease undergoing posterior fusion for scoliosis are nearly seven times more likely to lose >50% estimated total blood volume compared to similar demographic patients without underlying neuromuscular disease.[27] Amongst neuromuscular scoliosis patients, those with cerebral palsy and Duchenne muscular dystrophy appear to be most at risk for severe blood loss.[28,29] Approximately 35% to 37% of neuromuscular scoliosis patients require a blood transfusion in association with surgery, significantly greater than that reported for idiopathic scoliosis.[30–32] Preoperatively, the use of erythropoietin has been shown to improve postoperative hematocrit levels.[33] Intraoperatively, several techniques are available to decrease blood loss. Hypotension during approach and avoidance of intraoperative hypothermia both decrease intraoperative blood loss.[34,35] Intrathecal narcotic administration, antifibrinolytic drugs, use of bipolar sealer devices, and cell salvage devices have all repeatedly demonstrated decreases in intraoperative blood loss and need for transfusion.[36–42] Similarly, staged surgery in anterior-posterior fusions and use of two attending surgeons have also demonstrated decreased intraoperative blood loss in this patient population.[43–45]

Pulmonary Complications

Pulmonary complications are the most common complication amongst neuromuscular scoliosis patients undergoing surgery, occurring in up to 25% of patients.[42,46–49] Poor preoperative pulmonary function (forced vital capacity <40% and/or forced expiratory volume in 1 second <40% predicted value) in the neuromuscular patient increases the risk of postoperative pulmonary complication and prolonged intubation.[50–52] Patients with implanted gastrointestinal tube, history of previous pneumonia, and greater primary curve Cobb angle are also at risk of increased postoperative pulmonary complications.[48,50,53] Need for prolonged intubation is an independent predictor of increased perioperative and postoperative respiratory, cardiovascular, gastrointestinal, and surgical site complications, as well as prolonged intensive care unit and overall hospitalization stay duration.[54] Preexisting pulmonary disease is also an independent risk factor for 90-day readmission after spinal surgery.[30]

Thoughtful preoperative evaluation and optimization of pulmonary status can help reduce pulmonary complications. Preoperative pulmonary consultation should be done for any congenital scoliosis patients with preoperative pulmonary symptoms or history of recurrent pulmonary infections and all patients with neuromuscular scoliosis planned for spinal surgery. Using at-home noninvasive oxygen supplementation prior to surgery may decrease perioperative pulmonary complications in these patients.[55–57] Attempts should be made to reduce the need for prolonged intubation postoperatively by early transition to noninvasive positive pressure ventilation in the acute postoperative period.[58,59] Management of pulmonary complications postoperatively should be done in partnership with specialists in pediatric intensive care, hospital medicine, and pulmonary medicine.

Gastrointestinal Complications

Patients with neuromuscular scoliosis often have underlying nutritional and digestive deficiencies.[60] Baseline albumin <3.5 g/dL and total body lymphocyte count <1.5 g/dL increase risk of postoperative complications including infection, prolonged intubation, and longer hospitalization.[61] Reports of postoperative gastrointestinal complications in the neuromuscular scoliosis patient range between 13% and 17%[62–64] and include gastric dysmotility, prolonged paralytic ileus, acute pancreatitis, and superior mesenteric artery (SMA) syndrome. Patients with prolonged gastric dysmotility often require jejunal feeding to facilitate improved nutrition and return to preoperative weight.[65] Those with prolonged paralytic ileus commonly require nasogastric decompression until resolution of the ileus, resulting in prolonged hospital stay.[63] Postoperative pancreatitis has been described in up to 30.1% of cerebral palsy (CP) patients undergoing spine fusion for scoliosis,[66] more than three times that reported in idiopathic scoliosis cases.[67] Neuromuscular patients with preoperative gastroesophageal reflux disease (GERD) and reactive airway disease (RAD) are significantly more at risk for postoperative pancreatitis, and therefore treatment of those conditions should be optimized perioperatively.[66] SMA syndrome is a rare but serious complication of scoliosis correction surgery, occurring in up to 2.4% to 4.7% of cases; there does not appear to be an increased risk in congenital and neuromuscular scoliosis patients. Risk factors for development of SMA syndrome include decreased body mass index (BMI), increased lumbar lateralization of spinal curvature, and increased stiffness of the curve on bending films.[68] Goal BMI to decrease risk of SMA syndrome should be greater than 18.[69] Preoperative optimization of oral diet and supplemental tube feeds should be considered for patients with neuromuscular or congenital scoliosis who have low BMI and/or low preoperative nutritional lab markers. Most gastrointestinal complications following spine surgery, if caught early, can be treated with conservative measures and demonstrate a high rate of resolution; awareness is key. Partnership with pediatric hospital medicine and/or gastrointestinal medicine should be utilized if complications occur postoperatively.

Genitourinary Complications

Urinary tract infections (UTI) occur in surgical correction of neuromuscular scoliosis in 4.6% to 10.8% of cases.[30,70] Obesity increases the risk of UTI in neuromuscular scoliosis patients compared to those of normal weight.[71] Patients with cerebral palsy are nearly three times more likely to have their postoperative course complicated by UTI than similar patients with idiopathic scoliosis.[72] In patients with myelomeningocele, recurrent urinary tract infections are common due to neurogenic bladders. In these patients with positive urinary cultures at time of scoliosis surgery, perioperative wound infection occurs in up to 80% of patients with adequate preoperative nutrition and 100% of patients with inadequate nutrition.[73] Preoperative urine cultures should be obtained in patients with history of frequent UTI or baseline incontinence. Any identified positive cultures should be treated appropriately prior to surgery. Postoperatively, urinary catheters should be removed within 48 hours to reduce the risk of catheter-associate urinary tract infection.[74]

Surgical Complications

Surgical Site Infections

Infection is a concerning and serious complication in spine surgery, especially for those with neuromuscular disorders.[75] Patients with nonidiopathic scoliosis have higher rates of surgical site infection (5%–15%) than patients with idiopathic scoliosis (1%–3%).[76–80] Preoperative optimization of nutritional status, including albumin >3.5 g/dL and total blood lymphocyte count >1.5 g/dL, decreases risk of postoperative infection in CP patients.[62] Adherence to published antibiotic protocols, use of antibiotic-infused allograft, and postoperative drains may decrease postoperative infection.[81] Topically applied vancomycin powder in pediatric spine patients has been proven to be a safe option.[82,83] In complex cases, use of plastic surgery colleagues for a multilayered closure has shown a dramatic decrease in wound complication and postoperative infection.[84–86] Preoperative nasal swab screening for *Staphylococcus aureus* may be useful for modification of perioperative antibiotic regimens in the setting of colonization of resistant organisms.[87,88] Perhaps most importantly, a standardized and encompassing preoperative approach coupled with routine postoperative monitoring is recommended to prevent surgical site infection in a higher-risk population such as congenital and neuromuscular scoliosis is prudent and recommended.[89,90]

Unfortunately, infections may still occur. Use of antibiotics and vacuum-assisted wound closure has demonstrated success in treatment of early (<90 days) deep surgical site infection without need for implant removal.[91–93] Incisional vacuum-assisted closure, especially in constructs extending to the pelvis, may help to prevent soiling of the incision.[94] With appropriate early treatment and eradication of infection, recurrence is low.[95] Late appearing infections (>90 days) are often more resistant to simple debridement and may necessitate multiple surgeries and ultimate removal of implants to resolve the infection.[96,97]

Neurologic Injury

Patients with congenital and neuromuscular scoliosis are at higher risk of intraoperative neurologic complications, with reports between 2% and 3% and 1% and 5% of cases, respectively.[18,98,99] Cases utilizing osteotomies, including posterior column (e.g., Smith-Peterson, Ponte), pedicle subtraction, and vertebral column resection, have a sequentially greater risk of neurologic injury than cases not involving osteotomy. Intraoperative neuromonitoring (IONM) has become standard of care for spinal deformity surgery. However, baseline value of IONM in congenital and neuromuscular scoliosis patients are often lower and more difficult to reliably obtain than those in idiopathic patients.[100–102] False-positive changes are more frequent in neuromuscular scoliosis patients, occurring in up to 13.8% of cases.[103] Changes in IONM are most frequently noted during corrective maneuvers.[104] Best Practice Guidelines have been established by Vitale et al. to prevent and address IONM changes, centered around a team approach that involves all members of the operating room.[105]

Implant Malposition

Symptomatic screw malposition is a relatively rare complication but can have serious consequences. Patients with congenital and neuromuscular scoliosis are frequently younger, smaller, and have smaller and abnormally shaped pedicles; these factors increase the risk of screw malposition in congenital and neuromuscular scoliosis compared to idiopathic patients.[106,107] Use of freehand technique in neuromuscular scoliosis patients may result in up to 6.7% of screws being placed outside of a defined "safe zone."[108] The advent of three-dimensional (3D) printed guides has shown improved accuracy of screw placement, especially in complex congenital spine deformities.[109–112] Similarly, computed tomography (CT)-guided navigation for pedicle screw placement results in fewer malpositioned screws and less return to OR for screw revision.[113] This technique has specifically been shown to improve pedicle screw accuracy in patients less than 10 years of age.[114] CT-guided navigation may better identify anomalous pedicles in the congenital scoliosis patient, preventing attempt at a pedicle unfit for screw insertion.[115] CT-guided and robot-assisted pedicle screw placement technologies are not perfect, however; congenital scoliosis remains an independent risk factor for pedicle screw misplacement even in the setting of CT-guided and robot-assisted screw placement.[116,117] Careful study of the deformity and attention to detail while utilizing these technologies is still paramount to successful pedicle screw insertion.

Implant-Related Complications

Implant-related complications are common in congenital and neuromuscular scoliosis patients, occurring in 1.5% to 56% of cases.[18,50,118–120] These include screw back out, implant breakage, disengagement of set plugs/connectors, and implant prominence. Risk of implant breakage is increased in nonambulatory and spastic neuromuscular patients,[118,121] as well as in thoracic-level paralysis myelomeningocele patients.[120]

Pedicle screw constructs are preferred over sublaminar wires and hooks due to their lower risk of implant breakage, increased deformity correction, reduced bleeding, and increased safety.[122,123] Smaller diameter rods have increased risk of fracture, especially in skeletally mature neuromuscular patients.[119] Use of pedicle screw constructs and larger diameter rods can help reduce implant-related complications in neuromuscular and congenital scoliosis.

Implant failure at the pelvis is a common problem in patients with neuromuscular scoliosis. In the nonambulatory patient, extension of fixation to the pelvis improves correction of primary curve and pelvic obliquity, with decreased loss of pelvic obliquity correction over time.[124] Extension to the pelvis may improve functional results in these patients as well.[125] Traditional iliac screws have a reported rate of implant failure between 5% and 57%.[126–129] Techniques have been developed to decrease risk of these failures including bilateral high density screw fixation at L5, S1 and S2 alar iliac or iliac[125] and use of inter-rod/cross-link connectors at the caudal instrumentation.[121,130,131]

Implementation of the S2 alar iliac (SAI) screw technique has further decreased risk of implant failure, as well as decreased risk of symptomatic screw prominence and subsequent need for revision surgery.[128,129,131–133] SAI screws show decreased toggle compared to traditional iliac screws, as well as ability to accommodate larger diameter and longer screw lengths, which may contribute to further improvement in stability and decreased implant failure.[131,134]

Proximal Junctional Kyphosis

Development of proximal junctional kyphosis (PJK) is a concern in spinal surgery, especially in congenital and neuromuscular patients undergoing surgery at a young age. PJK occurs more frequently in congenital scoliosis than either neuromuscular or idiopathic scoliosis.[135] Rates of PJK in patients with congenital scoliosis undergoing instrumented fusion range from 11.6% and 48.9%. Risk is significantly increased in patients with disruption of proximal posterior elements, preoperative thoracic hyperkyphosis, longer fusions, and increased kyphosis correction at time of surgery.[135–139] Unfortunately, there are no evidence-based strategies identified to reduce the rate of PJK in the surgical treatment of patients with neuromuscular and congenital scoliosis. We recommend careful evaluation of the preoperative sagittal parameters of each patient and using this information to guide planned deformity correction.

Complications Specific to Growing-Rod Constructs

Growing-rod constructs are occasionally used in congenital scoliosis and young patients with neuromuscular scoliosis. Goals of these constructs include stabilization of the spine and prevention of deformity progression, while allowing for further growth and development of the thoracic cavity.[140] Results of early definitive fusion prior to development of the thoracic cavity can be devastating.[8] Complications in growing-rod constructs occur in 33% to 50% of cases.[141,142] Risk of complication increases by 24% with each additional surgery.[143] Rod fractures occur in approximately 15% of cases. Single rod constructs, smaller diameter rods, and smaller tandem connectors all increase risk of rod fracture.[144,145] Wound complications occur in 5.3% to 14% of cases.[143,146,147] Use of stainless steel rods have shown a 5.7 times higher risk of infection than titanium implants.[148] Nonambulatory status and subcutaneous rod placement has shown increased risk of deep infection as well.[143] As stated in the previous section, PJK is a possible complication with growing-rod constructs; preoperative hyperkyphosis, spine-based instrumentation, and dramatic changes in pelvic parameters all increases risk.[149,150] Use of five or more proximal anchors and including the upper end vertebra of kyphosis significantly decreases risk of PJK requiring revision surgery.[151] Magnetically based growing-rod constructs are specifically at risk of distraction failure,[152–155] as well as development of significant tissue metallosis in up to 86% of cases.[156] Use of >5 anchors proximally, large diameter rods, submuscular placement of rods, and careful attention to soft tissue exposure and closure can help reduce complications with growing rod treatment.

Complications of Hemivertebra Excision

Hemivertebra excision is a common surgical treatment for progressive congenital scoliosis in patients with an isolated hemivertebra. The surgery is technically demanding with an overall complication rate up to 30% to 40% of cases.[157,158] Common complications include implant failure, implant malposition, pseudarthrosis, and progressive deformity. Implant failure and subsequent pseudarthrosis has been observed in 6% to 9% of total cases.[157,159,160] Novel techniques such as the "three-rod technique" and extension of fixation to the pelvis in lumbosacral hemivertebrectomy may decrease rates of implant failure.[161,162] In cases of small or anomalous pedicles, asymmetric constructs may be used to maximize fixation in best-fit pedicles.[163]

With patients commonly undergoing operation at a young age, loss of correction is a significant concern. Radiographic loss of coronal and sagittal correction has been reported in 9% to 18.5% of cases,[137,138] frequently requiring revision surgery for extension of the construct to control either proximal or distal junctional kyphosis. Patients with larger preoperative kyphotic deformity and longer surgical constructs are especially at risk for PJK.[137] Overall, centers performing higher volumes of hemivertebrectomy surgeries appear to have decreased complications.[157]

Conclusion

Congenital and neuromuscular scoliosis patients present with complex deformities and are at increased risk for complication following surgery.[18] Careful attention and planning should be executed in the preoperative, intraoperative, and postoperative settings in order to achieve the most optimal results. Knowledge of the most common complications, along with techniques to avoid them and solutions if they do occur, should allow the surgeon to approach these cases with thoughtful yet cautious confidence.

References

1. McMaster MJ. Congenital scoliosis. In: Weinstein SL, ed. *The Pediatric Spine: Principles and Practice*. New York: Raven Press; 1994:229.
2. Richards BS, Sucato DJ, Johnston CE. Scoliosis. In: Herring JA, ed. *Tachdjian's Pediatrtic Orthopaedics: From the Texas Scottish Rite Hospital for Children*. 6th ed. Philadelphia: Elselvier; 2022:177181.
3. Basu PS, Elsebaie H, Noordeen MH. Congenital spinal deformity: a comprehensive assessment at presentation. *Spine*. 2002;27(20):2255–2259.
4. Beals RK, Robbins JR, Rolfe B. Anomalies associated with vertebral malformations. *Spine*. 1993;18(10):1329–1332.
5. Johnston CE, McClung AM, Thompson GH, et al. Comparison of growing rod instrumentation versus serial cast treatment for early-onset scoliosis. *Spine Deform*. 2013;1(5):339–342.

6. McMaster MJ, Ohtsuka K. The natural history of congenital scoliosis. *J Bone Joint Surg Am.* 1982;64:1128–1147.
7. Goldberg CJ, Moore DP, Fogarty EE, et al. Long-term results from in situ fusion for congenital vertebral deformity. *Spine.* 2002;27:619–628.
8. Karol LA, Johnston C, Mladenov K, et al. Pulmonary function following early thoracic fusion in non-neuromuscular scoliosis. *J Bone Joint Surg Am.* 2008;90:1272–1281.
9. Demirkiran HG, Bekmez S, Celilov R, et al. Serial derotational casting in congenital scoliosis as a time-buying strategy. *J Pediatr Orthop.* 2015;35:43–49.
10. Baulesh DM, Huh J, Judkins T, et al. The role of serial casting in early-onset scoliosis (EOS). *J Pediatr Orthop.* 2012;32:658–663.
11. Bradford DS, Hu SS. Neuromuscular spinal deformity. In: Lonstein JE, Bradford DS, Winter RB, Oglivie JW, eds. *Moe's Textbook of Scoliosis and Other Spinal Deformities.* 3rd ed. Philadelphia: WB Saunders; 1987:295–322.
12. Persson-Bunke M, Hagglund G, Lauge-Pedersen H, Wagner P, Westbom L. Scoliosis in a total population of children with cerebral palsy. *Spine.* 2012;37:E708–713.
13. Fujak A, Raab W, Schuh A, Richter S, Forst R, Forst J. Natural course of scoliosis in proximal spinal muscular atrophy type II and IIIa: descriptive clinical study with retrospective data collection of 126 patients. *BMC Musculoskelet Disord.* 2013;14:283.
14. Gu Y, Shelton JE, Ketchum JM, et al. Natural history of scoliosis in nonambulatory spastic tetraplegic cerebral palsy. *PM R.* 2011;3:27–32.
15. Mulcahey MJ, Gaughan JP, Betz RR, Samdani AF, Barakat N, Hunter LN. Neuromuscular scoliosis in children with spinal cord injury. *Top Spinal Cord Inj Rehabil.* 2013;19:96–110.
16. Bohtz C, Meyer-Heim A, Min K. Changes in health-related quality of life after spinal fusion and scoliosis correction in patients with cerebral palsy. *J Pediatr Orthop.* 2011;31:668–673.
17. Jones KB, Sponseller PD, Shindle MK, McCarthy ML. Longitudinal parental perceptions of spinal fusion for neuromuscular spine deformity in patients with totally involved cerebral palsy. *J Pediatr Orthop.* 2003;23:143–149.
18. Reames DL, Smith JS, Fu KM, et al. Complications in the surgical treatment of 19,360 cases of pediatric scoliosis: a review of the Scoliosis Research Society Morbidity and Mortality database. *Spine.* 2011;36:1484–1491.
19. Miyanji F, Nasto LA, Sponseller PD, et al. Assessing the risk-benefit ratio of scoliosis surgery in cerebral palsy: Surgery is worth it. *J Bone Joint Surg Am.* 2018;100(7):556–563. https://doi.org/10.2106/JBJS.17.00621. PMID: 29613924.
20. Practice Advisory for Perioperative Visual Loss Associated with Spine Surgery 2019 An Updated Report by the American Society of Anesthesiologists Task Force on Perioperative Visual Loss, the North American Neuro-Ophthalmology Society, and the Society for Neuroscience in Anesthesiology and Critical Care. *Anesthesiology.* 2019;130(1):12–30.
21. Schwartz DM, Drummond DS, Hahn M, Ecker ML, Dormans JP. Prevention of positional brachial plexopathy during surgical correction of scoliosis. *J Spinal Disord.* 2000;13(2):178–182. https://doi.org/10.1097/00002517-200004000-00015. PMID: 10780696.
22. O'Brien MF, Lenke LG, Bridwell KH, et al. Evoked potential monitoring of the upper extremities during thoracic and lumbar spinal deformity surgery: A prospective study. *J Spinal Dis.* 1994;7:277–284.
23. Uribe JS, Kolla J, Omar H, et al. Brachial plexus injury following spinal surgery. *J Neurosurg Spine.* 2010;13(4):552–558. https://doi.org/10.3171/2010.4.SPINE09682. PMID: 20887154.
24. Labrom RD, Hoskins M, Reilly CW, Tredwell SJ, Wong PK. Clinical usefulness of somatosensory evoked potentials for detection of brachial plexopathy secondary to malpositioning in scoliosis surgery. *Spine (Phila Pa 1976).* 2005;30(18):2089–2093. https://doi.org/10.1097/01.brs.0000179305.89193.46. PMID: 16166901.
25. Joiner ER, Andras LM, Skaggs DL. Mechanisms and risk factors of brachial plexus injury in the treatment of early-onset scoliosis with distraction-based growing implants. *J Bone Joint Surg Am.* 2013;95(21):e161 https://doi.org/10.2106/JBJS.M.00222.PMID: 24196473.
26. Mineiro J, Yazici M. Technical aspects of surgical correction of spinal deformities in cerebral palsy. *J Child Orthop.* 2020; 14(1):30–40. https://doi.org/10.1302/1863-2548.14.190167. PMID: 32165979; PMCID: PMC7043119.
27. Edler A, Murray DJ, Forbes RB. Blood loss during posterior spinal fusion surgery in patients with neuromuscular disease: is there an increased risk? *Paediatr Anaesth.* 2003;13(9):818–822. https://doi.org/10.1046/j.1460-9592.2003.01171.x. PMID: 14617124.
28. Jain A, Njoku DB, Sponseller PD. Does patient diagnosis predict blood loss during posterior spinal fusion in children? *Spine (Phila Pa 1976).* 2012;37(19):1683–1687. https://doi.org/10.1097/BRS.0b013e318254168f. PMID: 22426452.
29. Shapiro F, Sethna N. Blood loss in pediatric spine surgery. *Eur Spine J.* 2004;13(Suppl 1):S6–17. https://doi.org/10.1007/s00586-004-0760-y.Epub 2004 Aug 13. PMID: 15316883; PMCID: PMC3592180.
30. Lee NJ, Fields M, Boddapati V, et al. Spinal deformity surgery in pediatric patients with cerebral palsy: A national-level analysis of inpatient and postdischarge outcomes. *Global Spine J.* 20202192568220960075. https://doi.org/10.1177/2192568220960075. Epub ahead of print. PMID: 329 64747.
31. Lu MZH, Reid SM, Lundine K, Crighton G. Blood transfusion following major orthopaedic surgery in cerebral palsy: a retrospective analysis. *ANZ J Surg.* 2021;91(3):409–414. https://doi.org/10.1111/ans.16288. Epub 2020 Sep 6. PMID: 32893430.
32. van Popta D, Stephenson J, Patel D, Verma R. The pattern of blood loss in adolescent idiopathic scoliosis. *Spine J.* 2014;14(12):2938–2945. https://doi.org/10.1016/j.spinee.2014.05.022. Epub 2014 Jun 7. PMID: 24912120.
33. Rosencher N, Poisson D, Albi A, Aperce M, Barre J, Samama CM. Two injections of erythropoietin correct moderate anemia in most patients awaiting orthopedic surgery. *Can J Anaesth.* 2005; 52(2):160–165.
34. Lenke LG, Sides BA, Koester LA, Hensley M, Blanke KM. Vertebral column resection for the treatment of severe spinal deformity. *Clin Orthop Relat Res.* 2010;468(3):687–699. Epub 2009 Sep 1.
35. Rajagopalan S, Mascha E, Na J, Sessler DI. The effects of mild perioperative hypothermia on blood loss and transfusion requirement. *Anesthesiology.* 2008;108(1):71–77.
36. Lesniak AB, Tremblay P, Dalens BJ, Aucoin M, Mercier P. Intrathecal morphine reduces blood loss during idiopathic scoliosis surgery: retrospective study of 256 pediatric cases. *Paediatr Anaesth.* 2013;23(3):265–270. Epub 2013 Jan 10.
37. Chou SH, Lin SY, Wu MH, et al. Intravenous tranexamic acid reduces blood loss and transfusion volume in scoliosis surgery for spinal muscular atrophy: Results of a 20-year retrospective analysis. *Int J Environ Res Public Health.* 2021;18(19):9959 https://doi.org/10.3390/ijerph18199959. PMID: 34639259; PMCID: PMC8507662.

38. Dhawale AA, Shah SA, Sponseller PD, et al. Are antifibrinolytics helpful in decreasing blood loss and transfusions during spinal fusion surgery in children with cerebral palsy scoliosis? *Spine (Phila Pa 1976)*. 2012;37:E549–E555.
39. Thompson GH, Florentino-Pineda I, Poe-Kochert C, Armstrong DG, Son-Hing J. Role of Amicar in surgery for neuromuscular scoliosis. *Spine (Phila Pa 1976)*. 2008;33(24):2623–2629. https://doi.org/10.1097/BRS.0b013e318187c046. PMID: 18981961.
40. Shapiro F, Zurakowski D, Sethna NF. Tranexamic acid diminishes intraoperative blood loss and transfusion in spinal fusions for duchenne muscular dystrophy scoliosis. *Spine (Phila Pa 1976)*. 2007;32(20):2278–2283. https://doi.org/10.1097/BRS.0b013e31814cf139.PMID: 17873823.
41. Michelet D, Julien-Marsollier F, Hilly J, Diallo T, Vidal C, Dahmani S. Predictive factors of intraoperative cell salvage during pediatric scoliosis surgery. Cell saver during scoliosis surgery in children. *Anaesth Crit Care Pain Med*. 2018;37(2):141–146. https://doi.org/10.1016/j.accpm.2017.03.003. Epub 2017 May 22. PMID: 28546128.
42. Liang J, Shen J, Chua S, et al. Does intraoperative cell salvage system effectively decrease the need for allogeneic transfusions in scoliotic patients undergoing posterior spinal fusion? A prospective randomized study. *Eur Spine J*. 2015;24(2):270–275. Epub 2014 Mar 30.
43. Tsirikos AI, Chang WN, Dabney KW, Miller F. Comparison of one-stage versus two-stage anteroposterior spinal fusion in pediatric patients with cerebral palsy and neuromuscular scoliosis. *Spine (Phila Pa 1976)*. 2003;28(12):1300–1305. https://doi.org/10.1097/01.BRS.0000065572.10824.AB.PMID: 12811275.
44. McDonald TC, Gnam AL, Brooks JT, Sukkarieh H, Replogle WH, Wright PB. The value-added benefit of utilizing two attending surgeons for patients with scoliosis secondary to cerebral palsy. *Spine Deform*. 2021;9(4):1145–1150. https://doi.org/10.1007/s43390-021-00301-x. Epub 2021 Feb 15. PMID: 33587269.
45. Shrader MW, Wood W, Falk M, Segal LS, Boan C, White G. The effect of two attending surgeons on the outcomes of posterior spine fusion in children with cerebral palsy. *Spine Deform*. 2018;6(6):730–735. https://doi.org/10.1016/j.jspd.2018.03.002. PMID: 30348351.
46. Yaszay B, Bartley CE, Sponseller PD, et al. Major complications following surgical correction of spine deformity in 257 patients with cerebral palsy. *Spine Deform*. 2020;8(6):1305–1312. https://doi.org/10.1007/s43390-020-00165-7.Epub 2020 Jul 27. PMID: 32720268; PMCID: PMC7384279.
47. Samdani AF, Belin EJ, Bennett JT, et al. Major perioperative complications after spine surgery in patients with cerebral palsy: assessment of risk factors. *Eur Spine J*. 2016;25(3):795–800. https://doi.org/10.1007/s00586-015-4054-3. Epub 2015 Jul 7. PMID: 26148567.
48. Matsumoto M, Miyagi M, Saito W, et al. Perioperative complications in posterior spinal fusion surgery for neuromuscular scoliosis. *Spine Surg Relat Res*. 2018;2(4):278–282. https://doi.org/10.22603/ssrr.2017-0075. PMID: 31435534; PMCID: PMC6690101.
49. Luhmann SJ, Furdock R. Preoperative variables associated with respiratory complications after pediatric neuromuscular spine deformity surgery. *Spine Deform*. 2019;7:107–111.
50. Sharma S, Wu C, Andersen T, et al. Prevalence of complications in neuromuscular scoliosis surgery: a literature meta-analysis from the past 15 years. *Eur Spine J*. 2013;22:1230–1249.
51. Kang GR, Suh SW, Lee IO. Preoperative predictors of postoperative pulmonary complications in neuromuscular scoliosis. *J Orthop Sci*. 2011;16(2):139–147. https://doi.org/10.1007/s00776-011-0028-4. Epub 2011 Feb 11. PMID: 21311930.
52. Yuan N, Skaggs DL, Dorey F, Keens TG. Preoperative predictors of prolonged postoperative mechanical ventilation in children following scoliosis repair. *Pediatr Pulmonol*. 2005;40(5):414–419. https://doi.org/10.1002/ppul.20291. PMID: 16145695.
53. Toll BJ, Samdani AF, Janjua MB, Gandhi S, Pahys JM, Hwang SW. Perioperative complications and risk factors in neuromuscular scoliosis surgery. *J Neurosurg Pediatr*. 2018;22(2):207–213. https://doi.org/10.3171/2018.2.PEDS17724. Epub 2018 May 11. PMID: 29749884.
54. Wang Y, Hai Y, Liu Y, Guan L, Liu T. Risk factors for postoperative pulmonary complications in the treatment of non-degenerative scoliosis by posterior instrumentation and fusion. *Eur Spine J*. 2019;28(6):1356–1362. https://doi.org/10.1007/s00586-019-05968-5. Epub 2019 Apr 8. PMID: 30963290.
55. LaValva SM, Baldwin K, Swarup I, et al. Harms Study Group. Prolonged postoperative intubation after spinal fusion in cerebral palsy: Are there modifiable risk factors and associated consequences? *J Pediatr Orthop*. 2020;40(8):431–437. https://doi.org/10.1097/BPO.0000000000001566. PMID: 32301849.
56. Al-Iede MM, Al-Zayadneh E, Bridge C, Alqutawneh B, Waters K. Risk factors for postoperative pulmonary complications in children with severely compromised pulmonary function secondary to severe scoliosis. *Pediatr Pulmonol*. 2020;55(10):2782–2790. https://doi.org/10.1002/ppul.24997. Epub 2020 Aug 7. PMID: 32729967.
57. Eagle M, Bourke J, Bullock R, et al. Managing Duchenne muscular dystrophy--the additive effect of spinal surgery and home nocturnal ventilation in improving survival. *Neuromuscul Disord*. 2007;17(6):470–475. https://doi.org/10.1016/j.nmd.2007.03.002. Epub 2007 May 8. PMID: 17490881.
58. Khirani S, Bersanini C, Aubertin G, Bachy M, Vialle R, Fauroux B. Non-invasive positive pressure ventilation to facilitate the post-operative respiratory outcome of spine surgery in neuromuscular children. *Eur Spine J*. 2014;23(Suppl 4):S406–411. https://doi.org/10.1007/s00586-014-3335-6. Epub 2014 May 10. PMID: 24816609.
59. Bach JR, Sabharwal S. High pulmonary risk scoliosis surgery: role of noninvasive ventilation and related techniques. *J Spinal Disord Tech*. 2005;18(6):527–530. https://doi.org/10.1097/01.bsd.0000154457.62714.4b. PMID: 16306844.
60. Mills B, Bach JR, Zhao C, Saporito L, Sabharwal S. Posterior spinal fusion in children with flaccid neuromuscular scoliosis: the role of noninvasive positive pressure ventilatory support. *J Pediatr Orthop*. 2013;33(5):488–493. https://doi.org/10.1097/BPO.0b013e318287058f. PMID: 23752144.
61. Sullivan PB. Gastrointestinal disorders in children with neurodevelopmental disabilities. *Dev Disabil Res Rev*. 2008;14(2):128–136. https://doi.org/10.1002/ddrr.18. PMID: 18646021.
62. Jevsevar DS, Karlin LI. The relationship between preoperative nutritional status and complications after an operation for scoliosis in patients who have cerebral palsy. *J Bone Joint Surg Am*. 1993;75:880–884. Erratum in: *J Bone Joint Surg Am*. 1993;75:1256.
63. Master DL, Son-Hing JP, Poe-Kochert C, Armstrong DG, Thompson GH. Risk factors for major complications after surgery for neuromuscular scoliosis. *Spine (Phila Pa 1976)*. 2011;36(7):564–571. https://doi.org/10.1097/BRS.0b013e3181e193e9. PMID: 20683386.

64. Jalanko T, Helenius I, Pakarinen M, Koivusalo A. Gastrointestinal complications after surgical correction of neuromuscular scoliosis: A retrospective cohort study. *Scand J Surg.* 2018;107(3):252–259. https://doi.org/10.1177/1457496917748223.Epub 2017 Dec 21. PMID: 29268665.
65. Verhofste BP, Berry JG, Miller PE, et al. Harms Study Group. Risk factors for gastrointestinal complications after spinal fusion in children with cerebral palsy. *Spine Deform.* 2021;9(2):567–578. https://doi.org/10.1007/s43390-020-00233-y. Epub 2020 Nov 17. PMID: 33201495.
66. Vande Velde S, Van Biervliet S, De Bruyne R, Van Renterghem K, Plasschaert F, Van Winckel M. Gastric dysmotility following orthopaedic scoliosis surgery in patients with cerebral palsy: a case series. *Neuropediatrics.* 2010;41(4):182–185. https://doi.org/10.1055/s-0030-1265227. Epub 2010 Nov 17. PMID: 21086223.
67. Borkhuu B, Nagaraju D, Miller F, et al. Prevalence and risk factors in postoperative pancreatitis after spine fusion in patients with cerebral palsy. *J Pediatr Orthop.* 2009;29(3):256–262. https://doi.org/10.1097/BPO.0b013e31819bcf0a. PMID: 19305276.
68. Laplaza FJ, Widmann RF, Fealy S, et al. Pancreatitis after surgery in adolescent idiopathic scoliosis: incidence and risk factors. *J Pediatr Orthop.* 2002;22(1):80–83. PMID: 11744859.
69. Tsirikos AI, Jeans LA. Superior mesenteric artery syndrome in children and adolescents with spine deformities undergoing corrective surgery. *J Spinal Disord Tech.* 2005;18(3):263–271. PMID: 15905772.
70. Smith BG, Hakim-Zargar M, Thomson JD. Low body mass index: a risk factor for superior mesenteric artery syndrome in adolescents undergoing spinal fusion for scoliosis. *J Spinal Disord Tech.* 2009;22(2):144–148. https://doi.org/10.1097/BSD.0b013e31816b6b9a. PMID: 19342937.
71. Sarwahi V, Sarwark JF, Schafer MF, et al. Standards in anterior spine surgery in pediatric patients with neuromuscular scoliosis. *J Pediatr Orthop.* 2001;21(6):756–760. PMID: 11675549.
72. Malik AT, Tamer R, Yu E, Kim J, Khan SN. The impact of body mass index (BMI) on 30-day outcomes following posterior spinal fusion in neuromuscular scoliosis. *Spine (Phila Pa 1976).* 2019;44(19):1348–1355. https://doi.org/10.1097/BRS.0000000000003084. PMID: 31261270.
73. Anastasio AT, Guisse NF, Farley KX, Rhee JM. Hospital burdens of patients with cerebral palsy undergoing posterior spinal fusion for scoliosis. *Global Spine J.* 2020219256822096854 2. doi: 10.1177/2192568220968542. Epub ahead of print. PMID: 33203253.
74. Wald HL, Ma A, Bratzler DW, Kramer AM. Indwelling urinary catheter use in the postoperative period: analysis of the national surgical infection prevention project data. *Arch Surg.* 2008;143(6):551–557. https://doi.org/10.1001/archsurg.143.6.551. PMID: 18559747.
75. Eguia F, Nhan DT, Shah SA, et al. Harms Study Group. Of major complication types, only deep infections after spinal fusion are associated with worse health-related outcomes in children with cerebral palsy. *Spine (Phila Pa 1976).* 2020;45(14):993–999. https://doi.org/10.1097/BRS.0000000000003463. PMID: 32150131.
76. Mackenzie WG, Matsumoto H, Williams BA, et al. Surgical site infection following spinal instrumentation for scoliosis: a multicenter analysis of rates, risk factors, and pathogens. *J Bone Joint Surg Am.* 2013;95(9):800–806, S1-2. https://doi.org/10.2106/JBJS.L.00010. PMID: 23636186.
77. Aleissa S, Parsons D, Grant J, Harder J, Howard J. Deep wound infection following pediatric scoliosis surgery: incidence and analysis of risk factors. *Can J Surg.* 2011;54(4):263–269. https://doi.org/10.1503/cjs.008210. PMID: 21658334; PMCID: PMC3191901.
78. Sponseller PD, Jain A, Shah SA, et al. Deep wound infections after spinal fusion in children with cerebral palsy: a prospective cohort study. *Spine (Phila Pa 1976).* 2013;38(23):2023–2027. https://doi.org/10.1097/BRS.0b013e3182a83e59.PMID: 23963019.
79. Ramo BA, Roberts DW, Tuason D, et al. Surgical site infections after posterior spinal fusion for neuromuscular scoliosis: a thirty-year experience at a single institution. *J Bone Joint Surg Am.* 2014;96(24):2038–2048. https://doi.org/10.2106/JBJS.N.00277. PMID: 25520337.
80. Minkara AA, Matsumoto H, Glotzbecker M, et al. Children's Spine Study Group. A multicenter study of the epidemiology of deep surgical site infections in children with nonidiopathic early-onset scoliosis including associated pathogens. *Spine Deform.* 2019;7(4):647–651. https://doi.org/10.1016/j.jspd.2018.11.015. PMID: 31202384.
81. Glotzbecker MP, Riedel MD, Vitale MG. What's the evidence? Systematic literature review of risk factors and preventive strategies for surgical site infection following pediatric spine surgery. *J Pediatr Orthop.* 2013;33(5):479–487. https://doi.org/10.1097/BPO.0b013e318285c507. PMID: 23752143.
82. Armaghani SJ, Menge TJ, Lovejoy SA, Mencio GA, Martus JE. Safety of topical vancomycin for pediatric spinal deformity: nontoxic serum levels with supratherapeutic drain levels. *Spine (Phila Pa 1976).* 2014;39(20):1683–1687. https://doi.org/10.1097/BRS.0000000000000465. PMID: 24921849.
83. Gans I, Dormans JP, Spiegel DA, et al. Adjunctive vancomycin powder in pediatric spine surgery is safe. *Spine (Phila Pa 1976).* 2013;38(19):1703–1707. https://doi.org/10.1097/BRS.0b013e31829e05d3. PMID: 23759805.
84. Ward JP, Feldman DS, Paul J, et al. Wound closure in nonidiopathic scoliosis: Does closure matter? *J Pediatr Orthop.* 2017;37(3):166–170. https://doi.org/10.1097/BPO.0000000000000610. PMID: 26214326.
85. Imahiyerobo T, Minkara AA, Matsumoto H, Vitale MG. Plastic multilayered closure in pediatric nonidiopathic scoliosis is associated with a lower than expected incidence of wound complications and surgical site infections. *Spine Deform.* 2018;6(4):454–459. https://doi.org/10.1016/j.jspd.2017.12.009. PMID: 29886919.
86. Garg S, Khechoyan D, Kim EB, French B. Multilayered and flap closure technique for pediatric spinal deformity surgery. *J Am Acad Orthop Surg.* 2020;28((3):e92–e99. https://doi.org/10.5435/JAAOS-D-18-00601. PMID: 31977607.
87. Luhmann SJ, Smith JC. Preoperative MRSA screening in pediatric spine surgery: A helpful tool or a waste of time and money? *Spine Deform.* 2016;4(4):272–276. https://doi.org/10.1016/j.jspd.2015.12.006. Epub 2016 Jun 16. PMID: 27927516.
88. Luhmann SJ, Smith JC. Nasal swab screening for Staphylococcus aureus in spinal deformity patients treated with growing rods. *J Pediatr Orthop.* 2019;39(9):e694–e697. https://doi.org/10.1097/BPO.0000000000001015. PMID: 31503226.
89. Poe-Kochert C, Shimberg JL, Thompson GH, Son-Hing JP, Hardesty CK, Mistovich RJ. Surgical site infection prevention protocol for pediatric spinal deformity surgery: does it make a difference? *Spine Deform.* 2020;8(5):931–938. https://doi.org/10.1007/s43390-020-00120-6. Epub 2020 Apr 30. PMID: 32356280.

90. Vitale MG, Riedel MD, Glotzbecker MP, et al. Building consensus: development of a Best Practice Guideline (BPG) for surgical site infection (SSI) prevention in high-risk pediatric spine surgery. *J Pediatr Orthop*. 2013;33(5):471–478. https://doi.org/10.1097/BPO.0b013e3182840de2. PMID: 23752142.
91. Ghattas PJ, Mehlman CT, Eichten D. Treatment of postoperative infection after posterior spinal fusion and instrumentation in a patient with neuromuscular scoliosis. *Am J Orthop (Belle Mead NJ)*. 2014;43(2):89–93. PMID: 24551867.
92. van Rhee MA, de Klerk LW, Verhaar JA. Vacuum-assisted wound closure of deep infections after instrumented spinal fusion in six children with neuromuscular scoliosis. *Spine J*. 2007;7(5):596–600. https://doi.org/10.1016/j.spinee.2006.09.002. Epub 2007 Jan 2. PMID: 17905322.
93. Canavese F, Gupta S, Krajbich JI, Emara KM. Vacuum-assisted closure for deep infection after spinal instrumentation for scoliosis. *J Bone Joint Surg Br*. 2008;90(3):377–381. https://doi.org/10.1302/0301-620X.90B3.19890. PMID: 18310764.
94. Suresh KV, Ikwuezunma I, Margalit A, Sponseller PD. Spinal fusion with sacral alar iliac pelvic fixation in severe neuromuscular scoliosis. *JBJS Essent Surg Tech*. 2021;11(3):e20.00060 https://doi.org/10.2106/JBJS.ST.20.00060. PMID: 34650826; PMCID: PMC8505341.
95. Jain A, Modhia UM, Njoku DB, et al. Recurrence of deep surgical site infection in cerebral palsy after spinal fusion is rare. *Spine Deform*. 2017;5:208–212.
96. Sponseller PD, LaPorte DM, Hungerford MW, Eck K, Bridwell KH, Lenke LG. Deep wound infections after neuromuscular scoliosis surgery: a multicenter study of risk factors and treatment outcomes. *Spine (Phila Pa 1976)*. 2000;25(19):2461–2466. https://doi.org/10.1097/00007632-200010010-00007. PMID: 11013497.
97. Master DL, Poe-Kochert C, Son-Hing J, Armstrong DG, Thompson GH. Wound infections after surgery for neuromuscular scoliosis: risk factors and treatment outcomes. *Spine (Phila Pa 1976)*. 2011;36(3):E179–185. https://doi.org/10.1097/BRS.0b013e3181db7afe. PMID: 21248588.
98. Qiu Y, Wang S, Wang B, Yu Y, Zhu F, Zhu Z. Incidence and risk factors of neurological deficits of surgical correction for scoliosis: analysis of 1373 cases at one Chinese institution. *Spine (Phila Pa 1976)*. 2008;33(5):519–526. https://doi.org/10.1097/BRS.0b013e3181657d93. PMID: 18317197.
99. Mohamad F, Parent S, Pawelek J, et al. Perioperative complications after surgical correction in neuromuscular scoliosis. *J Pediatr Orthop*. 2007;27(4):392–397. https://doi.org/10.1097/01.bpb.0000271321.10869.98. PMID: 17513958.
100. Krishnakumar R, Srivatsa N. Multimodal intraoperative neuromonitoring in scoliosis surgery: A two-year prospective analysis in a single centre. *Neurol India*. 2017;65(1):75–79. https://doi.org/10.4103/0028-3886.198189. PMID: 28084243.
101. Krishnakumar R, Srivatsa N. Multimodal intraoperative neuromonitoring in scoliosis surgery: A two-year prospective analysis in a single centre. *Neurol India*. 2017;65(1):75–79. https://doi.org/10.4103/0028-3886.198189. PMID: 28084243.
102. DiCindio S, Theroux M, Shah S, Miller F, Dabney K, Brislin RP, Schwartz D. Multimodality monitoring of transcranial electric motor and somatosensory-evoked potentials during surgical correction of spinal deformity in patients with cerebral palsy and other neuromuscular disorders. *Spine (Phila Pa 1976)*. 2003;28(16):1851–1855. discussion 1855-1856. https://doi.org/10.1097/01.BRS.0000083202.62956.A8. PMID: 12923474.
103. Pastorelli F, Di Silvestre M, Vommaro F, et al. Intraoperative monitoring of somatosensory (SSEPs) and transcranial electric motor-evoked potentials (tce-MEPs) during surgical correction of neuromuscular scoliosis in patients with central or peripheral nervous system diseases. *Eur Spine J*. 2015;24(Suppl 7):931–936. https://doi.org/10.1007/s00586-015-4282-6. Epub 2015 Oct 19. PMID: 26482497.
104. Ando K, Kobayashi K, Ito K, et al. Wave change of intraoperative transcranial motor-evoked potentials during corrective fusion for syndromic and neuromuscular scoliosis. *Oper Neurosurg (Hagerstown)*. 2019;16(1):53–58. https://doi.org/10.1093/ons/opy045. PMID: 29617870.
105. Vitale MG, Skaggs DL, Pace GI, et al. Best practices in intraoperative neuromonitoring in spine deformity surgery: Development of an intraoperative checklist to optimize response. *Spine Deform*. 2014;2(5):333–339. https://doi.org/10.1016/j.jspd.2014.05.003. Epub 2014 Aug 27. PMID: 279 27330.
106. Dede O, Ward WT, Bosch P, Bowles AJ, Roach JW. Using the freehand pedicle screw placement technique in adolescent idiopathic scoliosis surgery: what is the incidence of neurological symptoms secondary to misplaced screws? *Spine (Phila Pa 1976)*. 2014;39(4):286–290. https://doi.org/10.1097/BRS.0000000000000127. PMID: 24553446.
107. Baghdadi YM, Larson AN, McIntosh AL, Shaughnessy WJ, Dekutoski MB, Stans AA. Complications of pedicle screws in children 10 years or younger: a case control study. *Spine (Phila Pa 1976)*. 2013;38(7):E386–393. https://doi.org/10.1097/BRS.0b013e318286be5d. PMID: 23324942.
108. Modi HN, Suh SW, Fernandez H, Yang JH, Song HR. Accuracy and safety of pedicle screw placement in neuromuscular scoliosis with free-hand technique. *Eur Spine J*. 2008;17(12):1686–1696. https://doi.org/10.1007/s00586-008-0795-6. Epub 2008 Oct 1. PMID: 18830636; PMCID: PMC2587671.
109. Garg B, Gupta M, Singh M, Kalyanasundaram D. Outcome and safety analysis of 3D-printed patient-specific pedicle screw jigs for complex spinal deformities: a comparative study. *Spine J*. 2019;19(1):56–64. https://doi.org/10.1016/j.spinee.2018.05.001. Epub 2018 May 3. PMID: 29730456.
110. Cao J, Zhang X, Liu H, Yao Z, Bai Y, Guo D, Feng L. 3D printed templates improve the accuracy and safety of pedicle screw placement in the treatment of pediatric congenital scoliosis. *BMC Musculoskelet Disord*. 2021;22(1):1014 https://doi.org/10.1186/s12891-021-04892-4. PMID: 34863150; PM CID: PMC8645104.
111. Vissarionov SV, Kokushin DN, Khusainov NO, et al. Comparing the treatment of congenital spine deformity using free-hand techniques in vivo and 3D-printed templates in vitro (prospective-retrospective single-center analytical single-cohort study). *Adv Ther*. 2020;37(1):402–419. https://doi.org/10.1007/s12325-019-01152-9. Epub 2019 Nov 21. PMID: 31755038.
112. Luo M, Wang W, Yang N, Xia L. Does Three-dimensional printing plus pedicle guider technology in severe congenital scoliosis facilitate accurate and efficient pedicle screw placement? *Clin Orthop Relat Res*. 2019;477(8):1904–1912. https://doi.org/10.1097/CORR.0000000000000739. PMID: 31107327; PMCID: PMC6999999.
113. Baky FJ, Milbrandt T, Echternacht S, Stans AA, Shaughnessy WJ, Larson AN. Intraoperative computed tomography-guided navigation for pediatric spine patients reduced return to operating room for screw malposition compared with freehand/

fluoroscopic techniques. *Spine Deform.* 2019;7(4):577–581. https://doi.org/10.1016/j.jspd.2018.11.012.PMID:31202374; PMCID: PMC6578871.

114. Luo TD, Polly Jr DW, Ledonio CG, Wetjen NM, Larson AN. Accuracy of pedicle screw placement in children 10 years or younger using navigation and intraoperative CT. *Clin Spine Surg.* 2016;29(3):E135–138. https://doi.org/10.1097/BSD.0000000000000230. PMID: 27007788.
115. Larson AN, Polly Jr DW, Guidera KJ, et al. The accuracy of navigation and 3D image-guided placement for the placement of pedicle screws in congenital spine deformity. *J Pediatr Orthop.* 2012;32(6):e23–29. https://doi.org/10.1097/BPO.0b013e318263a39e. PMID: 22892631.
116. Zhang JN, Fan Y, Hao DJ. Risk factors for robot-assisted spinal pedicle screw malposition. *Sci Rep.* 2019;9(1):3025 https://doi.org/10.1038/s41598-019-40057-z. PMID: 30816334; PMCID: PMC6395613.
117. Jin M, Liu Z, Qiu Y, Yan H, Han X, Zhu Z. Incidence and risk factors for the misplacement of pedicle screws in scoliosis surgery assisted by O-arm navigation-analysis of a large series of one thousand, one hundred and forty five screws. *Int Orthop.* 2017;41(4):773–780. https://doi.org/10.1007/s00264-016-3353-6. Epub 2016 Dec 21. PMID: 27999927.
118. Nectoux E, Giacomelli MC, Karger C, Herbaux B, Clavert JM. Complications of the Luque-Galveston scoliosis correction technique in paediatric cerebral palsy. *Orthop Traumatol Surg Res.* 2010;96(4):354–361. https://doi.org/10.1016/j.otsr.2010.01.004. Epub 2010 May 13. PMID: 20471343.
119. Comstock CP, Leach J, Wenger DR. Scoliosis in total-body-involvement cerebral palsy. Analysis of surgical treatment and patient and caregiver satisfaction. *Spine (Phila Pa 1976).* 1998;23(12):1412–1424. discussion 1424-1425. https://doi.org/10.1097/00007632-199806150-00022. PMID: 9654634.
120. Parsch D, Geiger F, Brocai DR, Lang RD, Carstens C. Surgical management of paralytic scoliosis in myelomeningocele. *J Pediatr Orthop B.* 2001;10(1):10–17. PMID: 11269805.
121. Garg S, Holland C, LaGreca J, McNair B, Erickson M. Predicting failure of iliac fixation in neuromuscular spine deformity. *Spine Deform.* 2014;2(3):214–218. https://doi.org/10.1016/j.jspd.2014.01.002. Epub 2014 May 8. PMID: 27927421.
122. Watanabe K, Lenke LG, Bridwell KH, et al. Comparison of radiographic outcomes for the treatment of scoliotic curves greater than 100 degrees: wires versus hooks versus screws. *Spine (Phila Pa 1976).* 2008;33(10):1084–1092. https://doi.org/10.1097/BRS.0b013e31816f5f3a. PMID: 18449042.
123. Funk S, Lovejoy S, Mencio G, Martus J. Rigid instrumentation for neuromuscular scoliosis improves deformity correction without increasing complications. *Spine (Phila Pa 1976).* 2016;41(1):46–52. https://doi.org/10.1097/BRS.0000000000001170. PMID: 26352742.
124. Tøndevold N, Lastikka M, Andersen T, Gehrchen M, Helenius I. Should instrumented spinal fusion in nonambulatory children with neuromuscular scoliosis be extended to L5 or the pelvis? *Bone Joint J.* 2020;102-B(2):261–267. https://doi.org/10.1302/0301-620X.102B2.BJJ-2019-0772.R2.PMID: 32009441.
125. Akesen B, Atici T, Eken G, Ulusaloglu AC. The comparison of the results after spinal fusion with or without iliac screw insertion in the treatment of neuromuscular scoliosis. *Acta Orthop Traumatol Turc.* 2018;52(6):435–437. https://doi.org/10.1016/j.aott.2017.12.005. Epub 2018 Sep 25. PMID: 30266422; PMCID: PMC6318476.
126. Peelle MW, Lenke LG, Bridwell KH, Sides B. Comparison of pelvic fixation techniques in neuromuscular spinal deformity correction: Galveston rod versus iliac and lumbosacral screws. *Spine (Phila Pa 1976).* 2006;31(20):2392–2398. discussion 2399. https://doi.org/10.1097/01.brs.0000238973.13294.16. PMID: 16985470.
127. Myung KS, Lee C, Skaggs DL. Early pelvic fixation failure in neuromuscular scoliosis. *J Pediatr Orthop.* 2015;35(3):258–265. https://doi.org/10.1097/BPO.0000000000000254. PMID: 24992353.
128. Shabtai L, Andras LM, Portman M, et al. Sacral alar iliac (SAI) screws fail 75% less frequently than aliac screws in neuromuscular scoliosis. *J Pediatr Orthop.* 2017;37(8):e470–e475. https://doi.org/10.1097/BPO.0000000000000720. PMID: 26756987.
129. Wu Z, Schwend RM, Anderson JT, Marasigan JAM, Price NJ. Iliac screw instrumentation to the pelvis in children with neuromuscular and syndromic scoliosis. No lateral connectors and respect sagittal balance. *Spine Deform.* 2021;9(4):1115–1123. https://doi.org/10.1007/s43390-021-00287-6. Epub 2021 Jan 25. PMID: 33492654.
130. Perrault FD, Aubin CE, Wang X, Schwend RM. Biomechanical analysis of forces sustained by iliac screws in spinal instrumentation for deformity treatment: preliminary results. *Stud Health Technol Inform.* 2012;176:307–310. PMID: 22744516.
131. Lee MC, Jarvis C, Solomito MJ, Thomson JD. Comparison of S2-Alar and traditional iliac screw pelvic fixation for pediatric neuromuscular deformity. *Spine J.* 2018;18(4):648–654. https://doi.org/10.1016/j.spinee.2017.08.253. Epub 2017 Sep 21. PMID: 28870838.
132. Sponseller PD, Zimmerman RM, Ko PS, et al. Low profile pelvic fixation with the sacral alar iliac technique in the pediatric population improves results at two-year minimum follow-up. *Spine (Phila Pa 1976).* 2010;35(20):1887–1892. https://doi.org/10.1097/BRS.0b013e3181e03881. PMID: 20802390.
133. Ravindra VM, Mazur MD, Brockmeyer DL, et al. Clinical effectiveness of S2-alar iliac screws in spinopelvic fixation in pediatric neuromuscular scoliosis: Systematic literature review. *Global Spine J.* 2020;10(8):1066–1074. https://doi.org/10.1177/2192568219899658. Epub 2020 Jan 7. PMID: 32875851; PMCID: PMC7645097.
134. Desrochers-Perrault F, Aubin CE, Wang X, Schwend RM. Biomechanical analysis of iliac screw fixation in spinal deformity instrumentation. *Clin Biomech (Bristol, Avon).* 2014;29(6):614–621. https://doi.org/10.1016/j.clinbiomech.2014.04.016. Epub 2014 May 20. PMID: 24906687.
135. Piantoni L, Remondino RG, Tello CA, Wilson IAF, Galaretto E, Noel MA. Proximal junction kyphosis after posterior spinal fusion for early-onset scoliosis. *Spine Deform.* 2020;8(2):311–316. https://doi.org/10.1007/s43390-020-00029-0. Epub 2020 Feb 24. PMID: 32096133.
136. Chen X, Chen ZH, Qiu Y, et al. Proximal junctional kyphosis after posterior spinal instrumentation and fusion in young children with congenital scoliosis: A preliminary report on its incidence and risk factors. *Spine (Phila Pa 1976).* 2017;42(20):E1197–E1203. https://doi.org/10.1097/BRS.0000000000002109. PMID: 28187070.
137. Chen X, Xu L, Qiu Y, et al. Incidence, risk factors, and evolution of proximal junctional kyphosis after posterior hemivertebra resection and short fusion in young children with congenital scoliosis. *Spine (Phila Pa 1976).* 2018;43(17):1193–1200. https://doi.org/10.1097/BRS.0000000000002593. PMID: 29419719.

138. Bao B, Su Q, Hai Y, et al. Posterior thoracolumbar hemivertebra resection and short-segment fusion in congenital scoliosis: surgical outcomes and complications with more than 5-year follow-up. *BMC Surg.* 2021;21(1):165 https://doi.org/10.1186/s12893-021-01165-8. PMID: 33765989; PMCID: PMC7993516.
139. Erkilinc M, Baldwin KD, Pasha S, Mistovich RJ. Proximal junctional kyphosis in pediatric spinal deformity surgery: a systematic review and critical analysis. *Spine Deform.* 2022;10(2):257–266. https://doi.org/10.1007/s43390-021-00429-w.
140. Fernandes P, Weinstein SL. Natural history of early onset scoliosis. *J Bone Joint Surg Am.* 2007;89(suppl 1):21–33.
141. Helenius IJ. Standard and magnetically controlled growing rods for the treatment of early onset scoliosis. *Ann Transl Med.* 2020;8(2):26.
142. Smith JT, Johnston C, Skaggs D, et al. A new classification system to report complications in growing spine surgery: a multicenter consensus study. *J Pediatr Orthop.* 2015;35:798–803.
143. Bess S, Akbarnia BA, Thompson GH, et al. Complications of growing-rod treatment for early-onset scoliosis: analysis of one hundred and forty patients. *J Bone Joint Surg Am.* 2010;92:2533–2543.
144. Yang JS, Sponseller PD, Thompson GH, et al. Growing rod fractures: risk factors and opportunities for prevention. *Spine (Phila Pa 1976).* 2011;36(20):1639–1644.
145. Smith JS, Shaffrey CI, Ames CP, et al. Assessment of symptomatic rod fracture after posterior instrumented fusion for adult spinal deformity. *Neurosurgery.* 2012;71(4):862–867.
146. Harrington PR. Treatment of scoliosis. Correction and internal fixation by spine instrumentation. *J Bone Joint Surg Am.* 1962; 44:591–610.
147. Helenius IJ. Standard and magnetically controlled growing rods for the treatment of early onset scoliosis. *Ann Transl Med.* 2020;8(2):26.
148. Kabirian N, Akbarnia BA, Pawelek JB, et al. Growing Spine Study Group. Deep surgical site infection following 2344 growing-rod procedures for early-onset scoliosis: Risk factors and clinical consequences. *J Bone Joint Surg Am.* 2014;96(15):e128 https://doi.org/10.2106/JBJS.M.00618. PMID: 25100781.
149. Gomez JA, Kubat O, Tovar Castro MA, et al. Pediatric Spine Study Group (PSSG). The effect of spinopelvic parameters on the development of proximal junctional kyphosis in early Oonset: Mean 4.5-year follow-up. *J Pediatr Orthop.* 2020;40(6):261–266. https://doi.org/10.1097/BPO.0000000000001516. PMID: 32501899.
150. Li Y, Gold M, Karlin L. Proximal junctional kyphosis after vertical expandable prosthetic titanium rib insertion. *Spine Deform.* 2013;1(6):425–433. https://doi.org/10.1016/j.jspd.2013.07.013. Epub 2013 Nov 21. PMID: 27927368.
151. Watanabe K, Uno K, Suzuki T, et al. Risk factors for proximal junctional kyphosis associated with dual-rod growing-rod surgery for early-onset scoliosis. *Clin Spine Surg.* 2016;29(8): E428–E433.
152. Kwan KYH, Alanay A, Yazici M, et al. Unplanned reoperations in magnetically controlled growing rod surgery for early onset scoliosis with a minimum of two-year follow-up. *Spine.* 2017;42:E1410–E1414.
153. Rushton PRP, Smith SL, Kandemir G, et al. Spinal lengthening with magnetically controlled growing rods: Data from the largest series of explanted devices. *Spine (Phila Pa 1976).* 2020; 45(3):170–176.
154. Agarwal A, Kelkar A, Garg Agarwal A, Jayaswal D, Jayaswal A, Shendge V. Device-related complications associated with Magec rod usage for distraction-based correction of scoliosis. *Spine Surg Relat Res.* 2019;4(2):148–151.
155. Akbarnia BA, Mundis GM. Magnetically controlled growing rods in early onset scoliosis: Indications, timing and treatment. *Orthopade.* 2019;48(6):477–485.
156. Teoh KH, von Ruhland C, Evans SL, et al. Metallosis following implantation of magnetically controlled growing rods in the treatment of scoliosis: a case series. *Bone Joint J.* 2016;98-B(12): 1662–1667. https://doi.org/10.1302/0301-620X.98B12.38061. PMID: 27909129.
157. Yaszay B, O'Brien M, Shufflebarger HL, et al. Efficacy of hemivertebra resection for congenital scoliosis: a multicenter retrospective comparison of three surgical techniques. *Spine (Phila Pa 1976).* 2011;36(24):2052–2060. https://doi.org/10.1097/BRS.0b013e318233f4bb. PMID: 22048650.
158. Jalanko T, Rintala R, Puisto V, Helenius I. Hemivertebra resection for congenital scoliosis in young children: comparison of clinical, radiographic, and health-related quality of life outcomes between the anteroposterior and posterolateral approaches. *Spine (Phila Pa 1976).* 2011;36(1):41–49. https://doi.org/10.1097/BRS.0b013e3181ccafd4. PMID: 20622749.
159. Guo J, Zhang J, Wang S, et al. Risk factors for construct/implant related complications following primary posterior hemivertebra resection: Study on 116 cases with more than 2 years' follow-up in one medical center. *BMC Musculoskelet Disord.* 2016; 17(1):380 https://doi.org/10.1186/s12891-016-1229-y. PMID: 27589864; PMCID: PMC5010738.
160. Holte DC, Winter RB, Lonstein JE, Denis F. Excision of hemivertebrae and wedge resection in the treatment of congenital scoliosis. *J Bone Joint Surg Am.* 1995;77(2):159–171. https://doi.org/10.2106/00004623-199502000-00001. PMID: 7844121.
161. Hedequist D, Emans J, Proctor M. Three rod technique facilitates hemivertebra wedge excision in young children through a posterior only approach. *Spine (Phila Pa 1976).* 2009;34(6):E225–229. https://doi.org/10.1097/BRS.0b013e3181997029. PMID: 19282729.
162. Hosalkar HS, Luedtke LM, Drummond DS. New technique in congenital scoliosis involving fixation to the pelvis after hemivertebra excision. *Spine (Phila Pa 1976).* 2004;29(22):2581–2587. https://doi.org/10.1097/01.brs.0000145414.43650.62. PMID: 15543077.
163. Wang C, Meng Z, You DP, et al. Individualized study of posterior hemivertebra excision and short-segment pedicle screw fixation for the treatment of congenital scoliosis. *Orthop Surg.* 2021;13(1):98–108. https://doi.org/10.1111/os.12838. Epub 2020 Nov 30. PMID: 33258309; PMCID: PMC7862179.

29

Long-Term Complications in Pediatric Spine Surgery

JOHN NGO AND AFSHIN AMINIAN

CHAPTER OUTLINE

Delayed Postoperative Neurologic Deficit

In the first significant analysis of the Scoliosis Research Society (SRS) Morbidity and Mortality data in 1975 analyzing 7885 scoliosis cases, most of whom underwent posterior spinal fusion with Harrington rods, MacEwen et al. noted a neurologic complication rate of 0.72%.[1] Coe et al. presented an update on complication rates using the SRS Morbidity and Mortality data for the years 2001, 2002, and 2003 in 6334 patients undergoing corrective surgery for adolescent idiopathic scoliosis (AIS). In their analysis, neurologic complication rates for anterior, posterior, and combined anterior-posterior procedures were 0.26%, 0.32%, and 1.75%, respectively, with the combined procedures statistically significant for increased risk.[2] Though there are no details on whether these neurologic complications were intraoperative or delayed presentations.

Delayed postoperative neurologic deficit (DPND) is described as neurologic deficits that arise hours to days after corrective surgery. Intraoperative neuromonitoring (IONM) with somatosensory evoked potentials (SSEP) and motor evoked potentials (MEP) has given surgeons the ability to adjust accordingly to neurologic insult or changes during surgery and correction maneuvers.[3] There are guidelines and recommendations for timely remedy of intraoperative alerts, such as certain inhalational anesthetics, modulation of mean arterial pressure, positioning, etc. Despite utilization of IONM, uneventful surgeries without alerts, and a normal postoperative exam, it is still possible to develop delayed neurologic deficits after corrective surgery.

Fortunately, these cases are rare and the incidence is estimated to be at 1 of 9910 cases (0.01%) in a cross-sectional study of spinal deformity patients by Auerbach.[4] In this study, the most common cited problems were spinal cord ischemia and compression, 38% and 15%, respectively. Due to the low incidence of these cases, literature on this complication mainly consists of case series and reports. There are no multicenter studies available on this phenomenon.

A recent case was detailed in 2021 in a 12-year-old patient with AIS undergoing posterior fusion and correction for a severe 125 degree thoracolumbar curve. IONM alerts were noted during surgery that improved with increasing mean arterial pressure (MAP) and relaxing bending correction with rod removal. Immediate postoperative exam was normal; however, the patient was found to have ASIA B impairment with nearly complete paraplegia of the lower extremities on postoperative day 2 after transient decrease in MAP at 36 hours after surgery. Transcutaneous motor evoked potentials (TcMEP) improved and return of function was achieved after emergent exploration and removal of apical pedicles.[5] The authors believed that the DPND in this case was due to transient hypoperfusion and compression on the apical concave pedicles.

Another case in 2006 involved a delayed epidural hematoma causing paralysis of the left lower extremity 24 hours after surgery. This was a 12-year-old patient with AIS undergoing anterior and posterior correction with posterior spinal fusion for an 80 degree lower thoracic curve. The patient underwent emergent decompression with partial removal of hardware and re-insertion of segmental hardware 2 weeks later. The patient had full return of function and correction was maintained at 85% at 4 months follow-up.[6] Auerbach noted that 63% of DPND cases were identified within the first 24 hours postoperatively, and 90% of cases were detected within the first 48 hours, emphasizing the importance of vigilance during physical exams after surgery.[4] Other cited causes of DPND include compression of the cord due to kinking after correction of vertebral column or residual angular deformity. Advanced imaging, such as magnetic resonance imaging (MRI), is recommended in localizing pathology if there is no significant delay to intervention.

Auerbach also investigated the recovery and long-term course after DPND, though this population was heterogeneous in diagnosis, including cervical, kyphosis, spondylolisthesis cases and not specifically on corrective surgery. He reported complete neurologic recovery in 41% of patients, with 26% achieving a partial neurologic recovery. However, 33% had no neurologic recovery despite corrective measures.[4] These patients appeared to have better improvement if the etiology was compression, hematoma, or instrumentation, with recovery of at least one American Spinal Injury Association (ASIA) grade when compared to patients with etiology of ischemia. Recovery of neurologic function may also be seen as far as 6 months after surgery, with only 22% of patients demonstrating their final neurologic status at 1 week after surgery. These authors recommend optimizing MAP to at least 90 if DPND develops with subsequent emergent advanced imaging, MRI, computed tomography (CT), or CT myelogram, to identify areas of compression. For the neurologic complications in Coe et al.'s patient population, complete recovery was seen in 11 patients (61%), and incomplete recovery was noted in 6 patients (33%).[2]

Late neurologic presentations have been observed as late as 2 to 3 years after posterior spinal fusion with pedicle screws. Mac-Thiong et al. presented a series of nine patients who were referred to their institution for medially malpositioned pedicle screws breaching the spinal canal during corrective surgery for AIS.[7] Two of the nine patients in this series developed neurologic deficits 2 and 3 years after index surgery and CT scan demonstrated pedicle intrusion of the spinal canal. One patient had onset of symptoms after kicking a ball with subsequent midback pain. Intraoperative findings demonstrated solid fusion mass of the spine; however, the malpositioned screws were loose. This suggests that poorly placed pedicle screws have suboptimal purchase and can migrate despite solid fusion, causing late neurologic deficits as the screws migrate and impinge on the spinal cord. Both of these patients had no neuromonitoring alerts intraoperatively, therefore one must understand that spinal canal intrusion may still be possible in uneventful surgeries. One patient was seen 1 year and 11 months after complete implant removal with return of full neurologic function, while the other had persistent hypoesthesia and abnormal proprioception 6 and a half years after implant removal. Mac-Thiong et al. strongly recommends the removal of the malpositioned screws when detected, with attention to any cerebrospinal fluid leaks to perform dural repair when found. There are other patients, specifically three, in this series that have no neurological deficits despite complete intrusion of the pedicle screw even with 9, 7, and 5 years of follow up after initial surgery.

Delayed Infections

Early postoperative spinal infections are usually caused by virulent pathogens, such as *Staphylococcus aureus*, B-hemolytic streptococci, and aerobic gram-negative bacilli. Postoperative spinal implant infection (PSII) manifests at different time periods based on microbial virulence, either early within 4 weeks or later after 4 weeks.[8] Delayed infection in PSII most commonly has been defined as an infection occurring greater than 3 months after index surgery,[9] with symptoms and signs of chronic pain, implant failure, or lack of adequate fusion several months to years after surgery. Other common presentations include nonspecific vague back pain, with fevers occurring less reliably in 16% to 65% of patients.[10] As with all infection workups, studies should include blood cultures, complete blood count (CBC) with diff, erythrocyte sedimentation rate (ESR), and C-reactive protein (CRP). However, a recent study showed low sensitivity, at only 64%, and low specificity, at 68%, for serum CRP in detecting delayed PSII especially in pathogens with low virulence.[11] Hanh et al.'s[12] series of 101 consecutive adolescent scoliosis patients, with minimum of 24 months follow up, with posterior fusion using pedicle screws demonstrated no early infections but did identify 7 patients with late infections (6.9%). In this population, indicators for infection were sudden onset of local pain without fever after an initial pain-free interval. Normal CRP and ESR did not rule out late infection, suggesting no reliable laboratory markers. None of the seven patients presented with fever, but all had pain after a pain-free interval. None of the seven had preoperative risks for infection. Extended cultures were done from intraoperative samples; six patients yielded *Propionibacterium acnes*. The one without *P. acnes* had no organism growth in culture.[12] Imaging can be with x-ray, CT, MRI, but the gold standard for diagnosing PSII is intraoperatively obtained tissue cultures.

In delayed PSII, low-virulent pathogens are more commonly found, such as coagulase-negative *staphylococci* (*S. epidermidis*), *Cutibacterium species,* and *C. acnes.*[13] These organisms are known to develop biofilm and remain dormant, which allows for avoidance of the host's immune system and lack of systemic inflammation during presentation. Though not in pediatric patients, Pumberger et al. in 2019 showed sonication cultures in presumed aseptic spine revision surgeries in adults, at an average of 39 months from index surgery, were positive in 45.2% of cases,[14] with *Cutibacterium acnes* and *S. epidermidis* as the most commonly isolated microorganisms, observed in 45% and 31% of cases, respectively.

With the increased recognition of low-virulence skin flora, *S. epidermidis* and *C. acnes,* in delayed infections of pediatric spinal deformity surgery,[15,16] it is imperative to understand the causes, risk factors, and management plans to provide optimal care. There are two theories for delayed infections in AIS surgery, hematogenous spread and inoculation during the index surgery. Hematogenous spread was first described by Heggeness et al. They reported six cases of spinal infections at 10 months or more after surgery, of which five patients had a distant focus of infection before clinical symptoms of a spinal infection occurred.[17] However, recent literature supports the latter theory as low-virulence skin flora have been the most commonly cited culprits, *S. epidermidis* and *C. acnes*.[12,15,16,18,19] Dietz et al. found positive wound cultures in >50% of patients undergoing clean, elective orthopedic procedures with no antibiotic prophylaxis. Coagulase-negative *Staphylococcus* was found in 58% of the cultures and *C. acnes* was found in 24%, suggesting introduction of skin flora during surgery.[20] Nandyala and Schwend demonstrated that *C. acnes* was the most common organism (69%), followed by *Staphylococcus* species in 114 cases of pediatric posterior instrumented deformity surgery. All of the cases of *C. acnes* involved adolescents 11 years and older, and back acne was a significant association.[21] Acne is also associated more closely with the adolescent population. These authors also recommend preoperative showering with an antimicrobial wash and a dermatology consultation for adolescents with back acne to lower the risk of intraoperative seeding of skin organisms.

C. acnes, previously referred to as *Propionibacterium acnes*, is a gram-positive aerotolerant anaerobic organism that exists on skin flora and is associated with the skin condition of acne. In 1996, Jakab et al. identified the pathogenic potential of this organism in late surgical infections. The most common predisposing conditions were previous surgery preceding the infection from 2 weeks to 4 years, with an average of 4 to 5 months, and implantation of foreign bodies. Suggesting introduction of skin flora with retained hardware in the body.[22] *C. acnes* has a high affinity for deep skin structures, making it difficult to eradicate with commonly applied disinfectants.[23] Richards and Emara recommended using iodine-impregnated plastic adhesives to cover skin surfaces during surgery and culturing intraoperative samples for at least 10 days as *C. acnes* requires extended time for identification, and to not attribute a delayed positive result for *S. epidermidis* or *C. acnes* as a contaminated specimen.[16] Clark et al.[15] recommends the same extended time for identification of *C. acnes,* and also *S. epidermidis,* with culturing for delayed infections. Cultures were continued for only 72 h in their first 10 patients and 90% of these were negative. Cultures were subsequently continued for 7 days in their last 12 patients and 92% of these were positive. *S. epidermidis* was found in six cultures and *P. acnes* was found in three cultures.[15] Identification of the most common organisms in delayed infections at each institution allows for institutional practices for appropriate coverage with surgical prophylaxis. For example, Texas Scottish Rite Hospital (TSRH) changed their antibiotic prophylaxis from Ancef to vancomycin and ceftazidime to cover *S. epidermidis* and other organisms.[24]

In a review of all publications between 1973 and 2012 to study postoperative spine infections, risk factors were grouped into patient-specific and surgery-specific factors, though this study was not limited to just pediatric patients. Patient-related risk factors included age, American Society of Anesthesiologists (ASA) score, diabetes mellitus, cardiovascular disease, obesity, smoking, malignancy, steroid use, previous lumbar surgery, nutritional status, chronic obstructive pulmonary disease, and immunologic competency. Surgery-related risk factors included duration of surgery, blood loss and blood transfusion, use of instrumentation, number of levels fused, surgical approach, and prolonged hospital stay.[25] Bose suggested decreasing the size and number of components in the fusion construct to minimize the irritation and inflammation that provide a favorable environment for low-virulence bacteria.[18] Considering the long levels of fusion during AIS surgery, surgeons should be conscientious of this possible risk factor. In a retrospective case control study by Nandyala and Schwend evaluating bacterial contamination in intraoperative tissue during posterior pediatric spinal deformity surgery, they reported a 23% rate of positive tissue cultures from pediatric patients undergoing posterior spinal fusion (PSF). Significant risk factors for intraoperative wound contamination were neuromuscular scoliosis with fusion to the pelvis, duration of surgery greater than 6 hours, and patients over 11 years of age.[21] Surgeons can use this information to stratify the risks in their patients and prepare accordingly.

As with other cases of infected hardware, there is a general consensus in the management of delayed PSII that includes irrigation, debridement, removal of hardware, and a course of antibiotics. Richards and Emara had success with implant removal, primary closure, and short course of antibiotics in 23 patients who underwent TSRH instrumentation for adolescent idiopathic scoliosis who subsequently presented with delayed infection.[16,19] Clark and Shufflebarger reported similar results with a similar protocol in their series of 22 patients undergoing posterior instrumentation for AIS deformity surgery.[15] Soultanis et al. added continuous antibiotic irrigation for 5 days after removal of implants in addition to postoperative antibiotics to eradicate delayed infections in five patients who had spinal instrumentation for correction of scoliosis.[26]

Considering the prevalence of low virulence organisms in delayed infections, and their ability to form biofilm, the removal of implants appears to be a logical procedure. It is commonly understood that irrigation and retention of implants are not effective in eradicating microorganisms that have seeded hardware.[27] Ho et al. retrospectively reviewed 622 patients who had posterior instrumented fusion for pediatric scoliosis and identified 53 patients who presented with delayed infection at or greater than 6 months after index surgery. They found that retention of hardware was the only significant predictor of necessity for repeat irrigation and debridements.[24] The isolated bacteria from intraoperative cultures was not a significant indicator of need for further irrigation and debridement after first washout. Despite other studies citing increased infection risks in patients with cerebral palsy and paraplegia,[28] Ho and Skaggs et al. demonstrated that idiopathic scoliosis patients did not clear infection any better than other diagnoses. Overall, they predicted a 50% need for repeat irrigation and debridement if hardware was retained after initial washout for delayed infection of spinal instrumentation.

One must consider the status of fusion prior to removing hardware in patients who underwent instrumentation in corrective deformity, though literature on this appears limited. In Hanh's 7 AIS patients, out of their series of 101 consecutive patients undergoing deformity surgery, who developed delayed infection, all were successfully treated with implant removal and antibiotic treatment for 4 to 9 weeks.[12] Despite no pseudoarthrosis found intraoperatively after implant removal, three patients had loss of correction, ranging from 10 to 26 degrees. Patients who had implant removal sooner after index surgery had the greatest loss of correction. One patient who had a period of 14 months from index surgery had 26 degrees loss of correction. In Ho et al., of the 10 patients who had removal of their hardware, 60% of them had 10 degrees of deformity progression in at least one plane. Muschik et al. retrospectively reviewed 45 scoliosis patients who had implant removal for late infections and reported an average loss of correction of 6 degrees for the thoracic curve, 5 degrees for the lumbar curve, and 11 degrees for thoracic kyphosis with average length of follow-up of 3.6 years.[29] The clinician must balance the need for implant removal against the risk of deformity progression. Alternatives include retention of implants, though this has been demonstrated with additional need for washout incurring more costs and additional surgeries, or use of suppression antibiotics until solid fusion, which can be difficult to assess.

Potter et al. performed a retrospective radiographic analysis of patients with AIS who had removal of their instrumentation for multiple etiologies. In their group of 15 patients, exploration of the fusion mass intraoperatively did not demonstrate evidence of pseudoarthrosis. Loss of correction after instrumentation removal occurred at all curves, main thoracic and thoracolumbar-lumbar, and not at just one segment or disc, suggesting that there are no underlying pseudoarthrosis. Interestingly, there were no significant differences in sagittal measures before and after removal of instrumentation.[30]

Adding on Phenomena

"Adding on" is a phenomenon that is seen in corrective spinal fusion for deformities. It was first noted by Suk et al. in 2003, characterizing it as progression of the curve after fusion.[31] The pooled prevalence of this phenomena is 14%, though it ranges between 2% to 21% in literature, in a recent meta-analysis by Yang et al.[32] Adding-on has been commonly defined as an increase in Cobb angle of at least 5 degrees and distalization of the end vertebrae, or a change in disc angulation of 5 degrees or greater below the lowest instrumented vertebra (LIV) from the first erect to the 2-year follow-up radiographs.[33–35] The incorrect selection of lowest instrumented vertebra is the most commonly cited risk factor for occurrence of adding on. Traditionally, the recommendation to fuse to the stable vertebrae (SV) by King et al. was done in the age of Harrington rods that provided uniplanar correction.[36] Selective thoracic fusion during this time with Harrington rods for S-shaped curves with a lumbar curve that is the same or smaller in size than the thoracic curve appeared to have satisfactory results. However, with the advent of pedicle screw systems, greater magnitude correction and de-rotational maneuvers were possible for selective fusion with goals of preserving motion segments, which led to observations of lumbar decompensations in a substantial number of patients. The reasons for curve progression have been attributed to inappropriate selection of the LIV, selective thoracic fusion,[31] postoperative lumbar Cobb angle, overcorrection of the thoracic curve,[34] rigid preoperative curves, severe rotation,[37] or hardware protrusion to facet joints.[38]

Decision-making on choosing the LIV during preoperative planning for AIS corrective surgery is controversial. This is important because the selection of LIV has been cited as an independent risk factor for adding on. From analyzing risk factors from numerous studies, Yang et al. listed the following recommendations that are consistent with others.[32] First, fusion should be extended to at least one level beyond the preoperative end vertebrae (EV). Second, the LIV should be within two levels of the preoperative SV. Lastly the authors recommend selecting a LIV that is the first vertebra cephalad from the sacrum that deviates from the central sacral vertical line (CSVL) by more than 10 mm. Characteristics of patients who experienced adding on were described as having smaller proximal thoracic curve, main thoracic curve, clavicular angle, T1 tilt angle, and radiographic shoulder height. Smaller curves tend to be more flexible, thus overcorrection of these proximal curves could lead to decompensations distally, which have been cited in other studies as well. Besides selection of LIV, additional risk factors in Yang et al.'s study include the commonly cited younger age and skeletal immaturity. Something to consider with these risk factors is that in younger patients, there could be tendency to perform more selective fusion to allow growth and preservation of motion segments thus leading to an inappropriately selected LIV.[34]

Suk et al. found that the relationship between the neutral vertebrae (NV) and EV in AIS patients with a major thoracic curve was an important factor in deciding the extent of distal fusion to prevent "adding on." Their analysis demonstrated a significantly higher chance of curve progression if the distal fusion were extended to the NV-2 and NV-3 as it led to unsatisfactory results in their study group. Fusion to the neutral vertebrae was recommended if the preoperative NV and EV showed no more than a 2-level difference. They concluded that in single thoracic curves, fusion can be performed down to NV-1 or NV instead of the stable vertebrae (SV) to allow for preservation of motion segments.[31]

Other risk factors for adding on associated with choosing the LIV also include the CSVL. Hosogane et al. analyzed 58 patients undergoing selective thoracic fusion with a minimum of 2-year follow up.[39] Age, Risser grade, coronal balance, sagittal parameters, and curve magnitudes were not significant risk factors in their study. However, if the preoperative LIV was translated more than 10 mm from the CSVL or choosing the LIV that was 2 or more levels cephalad to the preoperative NV, there was significant risk of adding on. Wang et al. utilized a parameter involving CSVL as well and observed that the spontaneous correction after selective thoracic fusion in Lenke 1 A curves may progress and decompensate if fusion is not extended distal enough to maintain this correction.[34] The risk factors for adding on in this group of 23, out of 45 included patients, were age, SV-LIV > 2, EV-LIV > 1, and deviation from the CSVL of the LIV + 1. These are similar to other studies for age, which relates to skeletal maturity and LIV selection. Their conclusion was if the preoperative LIV +1 deviated more than 10 mm from the CSVL, then it is very likely that the patient's distal curve would progress.

Investigations have been done to identify risk factors for adding on in specific curve types. Cho et al. reviewed 195 AIS patients, with Lenke 1 A curves with L4 tilted either left or right, to evaluate the risk factors for adding on in this population. Their data showed that age of fusion and skeletal maturity based on Risser grading for Lenke 1A-L curves were significant risk factors for adding on. There was a trend in this group that those who experienced adding on had a more proximal LIV compared to those who did not. For the Lenke 1A-R group, fusing too short of the neutral vertebrae was a significant risk factor, though fusing too short of the stable vertebrae also trended towards statistical significance.[35]

In Lenke 1 and 2 curves, Yang et al.[40] evaluated their group of 98 AIS patients with a minimum of 2-year follow up for risk factors related to adding on, and also to develop a model to predict the chances of this phenomena. In the group of 16 patients that experienced adding on, the length between LIV and EV, SV, and the number of unfused segments showed significant differences. Again, this is similar to other studies citing LIV selection. The main factors associated with adding on in this study were the number of unfused segments and postoperative lumbar curve Cobb angle. Spontaneous correction of the lumbar curve in Lenke 1 and 2 patients have been noted after selective fusion of the thoracic curve, thus the authors in this study concluded that the postoperative Cobb angle of the lumbar curve correlates to the degree of correction of the main thoracic curve. Their adding on index to predict the risk of decompensation is described as 4 x DnfS – postoperative lumbar curve angle.[40] The authors used this index to describe the importance of LIV selection and to not overcorrect the main thoracic curve. They also noted in this population that there was no significant difference in postoperative SRS scores, in total or any domains, between patients with or without add on, consistent with Matsumoto et al.[41]

In Lenke 5 and 6 curves, Chang et al. analyzed 28 patients with either of these curves undergoing posterior spinal fusion with the LIV in the stable zone and as horizontal as possible. Eleven out of eighteen (61.1%) patients fused to L3 demonstrated adding on, while one out of ten (10%) who were fused to L4 demonstrated adding on.[37] LIV disc angles improved in the immediate postoperative period in patients fused to L4; however, these deteriorated similarly to patients fused to L3 that there was no significant difference at last follow up. Decision-making on LIV is a delicate balance of correction and preserving motion segments, to avoid disc degeneration and low back pain; however, there are studies that show no significant differences in patient-reported outcomes, the Scoliosis Research Society-22, Oswestry Disability Index, Visual Analog Scale, or Short-Form 36 scores, of LIV at L3 or L4.[42]

Despite the importance of LIV in literature for adding on, there appears to be no significant association between LIV selection and adding on with low back pain (LBP). Numerous series with follow up ranging from at least 17 to 20 years concluded that operated AIS patients had no more LBP than normal straight controls.[43–46] In addition, recent meta-analysis found no significant association between the distal level of fusion, the LIV, and incidence of LBP.[47–49]

It is worth noting that in the selection of LIV using biplanar preoperative spine radiographs, surgeons should be aware of the variability that exists. Studies have shown the changes of LIV in serial radiographs of the same patient and was dependent on posture. Therefore, in preoperative planning surgeons should employ multiple parameters when deciding on the LIV.[50] In addition, Potter et al. reported poor reliability of the three landmarks commonly used in decision making of LIV, with kappa of 0.3 for the EV, kappa of 0.26 for NV, and kappa of 0.39 for SV.[51]

Sagittal Malalignment and Junctional Problems

Restoration of sagittal alignment is imperative for balance and decreased energy utilization in daily activities, but recent research has shown a relationship with adjacent segment disease. Evaluation of intervertebral discs using MRI has been the most efficient method of disc degeneration after spinal fusion. Studies have demonstrated that postoperative sagittal balance is more important that LIV selection at 5- to 10-year follow up and that postoperative imbalance was associated with greater disc degeneration on MRI at an average of 7.5 years follow up.[52,53] Another study noted that if sagittal balance was restored in AIS patients, then no differences were observed in terms of degenerative change, quality of life, and daily activity when compared to normal controls.[54] In addition to sagittal balance, Abelin-Genevois et al. evaluated the pelvic parameters as well in their analysis of intervertebral discs on MRI. In their study, pelvic incidence (PI) appeared to influence the condition of the discs, suggesting that restoration of lumbo-pelvic congruence may help limit early degenerative changes in the free-motion segment discs after AIS surgery. Despite the goal of many surgeons to preserve motion segments, Abelin-Genevois et al. recommends striking a balance with restoring sagittal alignment even if that means longer fusion constructs.[55]

The adding on phenomena is the loss of correction, progression of the deformity, and decompensation in the coronal plane. In the sagittal plane, similar effects are called proximal junctional kyphosis (PJK) and distal junctional kyphosis (DJK). Cho et al. eloquently describes PJK as a form of adjacent segment pathology associated with spinal fusion most often seen after correction of scoliosis or kyphosis. PJK often manifests as a kyphotic change in the disk space above the proximal fusion site in pediatric patients.[56] Numerous definitions have been proposed over the years; however, the most commonly referred measurement in literature was proposed by Glattes et al.[57] as a sagittal Cobb angle between the inferior end plate of the upper instrumented vertebrae (UIV) and the upper end plate of UIV-2 of greater than or equal to 10 degrees. Lee et al. first reported on the incidence of PJK, of 46%, in their analysis of AIS patients in 1999.[57] It is important to note that many studies use different criteria for what they define as PJK, thus the incidence has been reported ranging from 9.2% to as high as 46%.[58–61] In a recent multicenter study, the incidence of PJK was found to be 7.05% and varies based on Lenke classification. Their definition of PJK was a Cobb angle of cephalad end plate of UIV-1 and caudal end plate of UIV that is greater than or equal to 10 degrees at 2-year follow up compared to preoperative films.[62] There is no consensus on which value precisely defines PJK. Overall, there appears to be no significant correlation between the radiographic development of PJK and the clinical outcome following surgery in children. SRS outcome scores for patients with PJK and those without PJK have no significant differences. In three different study groups with up to an average of 5 years follow up, there were no significant differences in any of the SRS subdomain scores and none of their patients with PJK required revision surgery.[59–61]

Numerous risk factors have been cited for PJK, from intrinsic and extrinsic factors related to AIS and spinal fusion. Lee et al. found that a preoperative one-level junctional kyphosis of greater than or equal to 5 degrees above the UIV was both sensitive and specific for PJK development.[57] Kim et al. identified three risk factors: performing thoracoplasty, preoperative thoracic hyperkyphosis, and hybrid instrumentation of proximal hooks and distal fixation of pedicle screws. The authors believed that thoracoplasty compromises the spine-chest cage structure leading to additional stress on the instrumentation. Preoperative hyperkyphosis of greater than or equal to 40 degrees was identified as a significant risk factor. Kim et al. noticed that these hyperkyphotic patients undergo substantial reduction of thoracic kyphosis during posterior spinal fusion, and this acute change may lead to reciprocal kyphosis at the proximal junction. They also theorized that distal pedicle screw fixation with proximal hooks versus all hook constructs may be more rigid, thus leading to increased junctional stress.[59] Kim et al. also evaluated for PJK risk factors in three different types of PSF constructs. The authors found the highest prevalence of PJK in all pedicle screw fixation constructs at 35%, compared to hooks only at 22% and hybrid constructs at 29%, trending towards significance ($P = 0.058$).[60] These findings were corroborated by Helgeson et al. where authors found a significantly high prevalence of PJK in the all pedicle screws construct when compared to the hybrid construct and all hooks group. They also reported that preoperative hyperkyphosis, greater than or equal to 40 degrees, and reducing thoracic kyphosis by greater than or equal to 5 degrees to be significant risk factors for developing DJK. Their study also showed male gender to be a risk factor without explanation.[63] Ferrero et al. defined PJK as a 10 degree increase in sagittal Cobb angle measured between the UIV and UIV-2 between postoperative and 2 years follow-up x-rays, and found that patients with PJK had significantly larger preoperative PI, lumbar lordosis, and C7 slope.[64] Rhee et al. attributed the greater incidence of PJK following posterior instrumentation to dissection of soft tissue, correction of proximal thoracic scoliosis, and reciprocal kyphosis in response to reduction in thoracic kyphosis associated with posterior instrumentation.[58] Contrary to these studies, Hollenbeck et al. analyzed 15 risk factors and found none of them to be significant.[61] In our approach to prevent PJK, we employ a hybrid of pedicle screws, sublaminar bands at the apex of thoracic kyphosis, and hooks at the cephalad segment. Helgeson et al.[63] reported a decrease in proximal kyphosis in constructs of all pedicle screws with hooks at the UIV, though not statistically significant when compared to all screws and all hook constructs. We believe using hooks at the UIV allows for a "softer landing" spot with aims to decrease disruption of the posterior complex.

Lonner et al.[62] analyzed different Lenke types in AIS and found specific risk factors for each curve. In Lenke 1 patients, risk factors for PJK included loss of kyphosis after fusion and choosing the UIV caudal to the upper end vertebra (UEV). Risk of developing PJK increased by 7.1% with each degree of kyphosis lost compared to preoperative films. Fusion should not be caudal to the UEV in Lenke 1 curves, and one should attempt to restore kyphosis. In Lenke 2 and 4 curves, loss of kyphosis and less kyphotic rod contour angle (RCA) were risk factors for PJK. In Lenke 3 and 6 curves, larger preoperative T5-T12 kyphosis was the only significant risk factor for PJK. Fusions should be extended more proximally and aim to maintain kyphosis to avoid reciprocal kyphosis of the proximal junction after fusion. In Lenke 5 curves, UIV at or cephalad to the UEV was associated with increased risk for PJK. Fusion should not extend more proximally than the UEV. In contrast to Ferrero et al., the authors found no significant correlation between sagittal pelvis parameters and development of PJK.[62]

Unlike PJK, DJK has been cited to be clinically significant with symptoms such as low back pain distal to the fusion construct in hyperkyphosis. DJK also appears to have a more uniformed definition as the angle, of greater than or equal 10 degrees, between the cephalad end plate of the LIV and the caudal end plate of LIV+1. The overall incidence of DJK ranges from 6% to 10%.[65–67] Early observations by Lowe et al.[65] reported higher risk of DJK development in posterior spinal fusion versus anterior spinal fusion. This could possibly be explained by earlier theories of soft tissue dissection and disruption seen in PJK. The authors found higher rates of PJK in those with posterior fusion, and greater deformity changes in that group as well. From their study, they recommended including the junctional level in the fusion construct, as well as maintaining normal sagittal profile over the main thoracic region (T5–T12) and thoracolumbar junction (T10–L2). As sagittal alignment garnered more attention due to the possibility of low back pain and adjacent segment disease, more research was directed to prevent these decompensations.

As with the adding on phenomena, selection of LIV to prevent DJK is complex; however, unlike LIV selection in the coronal plane, the literature for LIV selection in the sagittal plane is not as robust. Recent attention has been focused on the concept of the sagittal stable vertebra first described by Cho et al. in 2009, defined as the most proximal lumbar vertebral body touched by the vertical line from the posterior-superior corner of the sacrum.[68] Their study included patients who presented with thoracic hyperkyphosis and found that those with the LIV cephalad to the stable sagittal vertebra (SSV), which simply means the fusion mass is not well centered over the sacrum in the sagittal plane, developed DJK to a greater extent. The authors described that DJK occurred as a compensatory mechanism for a negatively balanced distal fusion mass. Therefore, for conditions of hyperkyphosis, Cho et al. recommend including the SSV in the fusion construct, having the posterior sacral vertical line (PSVL) touching the LIV, with pedicle screws distally to prevent loosening.

In 2017, Yang et al.[66] further defined the SSV as the vertebral level at which 50% of the vertebral body was in front of the PSVL on a standing lateral radiograph in their study on AIS patients undergoing selective thoracic fusion above L2. They investigated the relationship between LIV and the development of DJK and associated risk factors. They reported that when the LIV was proximal to the SSV, the rate of DJK was 17% (8/46) versus 0% (0/67) when the LIV was at or distal to the SSV. The authors found no significant association between preoperative maximum kyphosis, thoracic kyphosis, thoracolumbar kyphosis, PI, sagittal or coronal balance, skeletal maturity, and the development of DJK. The revision rate for DJK in this study was 1%. The authors recommended extending the fusion construct to the SSV or distal.

Rod Fractures and Pseudoarthrosis

Unlike the adult population, hardware failure and pseudoarthrosis is less common in pediatric patients. The incidence of hardware failure has been estimated to be at 0.5%.[69] In a study of 1046 pediatric patients undergoing spinal fusion for idiopathic scoliosis, the rates of pseudoarthrosis was 3.1% in the anterior fusion group and 2.5% in the posterior fusion group, which were not significantly different. Of the 172 re-operations in the group of 1046 patients, 15 of those surgeries, 8.7%, were due to dislodged or broken implants. Revision surgery for broken and dislodged implants occurred within the first 3 months, at an average of 1.3 months.[70] Patients may present with progressive pain within the fusion construct, obvious evidence of failure on orthogonal radiographs, soft tissue mass and inflammation from metal debris,[71] and deformity progression.

Pertinent imaging in addition to orthogonal radiographs may include flexion-extension films to detect gross motion, bone scan, or three-dimensional CT that can also assist with surgical planning.[72] The gold standard for diagnosing pseudoarthrosis is still surgical exploration of the fusion mass. Goals of treatment are to identify the etiology of failure and to create a solid fusion construct that usually requires posterior revision instrumentation. In summary, complications after corrective spine surgery are well documented in literature. Understanding these issues allows for improved preventive strategies and implementation of protocols for these complications when they arise.

Conclusion

Vigilance in postoperative examination in the first 48 hours should be practiced for detection of DPND. Treatment algorithms should be established to address the more common causes of DPND, such as cord ischemia or compression from epidural hematomas or apical pedicles.

Delayed infections are most commonly attributed to low virulence bacteria that exist on skin flora. Diagnosis may not be obvious due to lack of systemic symptoms and difficulty obtaining positive cultures. Attention should be given patients with acute onset of pain after a pain-free interval as normal laboratory studies were not shown to rule out delayed infections. Cultures should be held for at least 10 days for identification of fastidious bacteria. Commonly accepted treatment recommendations include removal of hardware with irrigation and debridement, followed by a course of antibiotics.

Regarding the adding on phenomena in AIS corrective surgery, the incorrect selection of the LIV was found to be an independent risk factor. There are many studies that analyze the relationship between the LIV, CSVL, NV, and EV to assist with preoperative planning. Studies also evaluated these relationships in different Lenke curve types. However, there are no studies that demonstrate a significant association between LIV selection and adding on, with low back pain.

PJK and DJK are decompensations that can be seen in the sagittal plane. Radiographic evidence of PJK does not appear to have any clinical effects on patients, but the development of DJK has been cited to be clinically significant with symptoms of low back pain. MRI studies demonstrated greater disc degeneration in patients with poor sagittal alignment. Risk factors for PJK include preoperative hyperkyphosis, dissection of the posterior soft tissue, and types of fusion constructs. Recommendations to prevent DJK are including the SSV and junctional level in the fusion construct, and restoring normal sagittal alignment through the thoracic and thoracolumbar junction.

We are optimistic that improved sagittal planning and use of technology, such as customized precontoured, could lessen the risk of sagittal malalignment in patients with adolescent idiopathic scoliosis. Although to this date, there are no reported studies on the efficacy of precontoured rods use in AIS corrective surgery.

References

1. MacEwen GD, Bunnell WP, Siriam K. Acute neurological complications in the treatment of scoliosis. A report of the Scoliosis Research Society. *J Bone Joint Surg Am.* 1975;57:404–408.
2. Coe JD, Arlet V, Donaldson W, et al. Complications in spinal fusion for adolescent idiopathic scoliosis in the new millennium. A report of the Scoliosis Research Society Morbidity and Mortality Committee. *Spine (Phila Pa 1976).* 2006;31(3):345–349. https://doi.org/10.1097/01.brs.0000197188.76369.13.
3. Vitale MG, Skaggs DL, Pace GI, et al. Best practices in intraoperative neuromonitoring in spine deformity surgery: Development of an intraoperative checklist to optimize response. *Spine Deform.* 2014;2(5):333–339. https://doi.org/10.1016/j.jspd.2014.05.003.
4. Auerbach JD, Kean K, Milby AH, et al. Delayed postoperative neurologic deficits in spinal deformity surgery. *Spine (Phila Pa 1976).* 2016;41(3):E131–E138. https://doi.org/10.1097/BRS.0000000000001194.
5. Quinonez A, Pahys JM, Samdani AF, et al. Complete paraplegia 36h after attempted posterior spinal fusion for severe adolescent idiopathic scoliosis: a case report. *Spinal Cord Ser Cases.* 2021;7:33. https://doi.org/10.1038/s41394-021-00386-6.
6. Chang JH, Hoernschemeyer DG, Sponseller PD. Delayed postoperative paralysis in adolescent idiopathic scoliosis: management with partial removal of hardware and staged correction. *J Spinal Disord Tech.* 2006;19(3):222–225. https://doi.org/10.1097/01.bsd.0000168323.58576.2f.
7. Mac-Thiong JM, Parent S, Poitras B, Joncas J, Hubert L. Neurological outcome and management of pedicle screws misplaced totally within the spinal canal. *Spine (Phila Pa 1976).* 2013;38(3):229–237. https://doi.org/10.1097/BRS.0b013e31826980a9).
8. Schömig F, Putzier M. Clinical presentation and diagnosis of delayed postoperative spinal implant infection. *J Spine Surg.* 2020;6(4):772–776. https://doi.org/10.21037/jss-20-499.
9. Hedequist D, Haugen A, Hresko T, Emans J. Failure of attempted implant retention in spinal deformity delayed surgical site infections. *Spine (Phila Pa 1976).* 2009;34(1):60–64.
10. Carragee EJ. Pyogenic vertebral osteomyelitis. *J Bone Joint Surg Am.* 1997;79:874–880.
11. Akgün D, Bürger J, Pumberger M, et al. C-reactive protein misdiagnoses delayed postoperative spinal implant infections in patients with low-virulent microorganisms. *Eur Spine J.* 2019;28:2990–2995.
12. Hahn F, Zbinden R, Min K. Late implant infections caused by Propionibacterium acnes in scoliosis surgery. *Eur Spine J.* 2005;14(8):783–788. https://doi.org/10.1007/s00586-004-0854-6.
13. Kowalski TJ, Berbari EF, Huddleston PM, et al. The management and outcome of spinal implant infections: contemporary retrospective cohort study. *Clin Infect Dis.* 2007;44:913–920.
14. Pumberger M, Bürger J, Strube P, et al. Unexpected positive cultures in presumed aseptic revision spine surgery using sonication. *Bone Joint J.* 2019;101-B:621–624.
15. Clark CE, Shufflebarger HL. Late-developing infection in instrumented idiopathic scoliosis. *Spine.* 1999;24:1909–1912. https://doi.org/10.1097/00007632-199909150-00008.
16. Richards BS, Emara KM. Delayed infections after posterior TSRH spinal instrumentation for idiopathic scoliosis: revisited. *Spine.* 2001;26:1990–1996. https://doi.org/10.1097/00007632-200109150-00009.
17. Heggeness MH, Esses SI, Errico T, Yuan HA. Late infection of spinal instrumentation by hematogenous seeding. *Spine.* 1993;18:492–496.
18. Bose B. Delayed infection after instrumented spine surgery: case reports and review of the literature. *Spine J.* 2003;3(5):394–399. https://doi.org/10.1016/s1529-9430(03)00023-8.
19. Richards BS. Delayed infections following posterior spinal instrumentation for the treatment of idiopathic scoliosis. *J Bone Joint Surg Am.* 1995;77(4):524–529.
20. Dietz FR, Koontz FP, Found EM, et al. The importance of positive bacterial cultures of specimens obtained during clean orthopaedic operations. *J Bone Joint Surg Am.* 1991;73:1200–1207.
21. Nandyala SV, Schwend RM. Prevalence of intraoperative tissue bacterial contamination in posterior pediatric spinal deformity surgery. *Spine (Phila Pa 1976).* 2013;38(8):E482–E486. https://doi.org/10.1097/BRS.0b013e3182893be1.
22. Jakab E, Zbinden R, Gubler J, Ruef C, von Graevenitz A, Krause M. Severe infections caused by Propionibacterium acnes: an underestimated pathogen in late postoperative infections. *Yale J Biol Med.* 1996;69(6):477–482.
23. Brook I, Frazier EH. Infections caused by Propionibacterium species. *Rev Infect Dis.* 1991;13(5):819–822. https://doi.org/10.1093/clinids/13.5.819).
24. Ho C, Skaggs DL, Weiss JM, Tolo VT. Management of infection after instrumented posterior spine fusion in pediatric scoliosis. *Spine (Phila Pa 1976).* 2007;32(24):2739–2744. https://doi.org/10.1097/BRS.0b013e31815a5a86.
25. Parchi PD, Evangelisti G, Andreani L, et al. Postoperative spine infections. *Orthop Rev (Pavia).* 2015;7:5900..
26. Soultanis K, Mantelos G, Pagiatakis A, et al. Late infection in patients with scoliosis treated with spinal instrumentation. *Clin Orthop Relat Res.* 2003;411:116–123.
27. Ribeiro M, Monteiro FJ, Ferraz MP. Infection of orthopedic implants with emphasis on bacterial adhesion process and techniques used in studying bacterial-material interactions. *Biomatter.* 2012;2(4):176–194. https://doi.org/10.4161/biom.22905.
28. Lonstein J, Winter R, Moe J, et al. Wound infection with Harrington instrumentation and spine fusion for scoliosis. *Clin Orthop Relat Res.* 1973;96:222–233.
29. Muschik M, Luck W, Schlenzka D. Implant removal for late-developing infection after instrumented posterior spinal fusion for scoliosis: reinstrumentation reduces loss of correction. A retrospective analysis of 45 cases. *Eur Spine J.* 2004;13:645–651.
30. Potter BK, Kirk KL, Shah SA, Kuklo TR. Loss of coronal correction following instrumentation removal in adolescent idiopathic scoliosis. *Spine (Phila Pa 1976).* 2006;31(1):67–72. https://doi.org/10.1097/01.brs.0000192721.51511.fe.
31. Suk SI, Lee SM, Chung ER, Kim JH, Kim WJ, Sohn HM. Determination of distal fusion level with segmental pedicle screw fixation in single thoracic idiopathic scoliosis. *Spine (Phila Pa 1976).* 2003;28(5):484–491. https://doi.org/10.1097/01.BRS.0000048653.75549.40.

32. Yang M, Zhao Y, Yin X, Chen Z, Yang C, Li L, Li M. Prevalence, risk factors, and characteristics of the "adding-on" phenomenon in idiopathic scoliosis after correction surgery: A systematic review and meta-analysis. *Spine (Phila Pa 1976)*. 2018;43(11):780–790. https://doi.org/10.1097/BRS.0000000000002423. PMID: 28937532.
33. Lakhal W, Loret JE, de Bodman C, et al. The progression of lumbar curves in adolescent Lenke 1 scoliosis and the distal adding-on phenomenon. *Orthop Traumatol Surg Res*. 2014;100(4 Suppl):S249–S254. https://doi.org/10.1016/j.otsr.2014.03.012.
34. Wang Y, Hansen ES, Høy K, Wu C, Bünger CE. Distal adding-on phenomenon in Lenke 1A scoliosis: risk factor identification and treatment strategy comparison. *Spine (Phila Pa 1976)*. 2011;36(14):1113–1122. https://doi.org/10.1097/BRS.0b013e3181f51e95.
35. Cho RH, Yaszay B, Bartley CE, Bastrom TP, Newton PO. Which Lenke 1A curves are at the greatest risk for adding-on... and why? *Spine (Phila Pa 1976)*. 2012;37(16):1384–1390. https://doi.org/10.1097/BRS.0b013e31824bac7a.
36. King HA, Moe JH, Bradford DS, et al. The selection of fusion levels in thoracic idiopathic scoliosis. *J Bone Joint Surg Am*. 1983;65:1302–1313.
37. Chang DG, Suk SI, Song KS, et al. How to avoid distal adding-on phenomenon for rigid curves in major thoracolumbar and lumbar adolescent idiopathic scoliosis? Identifying the incidence of distal adding-on by selection of lowest instrumented vertebra. *World Neurosurg*. 2019;132:e472–e478. https://doi.org/10.1016/j.wneu.2019.08.110.
38. Siala M., N'Dele D., Accadbled F., Sales De Gauzy J. Postoperative adding-on in adolescent idiopathic scoliosis, a particular etiology: Conflict between the upper articular process and the instrumentation material: A case report. https://www.hilarispublisher.com/abstract/postoperative-addingon-in-adolescent-idiopathic-scoliosis-a-particular-etiology-conflict-between-the-upper-articular-pro-37740.html. Accessed October 1, 2021.
39. Hosogane N, Widmann R, Kim Y. *The risk factors for adding-on phenomenon after thoracic fusion in adolescent idiopathic scoliosis*. San Francisco, CA: American Academy Of Orthopedic Surgeons; 2008.
40. Yang C, Li Y, Yang M, et al. Adding-on phenomenon after surgery in Lenke type 1, 2 adolescent idiopathic scoliosis: Is it predictable. *Spine (Phila Pa 1976)*. 2016;41(8):698–704. https://doi.org/10.1097/BRS.0000000000001303.
41. Matsumoto M, Watanabe K, Hosogane N, et al. Postoperative distal adding-on and related factors in Lenke type 1A curve. *Spine (Phila Pa 1976)*. 2013;38(9):737–744. https://doi.org/10.1097/BRS.0b013e318279b666.
42. Ding R, Liang J, Qiu G, Shen J, Li Z. Evaluation of quality of life in adolescent idiopathic scoliosis with different distal fusion level: a comparison of L3 versus L4. *J Spinal Disord Tech*. 2014;27(5):E155–E161. https://doi.org/10.1097/BSD.0000000000000073.
43. Takayama K, Nakamura H, Matsuda H. Low back pain in patients treated surgically for scoliosis: longer than sixteen-year follow-up. *Spine (Phila Pa 1976)*. 2009;34(20):2198–2204.
44. Akazawa T, Minami S, Kotani T, Nemoto T, Koshi T, Takahashi K. Long-term clinical outcomes of surgery for adolescent idiopathic scoliosis 21 to 41 years later. *Spine (Phila Pa 1976)*. 2012;37(5):402–405.
45. Danielsson AJ, Nachemson AL. Back pain and function 23 years after fusion for adolescent idiopathic scoliosis: a case–control study-part II. *Spine (Phila Pa 1976)*. 2003;28(18):E373–E383.
46. Delfno R, Pizones J, Ruiz-Juretschke C, Sánchez-Mariscal F, Zúñiga L, Izquierdo E. Selective anterior thoracolumbar fusion in adolescent idiopathic scoliosis: long-term results after 17-year follow-up. *Spine (Phila Pa 1976)*. 2017;42(13):E788–E794.
47. Lavelle WF, Beltran AA, Carl AL, Uhl RL, Hesham K, Albanese SA. Fifteen to twenty-fve year functional outcomes of twenty-two patients treated with posterior Cotrel-Dubousset type instrumentation: a limited but detailed review of outcomes. *Scoliosis Spinal Disord*. 2016;8(11):18..
48. Merriman M, Hu C, Noyes K, Sanders J. Selection of the lowest level for fusion in adolescent idiopathic scoliosis-a systematic review and meta-analysis. *Spine Deform*. 2015;3(2):128–135.
49. Larson AN, Fletcher ND, Daniel C, Richards BS. Lumbar curve is stable after selective thoracic fusion for adolescent idiopathic scoliosis: a 20-year follow-up. *Spine (Phila Pa 1976)*. 2012;37(10):833–839.
50. Ball JR, Konigsberg MW, Plachta S, et al. Variability in stable sagittal vertebra (SSV) during full-length biplanar x rays can affect the choice of fusion levels in patients with adolescent idiopathic scoliosis (AIS). *Spine Deform*. 2020;8(6):1261–1267. https://doi.org/10.1007/s43390-020-00166-6.
51. Potter BK, Rosner MK, Lehman Jr Jr RA, Polly Jr Jr DW, Schroeder TM, Kuklo TR. Reliability of end, neutral, and stable vertebrae identification in adolescent idiopathic scoliosis. *Spine (Phila Pa 1976)*. 2005;30(14):1658–1663. https://doi.org/10.1097/01.brs.0000170290.05381.9a.
52. Bernstein P, Hentschel S, Platzek I, Hühne S, Ettrich U, Hartmann A, Seifert J. Thoracal flat back is a risk factor for lumbar disc degeneration after scoliosis surgery. *Spine J*. 2014;14(6):925–932.
53. Enercan M, Kahraman S, Cobanoglu M, et al. Selective thoracic fusion provides similar health-related quality of life but can cause more lumbar disc and facet joint degeneration: a comparison of adolescent idiopathic scoliosis patients with normal population 10 years after surgery. *Spine Deform*. 2015;3(5):469–475.
54. Pérez-Grueso FS, Fernández-Baíllo N, Arauz de Robles S, García Fernández A. The low lumbar spine below Cotrel-Dubousset instrumentation: long-term findings. *Spine (Phila Pa 1976)*. 2000;25(18):2333–2341.
55. Abelin-Genevois K, Estivalezes E, Briot J, Sévely A, Sales de Gauzy J, Swider P. Spino-pelvic alignment influences disc hydration properties after AIS surgery: a prospective MRI-based study. *Eur Spine J*. 2015;24(6):1183–1190. https://doi.org/10.1007/s00586-015-3875-4.
56. Cho SK, Kim YJ, Lenke LG. Proximal junctional kyphosis following spinal deformity surgery in the pediatric patient. *J Am Acad Orthop Surg*. 2015;23(7):408–414. https://doi.org/10.5435/JAAOS-D-14-00143.
57. Lee GA, Betz RR, Clements 3rd DH, Huss GK. Proximal kyphosis after posterior spinal fusion in patients with idiopathic scoliosis. *Spine (Phila Pa 1976)*. 1999;24(8):795–799. https://doi.org/10.1097/00007632-199904150-00011.
58. Rhee JM, Bridwell KH, Won DS, Lenke LG, Chotigavanichaya C, Hanson DS. Sagittal plane analysis of adolescent idiopathic scoliosis: The effect of anterior versus posterior instrumentation. *Spine (Phila Pa 1976)*. 2002;27(21):2350–2356.
59. Kim YJ, Bridwell KH, Lenke LG, Kim J, Cho SK. Proximal junctional kyphosis in adolescent idiopathic scoliosis following segmental posterior spinal instrumentation and fusion: minimum 5-year follow-up. *Spine (Phila Pa 1976)*. 2005;30(18):2045–2050. https://doi.org/10.1097/01.brs.0000179084.45839.ad.

60. Kim YJ, Lenke LG, Bridwell KH, et al. Proximal junctional kyphosis in adolescent idiopathic scoliosis after 3 different types of posterior segmental spinal instrumentation and fusions: incidence and risk factor analysis of 410 cases. *Spine (Phila Pa 1976).* 2007;32(24):2731–2738. https://doi.org/10.1097/BRS.0b013e31815a7ead.
61. Hollenbeck SM, Glattes RC, Asher MA, Lai SM, Burton DC. The prevalence of increased proximal junctional flexion following posterior instrumentation and arthrodesis for adolescent idiopathic scoliosis. *Spine (Phila Pa 1976).* 2008;33(15):1675–1681. https://doi.org/10.1097/BRS.0b013e31817b5bea.
62. Lonner BS, Ren Y, Newton PO, et al. Risk factors of proximal junctional kyphosis in adolescent idiopathic scoliosis-the pelvis and other considerations. *Spine Deform.* 2017;5(3):181–188. https://doi.org/10.1016/j.jspd.2016.10.003.
63. Helgeson MD, Shah SA, Newton PO, et al. Evaluation of proximal junctional kyphosis in adolescent idiopathic scoliosis following pedicle screw, hook, or hybrid instrumentation. *Spine (Phila Pa 1976).* 2010;35(2):177–181. https://doi.org/10.1097/BRS.0b013e3181c77f8c.
64. Ferrero E, Bocahut N, Lefevre Y, et al. Proximal junctional kyphosis in thoracic adolescent idiopathic scoliosis: risk factors and compensatory mechanisms in a multicenter national cohort. *Eur Spine J.* 2018;27(9):2241–2250. https://doi.org/10.1007/s00586-018-5640-y.
65. Lowe TG, Lenke L, Betz R, et al. Distal junctional kyphosis of adolescent idiopathic thoracic curves following anterior or posterior instrumented fusion: incidence, risk factors, and prevention. *Spine (Phila Pa 1976).* 2006;31(3):299–302. https://doi.org/10.1097/01.brs.0000197221.23109.fc).
66. Yang J, Andras LM, Broom AM, et al. Preventing distal junctional kyphosis by applying the stable sagittal vertebra concept to selective thoracic fusion in adolescent idiopathic scoliosis. *Spine Deform.* 2018;6(1):38–42. https://doi.org/10.1016/j.jspd.2017.06.007.
67. Segal DN, Orland KJ, Yoon E, Bastrom T, Fletcher ND. Harms Study Group. Fusions ending above the sagittal stable vertebrae in adolescent idiopathic scoliosis: does it matter? *Spine Deform.* 2020;8(5):983–989. https://doi.org/10.1007/s43390-020-00118-0.
68. Cho KJ, Lenke LG, Bridwell KH, Kamiya M, Sides B. Selection of the optimal distal fusion level in posterior instrumentation and fusion for thoracic hyperkyphosis: the sagittal stable vertebra concept. *Spine (Phila Pa 1976).* 2009;34(8):765–770. https://doi.org/10.1097/BRS.0b013e31819e28ed.
69. Mendenhall S, Mobasser D, Relyea K, Jea A. Spinal instrumentation in infants, children, and adolescents: a review. *J Neurosurg Pediatr.* 2019;23(1):1–15. https://doi.org/10.3171/2018.10.PEDS18327.
70. Richards BS, Hasley BP, Casey VF. Repeat surgical interventions following "definitive" instrumentation and fusion for idiopathic scoliosis. *Spine (Phila Pa 1976).* 2006;31(26):3018–3026.
71. Botolin S, Merritt C, Erickson M. Aseptic loosening of pedicle screw as a result of metal wear debris in a pediatric patient. *Spine (Phila Pa 1976).* 2013;38(1):E38–E42. https://doi.org/10.1097/BRS.0b013e3182793e51.
72. Kim HJ, Cunningham ME, Boachie-Adjei O. Revision spine surgery to manage pediatric deformity. *J Am Acad Orthop Surg.* 2010;18(12):739–748. https://doi.org/10.5435/00124635-201012000-00004.

30 When to Operate on Adult Spine Deformity

MUNISH C. GUPTA AND SHYAM AJIT PATEL

CHAPTER OUTLINE

Introduction

Adult spinal deformity (ASD) refers to abnormal spinal curvature in the coronal or sagittal plane. It presents de novo consequent to degenerative processes in adults or iatrogenically after a prior decompression or fusion. In either scenario, this is termed degenerative scoliosis and is in contrast to when ASD occurs as a progression of untreated adolescent idiopathic scoliosis that is termed adult idiopathic scoliosis. Regardless of pathoetiology, while many patients may tolerate such scoliosis, many develop pain, muscular fatigue, and neurologic symptoms leading to disability. Surgical intervention can help these individuals resume a more active, comfortable lifestyle. But first, these patients need a full preoperative assessment and need to be optimized for surgery to avoid complications. Furthermore, when complications do occur, they need to be identified and addressed expediently and appropriately.

Treatment of Adult Spinal Deformity: Nonoperative Management

The goal of ASD treatment is to improve quality of life by decreasing pain and disability. Given the high overall risk associated with surgery, prior to pursuing surgical intervention, nonoperative measures should be trialed as ASD surgeries carry a complication rate as high as 55% or greater despite advances in both surgical instrumentation and perioperative medical and surgical care.[1–4] Recommended measures include physical therapy, exercise, epidural steroid injections (ESI), aquatic-based rehabilitation, and chiropractic manipulation.[5,6] A referral to pain management services may be beneficial for opioid weaning and multimodal medication treatment (e.g., nonsteroidal anti-inflammatory drugs and nerve stabilizers such as gabapentin); however, these should be used judiciously due to toxic side effect profiles. Long-term narcotic use is not routinely recommended secondary to dangerous side effect profiles and risk of addiction.[7,8]

Still, the literature on nonoperative management of ASD is limited.[7–10] Glassman et al.[10] reviewed 123 cases of adults with scoliosis who underwent nonoperative management consisting of physical therapy, exercise, pain management, injections, bracing, and bedrest. The mean cost of treatment was $10,815 with no improvement of pain or disability. Predictors of improvement were assessed in a retrospective review of 215 patients with ASD followed for 2 years. Nonoperative patients who achieved a minimal clinically important difference in Scoliosis Research Society (SRS) Activity or Pain scores had a lower baseline SRS Pain score and less coronal deformity in the thoracolumbar region. They proposed that patients with coronal deformities in the thoracolumbar region may not do as well with nonoperative management.[1]

Treatment of Adult Spinal Deformity: Operative Management

Preoperative Evaluation & Patient Selection

The number of ASD surgeries performed each year is increasing with the growing geriatric population and our improved ability to manage complex surgical patients.[2] The surgical indications for ASD are debated; however, the general recommendation is that operative intervention should be pursued for those with pain refractory to nonoperative management, decline in functional status or inability to perform activities of daily living, progressive deformity, and/or neurologic symptoms due to nerve/spinal cord compression.[3]

Unfortunately, the presence of medical comorbidities presents challenges. Fu et al.[4] found an incremental increase in rate of complications in patients that are American Society of Anesthesiologists (ASA) grade 1 (5.4%) to grade 5 (50%). Hence, these conditions should be optimized.

The highest mortality of all cardiopulmonary complications is with myocardial infarction and cardiac arrest.[11] After ASD, the 1 month incidence of these complications has been reported as anywhere from 0.13% to 1.6%.[12] Given this risk, all ASD patients should be assessed for cardiac risk factors including older age, chronic kidney disease, need for multilevel fusion, longer operative times, increased postoperative stay, and need for intraoperative blood transfusions.[11] Preoperative stress testing should be performed on patients with known coronary artery disease. Excessive blood loss during deformity surgery can decrease coronary artery perfusion, leading to MI. It is important to preoperatively risk stratify and identify patients at risk for such an event and make sure they have a thorough evaluation by their primary care doctor or cardiologist. Due to the severity of these complications, there should be a low threshold for cardiac workup in the postoperative period. The use of perioperative beta blockers has been shown to cause significant reduction in cardiac events at 30 days post surgery and also demonstrated mortality benefit at 1 and 2 year postop.[13] Smoking cessation 6 to 8 weeks prior to surgery has also been shown to decrease both cardiac and pulmonary complications.[11]

Pulmonary complications after ASD surgery are common and can be fatal. Risk factors that should be assessed include older age, smoking, diabetes, malnutrition, poor dental hygiene, surgical duration, poor mobility, thoracoplasty, and a greater number of spinal levels.[14,15] Some of the more common pulmonary complications include pneumonia, atelectasis, acute respiratory distress syndrome (ARDS), and pulmonary embolism (PE).[16] Preoperatively, every patient's lung function should be assessed. Preoperative lung function remains the most significant risk factor for postoperative pulmonary complications.[14] The more severe a patient's lung disease, the more postoperative pulmonary complications a patient is likely to have.[15]

Thromboembolic events and their prevention are of particular interest when it comes to spine surgery. These include deep venous thrombosis (DVT) and PE, which can be fatal. In spine, the prevalence of venous thromboembolisms (VTEs) is 0.5%—particularly with operations in the thoracic and thoracolumbar regions. This is likely secondary to decreased mobility in patients after surgery. Preoperatively, prehab and strengthening prior to surgery may improve postoperative mobility and ultimately decrease the risk of VTEs, although this has not been studied. Postoperatively, the use of incentive spirometry, elevating the head of the bed, early mobilization, and in-hospital oral care should be utilized as appropriate.[15] Additionally, mechanical prophylaxis in the form of pneumatic compression devices should be employed, routinely barring any contraindication such as lower extremity fracture, infection, or other trauma.[17] Chemical prophylaxis is controversial. At this time, its utility and timing of use are controversial due to concerns of postoperative epidural hematoma amongst other bleeding complications.[18,19] Generally speaking, however, risk of VTE in a standard posterior approach is low, and chemical prophylaxis may not be warranted.

Postoperative pneumonia should also be considered. Prior to surgery, dental hygiene can help decrease total perioral bacterial load, which may decrease risk of postoperative pneumonia.[15] Dental hygiene can include smoking cessation as it improves overall oral health.[15] Patients usually present with fever and shortness of breath. Typically, diagnosis is made with a combination of chest x-ray and physical exam. Treatment and resolution of infection requires antibiotics, chest physiotherapy, and analgesia.[14]

Medically, diabetes is associated with many complications including need for reoperation,[20] recurrent disc herniation,[21] and infection.[14,16] Medical consultation with an endocrinologist can be beneficial in controlling perioperative as well as postoperative blood glucose.[14,16,20,21] Reducing HgA1c to less than 7.0 has been shown to decrease diabetes-related complications.

Osteoporosis presents a significant management challenge in these patients, as poor bone quality may lead to pedicle screw loosening and graft subsidence.[15] Referral to a bone endocrinologist can be useful to optimize bone quality via parathyroid hormone analogues, antiresorptive agents, and bisphosphonates.[15] Surgical technique considerations in these patients include preservation of endplate integrity, multiple sites of fixation, bicortical screws, cement augmentation with polymethylmethacrylate, and the use of both anterior column support and posterior column support.[22]

Intraoperative Considerations

Muscle relaxants and general anesthetic agents can interfere with neuromonitoring potentials. Halogenated inhalational agents and nitrous oxide decrease amplitude and increase latency of somatosensory evoked potentials (SSEP).[23] Muscle relaxants prevent proper acquisition of motor-evoked potentials (MEPs). The preferred agents are ketamine and etomidate, as both increase cortical amplitudes of SSEP and MEP.[17] Improper patient positioning can also result in neuromonitoring abnormalities. The arms should not be extended, externally rotated, or abducted greater than 90 degrees because these movements stretch the brachial plexus.[18] Intraoperative blood salvage devices have been shown to decrease the requirements of allogeneic blood transfusion.[12,19,24] Liang et al. performed a randomized, prospective study in 110 scoliosis patients undergoing posterior spinal fusion. They reported blood transfusion requirements with the use of a blood salvage device was 14.5% versus 33% in the controls.[12] The use of antifibrinolytic agents such as tranexamic acid has been shown to decrease blood loss in major spine surgery.[25]

Operative Technique

Patient positioning is critical: all bony prominences should be well padded to protect pressure sensitive areas. We routinely use Gardner-Wells tongs and position the patient in a slight bit of reverse Trendelenburg to prevent ocular complications such as permanent, partial, or complete loss of vision. Although the causes are multifactorial, extended lengths of time in the prone position can adversely affect the eyes via optic ischemia or compartment syndrome. These complications are rare but irreversible and so every measure should be undertaken to prevent them.

A meticulous surgical dissection during exposure should be performed to prevent blood loss. Earlier we mentioned the risk of MI in patients with a cardiac history who sustained excessive blood loss during surgery. We routinely use an epinephrine solution in the dermis as a vasoconstrictive agent to reduce dermal oozing. Meticulous use of electrocautery and a subperiosteal dissection are also critical. The addition of osteotomies to an index operation increases surgical time, bleeding, and rates of complications. In a retrospective study of 33 patients undergoing pedicle subtraction osteotomies (PSOs), five patients (15%) developed transient neurologic deficits.[26]

In a retrospective multicenter study, Charosky et al. reported on 306 patients undergoing adult deformity surgery. They report a 7.5% incidence of postoperative neurologic complication.[27] Carreon et al. found increasing age and number of levels fused to be significant risk factors for complications in patients greater than 65 years old undergoing lumbar decompression and arthrodesis.[28] Daubs et al. found an overall perioperative complication rate of 37% in patients older than 60 years undergoing an average of nine levels of fusion and instrumentation.[29]

Buchowski et al.[30] reported on the neurologic complications following 108 PSOs. Neurologic deficits were seen in 12 patients (11.1%). These deficits were permanent in three patients (2.8%).[26] Auerbach et al. reported on 105 consecutive three-column osteotomies. A total of 87 patients underwent a PSO and 18 had a vertebral column resection (VCR). The overall rate of neurologic deficit with PSO procedures was 5.7% major permanent, 5.7% minor permanent, and 9.2% transient impairment. With VCR, one patient (5.6%) awoke with a transient sensory deficit.[31]

Vascular Complications

Vascular complications are rare but can have devastating consequences. When larger vessels such as the aorta are involved, rapid recognition and involvement of the appropriate services is necessary. Cardiothoracic or vascular surgery should be involved early if necessary in the setting of injury. Careful evaluation of preoperative imaging can help to identify anatomic variants and prevent injury.

Even with posterior approaches to the spine, the aorta, vena cava, and common iliac vessels can all be injured. Posterior injuries can be lethal as they can lead to hemorrhage, hypovolemic shock, and death. Aortic injury from pedicle screw placements is not common but has been repeatedly published. Aggressive use of instruments in the anterior disc space during a lumbar discectomy or posterior interbody procedure can result in injury to the major vessels. Most commonly at L4-5 the left common iliac vessels are injured; however, injury to the aorta, vena cava, and common iliacs are also possible. The risk of vascular injury can be minimized with careful surgical technique and positioning with the abdomen free, avoiding blind use of the pituitary in the anterior disc space, and careful positioning and trajectories of pedicle screws. Less than 50% of vascular injuries are recognized initially and surgeons should be well aware of signs of an injury include bleeding, hypotension, tachycardia, and abdominal rigidity.

Proximal Junctional Kyphosis

Proximal junctional kyphosis (PJK) is a type of adjacent segment disease that affects the cranial level next to the upper most instrumented segment. It has been defined as a proximal junctional Cobb angle between 10 and 20 degrees in the sagittal plane.[32,33] PJK can occur early (within 6 weeks of surgery) or delayed (approx. 2 years postoperatively). It can present as fracture, spondylolisthesis, ligamentous failure, mechanical instability, or a combination of these factors. The development of PJK has been associated with poor long-term outcomes,[34] and has been associated with neurologic injury, increasing pain, and functional limitations that often require revision surgery.[35] When requiring additional surgery, this condition is referred to as proximal junctional failure (PJF).[35] Patient risk factors for this condition include smokers, age over 55 years, poor bone quality. Surgery-related risk factors include disruption of posterior soft tissues, combined anterior and posterior approach, fusion to pelvis, and increased magnitude of deformity correction.[36]

Pseudarthrosis

ASD surgery is an independent risk factor for pseudarthrosis (PSAR) and nonunion.[37] Patients can present with new pain and/or neurologic symptoms or persistent symptoms months to years after surgery.[37] Instrumentation failure such as rod fracture can occur in PSAR leading to pain, poor outcomes, and the need for revision surgery.[38] The incidence of PSAR varies between 5% to 27%. The most common site for PSAR is in the thoracolumbar and lumbosacral junction. Risk factors include number of levels fused, over 20 degrees of kyphosis, hip osteoarthritis, positive sagittal balance, thoracolumbar kyphosis, and age.[39]

PSAR presents a diagnostic challenge.[38] Flexion and extension standing imaging can be performed to assess for motion; however, this can be difficult to determine on x-ray.[38] If clinically suspected, a CT scan is recommended to assess for the presence of PSAR.[38,39] Treatment for these patients requires identification of modifiable risk factors as well as revision surgery with or without the use of osteobiologics and interbody fusion.[38,39]

Mortality

ASD surgery has reported mortality rates ranging from 1% to 3.5% at 1 year postop.[13] A study by Zuckerman et al. identified 6158 patients undergoing ASD surgery from the National Surgical Quality Improvement Program (NSQIP) database and assessed for risk factors for all-cause mortality at 1 year.[40] Preoperative risk factors include increased age, history of cancer, high ASA score, and unintentional weight loss. It was recommended that age should not be regarded as an absolute cutoff, but rather be taken in the context of general overall health.[40] The authors cited higher ASA scores as an independent risk factor for death at 1 year; however, designation of ASA grade varies between anesthesiologists. Additional postoperative risk factors for mortality include DVT, pneumonia, and unplanned intubation.[40] De la Garza Ramos et al. performed a retrospective study and found that patients who had postoperative reintubation had a mortality risk that was 9.8 times higher than their peers. Risk factors for reintubation included fusion of 8 or more levels, history of chronic lung disease, sepsis, and DVT.[41]

Case 1

73-year-old female who presented with debilitating back pain as well as weakness and fatigue that was worse with prolonged standing and walking secondary to iatrogenic flatback deformity with proximal junctional kyphosis and positive sagittal balance. She initially underwent L3 to S1 posterior spinal fusion in 2006. This was extended to L2 a year later followed by a revision fusion from T11 to the pelvis in 2015. Her medical comorbidities included well-controlled type 2 diabetes, obesity (BMI 40), obstructive sleep apnea (OSA), anxiety, and hypertension. She was a nonsmoker. On exam she had a very flat lumbar spine with positive sagittal balance but had normal sensation and strength throughout bilateral upper and lower extremities without long tract signs.

Given her cardiopulmonary risk factors she underwent a cardiac stress test that demonstrated normal perfusion. We obtained a baseline EKG that demonstrated normal sinus rhythm. She was also noted to be high risk for pneumonia and other respiratory complications because of her weight and OSA so care was taken to keep the head of bed elevated at 30 degrees and the patient was mobilized several times per day in the postoperative period. This additionally decreased the likelihood of skin complications and decubitus ulcers. Her starting hemoglobin was slightly low (11.6 g/dL), and there was the potential for significant blood loss during her procedure, so meticulous attention to surgical dissection was necessary. Epinephrine solution was used during the exposure as well as the aquamantis cautery. Hemosorb and the bone scalpel helped limit blood loss during facetectomies. A diamond burr during the pedicle subtraction osteotomy is also helpful in limiting bony bleeding.

During her case, there was a complete loss of motor-evoked potentials and the SSEPs were dissipating after prior instrumentation was removed. The prior fusion mass was thoroughly explored and was stable from T11-sacrum. Her PJK was above the level of her prior instrumented fusion so a large decompression was performed with laminectomy and partial facetectomies at T9, T10, and T11. There was severe compression at these levels and after thorough decompression the SSEPs returned but motor-evoked potentials did not. At this point, a wake-up test was performed and mean arterial pressure was increased to 90. The patient was able to wiggle her toes but there was no return of motor-evoked potentials so the pedicle subtraction osteotomy was aborted. Pedicle screws were placed at T7-8 bilaterally and a provisional T7-pelvis posterior spinal fusion (PSF) was performed. The patient was taken for a CT myelogram to evaluate for ongoing compression but there was no evidence on spinal cord compression and the patient had a normal neurological exam. After resuscitation and recovery on the orthopedic floor she was taken back to the OR the following week for the pedicle subtraction osteotomy and completion of the planned T4- pelvis posterior spinal fusion without complication (Fig. 30.1).

Conclusion

ASD surgery can significantly improve the quality of a patient's life. Although advances in medical and surgical care have allowed for more patients to qualify than ever before, complication rates still remain high. It is important that the deformity surgeon be aware of these complications so that they may be prevented or treated expediently in the event that they occur.

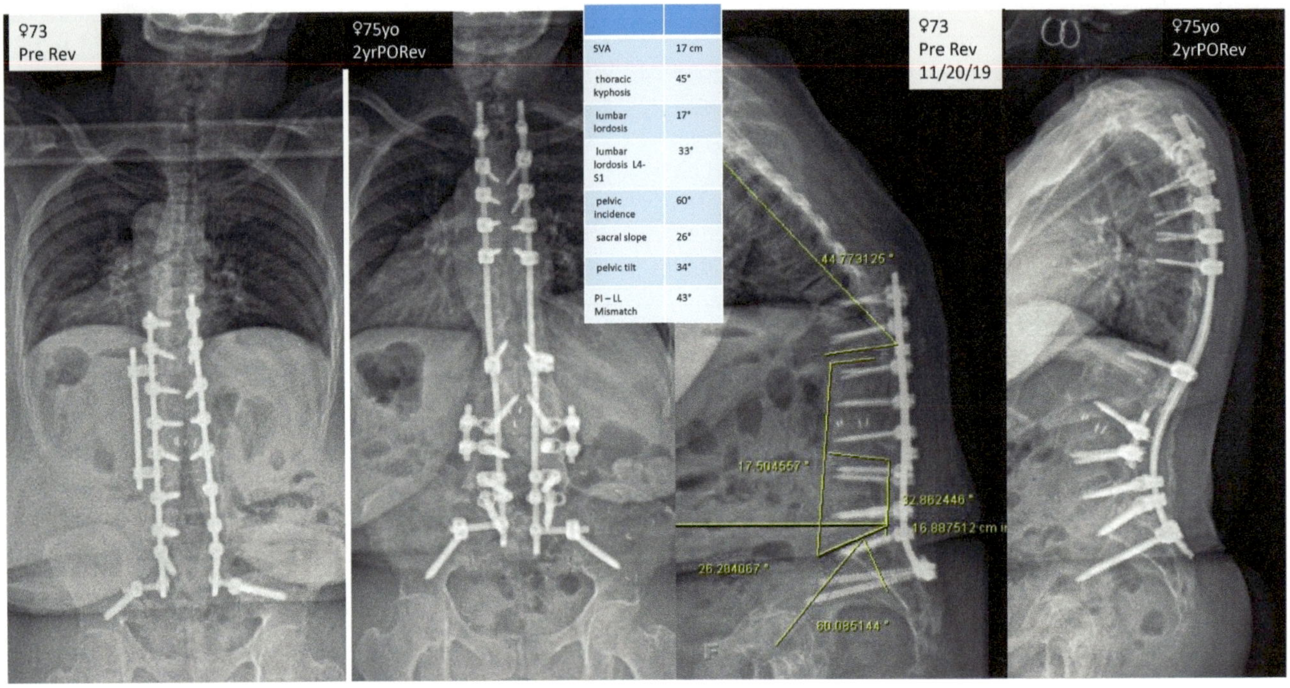

• **Fig. 30.1** Standing saggital profile. Before and 2 years after surgery.

References

1. Liu S, Diebo BG, Henry JK, et al. The benefit of nonoperative treatment for adult spinal deformity: identifying predictors for reaching a minimal clinically important difference. *Spine J*. 2016;16(2):210–218.
2. Deyo RA, Mirza SK, Martin BI. Error in trends, major medical complications, and charges associated with surgery for lumbar spinal stenosis in older adults. *JAMA*. 2011;306(10):1088.
3. Garfin SR, Eismont FJ, Bell GR, Bono CM, Fischgrund J. *Rothman and Simeone's The Spine*. Elsevier Health Sciences; 2017.
4. Fu KMG, Smith JS, Polly DW Jr, et al. Correlation of higher preoperative American Society of Anesthesiology grade and increased morbidity and mortality rates in patients undergoing spine surgery. *J Neurosurg Spine*. 2011;14(4):470–474.
5. Lonstein JE, Winter RB. Adolescent idiopathic scoliosis Nnonoperative treatment. *Orthop Clin North Am*. 1988;19(2):239–246.
6. Fast A. Low back disorders: conservative management. *Arch Phys Med Rehabil*. 1988;69(10):880–891.
7. Bridwell KH, Glassman S, Horton W, et al. Does treatment (nonoperative and operative) improve the two-year quality of life in patients with adult symptomatic lumbar scoliosis: A prospective multicenter evidence-based medicine study. *Spine*. 2009;34(20):2171.
8. van Dam BE. Nonoperative treatment of adult scoliosis. *Orthop Clin North Am*. 1988;19(2):347–351.
9. Smith JS, Shaffrey CI, Berven S, et al. Operative versus conservative treatment of back pain in adults with scoliosis. *Neurosurgery*. 2008;62(6):1406.
10. Glassman SD, Carreon LY, Shaffrey CI, et al. The costs and benefits of nonoperative management for adult scoliosis. *Spine*. 2010;35(5):578–582.
11. Warner MA, Offord KP, Warner ME, Lennon RL, Conover MA, Jansson-Schumacher U. Role of preoperative cessation of smoking and other factors in postoperative pulmonary complications: a blinded prospective study of coronary artery bypass patients. *Mayo Clin Proc*. 1989;64(6):609–616.
12. Liang J, Shen J, Chua S, et al. Does intraoperative cell salvage system effectively decrease the need for allogeneic transfusions in scoliotic patients undergoing posterior spinal fusion? A prospective randomized study. *Eur Spine J*. 2015;24(2):270–275.
13. Hu SS, Berven SH. Preparing the adult deformity patient for spinal surgery. *Spine*. 2006;31(19 Suppl):S126–S131.
14. Chen S, Anderson MV, Cheng WK, Wongworawat MD. Diabetes associated with increased surgical site infections in spinal arthrodesis. *Clin Orthop Relat Res*. 2009;467(7):1670–1673.
15. Birknes JK, White AP, Albert TJ, Shaffrey CI, Harrop JS. Adult degenerative scoliosis: a review. *Neurosurgery*. 2008;63(3 Suppl):94–103.
16. Hikata T, Iwanami A, Hosogane N, et al. High preoperative hemoglobin A1c is a risk factor for surgical site infection after posterior thoracic and lumbar spinal instrumentation surgery. *J Orthop Sci*. 2014;19(2):223–228.
17. Glassman SD, Shields CB, Linden RD, Zhang YP, Nixon AR, Johnson JR. Anesthetic effects on motor evoked potentials in dogs. *Spine*. 1993;18(8):1083–1089.
18. Uribe JS, Kolla J, Omar H, et al. Brachial plexus injury following spinal surgery: A review. *J Neurosurg Spine*. 2010;13(4):552–558.

19. Bélisle S, Hardy JF. Hemorrhage and the use of blood products after adult cardiac operations: myths and realities. *Ann Thorac Surg.* 1996;62(6):1908–1917.
20. Miller JA, Webb MR, Benzel EC, Mroz T, Mayer E. 320 association between hemoglobin A1c and reoperation following spine surgery. *Neurosurgery.* 2016;63(Suppl 1):193.
21. Huang W, Han Z, Liu J, Yu L, Yu X. Risk factors for recurrent lumbar disc herniation: A systematic review and meta-analysis. *Medicine.* 2016;95(2):e2378.
22. Ailon T, Smith JS, Shaffrey CI, et al. Degenerative spinal deformity. *Neurosurgery.* 2015;77(Suppl 4):S75–S91.
23. Sloan TB, Heyer EJ. Anesthesia for intraoperative neurophysiologic monitoring of the spinal cord. *J Clin Neurophysiol.* 2002;19(5):430–443.
24. Gause PR, Siska PA, Westrick ER, Zavatsky J, Irrgang JJ, Kang JD. Efficacy of intraoperative cell saver in decreasing postoperative blood transfusions in instrumented posterior lumbar fusion patients. *Spine.* 2008;33(5):571–575.
25. Elgafy H, Bransford RJ, McGuire RA, Dettori JR, Fischer D. Blood loss in major spine surgery: are there effective measures to decrease massive hemorrhage in major spine fusion surgery? *Spine.* 2010;35(9 Suppl):S47–S56.
26. Bridwell KH, Lewis SJ, Edwards C, et al. Complications and outcomes of pedicle subtraction osteotomies for fixed sagittal imbalance. *Spine.* 2003;28(18):2093–2101.
27. Charosky S, Guigui P, Blamoutier A, Roussouly P, Chopin D. Study Group on Scoliosis. Complications and risk factors of primary adult scoliosis surgery: a multicenter study of 306 patients. *Spine.* 2012;37(8):693–700.
28. Carreon LY, Puno RM, Dimar 2nd JR, Glassman SD, Johnson JR. Perioperative complications of posterior lumbar decompression and arthrodesis in older adults. *J Bone Joint Surg Am.* 2003;85(11):2089–2092.
29. Daubs MD, Lenke LG, Cheh G, Stobbs G, Bridwell KH. Adult spinal deformity surgery: complications and outcomes in patients over age 60. *Spine.* 2007;32(20):2238–2244.
30. Buchowski JM, Bridwell KH, Lenke LG Neurologic complications of lumbar pedicle subtraction osteotomy: a 10-year assessment. Spine (Phila Pa 1976). 2007;32(20):2245–2252. https://doi.org/10.1097/BRS.0b013e31814b2d52.
31. Auerbach JD, Lenke LG, Bridwell KH, et al. Major complications and comparison between 3-column osteotomy techniques in 105 consecutive spinal deformity procedures. *Spine.* 2012;37(14):1198–1210.
32. Glattes RC, Bridwell KH, Lenke LG, Kim YJ, Rinella A, Edwards 2nd. C. Proximal junctional kyphosis in adult spinal deformity following long instrumented posterior spinal fusion: incidence, outcomes, and risk factor analysis. *Spine.* 2005;30 (14):1643–1649.
33. Bridwell KH, Lenke LG, Cho SK, et al. Proximal junctional kyphosis in primary adult deformity surgery: evaluation of 20 degrees as a critical angle. *Neurosurgery.* 2013;72(6):899–906.
34. Schairer WW, Carrer A, Deviren V, et al. Hospital readmission after spine fusion for adult spinal deformity. *Spine.* 2013;38(19):1681.
35. Safaee MM, Deviren V, Dalle Ore C, et al. Ligament augmentation for prevention of proximal junctional kyphosis and proximal junctional failure in adult spinal deformity. *J Neurosurg Spine.* 2018;28(5):512–519.
36. Kim HJ, Iyer S. Proximal Junctional Kyphosis. *J Am Acad Orthop Surg.* 2016;24(5):318–326.
37. Raizman NM, O'Brien JR, Poehling-Monaghan KL, Yu WD. Pseudarthrosis of the spine. *J Am Acad Orthop Surg.* 2009;17 (8):494–503.
38. Daniels AH, DePasse JM, Durand W, et al. Rod fracture after apparently solid radiographic fusion in adult spinal deformity patients. *World Neurosurg.* 2018;117:e530–e537.
39. Kim Y, Bridwell K, Lenke L, Cheh G. P101. Pseudarthrosis in long adult spinal deformity instrumentation and fusions to the sacrum: incidence and risk factor analysis of 149 cases. *Spine J.* 2005;5(4):S160.
40. Zuckerman SL, Lakomkin N, Smith JS, Shaffrey CI, Devin CJ. Incidence and predictors of all-cause mortality within one year after adult spinal deformity surgery. *J Spine Surg.* 2018; 4(2):333–341.
41. De la Garza Ramos R, Passias PG, Schwab F, Bydon A, Lafage V, Sciubba DM. Incidence, risk factors, and mortality of reintubation in adult spinal deformity aurgery. *Clin Spine Surg.* 2017; 30(7):E896–E900.

31

Complications of Adult Deformity Surgery

ZACHARY T. SHARFMAN, AYUSH ARORA, AND SIGURD H. BERVEN

CHAPTER OUTLINE

Introduction

Adult spinal deformity (ASD) is a common pathology and has a significant and measurable impact on health-related quality of life.[1–3] ASD may occur as a de novo deformity of the aging spine or as an adult sequela of pediatric deformity. Both etiologies involve degenerative pathophysiology, and the prevalence of deformity, symptomatic and asymptomatic, increases with age.[2,4] The clinical impact of ASD on patients with symptoms is related to pathologies including symptomatic disc degeneration, facetogenic pain, mechanical instability related to their deformity, and neural symptoms including symptomatic spinal stenosis and radiculopathy.[2,3,5] The associated burden of disease for patients is significant based upon the prevalence of ASD and the impact of ASD on affected patients.[6] Therefore, the appropriate management of ASD is a priority for our healthcare system.[7]

Reconstructive surgery for the management of ASD imposes a large physiologic burden on patients due to the use of extensive exposures, multiple approaches, prolonged operative times, osteotomies, considerable blood loss, advanced ages, and associated preexisting medical comorbidities.[3] Consequently, there is significant risk of complications associated with ASD surgery. Many authors have studied the risk of perioperative complications following ASD surgeries, and results have been reported variably. The reported rates of postoperative complications vary greatly. Some studies report rates as low as 13.8% while others report rates up to 41% and higher.[8–13] The variability in the reported rates of complications in ASD is related to methodology of data collection. Studies utilizing prospective data collection with validated tools reliably identify more complications than retrospective investigation or voluntary databases.[14] Studies with prospective data collection have reported complications rates of 46%,[15] 52%,[16] and 69.8%[17] at up to 2-year follow-up. Furthermore, recent studies have concentrated on classifying complications to better understand the clinical impact, economic burden, and morbidity associated with complications of ASD surgery.[18]

Understanding the complication profile associated with ASD surgery is important for guiding appropriate care and for planning healthcare budgets. The predicted rates of major and minor complications, and the risk factors which predispose patients to those complications, is vital for informed choice and shared decision-making prior to ASD surgery.[19] It is also important to understand the economic implications of ASD surgery. As the world's population ages and patients expect greater functional abilities into their geriatric years, it can be expected that the number of ASD surgeries will continue to increase. Implementing appropriate planning for the greater number of these procedures and associated adverse events and their economic impact will become increasingly important. As our global healthcare economy changes towards a model with more outcome-based measures and bundled payments, there will be major implications for these healthcare economic models and their risk sharing strategies.[6,20] The rest of this chapter will review the classification, prevalence, and impact of complications in adult deformity surgery.

Challenges in Classifying Complications and Current Classification Systems

Accurate classification of complications following ASD surgery requires a systematic approach and is important for clinical research and translation of results between centers. Many proposed methods of categorizing complications have fallen short of capturing the heterogeneity and impact of the ASD surgery complication profile. The gap may be due to limited follow-up in existing studies and failure to capture the implications of complications on patient outcomes.[21] For example, certain systems categorize complications by severity while others use "major" and "minor" criteria.[22,23] As individual institutions often self-report complications, data derived from multiple sources lack standardization. Most studies focus on one category of complications with few studies capturing both medical and surgical complications.[5,24] Systematic classification systems are necessary to capture the complexity and heterogeneity of complications after ASD surgery and to develop data-driven risk reduction strategies. Better classification systems may enable better preoperative counseling and guidance of patient expectations with regards to postoperative outcomes.[25]

An ideal classification system for complications of ASD surgery encompasses the full breadth of complications, the clinical impact of those complications, as well as the duration of impact and likelihood of resolution. The ASD-specific complications classification system was developed by the International Spine Study Group (ISSG), the AI Spine Deformity Knowledge Forum, and the European Spine Study Group. This system is known as the ISSG-AO Spine Complication System.[18] The framework of the ISSG-AO Spine Complications Classification System is outlined in Fig. 31.1.

The ISSG-AO complications system broadly categorizes complications as medical or surgical.[18] Medical complications include cardiopulmonary, central nervous system, gastrointestinal, infections (nonspine), musculoskeletal, oncologic, and renal complications. Surgical complications include implant-related events, radiographic events, intraoperative events, and wound events. For each medical or surgical event, a neural component is further delineated. The neural complication component was specifically included as these adverse events are highly debilitating to patients and can outweigh the benefit of surgery.[26] Components of neural complications include motor deficit, sensory disturbance, bowel/bladder deficit, and/or impact on ambulation. Each medical, surgical, and neural adverse event is stratified by time course, occurring in either the preoperative setting, in hospital, or at a 1-year follow-up. Then interventions to address complications are organized based on the modified Clavien-Dindo criteria, a robust tool for quality assessment in surgery adapted for ASD surgery patients.[27] Categories of intervention included none, mild (i.e., consultation, labs, radiographic imaging), moderate (i.e., angiography, cardioversion, chest tube), and severe (i.e., inpatient hospitalization, return to the operating room). Finally, outcomes of each complication are classified as resolved, partial resolution, unresolved, or death. Table 31.1 provides a summative view of the ISSG-AO classification system components.

Medical Complications

The overall rate of medical complications following ASD surgery has high variability, with rates ranging from 18% to 48%.[5,10,24] The prevalence of medical complications is likely underreported due to lack of standardized complication assessment and inadequate reporting of postoperative follow-up.[28] The impact of medical complications is important for understanding the risks of surgery as well as associated costs. The workup and treatment of medical complications can dramatically increase the costs of care and make spine surgery unsustainable for hospital systems under bundled health payment models.[29] Medical complications resulting in extended lengths of stay and discharge to postacute care facilities is highly indicative of catastrophic costs.[30,31] The remainder of this section will describe three important and common medical complications following ASD surgery including cardiopulmonary and gastrointestinal complications as well as delirium.

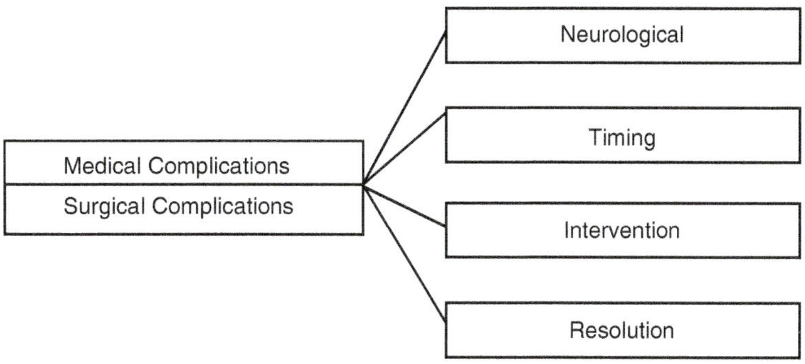

• **Fig. 31.1** Diagram of complication subcategories described by the ISSG-AO Spine Classification System[18].

TABLE 31.1 Modified Table of the Components Involved Within the ISSG-AO Classification System Outlined By Klineberg et al.[18]

Complication	*Medical*	-Cancer -Cardiopulmonary -Central nervous system -Gastrointestinal -Infectious (nonspine) -Musculoskeletal -Renal
	Surgical	-Implant-related event -Radiographic event -Neural event -Intraoperative event -Wound event
Neural Component	*Preop* *Operative* *Postop*	-Motor deficit -Spinal cord injury (myelopathy) -Impact on ambulation (requiring permanent assistive device) -Sensory disturbance -Bowel/bladder deficit
Intervention	*None*	-Monitoring alone
	Mild	-Consultation -Labs -Radiographic imaging -Epidural injections -Medication changes -Transfusions -Intraop dural repair -Nasogastric tube
	Moderate	-Angiography -Chemo/radiation therapy -Inferior vena cava filter -Cardioversion -Hemodialysis -Intensive care unit admission -Chest tube -Intubation/mechanical ventilation -Percutaneous endoscopic gastrostomy
	Severe	-Aborted surgical procedure -Inpatient hospitalization -Surgical operating room
Outcome	*Resolved*	–
	Partial resolution	
	Unresolved	
	Death	

Cardiopulmonary Complications

Cardiac and pulmonary complications are among the most reported medical complications following ASD surgery. In a retrospective literature review of 37 studies and a combined 26,207 patients by Akinturk et al., the average cardiac and pulmonary complication rate was 5.9% and 7.6%, respectively.[21] Cardiopulmonary complications following spine surgery may include arrhythmia, acute respiratory distress syndrome (ARDS), atelectasis, congestive heart failure (CHF), blood transfusion reaction, deep venous thrombosis (DVT), cardiac arrest/myocardial infarction, pulmonary effusion, pulmonary embolism (PE), or pneumothorax. Of these, myocardial infarction, or cardiac arrest, DVT, and PE comprise the majority of cases.[32,33] An underlying factor frequently cited is excessive bleeding, necessitating blood transfusions that cause fluid shifts and increase risk of myocardial infarction.[33,34] Preoperative efforts to optimize the patient and prevent cardiopulmonary complications would include a full cardiac workup prior to surgery, cardiac stress tests, statin therapy, anticoagulation, and echocardiography.[35]

Gastrointestinal Complications

Gastrointestinal (GI) complications are frequently encountered after ASD surgery. Gastrointestinal complications may include postoperative nausea and vomiting, dysphagia, ileus, bowel obstruction, cholecystitis, GI bleed, liver failure, pancreatitis, and superior mesenteric artery syndrome among others. The most reported GI complication is postoperative ileus, with an estimated incidence of 3% to 16% after surgery.[36–39] According to a retrospective study of 234 patients undergoing spinal fusion by Bahk et al., significant risk factors for both postoperative ileus and elevated bilirubin include duration of anesthesia, number of fused segments, and preexisting hepatobiliary disease.[38] Preoperative workup of the patient's bilirubin, liver functional tests, and radiologic scans may be considered to reveal underlying risk factors for gastrointestinal complications and mitigate risk. If gastrointestinal complications do occur, early consultation with gastroenterologists or general surgeons may prevent serious sequela.

Postoperative Delirium

Postoperative delirium is a frequent occurrence after ASD surgery with reported rates ranging between 12% to 24%.[40,41] Two patient characteristics that stand out as significant risk factors for delirium are preoperative cognitive impairment and depression. Lee et al. reported that 38% of patients undergoing lumbar spine surgery met criteria for cognitive impairment when assessed on the mini-mental state exam (MMSE), placing them at significant risk for postoperative delirium.[42] Routine preoperative screening for older adult patients undergoing ASD surgery may be beneficial for complication avoidance.[43] Depression is another significant risk factor associated with postoperative delirium. To avoid this adverse outcome, preoperative screenings and appropriate preventative measures such as limited narcotic use, good sleep hygiene, and exposure to sunlight may be implemented among others.[44]

Surgical Complications

Surgical complications following ASD surgery are common and are associated with dramatically increased healthcare costs. Authors have categorized surgical complications into mechanical and nonmechanical complications. Mechanical complications include proximal junction kyphosis and failure, distal junctional kyphosis, and implant-related complications. Nonmechanical complications include dural tear, wound dehiscence, and surgical site infection in addition to others.[45] In one study of 245 ASD patients with 2-year follow-up, nearly one-third of patients experienced a surgical complication with half of these requiring reoperation.[45] Patients with radiographic and implant-related complications have significantly worse health-related quality of life (HRQOL) outcomes when compared with those who do not incur surgical complications.[45] Three critical, common, and devastating surgical complications associated with ASD are surgical site infection, implant failure, and junctional kyphosis.

Surgical Site Infection

Surgical site infection (SSI) following ASD surgery is a devastating complication for patients and a common metric for measuring quality of care. SSI is of greater concern after ASD surgery as deformity patients often have prolonged procedures times, high blood loss, and fusion of multiple spinal levels, which are all risk factors for SSI.[46] The burden for patients associated with SSI is dependent on the timing of infection (acute vs delayed), the location of infection (superficial or deep), and associated abscess.[47] Rates of SSI are variable within the literature and are correlated with patient risk factors. In an analysis of 47,755 spine deformity procedures acquired from the Scoliosis Research Society Database, Shillingford et al. reported the rate of SSI to be 1.2%, with operative treatment required in 81.8% of cases.[48] Regarding delayed SSI, occurring 3 months following index procedure, a systematic review including 96 publications and 12,168 patients reports an aggregated incidence of 0.18%.[49] Given the devastating nature of this complication for patients, the high rates of reoperation, and the associated costs, the importance of mitigating risks for SSI is paramount. Preoperative risk factors for SSIs after ASD surgery include smoking, poor glycemic control, elevated body mass index, malnutrition, steroid use, advanced age, and radiation exposure.[50–52] Operative risk factors include duration of surgery, increased surgical invasiveness, and combined anterior and posterior approach.[53,54] Anterior-alone fusion and minimally invasive surgery have shown to reduce likelihood of SSI due to shorter procedure times and less blood loss.[15,55] With careful assessment of the patient's risk profile prior to surgery, clinicians can predict cases at risk for SSI and optimize patient factors such as malnutrition and glycemic control to prevent infectious complications.[21] Some strategies to prevent infection include limiting operative time, using minimally invasive techniques, using appropriate preoperative antibiotics, redosing antibiotics appropriately during surgery, using vancomycin in the wound, and having plastic surgery assist with a multilayered closure.

Implant Failure

Implant-related failures include implant prominence, painful hardware, screw loosening, screw malposition, and rod/screw breakage. Rod/screw breakage and screw loosening are the most common types of implant failure, with average rates of 13.5% and 11.1%, respectively, in ASD patients.[21] The reoperation rate associated with implant failures is high. Soroceanu et al. reported that in a cohort of 245 ASD surgical patients, one-third sustained an implant-related complication at 2-year follow-up, and 52.6% of these required a reoperation.[45] The prevalence of rod fracture is particularly high in patients undergoing pedicle subtraction osteotomy (PSO) compared to grade 1 or 2 osteotomies, with rates of 22% and 4.7%, respectively.[56] Patients at risk for implant failures include those with advanced age, high BMI, osteoporosis, rheumatological disease, and those who have undergone previous surgeries.[56,57] Some radiographic measurements that are associated with increased risk of implant failure include higher preoperative pelvic tilt (PT), high pelvic incidence/lumbar lordosis mismatch, as well as high postsurgical sagittal malalignment.[56] Multiple strategies to prevent implant failure exist. Certain studies have reported success with utilization of multiple rod constructs to distribute load bearing, while others report that three-rod constructs in osteoporotic patients have higher incidence of screw loosening when compared to two-rod constructs.[58–60] Mixed metal and same metal rod-screw constructs have not demonstrated significant differences in implant failure rates.[61] Optimization strategies to prevent implant failure include preoperative management of osteoporosis, use of sufficient bone grafts, achievement of proper sagittal balance, cement augmentation, and ligament augmentation among others.[21]

Junctional Kyphosis and Failure

Proximal junctional kyphosis (PJK) and proximal junctional failure (PJF) are often a late complication of ASD surgery and frequently requires revision surgery in symptomatic patients.[62,63] PJK is defined as a proximal junctional sagittal Cobb angle between the lower endplate of the upper instrumented vertebra (UIV) and the upper endplate of the two adjacent vertebrae of ≥10° while also being ≥10° from the preoperative measurement.[64] In an analysis of 1005 ASD surgical patients with 8-year follow-up, Segreto et al. discussed the rates of PJK during three postoperative time periods (<6 weeks of surgery, 6 weeks–1 year, and >1 year), reporting rates of 9.3%, 4.3%, and 1.8%, respectively.[65]

The clinical presentation of PJK is highly variable, as patients may be asymptomatic or may present with severe disability, neural deficits, and pain that requires intervention. Many studies have shown no significant difference in clinical symptoms between patients with and without PJK.[66–68] Park et al. and Bhagat et al. suggest that the PJK may be secondary to ligamentous failure, vertebral fracture, screw pullout, and proximal disc degeneration.[11,69] Risk factors for PJK include osteoporosis, advanced age (>55 years), smoking history, usage of pedicle screws, thoracoplasty procedures, large sagittal curve correction, combined anterior and posterior fusion, fusion of lumbar spine and sacrum, and overcorrection of lumbar lordosis or thoracic kyphosis.[63–65,70] The choice of UIV is important in PJK prevention and constructs should ideally end at a lordotic or neutral spinal segment.[71] Lafage et al. stipulates that orientation of the upper-most instrumented segment is crucial, finding that patients with PJK carry greater posterior construct inclination and implying that proper rod contouring (i.e., mild kyphosis) at the proximal end may mitigate PJK risk.[72] In constructs with the UIV located in the thoracolumbar spine, vertebral augmentation may prevent fracture at the UIV.[73,74] In constructs with the UIV at the upper thoracic spine where mechanism of PJK may be related to ligamentous failure, techniques to preserve the posterior tension band including use of hooks or ligamentous augmentation may prove useful.[75] Other optimization strategies to reduce PJK risk include bone density optimization, prophylactic vertebroplasty, and improving nutritional status (i.e., albumin and weight).[76–78]

Neural Complications

Neural complications following surgery for ASD can be debilitating for patients and difficult to treat. These complications are identified via clinical exam and can consist of motor deficits, sensory deficits, impact on ambulation, bowel/bladder dysfunction, or sympathetic changes. Most series report postoperative neural complication rates between 10% and 20%; however, few studies follow patients past the 2-year postoperative timepoint. Even fewer studies routinely track the progression of neurological exams to monitor for improvement or deterioration over time.[21,79] The Scoli-RISK-1 study is a notable initiative that examined 272 patients from 15 centers and monitored neurologic exams up to five years postoperatively.[80,81] The Scoli-RISK-1 study quantified neurological exams via the lower extremity motor score (LEMS). The study reported that patients with LEMS deterioration in the early postoperative period improved from 23% at discharge to 10% at 2 years. Within the 2 to 5 year postoperative period, one in five patients experienced a change in LEMS. Of these patients with postoperative changes, 11.1% deteriorated and 8.3% improved.[81]

Neural complications have a vast impact on HRQOL and there is substantial interest in understanding the risk factors that predispose patients to neurologic complications. Established risk factors and high-risk procedures include excessive neural tissue retraction during surgery, mispositioned screws, use of bone morphogenic protein (BMP), increased blood loss, preoperative neural deficits, advanced age, revision surgery, hypokyphosis, posterior spine fusion >5 levels, thoracic level 3-column osteotomies (compared to lumbar osteotomies), multilevel 3 column osteotomies, multilevel lateral lumbar interbody fusion (LLIF), LLIF at L4-L5, and prolonged surgery.[11,26,82] Additionally, patients with neural complications have significantly lower LEMS scores than those without at discharge, 6 months, and 5 years postoperatively.[81] Managing patient expectations, discussing the risks and benefits of complex osteotomies, and employing shared decision-making can help to manage expectations and better understand the trajectory for neural injury secondary to ASD surgery.

Case Example

A 68-year-old male presented to clinic reporting intractable back pain 18 months after undergoing an L1 to S1 posterior spinal instrumented fusion at a reputable outside

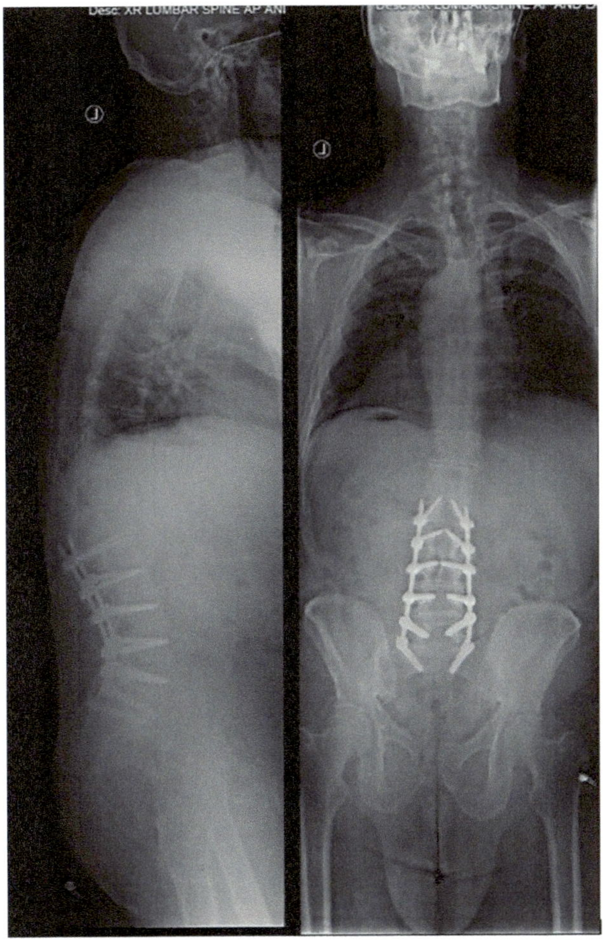

• **Fig. 31.2** Preoperative full-length radiographs demonstrating proximal junctional failure and sagittal malalignment.

institution. The patient reported mechanical back pain, limited ambulation, increasing deformity, and hunched stature. He was neurologically intact. The patient had failed an extensive trial of conservative management, and his goals and expectations were discussed.

Further workup revealed an L5/S1 pseudoarthrosis, loosening of the L1, L5, and S1 screws, as well as dynamic instability on flexion and extension radiographs. At the proximal end of the construct there was proximal junctional failure with 30 degrees of kyphosis between L1 and T11. Finally, the patient had a C7 sagittal vertical axis of 16 cm with considerable sagittal malalignment. In brief the patient had experienced multiple common complications associated with ASD surgery, including pseudoarthrosis, implant failure, and proximal junctional failure (Fig. 31.2).

The patient stated that he could no longer complete his activities of daily living (ADLs) such as caring for himself, grocery shopping, or living independently, and he could no longer play with his grandchildren. His goals were to regain self-efficacy in terms of his ADLs and to return to regular activity with his grandchildren (being able to pick them up and play with them).

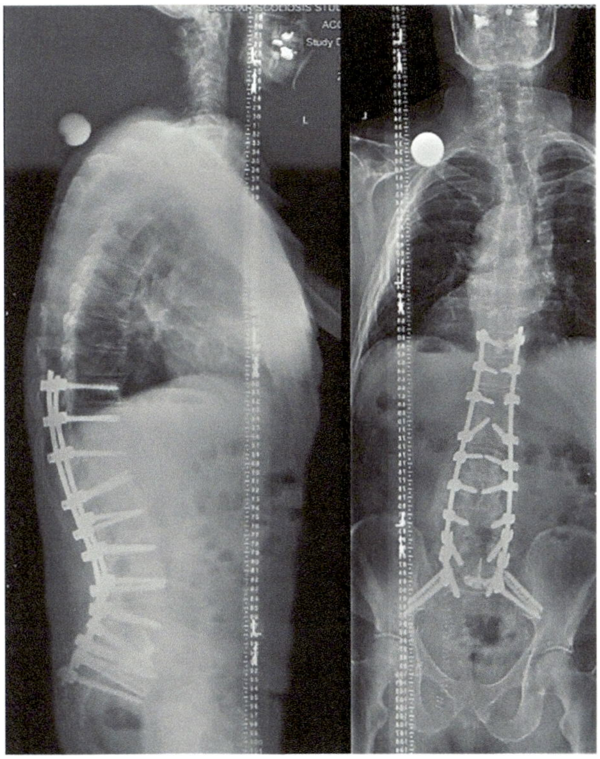

• **Fig. 31.3** Postoperative radiographs demonstrating improved sagittal alignment.

The patient was scheduled for an L5/S1 anterior lumbar interbody fusion and revision posterior spinal instrumented fusion from T10 to the pelvis with posterior column osteotomies, cement augmentation at the UIV, and bedrock of the sacroiliac joints (Fig. 31.3). Intraoperative cultures of the pseudoarthrosis were taken and were positive for staph epidermidis.

The patient was treated for his infection with input from the infectious disease team. The patient ultimately met and exceeded all his preoperative goals and was extremely pleased with his operative outcome.

Conclusion

Adult spinal deformity surgeries are associated with high complication rates. Despite this, patients obtain significant benefit from these procedures and report high satisfaction. Understanding the risk factors that predispose patients to complications after ASD surgery and implementing strategies to mitigate these risks is paramount to successful ASD surgery. Research classifying these complications and documenting the natural history of these complications helps surgeons to better inform patients and allows for improved shared decision-making and expectation management. Limiting healthcare expenditure by improving outcomes of ASD surgery will become increasingly important as the population ages and the number of these procedures increases.

References

1. Bess S, Schwab F, Lafage V, Shaffrey CI, Ames CP. Classifications for adult spinal deformity and use of the Scoliosis Research Society-Schwab Adult Spinal Deformity Classification. *Neurosurg Clin N Am.* 2013;24(2):185–193. https://doi.org/10.1016/j.nec.2012.12.008.
2. Kebaish KM, Neubauer PR, Voros GD, Khoshnevisan MA, Skolasky RL. Scoliosis in adults aged forty years and older: prevalence and relationship to age, race, and gender. *Spine (Phila Pa 1976).* 2011;36(9):731–736. https://doi.org/10.1097/BRS.0b013e3181e9f120.
3. Pellise F, Vila-Casademunt A, Ferrer M, et al. Impact on health related quality of life of adult spinal deformity (ASD) compared with other chronic conditions. *Eur Spine J.* 2015;24(1):3–11. https://doi.org/10.1007/s00586-014-3542-1.
4. Schwab F, Dubey A, Gamez L, et al. Adult scoliosis: prevalence, SF-36, and nutritional parameters in an elderly volunteer population. *Spine (Phila Pa 1976).* 2005;30(9):1082–1085. https://doi.org/10.1097/01.brs.0000160842.43482.cd.
5. Soroceanu A, Burton DC, Oren JH, et al. Medical complications after adult spinal deformity surgery: Incidence, risk factors, and clinical impact. *Spine (Phila Pa 1976).* 2016;41(22):1718–1723. https://doi.org/10.1097/BRS.0000000000001636.
6. Waldrop R, Cheng J, Devin C, McGirt M, Fehlings M, Berven S. The burden of spinal disorders in the elderly. *Neurosurgery.* 2015;77(Suppl 4):S46–50. https://doi.org/10.1227/NEU.0000000000000950.
7. Chen PG, Daubs MD, Berven S, et al. Surgery for degenerative lumbar scoliosis: The development of appropriateness criteria. *Spine (Phila Pa 1976).* 2016;41(10):910–918. https://doi.org/10.1097/BRS.0000000000001392.
8. Blamoutier A, Guigui P, Charosky S, Roussouly P, Chopin D. Groupe d'Étude de la Scoliose. Surgery of lumbar and thoracolumbar scolioses in adults over 50. Morbidity and survival in a multicenter retrospective cohort of 180 patients with a mean follow-up of 4.5 years. *Orthop Traumatol Surg Res.* 2012;98(5):528–535. https://doi.org/10.1016/j.otsr.2012.04.014.
9. Cho SK, Bridwell KH, Lenke LG, et al. Major complications in revision adult deformity surgery: risk factors and clinical outcomes with 2- to 7-year follow-up. *Spine (Phila Pa 1976).* 2012;37(6):489–500. https://doi.org/10.1097/BRS.0b013e3182217ab5.
10. Yadla S, Maltenfort MG, Ratliff JK, Harrop JS. Adult scoliosis surgery outcomes: a systematic review. *Neurosurg Focus.* 2010;28(3):E3. https://doi.org/10.3171/2009.12.FOCUS09254.
11. Bhagat S, Vozar V, Lutchman L, Crawford RJ, Rai AS. Morbidity and mortality in adult spinal deformity surgery: Norwich Spinal Unit experience. *Eur Spine J.* 2013;22(Suppl 1):S42–46. https://doi.org/10.1007/s00586-012-2627-y.
12. Charosky S, Guigui P, Blamoutier A, Roussouly P, Chopin D, Study Group on Scoliosis Complications and risk factors of primary adult scoliosis surgery: a multicenter study of 306 patients. *Spine (Phila Pa 1976).* 2012;37(8):693–700. https://doi.org/10.1097/BRS.0b013e31822ff5c1.
13. Schwab FJ, Hawkinson N, Lafage V, et al. Risk factors for major peri-operative complications in adult spinal deformity surgery: a multi-center review of 953 consecutive patients. *Eur Spine J.* 2012;21(12):2603–2610. https://doi.org/10.1007/s00586-012-2370-4.
14. Street JT, Thorogood NP, Cheung A, et al. Use of the Spine Adverse Events Severity System (SAVES) in patients with traumatic spinal cord injury. A comparison with institutional ICD-10 coding for the identification of acute care adverse events. *Spinal Cord.* 2013;51(6):472–476. https://doi.org/10.1038/sc.2012.173.
15. Uribe JS, Deukmedjian AR, Mummaneni PV, et al. Complications in adult spinal deformity surgery: an analysis of minimally invasive, hybrid, and open surgical techniques. *Neurosurg Focus.* 2014;36(5):E15. https://doi.org/10.3171/2014.3.FOCUS13534.
16. Acosta FL, Jr. McClendon J, Jr. O'Shaughnessy BA, et al. Morbidity and mortality after spinal deformity surgery in patients 75 years and older: complications and predictive factors. *J Neurosurg Spine.* 2011;15(6):667–674. https://doi.org/10.3171/2011.7.SPINE10640.
17. Smith JS, Klineberg E, Lafage V, et al. Prospective multicenter assessment of perioperative and minimum 2-year postoperative complication rates associated with adult spinal deformity surgery. *J Neurosurg Spine.* 2016;25(1):1–14. https://doi.org/10.3171/2015.11.SPINE151036.
18. Klineberg EO, Wick JB, Lafage R, et al. Development and validation of a multidomain surgical complication classification system for adult spinal deformity. *Spine (Phila Pa 1976).* 2021;46(4):E267–E273. https://doi.org/10.1097/BRS.0000000000003766.
19. Hassan FM, Lenke LG, Berven SH, et al. Independent prognostic factors associated with improved patient-reported outcomes in the prospective evaluation of elderly deformity surgery (PEEDS) study. *Global Spine J.* 2023:21925682231174182. https://doi.org/10.1177/21925682231174182.
20. Arutyunyan GG, Angevine PD, Berven S. Cost-effectiveness in adult spinal deformity surgery. *Neurosurgery.* 2018;83(4):597–601. https://doi.org/10.1093/neuros/nyx575.
21. Akinturk N, Zileli M, Yaman O. Complications of adult spinal deformity surgery: A literature review. *J Craniovertebr Junction Spine.* 2022;13(1):17–26. https://doi.org/10.4103/jcvjs.jcvjs_159_21.
22. Glassman SD, Hamill CL, Bridwell KH, Schwab FJ, Dimar JR, Lowe TG. The impact of perioperative complications on clinical outcome in adult deformity surgery. *Spine (Phila Pa 1976).* 2007;32(24):2764–2770. https://doi.org/10.1097/BRS.0b013e31815a7644.
23. McDonnell MF, Glassman SD, Dimar 2nd JR, Puno RM, Johnson JR. Perioperative complications of anterior procedures on the spine. *J Bone Joint Surg Am.* 1996;78(6):839–847. https://doi.org/10.2106/00004623-199606000-00006.
24. Dinizo M, Dolgalev I, Passias PG, Errico TJ, Raman T. Complications after adult spinal deformity surgeries: All are not created equal. *Int J Spine Surg.* 2021;15(1):137–143. https://doi.org/10.14444/8018.
25. Maitra S, Mikhail C, Cho SK, Daubs MD. Preoperative maximization to reduce complications in spinal surgery. *Global Spine J.* 2020;10(1 Suppl):45S–52S. https://doi.org/10.1177/2192568219882349.
26. Iorio JA, Reid P, Kim HJ. Neurological complications in adult spinal deformity surgery. *Curr Rev Musculoskelet Med.* 2016;9(3):290–298. https://doi.org/10.1007/s12178-016-9350-y.
27. Dindo D, Demartines N, Clavien PA. Classification of surgical complications: a new proposal with evaluation in a cohort of 6336 patients and results of a survey. *Ann Surg.* 2004;240(2):205–213. https://doi.org/10.1097/01.sla.0000133083.54934.ae.
28. Bohl DD, Russo GS, Basques BA, et al. Variations in data collection methods between national databases affect study results: a comparison of the nationwide inpatient sample and national

surgical quality improvement program databases for lumbar spine fusion procedures. *J Bone Joint Surg Am*. 2014;96(23):e193. https://doi.org/10.2106/JBJS.M.01490.

29. Theologis AA, Lau D, Dalle-Ore C, Tsu A, Deviren V, Ames CP. Costs and utility of post-discharge acute inpatient rehabilitation following adult spinal deformity surgery. *Spine Deform*. 2021; 9(3):817–822. https://doi.org/10.1007/s43390-020-00251-w.
30. Ames CP, Smith JS, Gum JL, et al. Utilization of predictive modeling to determine episode of care costs and to accurately identify catastrophic cost nonwarranty outlier patients in adult spinal deformity surgery: A step toward bundled payments and risk sharing. *Spine (Phila Pa 1976)*. 2020;45(5):E252–E265. https://doi.org/10.1097/BRS.0000000000003242.
31. Amin RM, Raad M, Jain A, et al. Risk factors for nonroutine discharge in adult spinal deformity surgery. *Spine J*. 2019;19(2): 357–363. https://doi.org/10.1016/j.spinee.2018.06.366.
32. Bovonratwet P, Bohl DD, Malpani R, et al. Cardiac complications related to spine surgery: Timing, risk factors, and clinical effect. *J Am Acad Orthop Surg*. 2019;27(7):256–263. https://doi.org/10.5435/JAAOS-D-17-00650.
33. Klineberg EO, Passias PG, Poorman GW, et al. Classifying complications: Assessing adult spinal deformity 2-year surgical outcomes. *Global Spine J*. 2020;10(7):896–907. https://doi.org/10.1177/2192568220937473.
34. Murray G, Beckman J, Bach K, Smith DA, Dakwar E, Uribe JS. Complications and neurological deficits following minimally invasive anterior column release for adult spinal deformity: a retrospective study. *Eur Spine J*. 2015;24(Suppl 3):397–404. https://doi.org/10.1007/s00586-015-3894-1.
35. Sweitzer B. Perioperative evaluation and optimization of patients at risk of cardiac complications for non-cardiac surgery. *Mo Med*. 2016;113(4):320–324.
36. Al Maaieh MA, Du JY, Aichmair A, et al. Multivariate analysis on risk factors for postoperative ileus after lateral lumbar interbody fusion. *Spine (Phila Pa 1976)*. 2014;39(8):688–694. https://doi.org/10.1097/BRS.0000000000000238.
37. Althausen PL, Gupta MC, Benson DR, Jones DA. The use of neostigmine to treat postoperative ileus in orthopedic spinal patients. *J Spinal Disord*. 2001;14(6):541–545. https://doi.org/10.1097/00002517-200112000-00014.
38. Bahk JH, Kim YH, Park HY, Min HK, Kim SI, Ha KY. Incidence and risk factors of gastrointestinal and hepatobiliary complications after spinal fusion surgery: a retrospective cohort study. *J Korean Med Sci*. 2020;35(40):e345. https://doi.org/10.3346/jkms.2020.35.e345.
39. Oh CH, Ji GY, Yoon SH, Hyun D, Park HC, Kim YJ. Paralytic ileus and prophylactic gastrointestinal motility medication after spinal operation. *Yonsei Med J*. 2015;56(6):1627–1631. https://doi.org/10.3349/ymj.2015.56.6.1627.
40. Adogwa O, Elsamadicy AA, Fialkoff J, et al. Effect of employment status on length of hospital stay, 30-day readmission and patient reported outcomes after spine surgery. *J Spine Surg*. 2017;3(1):44–49. https://doi.org/10.21037/jss.2017.03.08.
41. Seo JS, Park SW, Lee YS, Chung C, Kim YB. Risk factors for delirium after spine surgery in elderly patients. *J Korean Neurosurg Soc*. 2014;56(1):28–33. https://doi.org/10.3340/jkns.2014.56.1.28.
42. Lee YS, Kim YB, Lee SH, Park YS, Park SW. The Prevalence of undiagnosed presurgical cognitive impairment and its postsurgical clinical impact in older patients undergoing lumbar spine surgery. *J Korean Neurosurg Soc*. 2016;59(3):287–291. https://doi.org/10.3340/jkns.2016.59.3.287.
43. Adogwa O, Elsamadicy AA, Vuong VD, et al. Association between baseline cognitive impairment and postoperative delirium in elderly patients undergoing surgery for adult spinal deformity. *J Neurosurg Spine*. 2018;28(1):103–108. https://doi.org/10.3171/2017.5.SPINE161244.
44. Elsamadicy AA, Adogwa O, Lydon E, et al. Depression as an independent predictor of postoperative delirium in spine deformity patients undergoing elective spine surgery. *J Neurosurg Spine*. 2017;27(2):209–214. https://doi.org/10.3171/2017.4.SPINE161012.
45. Soroceanu A, Diebo BG, Burton D, et al. Radiographical and implant-related complications in adult spinal deformity surgery: Incidence, patient risk factors, and impact on health-related quality of life. *Spine (Phila Pa 1976)*. 2015;40(18):1414–1421. https://doi.org/10.1097/BRS.0000000000001020.
46. Pull ter Gunne AF, van Laarhoven CJ, Cohen DB. Incidence of surgical site infection following adult spinal deformity surgery: an analysis of patient risk. *Eur Spine J*. 2010;19(6):982–988. https://doi.org/10.1007/s00586-009-1269-1.
47. Wang M, Xu L, Yang B, et al. Incidence, management and outcome of delayed deep surgical site infection following spinal deformity surgery: 20-year experience at a single institution. *Global Spine J*. 2022;12(6):1141–1150. https://doi.org/10.1177/2192568220978225.
48. Shillingford JN, Laratta JL, Reddy H, et al. Postoperative surgical site infection after spine surgery: An update from the Scoliosis Research Society (SRS) morbidity and mortality database. *Spine Deform*. 2018;6(6):634–643. https://doi.org/10.1016/j.jspd.2018.04.004.
49. Zanirato A, Damilano M, Formica M, et al. Complications in adult spine deformity surgery: a systematic review of the recent literature with reporting of aggregated incidences. *Eur Spine J*. 2018;27(9):2272–2284. https://doi.org/10.1007/s00586-018-5535-y.
50. Aleem IS, Tan LA, Nassr A, Riew KD. Surgical site infection prevention following spine surgery. *Global Spine J*. 2020;10 (1 Suppl):92S–98S. https://doi.org/10.1177/2192568219844228.
51. Chahoud J, Kanafani Z, Kanj SS. Surgical site infections following spine surgery: eliminating the controversies in the diagnosis. *Front Med (Lausanne)*. 2014;1:7. https://doi.org/10.3389/fmed.2014.00007.
52. Yao R, Tan T, Tee JW, Street J. Prophylaxis of surgical site infection in adult spine surgery: A systematic review. *J Clin Neurosci*. 2018;52:5–25. https://doi.org/10.1016/j.jocn.2018.03.023.
53. Cizik AM, Lee MJ, Martin BI, et al. Using the spine surgical invasiveness index to identify risk of surgical site infection: a multivariate analysis. *J Bone Joint Surg Am*. 2012;94(4): 335–342. https://doi.org/10.2106/JBJS.J.01084.
54. Li G, Passias P, Kozanek M, et al. Adult scoliosis in patients over sixty-five years of age: outcomes of operative versus nonoperative treatment at a minimum two-year follow-up. *Spine (Phila Pa 1976)*. 2009;34(20):2165–2170. https://doi.org/10.1097/BRS.0b013e3181b3ff0c.
55. Lee NJ, Kothari P, Kim JS, et al. Early complications and outcomes in adult spinal deformity surgery: An NSQIP study based on 5803 patients. *Global Spine J*. 2017;7(5):432–440. https://doi.org/10.1177/2192568217699384.
56. Smith JS, Shaffrey E, Klineberg E, et al. Prospective multicenter assessment of risk factors for rod fracture following surgery for adult spinal deformity. *J Neurosurg Spine*. 2014;21(6): 994–1003. https://doi.org/10.3171/2014.9.SPINE131176.

57. Cruz A, Ropper AE, Xu DS, et al. Failure in lumbar spinal fusion and current management modalities. *Semin Plast Surg*. 2021;35(1):54–62. https://doi.org/10.1055/s-0041-1726102.
58. Banno T, Hasegawa T, Yamato Y, et al. Multi-rod constructs can increase the incidence of iliac screw loosening after surgery for adult spinal deformity. *Asian Spine J*. 2019;13(3):500–510. https://doi.org/10.31616/asj.2018.0209.
59. Guevara-Villazon F, Boissiere L, Hayashi K, et al. Multiple-rod constructs in adult spinal deformity surgery for pelvic-fixated long instrumentations: an integral matched cohort analysis. *Eur Spine J*. 2020;29(4):886–895. https://doi.org/10.1007/s00586-020-06311-z.
60. Hyun SJ, Lenke LG, Kim YC, Koester LA, Blanke KM. Comparison of standard 2-rod constructs to multiple-rod constructs for fixation across 3-column spinal osteotomies. *Spine (Phila Pa 1976)*. 2014;39(22):1899–1904. https://doi.org/10.1097/BRS.0000000000000556.
61. Denduluri SK, Koltsov JCB, Ziino C, et al. Rod-screw constructs composed of dissimilar metals do not affect complication rates in posterior fusion surgery performed for adult spinal deformity. *Clin Spine Surg*. 2021;34(2):E121–E125. https://doi.org/10.1097/BSD.0000000000001058.
62. Pellise F, Serra-Burriel M, Smith JS, et al. Development and validation of risk stratification models for adult spinal deformity surgery. *J Neurosurg Spine*. 2019:1–13. https://doi.org/10.3171/2019.3.SPINE181452.
63. Smith JS, Shaffrey CI, Ames CP, Lenke LG. Treatment of adult thoracolumbar spinal deformity: past, present, and future. *J Neurosurg Spine*. 2019;30(5):551–567. https://doi.org/10.3171/2019.1.SPINE181494.
64. Glattes RC, Bridwell KH, Lenke LG, Kim YJ, Rinella A, Edwards C. 2nd Proximal junctional kyphosis in adult spinal deformity following long instrumented posterior spinal fusion: incidence, outcomes, and risk factor analysis. *Spine (Phila Pa 1976)*. 2005;30(14):1643–1649. https://doi.org/10.1097/01.brs.0000169451.76359.49.
65. Segreto FA, Passias PG, Lafage R, et al. Incidence of acute, progressive, and delayed proximal junctional kyphosis over an 8-year period in adult spinal deformity patients. *Oper Neurosurg (Hagerstown)*. 2020;18(1):75–82. https://doi.org/10.1093/ons/opz128.
66. Kim HJ, Bridwell KH, Lenke LG, et al. Proximal junctional kyphosis results in inferior SRS pain subscores in adult deformity patients. *Spine (Phila Pa 1976)*. 2013;38(11):896–901. https://doi.org/10.1097/BRS.0b013e3182815b42.
67. Kim YJ, Bridwell KH, Lenke LG, Kim J, Cho SK. Proximal junctional kyphosis in adolescent idiopathic scoliosis following segmental posterior spinal instrumentation and fusion: minimum 5-year follow-up. *Spine (Phila Pa 1976)*. 2005;30(18):2045–2050. https://doi.org/10.1097/01.brs.0000179084.45839.ad.
68. Yagi M, Akilah KB, Boachie-Adjei O. Incidence, risk factors and classification of proximal junctional kyphosis: surgical outcomes review of adult idiopathic scoliosis. *Spine (Phila Pa 1976)*. 2011; 36(1):E60–68. https://doi.org/10.1097/BRS.0b013e3181eeaee2.
69. Park SJ, Park JS, Nam Y, Choi YT, Lee CS. Who will require revision surgery among neurologically intact patients with proximal junctional failure after surgical correction of adult spinal deformity? *Spine (Phila Pa 1976)*. 2021;46(8):520–529. https://doi.org/10.1097/BRS.0000000000003850.
70. Lee MJ, Konodi MA, Cizik AM, Bransford RJ, Bellabarba C, Chapman JR. Risk factors for medical complication after spine surgery: a multivariate analysis of 1,591 patients. *Spine J*. 2012; 12(3):197–206. https://doi.org/10.1016/j.spinee.2011.11.008.
71. Lee J, Park YS. Proximal junctional kyphosis: Diagnosis, pathogenesis, and treatment. *Asian Spine J*. 2016;10(3):593–600. https://doi.org/10.4184/asj.2016.10.3.593.
72. Lafage R, Line BG, Gupta S, et al. Orientation of the uppermost instrumented segment influences proximal junctional disease following adult spinal deformity surgery. *Spine (Phila Pa 1976)*. 2017;42(20):1570–1577. https://doi.org/10.1097/BRS.0000000000002191.
73. Ghobrial GM, Eichberg DG, Kolcun JPG, et al. Prophylactic vertebral cement augmentation at the uppermost instrumented vertebra and rostral adjacent vertebra for the prevention of proximal junctional kyphosis and failure following long-segment fusion for adult spinal deformity. *Spine J*. 2017;17(10):1499–1505. https://doi.org/10.1016/j.spinee.2017.05.015.
74. Ha Y, Maruo K, Racine L, et al. Proximal junctional kyphosis and clinical outcomes in adult spinal deformity surgery with fusion from the thoracic spine to the sacrum: a comparison of proximal and distal upper instrumented vertebrae. *J Neurosurg Spine*. 2013;19(3):360–369. https://doi.org/10.3171/2013.5.SPINE12737.
75. Safaee MM, Deviren V, Dalle Ore C, et al. Ligament augmentation for prevention of proximal junctional kyphosis and proximal junctional failure in adult spinal deformity. *J Neurosurg Spine*. 2018;28(5):512–519. https://doi.org/10.3171/2017.9.SPINE1710.
76. Hostin R, McCarthy I, O'Brien M, et al. Incidence, mode, and location of acute proximal junctional failures after surgical treatment of adult spinal deformity. *Spine (Phila Pa 1976)*. 2013;38(12):1008–1015. https://doi.org/10.1097/BRS.0b013e318271319c.
77. Martin CT, Skolasky RL, Mohamed AS, Kebaish KM. Preliminary results of the effect of prophylactic vertebroplasty on the incidence of proximal junctional complications after posterior spinal fusion to the low thoracic spine. *Spine Deform*. 2013;1(2): 132–138. https://doi.org/10.1016/j.jspd.2013.01.005.
78. Park SJ, Lee CS, Park JS, Lee KJ. Should thoracolumbar junction be always avoided as upper instrumented vertebra in long instrumented fusion for adult spinal deformity?: Risk factor analysis for proximal junctional failure. *Spine (Phila Pa 1976)*. 2020;45(10):686–693. https://doi.org/10.1097/BRS.0000000000003364.
79. Kim HJ, Iyer S, Zebala LP, et al. Perioperative neurologic complications in adult spinal deformity surgery: Incidence and risk factors in 564 patients. *Spine (Phila Pa 1976)*. 2017;42(6):420–427. https://doi.org/10.1097/BRS.0000000000001774.
80. Lenke LG, Shaffrey CI, Carreon LY, et al. Lower extremity motor function following complex adult spinal deformity surgery: Two-year follow-up in the Scoli-RISK-1 prospective, multicenter, international study. *J Bone Joint Surg Am*. 2018;100(8): 656–665. https://doi.org/10.2106/JBJS.17.00575.
81. Lenke LG, Zuckerman SL, Cerpa M, et al. The Scoli-RISK 1 results of lower extremity motor function 5 years after complex adult spinal deformity surgery. *Eur Spine J*. 2021;30(11): 3243–3254. https://doi.org/10.1007/s00586-021-06969-z.
82. Zeng Y, Chen Z, Guo Z, Qi Q, Li W, Sun C. Complications of correction for focal kyphosis after posterior osteotomy and the corresponding management. *J Spinal Disord Tech*. 2013;26(7):367–374. https://doi.org/10.1097/BSD.0b013e3182499237.

32

Osteotomy and Surgical Correction Related Complications

WYATT D. VANDER VOORT, HAI V. LE, AND ERIC O. KLINEBERG

CHAPTER OUTLINE

Introduction

Adult spinal deformity (ASD) refers to spinal malalignment in the coronal and/or sagittal planes. It is caused by a variety of conditions including untreated idiopathic adolescent scoliosis, degenerative spondylosis, iatrogenic instability and/or deformity from a prior surgery, or metabolic bone disease. Symptoms can include back pain, poor sitting and standing balance, radicular leg pain and weakness, neurogenic claudication, and decreased pulmonary function. Often, the treatment for ASD is surgical, with the aim to achieve neutral balance and prevent worsening deformity, relieve pain, and decompress areas of stenosis.[1] In cases where deformity correction cannot be achieved with facet or ligament releases alone, spinal osteotomies may be warranted.

The most common spinal osteotomies include Smith-Peterson osteotomy (SPO), pedicle subtraction osteotomy (PSO), and vertebral column resection (VCR) in order of increasing complexity and achievable degree of correction in the sagittal plane. The Schwab Classification is a commonly used anatomic classification system with excellent intra- and interobserver reliability.[2] It is comprised of six grades of resection, in order of increasing bone resection and degree of destabilization.[2] Grade 1 is classified as a partial facet resection that involves removal of the inferior facet and facet joint capsule. Grade 2 is a complete facet joint resection with removal of the ligamentum flavum. Additional posterior structures including the lamina and spinous process may also be removed. An SPO is considered a Grade 2 resection. Grade 3 involves partial wedge resection of the posterior vertebral body through the pedicles. A PSO would be classified as a Grade 3. In a Grade 4 resection, a larger wedge of vertebral body is removed with additional removal of an adjacent endplate and disc. Finally, a Grade 5 resection involves complete removal of the vertebral level, also known as a VCR.[2]

SPO, also referred to as a posterior column osteotomy (PCO), Ponte osteotomy, or Grade 2 osteotomy, involves resection of the posterior elements including the bilateral facet joints and posterior ligaments (supraspinous, infraspinous, and ligamentum flavum). The correction is achieved by hinging through the posterior aspect of the disc space; thus, adequate disc height and mobility are prerequisites for this procedure.[1,3] With an SPO, sagittal plane correction is achieved by lengthening the anterior column while shortening the posterior column across each mobile segment. The SPO offers 9.3 to 10.7 degrees of correction per level, and 1.0 degree of correction is achieved per millimeter of bone resected (Fig. 32.1).[1]

PSO, or Grade 3 or 4 osteotomy, is a three-column closing wedge osteotomy that involves resecting the posterior elements, pedicles, and a triangular segment of the vertebral body. Correction is achieved through the vertebral body, rather than the disc, and therefore, an immobile disc or anterior fusion is not a contraindication to this procedure.[1] A PSO offers 30 to 40 degrees of correction in the sagittal plane, depending if the resection is carried into the adjacent disc, and is often used for idiopathic or iatrogenic flatback deformity with fixed sagittal imbalance (FSI).[3–5] Ideal candidates for PSO are those with severe sagittal imbalance as determined by a spinal vertical axis (SVA) greater than 12 centimeters with a sharp, angular kyphotic deformity, and those with multilevel circumferential fusions precluding SPO or additional anterior release (Fig. 32.2).[1]

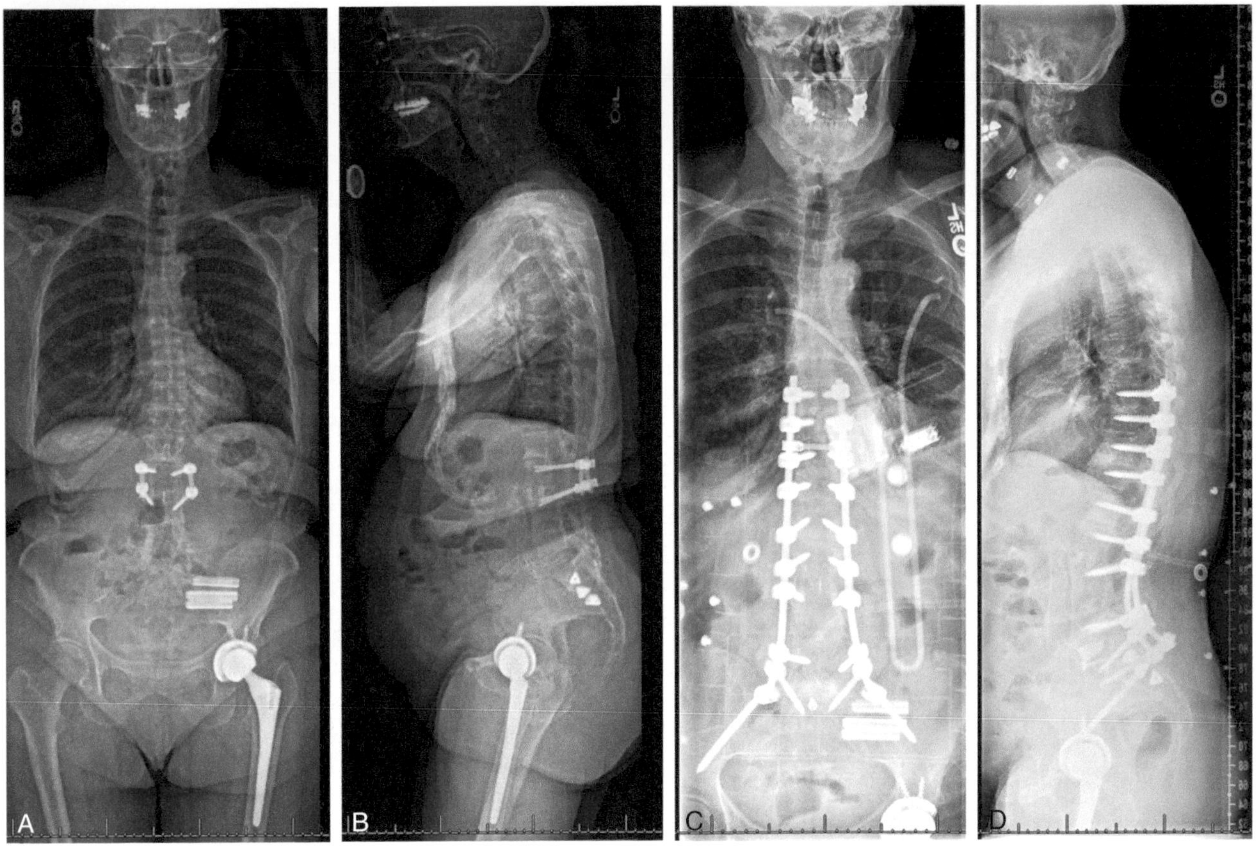

• **Fig. 32.1** Pre- (A, B) and postoperative (C, D) PA and lateral radiographs of a patient who underwent posterior column osteotomy.

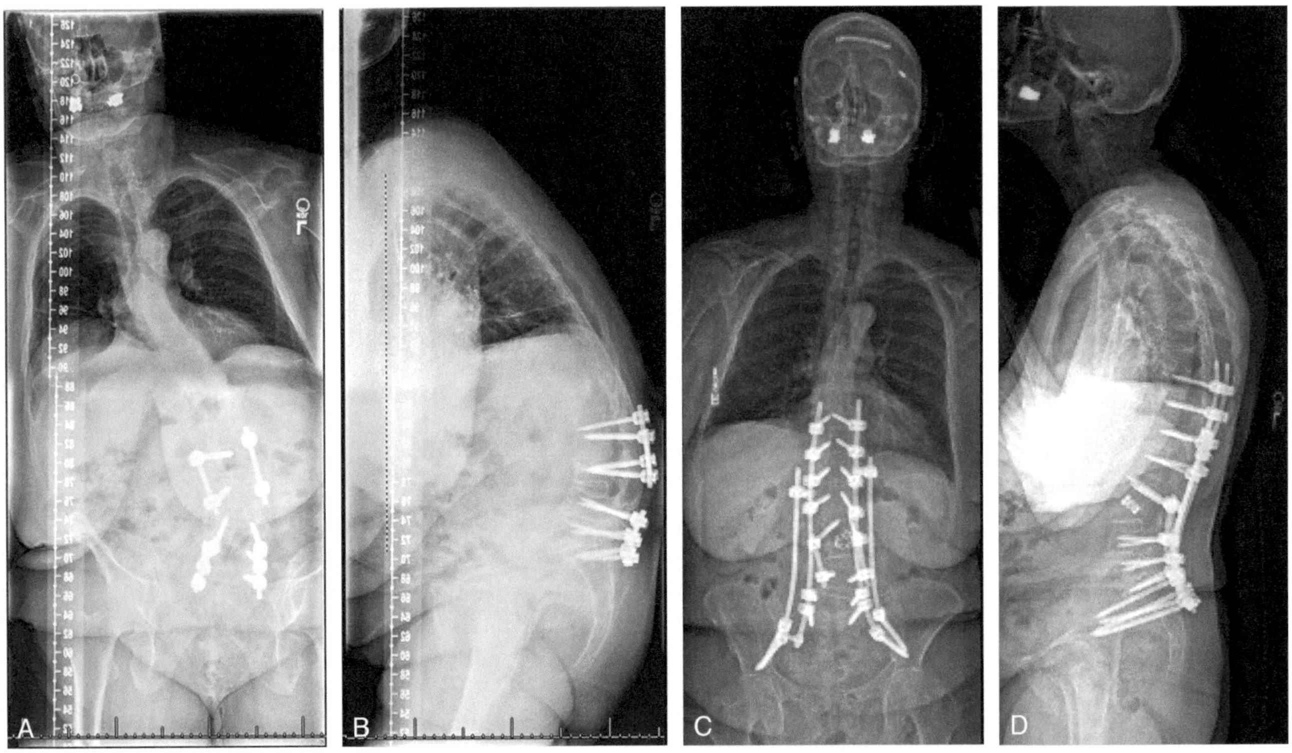

• **Fig. 32.2** Pre- (A, B) and postoperative (C, D) PA and lateral radiographs of a patient who underwent pedicle subtraction osteotomy.

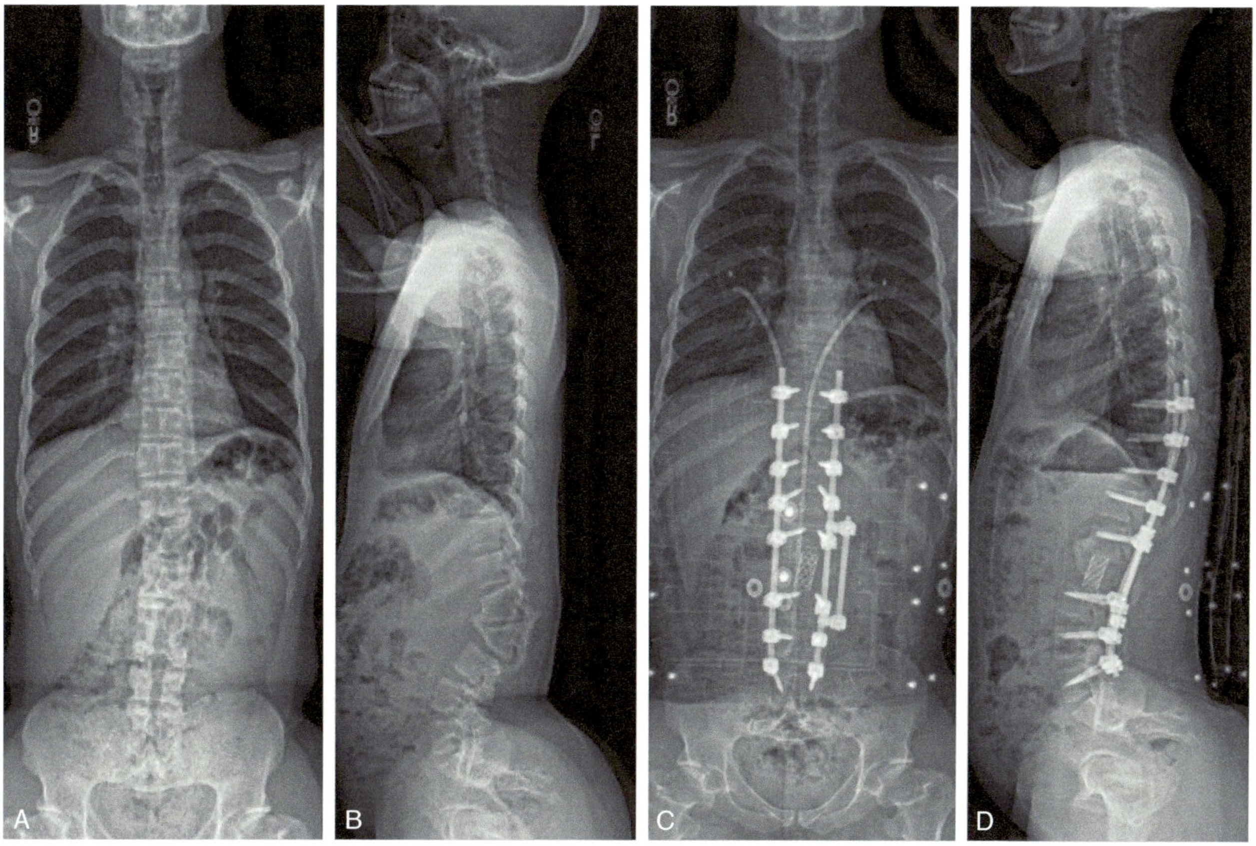

• **Fig. 32.3** Pre- (A, B) and postoperative (C, D) PA and lateral radiographs of a patient who underwent vertebral column resection.

VCR, or Grade 5 osteotomy, was traditionally used in the treatment of spinal tumors, severe spondylolisthesis and spondyloptosis, and congenital spinal abnormalities.[4] It is considered the most powerful osteotomy for deformity correction and entails complete resection of a vertebral level. Suk et al. reported a sagittal correction of 45.2 degrees and coronal correction of 61.9% with VCR.[6] VCR is indicated for severe, rigid, multiplanar deformities (Fig. 32.3).

Unfortunately, complications are not uncommon when performing these osteotomy procedures. The overall complication rate ranges between 13% and 55%.[3,7] Auerbach et al. found that major complications occurred in 35% of all three-column osteotomies.[4] Acute complications can be divided into surgical and medical. Common surgical complications include neurologic injury, dural tear, vascular injury, and excessive blood loss. Common medical complications include cardiopulmonary events, myocardial infarction, and optic neuropathy.[4] Many studies have identified risk factors for major complications, which include preoperative sagittal imbalance greater than 40 mm, age older than 60 years at the time of surgery, and the presence of three or more medical comorbidities.[4,6,8] Daubs et al. reported that patients over 60 years at the time of surgery were 7 times more likely to experience a major complication.[9] The purpose of this chapter is to discuss the complications specific to osteotomy and surgical correction in ASD cases and to provide strategies to avoid and/or effectively manage them.

Neurologic Deficit

Neurologic deficits, either transient or permanent, occur in approximately 10% to 20% of spinal osteotomy cases and are more common with three-column osteotomies. Buchowski et al. showed an intraoperative or postoperative neurological deficit rate of 11.1% after PSO. Only 2.8% of deficits were permanent over a 10-year period.[10] In their study, deficits were always unilateral and never proximal to the osteotomy. In addition, the neurologic injury did not occur at the site of the osteotomy and was not identified by intraoperative neuromonitoring.[10] After VCR, Suk et al. reported a neurological deficit rate of 17%. This included 2 complete cord deficits and 10 transient deficits, all of which recovered by 6 months.[6]

During SPO, nerve root compression may occur as a result of decreased foraminal height as the posterior column is shortened. After removal of the posterior elements, increased lordosis is introduced at the level of the osteotomy through the disc space. This results in a relative closure of the posterior structures and loss of foraminal height. It is critical to perform a wide facetectomy including removal of the superior articular process (SAP) at the level of the osteotomy in order to prevent nerve root compression and to inspect those nerves clinically to ensure that they are not entrapped.[1]

Transient neurologic deficit occurs in up to 20% of PSO cases.[1] This most commonly occurs during osteotomy closure. At this stage, the spinal column may become destabilized and result in unwanted translation and subsequent canal stenosis. A provisional unilateral rod can be used during osteotomy closure to provide stability and prevent this issue. Auerbach et al. noted that nerve roots at and distal to the level of the PSO on the concavity of a combined sagittal and coronal deformity are at particular risk during osteotomy closure.[4] Particular attention must be paid to these areas in order to prevent nerve root compression. In addition, during osteotomy closure, dural buckling and subsequent neurologic deficit may occur as a result of shortening the posterior elements. The risk of neurologic injury can be lowered with wide central and lateral recess decompression prior to osteotomy closure.[4] Dural buckling can also be managed with either duraplasty or by suturing the dura to one of the rods. This prevents the dura from creating any stenosis due to its redundancy.

During VCR, overshortening can result in buckling of the spinal cord, which can lead to neurologic deficit. Preventing overshortening and, if a deficit occurs, supporting and lengthening the anterior column may be necessary. This can be accomplished using a cage at the osteotomy site.[1] Like a PSO, a temporary rod can be used to prevent iatrogenic injury following destabilization of the spine.[1] Auerbach et al. noted that patients with preexisting thoracic myelopathy and prior fusion surgery with severe residual kyphosis or kyphoscoliosis have a higher risk of neurologic compromise during VCR. This deformity results in the spinal cord draping over the apex of the deformity, which causes tension and impairs blood flow.[4] In this situation, a large deformity correction may be more than what the spinal cord can tolerate. Maintaining a hemoglobin level >10 g/dL and mean arterial pressure (MAP) of 75 to 80 mmHg has been suggested during cases requiring extensive corrections.[1]

In all cases, neuromonitoring is required to aid in identification of an intraoperative neurologic deficit. Although previous literature has demonstrated that neuromonitoring fails to identify all insults, it remains a useful tool.[10] Upon identification of a neurologic deficit, the surgeon should cease further correction, confirm appropriate neuromonitoring lead connection, ensure maintenance of adequate MAP, and consider removing instrumentation and reversing the correction. If a persistent deficit remains, a wake-up test can be performed. Throughout the procedure, care must be taken to avoid direct and indirect impacts to the spinal cord, including impingement, compression, distraction, and shock. Additionally, excessive correction should be avoided in order to prevent extreme shortening or buckling of the spinal cord.[11] Vitale et al. developed a consensus-based checklist to guide surgeon response to intraoperative neuromonitoring changes (Table 32.1). The checklist consists of five headings (gain control of room, anesthetic/systemic, technical/neurophysiologic, surgical, and ongoing considerations) containing 26 factors to consider in response to neuromonitoring changes.[12] Implementation of this checklist may potentially improve outcomes and prevent complications.

Dural Tear

Incidental durotomies are a relatively common complication in the setting of adult deformity surgery. Previous studies have reported rates from 2% to 20%. Iyer et al. identified osteotomies as a risk factor for an incidental durotomy in patients undergoing ASD surgery.[13] When examining specific types of osteotomies, they found that those undergoing PSO were 2.8 times more likely to sustain a dural tear, whereas SPO and VCR did not significantly increase the risk.[13] An additional risk factor for incidental durotomy was the degree of preoperative sagittal deformity. Not surprisingly, these patients were more likely to require an osteotomy. The authors also found that patients undergoing revision surgery, decompression, and interbody fusion were at increased risk.[13]

Preventing incidental durotomies requires careful preoperative planning and meticulous surgical technique.[14] Patient selection and recognition of risk factors such as prior surgery are critical. In these patients, it is recommended to begin dissection in areas of unscarred tissue prior to exposing scarred area.[14] During decompression and deformity correction, avoid excessive traction on the dura and nerve roots as this can result in incidental durotomy.[14]

In the event of an incidental durotomy, prompt recognition and management are critical. One must first ensure adequate exposure of the durotomy, which may require expanding the bony resection.[14] Avoid aggressive suction in the area to prevent nerve root herniation through the dural defect. Placing the patient in a Trendelenburg position may allow the floating roots to drift anteriorly and relax the edges of the dura. Depending on the size and location of the tear, a combination of sutures, fibrin glue, fascial grafts, and tissue welding may be used to repair the defect.[14]

Dural tears have been associated with an increased rate of perioperative and postoperative complications including operative time, intraoperative blood loss, and length of inpatient stay.[15] However, Iyer et al. demonstrated that dural tears were not associated with poorer outcomes at any timepoint.[13] Similarly, Desai et al. demonstrated no difference in nerve root injury, mortality, need for additional surgery, or patient-reported outcomes at 4-year follow-up.[15]

Intraoperative Bleeding

Limiting intraoperative blood loss is imperative in patients undergoing osteotomy in order to prevent morbidity and mortality. Neurologic injuries can occur as a result of vascular insults and hypovolemia that limit perfusion to the spinal cord.[16] During anterior approaches, ligating multiple and/or bilateral segmental vessels places the cord at risk.

TABLE 32.1 Checklist for the response to intraoperative neuromonitoring changes in spine patients with a stable spine.

Gain Control of the Room	Anesthetic/ Systemic	Technical/ Neurophysiologic	Surgical

• Intraoperative pause: stop case and announce to the room
• Eliminate extraneous stimuli (e.g., music, conversations, etc.)
• Summon ATTENDING anesthesiologist, SENIOR neurologist or neurophysiologist, and EXPERIENCED nurse
• Anticipate need for intraoperative and/or perioperative imaging if not readily available
	• Optimize mean arterial pressure (MAP)
	• Optimize hematocrit
	• Optimize blood pH and pCO_2
	• Seek normothermia
	• Discuss POTENTIAL need for wake-up test with ATTENDING anesthesiologist
		• Discuss status of anesthetic agents
		• Check extent of neuromuscular blockade and degree of paralysis
		• Check electrodes and connections
		• Determine pattern and timing of signal changes
		• Check neck and limb positioning; check limb position on table especially if unilateral loss
			• Discuss events and actions just prior to signal loss and consider reversing actions:
			  • Remove traction (if applicable)
			  • Decrease/remove distraction or other corrective forces
			  • Remove rods
			  • Remove screws and probe for breach
			• Evaluate for spinal cord compression, examine osteotomy and laminotomy sites
			• Intraoperative and/or perioperative imaging (e.g. O-arm, fluoroscopy, x-ray) to evaluate implant placement

Ongoing Considerations			
• REVISIT anesthetic/systemic considerations and confirm that they are optimized • Wake-up test • Consultation with a colleague • Continue surgical procedure versus staging procedure • IV steroid protocol: methylprednisolone 30 mg/kg in first hr, then 5.4 mg/kg/hr for next 23 hrs			

Reproduced with permission from Vitale et al.: Best practices in intraoperative neuromonitoring in spine deformity surgery: Development of an intraoperative checklist to optimize response, *Spine Deform* 2(5):333–339, 2014.

Patel et al. recommend performing only unilateral ligation on the convexity of the curve at the mid-vertebral body.[16] Additionally, hypotensive anesthesia should be avoided.[16]

During correction of a coronal plane deformity, the spinal vessels on the concavity are placed on increased tension. This can result in spinal cord ischemia. Oftentimes, this may present as a delayed quadriplegia or paraplegia.[17] Close immediate postoperative monitoring is critical in order to identify this complication. Adequate postoperative resuscitation is necessary and provides potential for recovery.[17]

Increased blood loss has also been associated with cerebrovascular accidents (CVAs), particularly in patients with preexisting cardiac or vascular disease, hypertension, hyperlipidemia, previous cardiac events, and/or carotid stenosis.[18] Patients with signs and symptoms concerning for CVA should undergo immediate cross-sectional imaging of the head and neurology should be consulted.[16]

Spinal osteotomies, particularly PSO and VCR, have been associated with substantial blood loss. Cho et al. found that a single-level PSO resulted in almost twice as much bleeding as three consecutive SPOs.[19] During VCR, the mean estimated blood loss ranges from 820 to 3071 milliliters.[20] Familiarity with hemostasis techniques including the use of thrombin-soaked collagen sponges, gelfoam, bipolar electrocautery, and medical management with tranexamic acid (TXA) are necessary.[1] It is not uncommon to encounter profuse epidural bleeding during ligamentectomy and facetectomy, especially during the removal of the superior facet of the inferior vertebra.[1]

Although uncommon, vascular injuries represent a devastating complication. In the thoracic spine, the aorta can be injured during pedicle screw instrumentation. Careful and precise screw placement is necessary, and prompt recognition and involvement of cardiothoracic and/or surgery is mandatory.[16] In the lumbar spine, the most common vascular injuries include the left common iliac vein laceration, inferior vena cava laceration, and left common iliac artery or vein thrombosis during anterior approach.[16] Meticulous dissection and assistance from general or vascular surgery is recommended to prevent these injuries. Major vascular injury can also occur during lumbar discectomy, interbody instrumentation, or corpectomy. This can be avoided with adequate exposure and avoiding the blind use of grasping instruments in the anterior disc space.[16]

Medical Complications

Medical complications are common after spinal osteotomy procedures. Soroceanu et al. reported that approximately 26% of patients experience at least one medical complication.[21] Kim et al. reported that major, life-threatening medical complications occur in approximately 15% of cases.[5]

Major medical complications include cardiopulmonary events, myocardial infarction, and optical deficits. Other medical complications include respiratory distress, ileus, urinary tract infections, arrhythmias, deep vein thrombosis, and pulmonary embolism.[21]

Careful patient selection and medical optimization of comorbidities are essential to prevent or lower the risk of medical complications. Risk factors for medical complications include smoking, preoperative anemia, heart disease, hypertension, obesity, depression, longer duration of symptoms, and a higher American Society of Anesthesiologists (ASA) score.[21] In addition, minimizing operative time is critical. Patients who sustained at least one medical complication averaged 51 minutes longer operative time than those who had no medical complications.[21] Auerbach et al. analyzed the impact of major medical complications on clinical outcome scores separately and found that patients with medical complications still had a significant improvement from baseline to final follow-up with respect to stereotactic radiosurgery (SRS) pain, self-image, and subscore.[4]

Pearls and Pitfalls

- Surgical and medical complications are common with ASD surgery, especially when three-column osteotomies are performed. Therefore, it is important to medically optimize patients prior to surgery. Additionally, patients should be fully informed of these complications during the consent process.
- Neurologic injury can be identified with intraoperative neuromonitoring, adequate decompression of neural elements, and maintenance of MAP and hemoglobin level. Reliance on neuromonitoring alone is insufficient, and careful inspection of the neural elements during surgery is necessary.
- During SPO, bilateral SAP resection is recommended to create room for the exiting nerve roots as the posterior column is shortened for spinal correction.
- During PSO, the laminectomy should be one level above and below the previously planned osteotomy level. This is important to prevent acute buckling of the spinal cord. Normally, for a one-level resection procedure, a posterior column laminectomy will result in a 5 to 6 cm exposure of the dura and neural elements. Buckling becomes a more severe problem, especially in cases where a previous laminectomy or laminotomy has been performed and there is peridural fibrosis preventing the gliding movement of the dura as the osteotomy gap is closed. This should be removed prior to the closure of the PSO (Fig. 32.4). In addition to extending the laminectomy, laminar undercutting should be done to widen the spinal canal from within, again to prevent infolding of the ligamentum flavum and bony surfaces.[1] Duraplasty can be effective in decreasing recalcitrant buckling, but does increase the risk of CSF leak following surgery. Additionally, suture tenting of the dura may be an effective alternative.
- During VCR, because of vertebral rotation at the apex, even if the canal is identified using the location of the pedicles, the location and direction of the cord may be difficult to identify. All bone anterior to the posterior longitudinal ligament (PLL) must be resected to prevent buckling of the PLL and subsequent anterior compression of the spinal cord.[1] Shortening of the spinal cord should occur first before any correction is attempted.

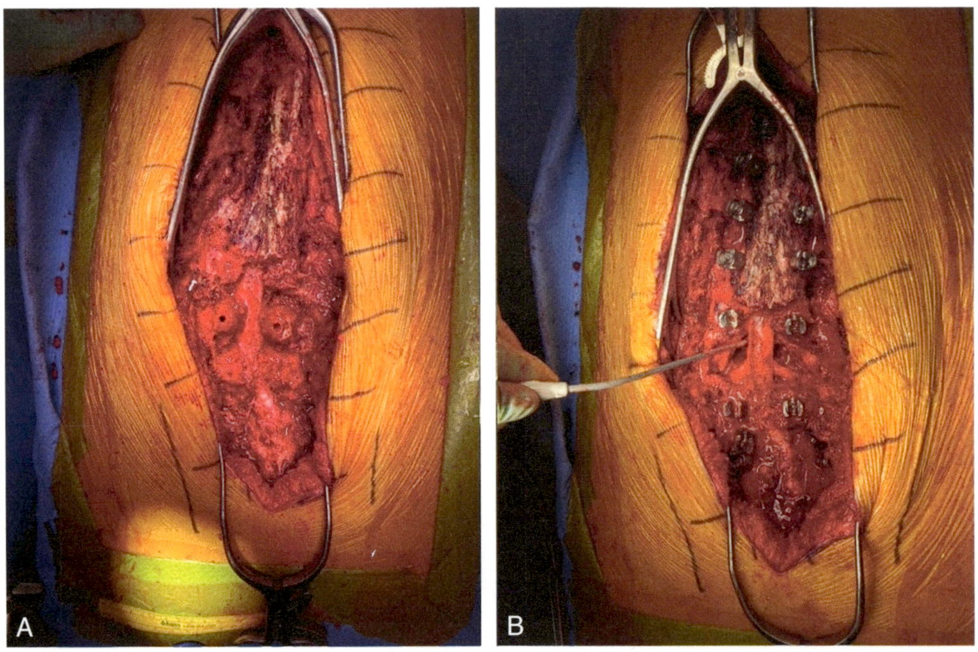

• **Fig. 32.4** Intraoperative clinical photo demonstrating isolation of the L3 pedicles (A), followed by L3 pedicle subtraction osteotomy (B).

- Provisional stabilization with a unilateral rod is recommended during closure of the PSO or VCR osteotomy gap to prevent translational instability.

Conclusion

Adult spinal deformity is a complex disorder of sagittal and coronal imbalance, and spinal osteotomies may be indicated in order to achieve adequate surgical correction. Complications following osteotomy and correction are not uncommon, ranging from 13% to 55%. Risk factors for complication include severe deformity, age over 60 years, and multiple medical comorbidities. Intraoperative complications include neurologic injury, incidental durotomy, and excessive blood loss. Postoperatively, medical complications include cardiopulmonary events, myocardial infarction, optical deficits, respiratory distress, ileus, urinary tract infections, arrhythmias, deep vein thrombosis, and pulmonary embolism. In order to both prevent and minimize the impact of complications in this population, appropriate patient selection and medical optimization is imperative. Intraoperative neuromonitoring, adequate decompression of neural elements, and maintenance of MAP and hemoglobin level during surgery minimizes neurologic injury. Precise surgical technique is required to ensure adequate decompression and maintain stability of the spine while performing the osteotomy and correction. Patients should be followed closely after surgery in order to prevent and/or quickly identify and treat postoperative medical complications.

Disclosures

No funding or other sources of support were used to aid this work. The authors declare that they have no potential or perceived conflicts of interest.

References

1. Kose KC, Bozduman O, Yenigul AE, Igrek S. Spinal osteotomies: indications, limits and pitfalls. *EFORT Open Rev*. 2017;2 (3):73–82.
2. Schwab F, Blondel B, Chay E, et al. The comprehensive anatomical spinal osteotomy classification. *Neurosurgery*. 2014;74(1): 112–120.
3. Hu WH, Wang Y. Osteotomy techniques for spinal deformity. *Chin Med J (Engl)*. 2016;129(21):2639–2641.
4. Auerbach JD, Lenke LG, Bridwell KH, et al. Major complications and comparison between 3-column osteotomy techniques in 105 consecutive spinal deformity procedures. *Spine*. 2012;37(14):1198–1210.
5. Kim YJ, Bridwell KH, Lenke LG, et al. Results of lumbar pedicle subtraction osteotomies for fixed sagittal imbalance: a minimum 5-year follow-up study. *Spine*. 2007;32:2189–2197.
6. Suk SI, Kim JH, Kim WJ, et al. Posterior vertebral column resection for severe spinal deformities. *Spine*. 2002;27:2374–2382.
7. Qian BP, Huang JC, Qiu Y, et al. Complications of spinal osteotomy for thoracolumbar kyphosis secondary to ankylosing spondylitis in 342 patients: incidence and risk factors. *J Neurosurg Spine*. 2018;30(1):91–98.
8. Acaroglu E. European Spine Study Group. Decision-making in the treatment of adult spinal deformity. *EFORT Open Rev*. 2017;1(5):167–176. https://doi.org/10.1302/2058-5241.1.000013.PMID: 28461944; PMCID: PMC5367523.
9. Daubs MD, Brodke DS, Annis P, Lawrence BD. Perioperative complications of pedicle subtraction osteotomy. *Global Spine J*. 2016;6(7):630–635.
10. Buchowski JM, Bridwell KH, Lenke LG, et al. Neurologic complications of lumbar pedicle subtraction osteotomy: a 10-year assessment. *Spine (Phila Pa 1976)*. 2007;32:2245–2252.
11. Zeng Y, Chen Z, Guo Z, Qi Q, Li W, Sun C. The posterior surgical treatment for focal kyphosis in upper-middle thoracic spine. *Eur Spine J*. 2014;23(11):2291–2298.
12. Vitale MG, Skaggs DL, Pace GI, et al. Best practices in intraoperative neuromonitoring in spine deformity surgery: Development of an intraoperative checklist to optimize response. *Spine Deform*. 2014;2(5):333–339.
13. Iyer S, Klineberg EO, Zebala LP, et al. International Spine Study Group (ISSG). Dural tears in adult deformity surgery: Incidence, risk factors, and outcomes. *Global Spine J*. 2018;8(1):25–31. https://doi.org/10.1177/2192568217717973.Epub 2017 Jul 20.
14. Bosacco SJ, Gardner MJ, Guille JT. Evaluation and treatment of dural tears in lumbar spine surgery: A review. *Clin Orthop Relat Res*. 2001;389:238–247.
15. Desai A, Ball PA, Bekelis K, et al. SPORT: Does incidental durotomy affect longterm outcomes in cases of spinal stenosis? *Neurosurgery*. 2015;76 Suppl 1(0 1):S57–S63.
16. Patel SA, McDonald CL, Reid DBC, et al. Complications of thoracolumbar adult spinal deformity surgery. *JBJS Rev*. 2020;8(5): e0214.
17. Taylor BA, Webb PJ, Hetreed M, Mulukutla RD, Farrell J. Delayed postoperative paraplegia with hypotension in adult revision scoliosis surgery. *Spine (Phila Pa 1976)*. 1994;19(4):470–474.
18. Nagre AS. Perioperative stroke - prediction, prevention, and protection. *Indian J Anaesth*. 2018;62(10):738–742.
19. Cho KJ, Bridwell KH, Lenke LG, Berra A, Baldus C. Comparison of Smith-Petersen versus pedicle subtraction osteotomy for the correction of fixed sagittal imbalance. *Spine (Phila Pa 1976)*. 2005;30(18):2030–2038.
20. Sorour I, Elhabashy AM, Fayed AA. Safety and efficacy of posterior vertebral column resection in complex pediatric deformities. *Egypt J Neurosurg*. 2022;37(1):10.
21. Soroceanu A, Burton DC, Oren JH, et al. Medical complications after adult spinal deformity surgery: Incidence, risk factors, and clinical impact. *Spine (Phila Pa 1976)*. 2016;41(22):1718–1723.

33

Long-Term Complications

ELIZABETH LORD

CHAPTER OUTLINE

Introduction

Adult spinal deformity (ASD) may affect up to 9% of the adult population, with incidence increasing with age.[1] Left untreated, ASD has a substantial negative impact on health-related quality of life outcomes. Surgical management of ASD in appropriately indicated patients has been shown to be beneficial.[2,3] Developments in instrumentation, biologics, and surgical technique in recent decades have allowed for more powerful correction of deformity with improved outcomes.[1,3,4] Nonetheless, surgery for ASD is technically challenging and is associated with high complication rates.[1,4] The complication profile of ASD can be divided into categories. Biological failure occurs when bony fusion does not occur due to poor biologic response, technical failures, or infection and is referred to as pseudoarthrosis. Failure of instrumentation refers to implant fracture, loosening, or pull-out, often resulting from or resulting in pseudoarthrosis. The abrupt transition from a mobile spine to a stiff, fused construct may lead to accelerated rates of degeneration cephalad and caudal to the fusion construct. In its advanced state, this can lead to proximal or distal junctional failure. The combination of the aforementioned mechanical complications as well as nonmechanical complications (e.g., wound infection, perioperative medical complications, chronic pain) negatively influence patient-reported outcomes.[5]

Biological Failure

The etymology of the word "pseudoarthrosis" comes from the Greek meaning "false joint" and is the most common iatrogenic complication following fusion surgery.[6–10] It is defined as significant motion in the area of fusion more than 1 year after index surgery.[11] It is hypothesized that fibrous soft tissue develops in the areas of attempted fusion and microfractures occur in cancellous bones leading to failure of fusion and pain postoperatively.[12] Patients with pseudoarthrosis may present with persistent or new back pain and radiographic evidence of loss of alignment of 10 degrees, no continuity in fusion mass, and >3 mm of sagittal motion on the lateral flexion-extension radiographs.[7,12–15] Heggeness and Esses described four categories of posterolateral lumbar pseudoarthrosis: atrophic, transverse, shingle, and complex.[16] An atrophic pattern displays no bone formation. Transverse patterns show a large mass of remodeled bone without continuous bridging. A shingle pattern has a defect within the fusion mass.[12] While this classification provides radiographic description of pseudoarthrosis, it does not address whether patients become symptomatic or remain asymptomatic.[9,13,17] Not all persistent low back pain and disability after adult spinal surgery is secondary to pseudoarthrosis.[7,14] Additionally, standard radiographs may miss pseudoarthrosis in symptomatic ASD patients.[18] Computed tomography (CT) scans are considered the most accurate imaging modality for assessing pseudoarthrosis but is limited in its use due to cost and radiation risk.[12,19]

Pseudoarthrosis risk is related to both surgeon and patient factors.[10,20,21] Generally, pseudoarthrosis is due to inadequate fixation or inadequate bone formation.[12] Certain factors lie in surgeons' hands.[10,15,17,20] As the number of fused levels increases, so does the rate of pseudoarthrosis—18% for one fused level, 26% for two, and up to 42% for a long ASD construct of three levels or more.[8,9,14,22] Although there is the hypothesized benefit of greater stability due to distribution of loading over more segments, longer constructs have more potential points of excessive motion and a decrease graft volume per level.[19] Greater lordosis correction, and the use of osteotomies, also increase the rate of pseudoarthrosis.[19,23]

Adult degenerative scoliosis often occurs with a combination of sagittal and coronal deformities; thus, there is no difference in pseudoarthrosis rates between these purely sagittal and coronal deformities.[19]

In ASD patients, the use of allograft has a reported pseudoarthrosis rate of 6%, while use of bone morphogenetic protein (BMP) use has a rate of 5.5%.[10,15,24] Iliac crest autograft is considered the gold standard for bone graft; however, many surgeons consider BMP a helpful adjuvant for the challenging fusion environment of long constructs.[12,15] Failure to properly prepare the graft bed through removal of soft tissue can increase fibrous ingrowth leading to an increased risk of fusion failure.[25] For example, small amounts of bone-related bleeding should be obtained, all articular surfaces should be cleaned of cartilage and other soft tissues, and graft surfaces need at least two-thirds endplate contact with the host.[10,25]

Patients older than 55 have an increased risk of developing pseudoarthrosis.[12,26] Endocrine abnormalities such as osteoporosis, low growth hormone, low thyroid hormone, compromised nutritional states, diabetes, and corticosteroid use all increased the risk of pseudoarthrosis due to abnormalities in bony formation metabolism.[7,12,19,23] Tobacco use is a well-documented risk of nonunion and it is recommended that patients stop smoking prior to fusion surgery.[12,14,19,27]

Knowing and recognizing the etiology of pseudoarthrosis plays a critical role in determining the need for and nature of revision spine surgery as outcomes for pseudoarthrosis revision surgery.[6,7,10] Options to address pseudoarthrosis include interbody fusion for anterior column support, up-sizing pedicle screw instrumentation, augmentation of posterolateral fusion mass with BMP, addition of pelvic fixation, or utilization of multiple spanning rods.[6,7,14,20] However, these adjuvants are not without its complications. For example, the use of a multiple rod construct can increase the risks of proximal junctional kyphosis or screw loosening.[28,29]

Late/indolent spinal surgery infections (LSSI) are defined as infections occurring at least 6 months after the index surgery and can manifest as back pain, wound drainage, and elevated inflammatory markers.[30,31] The incidence of LSSI ranges from 1.4% to 3.0%.[31] Patients with LSSI have worsened long-term outcomes, increased hospital stays, higher mortality, and rates of return to the operating room.[31–36] Risk factors that increase the risk for developing LSSI include patients with neuromuscular scoliosis, longer fusion lengths, increased surgical time and blood loss, and combined anterior-posterior approaches.[31,37,38] Although different studies have different definitions of "delayed presentation" (i.e., greater than 3 months, greater than 6 months, etc.), because of the prolonged time of infection development, the bacteria have developed biofilms that resist antibiotic penetration and host immune defense.[31,39]

Staphylococcus epidermidis and *Propionibacterium acnes* are the most common organisms found in implants that were removed from patients with LSSI in addition to *Escherichia coli* and *Pseudomonas aeruginosa*.[30,32,40–43] Because of their low-virulence state, these microorganisms can remain undetected early on leading to widespread biofilm formation.[44] In addition, hematoma formation, soft tissue reactions to hardware, and fretting corrosion promote bacterial growth within the surgical site.[45] It is posited that seeding occurs either hematogenously or intraoperatively, with the latter being harder to prove.[16,38,45,46] Heggeness et al. reported and described cases of hematogenous seeding, such as IV drug usage and pyelonephritis.[16] Other studies have demonstrated culture-positive implants after hardware removal pointing to an intraoperative cause of bacterial seeding.[38,45,46] Thus, hardware explantation is recommended to treat delayed infections.[31,39,47,48] However, with explantations, even in the setting of radiographic fusion, loss of correction and progression of kyphosis or scoliosis in the fusion area become evident.[49–51] Thus, surgeons should consider leaving the instrumentation in place for at least 2 years prior to removal with ongoing antibiotic suppression until osseous stability is achieved.[38,48] Even then there is the risk for continued curve progression secondary to underlying/occult pseudoarthrosis and pliability of immature fusion masses.[31,49,50,52] Both primary and delayed closure after hardware removal are effective and safe although the latter leads to discomfort for the patient.[38,48] An appropriate antibiotic course based on culture and sensitivity tests and consultation with infectious disease specialists should be utilized postoperatively.[53]

Instrumentation Failure

In addition to biological failure of achieving bony fusion, instrument-related failure is one of the most common complications encountered by adult spinal deformity surgeons. Implant-related complications include rod fracture, rod migration, screw fracture, screw loosening, and screw pull-out. Implant-related complications are a considerable source of morbidity after adult deformity correction. These complications may result in pain, loss of correction, neurologic deterioration, and poor patient-reported outcomes. Additionally, implant-related complications frequently require technically challenging revision surgery that is associated with high complication rates and increased health care costs.[54]

Rod fracture is the most common implant-related complication observed after ASD surgery.[1,3] Furthermore, rod fracture is the most common indication for revision surgery after ASD correction and is associated with lower overall patient satisfaction scores.[3,55] Published rates of rod fracture after ASD range from 6.5% to 18.4%.[1,3,4,54,56] Rod fracture is most commonly related to the development of pseudoarthrosis. Early rod fracture may potentiate the risk of pseudoarthrosis due to increased construct motion; however, late fracture may be caused by implant fatigue in the setting of pseudoarthrosis.[54,57] Most rod fractures occur early in the postoperative period, typically within the first 3 years.[3,54]

Multiple studies have identified potential risk factors for the development of rod fracture after ASD correction. Patients with larger preoperative deformities are more likely to suffer rod fracture after deformity correction. Increased preoperative sagittal vertical axis, thoracolumbar kyphosis, and pelvic incidence-lumbar lordosis mismatch have all been shown to be associated with rod fracture for adult deformity correction.[1–4,54–56,58] Fusion constructs that cross both the thoracolumbar and lumbosacral junctions have been shown to be associated with increased risk of postoperative rod fracture.[59] These constructs are at increased strain due to the elevated mechanical forces present at these junctions, particularly the lumbosacral junction.[3] Additionally, markedly higher rates of rod fracture are observed in cases involving a pedicle subtraction osteotomy compared to those without.[4] Rod fracture in these patients tends to occur at or immediately adjacent to the level of the osteotomy, typically early in the postoperative period prior to the onset of arthrodesis.[60,61]

Rod diameter may influence risk of fracture. Azakawa and colleagues reported that small diameter of rods <6 mm is associated with rod fracture, although this is an area of debate.[3,56] Similarly, there are conflicting reports on the effect of rod composition to fracture rates. Some have shown that cobalt chromium rods display lower rates of fracture compared to titanium alloy and stainless steel, while others have reported the opposite.[3,4,54] Intraoperative rod contouring has also been put forward as a risk factor for rod fracture, particularly with titanium or titanium alloy rods due to their notch sensitivity.[59,62,63] The risk of rod fracture increases as the postoperative change in sagittal vertical axis increases, lending credence to the hypothesis that instrumentation may be more likely to fatigue in the setting of excessive rod contouring and use of reduction devices for deformity correction.[4,64]

The lumbosacral junction is an area of high mechanical strain. Stiffer constructs are thus employed in this region to reduce the risk of pseudoarthrosis. Lumbopelvic fixation has been demonstrated to increase construct stiffness and to reduce the risk of pseudoarthrosis.[65] The use of iliac screws for lumbopelvic fixation has been shown to be a risk factor for rod fracture.[56] S2-alar-iliac screws have increased in prevalence for pelvic fixation, as they are associated with lower rates of implant prominence and wound complications compared to iliac screws.[66] The S2-alar-iliac screw head often requires aggressive angulation, however, in order to accommodate the rod. Additionally, this screw trajectory requires the head to be at an extreme angle relative to the shaft, introducing strain when the rod is reduced into the tulip. Thus, acute mechanical failure of S2-alar-iliac screws resulting in rod and/or set screw displacement from the screw head is an important consideration.[65,67] The magnitude of lumbar lordosis change is associated with failure risk. The considerable strain present at the lumbosacral junction from a large surgical correction may exceed the tolerance of the implant.[65]

For patients deemed to have high predicted risk of implant-related complication, potential intraoperative decisions can be made to protect against the risk of complication. Accessory supplemental rods or constructs with multiple rods have been shown to reduce the risk of rod fracture after ASD correction.[68,69] Multi-rod constructs may increase mechanical stability and decrease risk of rod fracture after ASD correction.[69] Interbody fusion is also predictive of rod fracture at the lumbosacral junction, particularly anterior lumbar interbody fusion and lateral lumbar interbody fusion compared to transforaminal interbody fusion.[55,70]

Adjacent Segment Disease, Proximal and Distal Junctional Failure

Rigid instrumentation is necessary to minimize the risk of pseudoarthrosis after deformity correction. This benefit, however, is inextricably linked to compensatory alterations in biomechanics of adjacent segments. Increased intradiscal pressure, increased facet loading, and increased mobility proximal and distal to the instrumented levels result in degenerative changes to adjacent segments.[71,72] This phenomenon is referred to as adjacent segment disease. The restoration of optimal sagittal alignment has been shown to slow the development of adjacent segment disease after instrumented lumbar fusion.[73,74] A related pathologic entity involving adjacent levels after deformity correction is proximal or distal junctional disease.

There are different definitions of proximal junctional kyphosis (PJK). Originally Bridwell et al. defined PJK as a proximal junctional sagittal Cobb angle between the lower endplate of uppermost instrumented vertebra (UIV) and the upper endplate of two supra-adjacent vertebra greater than or equal to 10 degrees or at least 10 degrees greater than the preoperative measurement.[75] However, Helgeson set the proximal junctional angle at 15 degrees while other authors used 20 degrees to define meaningful PJK leading to poor outcomes.[75–77] Today, at least a 10 degree increase in proximal sagittal cobb angle measurement compared to preoperative measurements is used as the definition of PJK.[78–80] Proximal junctional failure (PJF) refers to a symptomatic progressive form of PJK as a result of vertebral fracture, subluxation between vertebrae, failure of fixation, and neurological deficits leading to proximal extension of fusion surgery.[81–83] The reported incidence of PJK is between 17% to 61.7%.[81,84–86] Boachie-Adjei classified the grades and severity of PJK with three types and grades: type 1 is solely disc and ligamentous failure, type 2 includes bone failure, and 3 includes implant/bone interface failure; grade A has an increase in proximal junctional angle from 10 to 19 degrees, grade B has an increase in proximal junctional angle from 20 to 29 degrees, grade C has an increase greater than 30 degrees.[86]

There have been different reported risk factors for PJF and PJK. From the patient's perspective, older age (>55 years), high body mass index (BMI), osteoporosis or low bone density increased the risk for both PJK and PJF.[75,85,87] From the surgical aspect, damage to the posterior soft tissues (posterior tension band, facet capsules) intraoperatively will lead to decreased posterior strength and thus increased risk for

PJK and PJF.[79,86,88–91] Patients with anterior-posterior spinal fusion have a three times increased risk of PJK, and fusion extension to lower lumbar spine and sacrum also increased the incidence of PJK.[92,93] Pedicle screw–only constructs are linked with PJK as pedicle screws increase the rigidity of vertebrae leading to adjacent segment kyphosis.[76,94] Han et al. demonstrated that patients who received stiffer rods (i.e., use of cobalt chrome vs titanium alloy rod constructs) also had a higher risk of PJK.[90]

Currently there is no standardized guide in determining revision surgery, but there are several concepts that are agreed upon. Patients who are asymptomatic can generally be managed with reassurance and close monitoring.[95] Although those who are asymptomatic but with disruption of the posterior column can be considered for revision surgery as there is risk of progression and neurologic sequelae.[86,91] Those with significant symptoms and higher severity of deformity or instability can be considered for revision surgery. Hart et al. reported that surgeons are more likely to recommend revision in the setting of trauma and severe kyphosis.[96] Patients without rigid, severe kyphotic deformity proximal to the fusion construct can be treated with extension of fusion with or without decompression. Otherwise, Smith-Peterson osteotomies are often required to restore sagittal alignment, while more extensive procedures such as vertebral column resections or pedicle subtraction osteotomies are reserved for more rigid deformities or increased risks of neurological compromise.[95] Even with these concepts, there is a risk of up to 48% recurrence rate of PJK/PJF at the new UIV.[86]

Distal junctional failure (DJF) is rarer than PJK and the reported incidence of 6.8% was mostly in the pediatric population.[97] The main contributing factors for DJF are bone fragility, bony stress risers at LIV, screw loosening, and migration, although there have been reports of vertebral fractures.[98–100] However, given the specific L5 anatomy (wider and shorter pedicles) and biomechanics of L5/S1 interface revision surgery to the pelvis and sacrum have demonstrated unequivocal results as some studies demonstrated improvements in oswestry disability index (ODI) and Scoliosis Research Society (SRS) scores while others show high rates of major complications and revisions.[100–102] Thus, some have suggested extending the fixation to the ilium, which theoretically increases rigidity and pullout strength.[98,101,103]

Poor Patient-Reported Outcomes

Patient-reported outcomes (PRO) are important in providing insight to patient's assessment of their quality of life, function, pain, and satisfaction. Multiple studies have shown differing results concerning patient perceived effectiveness of surgery. The Scoli-RISK-1 study reported 5-year follow-up PRO on 77 ASD patients (including those with Cobb angles >80°, corrective osteotomy for congenital or revision deformity, and/or 3-column osteotomy) with significant improvements in all documented PROs (ODI, SF36-PCS, SF36-MCS, SRS-22-total, NRS-back pain, and NRS-leg pain).[104] Ryu et al. reported on 40 patients who underwent ASD surgery who had minimally clinical differences in back pain, leg pain, and functional status at the 12-month follow up.[105] Kyrölä et al. reported on 79 adult patients who underwent ASD surgeries and even those who suffered complications and reoperations still reported an overall improvement in ODI scores.[106] Hamilton et al. also found that patient satisfaction was not related to radiographic parameters or complications.[107] However, Scheer et al. found that in their cohort of 343 patients, at the 2-year postoperative mark those who had undercorrected in SVA (sagittal vertical axis) had worse health-related quality of life (HRQOL).[108] It is also shown that male sex, depression, and preoperative opiate use predicted poor outcomes.[106,109]

Conclusions

The surgical management of ASD is challenging. In addition to being technically challenging procedures to perform, these operations are associated with a high complication profile. Pseudoarthrosis, instrumentation failure, and proximal/distal junctional failure are serious complications that often require revision surgery that is itself associated with multiple complications and poor outcomes. Understanding the epidemiology, etiology, and risk factors for these adverse outcomes may allow for preoperative risk stratification and improved preoperative discussion of risks and benefits of surgery. Additionally, surgeons may choose to modify their surgical plan for patients with risk factors for mechanical failure to reduce the risk of these complications.

References

1. Soroceanu A, Diebo B, Burton D, et al. Radiographical and implant-related complications in adult spinal deformity surgery: incidence, patient risk factors, and impact on health-related quality of life. *Spine (Phila Pa 1976)*. 2015;40(18):1414–1421.
2. Hallager D, Karstensen S, Bukhari N, Gehrchen M, Dahl B. Radiographic predictors for mechanical failure after adult spinal deformity surgery. A retrospective cohort study in 138 patients. *Spine (Phila Pa 1976)*. 2017;42(14):E855–E863.
3. Lertudomphonwanit T, Kelly M, Bridwell K, et al. Rod fracture in adult spinal deformity surgery fused to the sacrum: prevalence, risk factors, and impact on health-related quality of life in 526 patients. *Spine J*. 2018;18(9):1612–1624.
4. Smith J, Shaffrey E, Klineberg E, et al. Prospective multicenter assessment of risk factors for rod fracture following surgery for adult spinal deformity. *J Neurosurg Spine*. 2014;21(6):994–1003.
5. Soroceanu A, Burton D, Oren J, et al. Medical complications after adult spinal deformity surgery: incidence, risk factors, and clinical impact. *Spine (Phila Pa 1976)*. 2016;41(22):1718–1723.
6. Dede O, Thuillier D, Pekmezci M, et al. Revision surgery for lumbar pseudoarthrosis. *Spine J*. 2015;15(5):977–982.
7. Lee Y-P, Farhan SA, Musa A, Bhatia N. Pseudoarthrosis in spine surgery: Diagnosis and treatment. *Contemp Spine Surg*. 2019;20(8):1–7.
8. Chun DS, Baker KC, Hsu WK. Lumbar pseudoarthrosis: A review of current diagnosis and treatment. *Neurosurg Focus*. 2015;39(4):E10.

9. DePalma AF, Rothman RH. The nature of pseudoarthrosis. *Clin Orthop Relat Res*. 1968;59:113–118.
10. Ondra SL, Marzouk S. Revision strategies for lumbar pseudoarthrosis. *Neurosurg Focus*. 2003;15(3):E9.
11. Raizman NM, O'Brien JR, Poehling-Monaghan KL, Yu WD. Pseudoarthrosis of the spine. *J Am Acad Orthop Surg*. 2009;17(8):494–503.
12. Kullar R, Klineberg E, Gupta M. Complications: Pseudoarthrosis/nonunion. In: Patel V, Patel A, Harrop J, Burger E, eds. *Spine Surgery Basics*. Springer. 2014:533–540.
13. Kornblum MB, Fischgrund JS, Herkowitz HN, Abraham DA, Berkower DL, Ditkoff JS. Degenerative lumbar spondylolisthesis with spinal stenosis: A prospective long-term study comparing fusion and pseudoarthrosis. *Spine (Phila Pa 1976)*. 2004;29(7):726–733; discussion 733–734.
14. Dinizo M, Passias P, Kebaish K, Errico TJ, Raman T. The approach to pseudoarthrosis after adult spinal deformity surgery: Is a multiple-rod construct necessary? *Global Spine J*. 2023;13(3):636–642.
15. Burkus JK, Dorchak JD, Sanders DL. Radiographic assessment of interbody fusion using recombinant human bone morphogenetic protein type 2. *Spine (Phila Pa 1976)*. 2003;28(4):372–377.
16. Heggeness MH, Esses SI, Errico T, Yuan HA. Late infection of spinal instrumentation by hematogenous seeding. *Spine (Phila Pa 1976)*. 1993;18(4):492–496. https://doi.org/10.1097/00007632-199318040-00013.
17. Carpenter CT, Dietz MJW, Leung KYK, Hanscom DA, Wagner TA. Repair of a pseudoarthrosis of the lumbar spine: A functional outcome study. *J Bone Joint Surg Am*. 1996;78(5):712–720.
18. Klineberg E, Gupta M, McCarthy I, Hostin R. Detection of pseudoarthrosis in adult spinal deformity: The use of health-related quality-of-life outcomes to predict pseudoarthrosis. *Clin Spine Surg*. 2016;29(8):318–322. https://doi.org/10.1097/BSD.0000000000000062.
19. Marques MF, Fiere V, Obeid I, et al. Pseudoarthrosis in adult spine deformity surgery: risk factors and treatment options. *Eur Spine J*. 2021;30(11):3225–3232.
20. Gertzbein SD, Hollopeter MR, Hall S. Pseudoarthrosis of the lumbar spine: Outcome after circumferential fusion. *Spine (Phila Pa 1976)*. 1998;23(21):2352–2356.
21. Bydon M, De La Garza-Ramos R, Abt NB, et al. Impact of smoking on complication and pseudoarthrosis rates after single- and 2-level posterolateral fusion of the lumbar spine. *Spine (Phila Pa 1976)*. 2014;39(21):1765–1770.
22. Cleveland M, Bosworth DM, Thompson FR. Pseudoarthrosis in the lumbosacral spine. *J Bone Joint Surg Am*. 1948;30A(2):302–312.
23. How NE, Street JT, Dvorak MF, et al. Pseudoarthrosis in adult and pediatric spinal deformity surgery: a systematic review of the literature and meta-analysis of incidence, characteristics, and risk factors. *Neurosurg Rev*. 2019;42(2):319–336.
24. Buttermann GR, Glazer PA, Hu SS, Bradford DS. Revision of failed lumbar fusions: A comparison of anterior autograft and allograft. *Spine (Phila Pa 1976)*. 1997;22(23):2748–2755.
25. Goldberg VM. The biology of bone grafts. *Orthopedics*. 2003;26(9):923–924.
26. Kim YJ, Bridwell KH, Lenke LG, Rhim S, Cheh G. Pseudoarthrosis in long adult spinal deformity instrumentation and fusion to the sacrum: prevalence and risk factor analysis in 144 cases. *Spine (Phila Pa 1976)*. 2006;31(20):2329–2336.
27. Brown CW, Orme TJ, Richardson HD. The rate of pseudoarthrosis (Surgical nonunion) in patients who are smokers and patients who are nonsmokers: A comparison study. *Spine (Phila Pa 1976)*. 1986;11(9):942–943.
28. Hyun SJ, Lenke LG, Kim YC, Koester LA, Blanke KM. Comparison of standard 2-rod constructs to multiple-rod constructs for fixation across 3-column spinal osteotomies. *Spine (Phila Pa 1976)*. 2014;39(22):1899–1904.
29. Banno T, Hasegawa T, Yamato Y, et al. Multi-rod constructs can increase the incidence of iliac screw loosening after surgery for adult spinal deformity. *Asian Spine J*. 2019;13(3):500–510.
30. Ikwuezunma I, Beutler GJ, Margalit A, Jain A, Kebaish KM, Sponseller PD. Late spinal infections are more common after pediatric than after adult spinal deformity surgery. *Spine Deform*. 2022;10(4):817–823.
31. Wang M, Xu L, Yang B, et al. Incidence, management and outcome of delayed deep surgical site infection following spinal deformity surgery: 20-year experience at a single institution. *Global Spine J*. 2022;12(6):1141–1150.
32. Kalfas F, Severi P, Scudieri C. Infection with spinal instrumentation: A 20-year, single-institution experience with review of pathogenesis, diagnosis, prevention, and management. *Asian J Neurosurg*. 2019;14(4):1181–1189.
33. Dowdell J, Brochin R, Kim J, et al. Postoperative spine infection: Diagnosis and management. *Global Spine J*. 2018;8(4Suppl):37S–43S.
34. Warner SJ, Uppstrom TJ, Miller AO, et al. Epidemiology of deep surgical site infections after pediatric spinal fusion surgery. *Spine (Phila Pa 1976)*. 2017;42(3):E163–E168.
35. Pesenti S, Pannu T, Andres-Bergos J, et al. What are the risk factors for surgical site infection after spinal fusion? A meta-analysis. *Eur Spine J*. 2018;27(10):2469–2480.
36. Garg S, LaGreca J, Hotchkiss M, Erickson M. Management of late (>1 y) deep infection after spinal fusion: a retrospective cohort study. *J Pediatr Orthop*. 2015;35(3):266–270.
37. Shen J, Liang J, Yu H, Qiu G, Xue X, Li Z. Risk factors for delayed infections after spinal fusion and instrumentation in patients with scoliosis. *J Neurosurg Spine*. 2014;21(4):648–652.
38. Soultanis K, Mantelos G, Pagiatakis A, Soucacos PN. Late infection in patients with scoliosis treated with spinal instrumentation. *Clin Ortho Relat Res*. 2003;411:116–123.
39. Silvestre M Di, Bakaloudis G, Lolli F, Giacomini S. Late-developing infection following posterior fusion for adolescent idiopathic scoliosis. *Eur Spine J*. 2011;20(Suppl 1):S121–127.
40. Abdul-Jabbar A, Berven SH, Hu SS, et al. Surgical site infections in spine surgery. *Spine (Phila Pa 1976)*. 2013;38(22):E1425–1431.
41. Agarwal A, Kelkar A, Agarwal AG, et al. Implant retention or removal for management of surgical site infection after spinal surgery. *Global Spine J*. 2020;10(5):640–646.
42. Li J, Zhu Y, Zhao K, et al. Incidence and risks for surgical site infection after closed tibial plateau fractures in adults treated by open reduction and internal fixation: A prospective study. *J Orthop Surg Res*. 2020;15(1):349.
43. Yin D, Liu B, Chang Y, Gu H, Zheng X. Management of late-onset deep surgical site infection after instrumented spinal surgery. *BMC Surg*. 2018;18(1):121.
44. Mhaidli HH, Der-Boghossian AH, Haidar RK. Propionibacterium acnes delayed infection following spinal surgery with instrumentation. *Musculoskelet Surg*. 2013;97(1):85–87.

45. Clark CE, Shufflebarger HL. Late-developing infection in instrumented idiopathic scoliosis. *Spine (Phila Pa 1976)*. 1999;24 (18):1909–1912.
46. Schofferman L, Schofferman J, Zucherman J, et al. Occult infections causing persistent low-back pain. *Spine (Phila Pa 1976)*. 1989;14(4):417–419.
47. Hedequist D, Haugen A, Hresko T, Emans J. Failure of attempted implant retention in spinal deformity delayed surgical site infections. *Spine (Phila Pa 1976)*. 2009;34(1):60–64.
48. Richards S. Delayed infections following posterior spinal instrumentation for the treatment of idiopathic scoliosis. *J Bone Joint Surg Am*. 1995;77(4):524–529.
49. Rathjen K, Wood M, McClung A, Vest Z. Clinical and radiographic results after implant removal in idiopathic scoliosis. *Spine (Phila Pa 1976)*. 2007;32(20):2184–2188.
50. Potter BK, Kirk KL, Shah SA, Kuklo TR. Loss of coronal correction following instrumentation removal in adolescent idiopathic scoliosis. *Spine (Phila Pa 1976)*. 2006;31(1):67–72.
51. Farshad M, Sdzuy C, Min K. Late implant removal after posterior correction of AIS with pedicle screw instrumentation - A matched case control study with 10-year follow-up. *Spine Deform*. 2013;1(1):68–71.
52. Kotani T, Akazawa T, Lumawig JMT, Sakuma T, Minami S. Reinstrumentation for rapid curve progression after implant removal following posterior instrumented fusion in adolescent idiopathic scoliosis: A case report. *Scoliosis*. 2013;8:15.
53. Hof H. *Miscellaneous Pathogenic Bacteria*. In: Baron S, ed. Medical Microbiology. 4th ed. Galveston (TX): University of Texas Medical Branch at Galveston. 1996. [Chapter 16].
54. Smith J, Shaffrey C, Ames C, et al. Assessment of symptomatic rod fracture after posterior instrumented fusion for adult spinal deformity. *Neurosurgery*. 2012;71:862–868.
55. Lee K, Lee J, Kang K, Im S, Lim H, Choi S. Strategies for prevention of rod fracture in adult spinal deformity: cobalt chrome rod, accessory rod techniqe, and lateral lumbar interbody fusion. *J Neurosurg Spine*. 2021;34:706–715.
56. Azakawa T, Kotani T, Sakuma T, Nemoto T, Minami S. Rod fracture after long construct fusion for spinal deformity: clinical and radiographic risk factors. *J Orthop Sci*. 2013;18: 926–931.
57. Daniels A, DePasse J, Durand W, et al. Rod fracture after apparently solid radiographic fusion in adult spinal deformity patients. *World Neurosurg*. 2018;117:e530–e537.
58. Kawabata A, Yoshii T, Sakai K, et al. Identification of predictive factors for mechanical complications after adult spinal deformity surgery. A multi-institutional retrospective study. *Spine (Phila Pa 1976)*. 2020;45(17):1185–1192.
59. Barton C, Noshchenko A, Patel V, Cain C, Kleck C, Burger E. Risk factors for rod fractre after posterior correction of adult spinal deformity with osteotomy: a retrospective case-series. *Scoliosis*. 2015;10:30.
60. Yang B, Ondra S, Chen L, Jung H, Koski T, Salehi S. Clinical and radiographic outcomes of thoracic and lumbar pedicle subtraction osteotomy for fixed sagittal imbalance. *J Neurosurg Spine*. 2006;5(1):9–17.
61. Bridwell K, Lewis S, Edwards C, et al. Complications and outcomes of pedicle subtraction osteotomies for fixed sagittal imbalance. *Spine (Phila Pa 1976)*. 2003;28(18):2093–2101.
62. Dick J, Bourgeault C. Notch sensitivity of titanium alloy, commercially pure titanium, and stainless steel spinal implants. *Spine (Phila Pa 1976)*. 2001;26:1668–1672.
63. Lindsey C, Deviren V, Xu Z, Yeh R, Puttlitz C. The effect of rod contouring on spinal constrct fatigue strength. *Spine (Phila Pa 1976)*. 2006;31(15):1680–1687.
64. Maruo K, Ha Y, Inoue S, et al. Predictive factors for proximal junctional kyphosis in long fusions to the sacrum in adult spinal deformity. *Spine (Phila Pa 1976)*. 2013;38(23):E1469–1476.
65. Martin C, Polly D, Holton K, et al. Acute failure of S2-alar-iliac screw pelvic fixation in adult spinal deformity: novel failure mechanism, case series, and review of the literature. *J Neurosurg Spine*. 2022;36:53–61.
66. De la Garza Ramos R, Nakhla J, Sciubba D, Yassari R. Iliac screw versus S2 alar-iliac screw fixation in adults: a meta-analysis. *J Neurosurg Spine*. 2018;30(2):253–258.
67. Guler U, Cetin E, Yaman O, et al. Sacropelvis fixation in adult spinal deformity (ASD); a very high rate of mechanical failure. *Eur Spine J*. 2015;24(5):1085–1091.
68. Rabinovich E, Buell T, Wang T. Reduced occurrence of primary rod fracture after adult spinal deformity surgery with accessory supplemental rods: retrospective analysis of 114 patients with minimum 2-year follow-up. *J Neurosurg Spine*. 2021;35(4):504–515.
69. Merrill R, Kim J, Leven D, Kim J, Cho S. Multi-rod constructs can prevent rod breakage and pseudoarthrosis at the lumbosacral junction in adult spinal deformity. *Global Spine J*. 2017;7(6):514–520.
70. Adogwa O, Buchowski J, Lenke L, et al. Comparison of rod fracture rates in long spinal deformity constructs after transforaminal versus anterior lumbar interbody fusions: a single-institution analysis. *J Neurosurg Spine*. 2019;11:1–8.
71. Park P, Garton H, Gala V, Hoff J, McGillicuddy J. Adjacent segment disease after lumbar or lumbosacral fusion: review of the literature. *Spine (Phila Pa 1976)*. 2004;29(17):1938–1944.
72. Anandjiwala J, Seo J, Ha K, Oh I, Shin D. Adjacent segment degeneration after instrumented posterolateral lumbar fusion: a prospective cohort study with a minimum five-year follow-up. *Eur Spine J*. 2011;20(11):1951–1960.
73. Wang M, Xu L, Chen X, et al. Optimal reconstruction of sagittal alignment according to global alignment and proportion score can reduce adjacent segment degeneration after lumbar fusion. *Spine (Phila Pa 1976)*. 2021;46(4):e257–e266.
74. Kim S, Min H, Hak K, et al. Effects of restoration of sagittal alignment on adjacent segment degeneration in instrumented lumbar fusion. *Spine (Phila Pa 1976)*. 2020;45(23):e1588–e1595.
75. Bridwell KH, Lenke LG, Cho SK, et al. Proximal junctional kyphosis in primary adult deformity surgery: Evaluation of 20 degrees as a critical angle. *Neurosurgery*. 2013;72(6):899–906.
76. Helgeson MD, Shah SA, Newton PO, et al. Evaluation of proximal junctional kyphosis in adolescent idiopathic scoliosis following pedicle screw, hook, or hybrid instrumentation. *Spine (Phila Pa 1976)*. 2010;35(2):177–181.
77. O'Shaughnessy BA, Bridwell KH, Lenke LG, et al. Does a long-fusion "t3-Sacrum" portend a worse outcome than a short-fusion "t10-Sacrum" in primary surgery for adult scoliosis? *Spine (Phila Pa 1976)*. 2012;37(10):884–890.
78. Cho SK, Kim YJ, Lenke LG. Proximal junctional kyphosis following spinal deformity surgery in the pediatric patient. *J Am Acad Orthop Surg*. 2015;23(7):408–414.
79. Glattes RC, Bridwell KH, Lenke LG, Kim YJ, Rinella A, Edwards C. Proximal junctional kyphosis in adult spinal deformity following long instrumented posterior spinal fusion: Incidence, outcomes, and risk factor analysis. *Spine (Phila Pa 1976)*. 2005;30(14):1643–1649.

80. Hart RA, McCarthy I, Ames CP, Shaffrey CI, Hamilton DK, Hostin R. Proximal junctional kyphosis and proximal junctional failure. *Neurosurg Clin N Am.* 2013;24(2):213–218.
81. Hyun S-J, Lee BH, Park J-H, Kim K-J, Jahng T-A, Kim H-J. Proximal junctional kyphosis and proximal junctional failure following adult spinal deformity surgery. *Korean J Spine.* 2017; 14(4):126–132.
82. Hostin R, McCarthy I, O'Brien M, et al. Incidence, mode, and location of acute proximal junctional failures after surgical treatment of adult spinal deformity. *Spine (Phila Pa 1976).* 2013;38(12):1008–1015.
83. Park SJ, Lee CS, Chung SS, Lee JY, Kang SS, Park SH. Different risk factors of proximal junctional kyphosis and proximal junctional failure following long instrumented fusion to the sacrum for adult spinal deformity: Survivorship analysis of 160 patients. *Neurosurgery.* 2017;80(2):279–286.
84. Hyun SJ, Rhim SC. Clinical outcomes and complications after pedicle subtraction osteotomy for fixed sagittal imbalance patients: A long-term follow-up data. *J Korean Neurosurg Soc.* 2010;47(2):95–101.
85. Kim YJ, Bridwell KH, Lenke LG, Glattes CR, Rhim S, Cheh G. Proximal junctional kyphosis in adult spinal deformity after segmental posterior spinal instrumentation and fusion: Minimum five-year follow-up. *Spine (Phila Pa 1976).* 2008;33(20):2179–2184.
86. Yagi M, King AB, Boachie-Adjei O. Incidence, risk factors, and natural course of proximal junctional kyphosis: Surgical outcomes review of adult idiopathic scoliosis. minimum 5 years of follow-up. *Spine (Phila Pa 1976).* 2012;37(17):1479–1489.
87. Kim HJ, Bridwell KH, Lenke LG, et al. Patients with proximal junctional kyphosis requiring revision surgery have higher postoperative lumbar lordosis and larger sagittal balance corrections. *Spine (Phila Pa 1976).* 2014;39(9):E576–580.
88. Denis F, Sun EC, Winter RB. Incidence and risk factors for proximal and distal junctional kyphosis following surgical treatment for Scheuermann kyphosis: Minimum five-year follow-up. *Spine (Phila Pa 1976).* 2009;34(20):E729–734.
89. Han S, Hyun SJ, Kim KJ, Jahng TA, Kim HJ. Comparative study between cobalt Chrome and titanium alloy rods for multilevel spinal fusion: Proximal junctional kyphosis more frequently occurred in patients having cobalt chrome rods. *World Neurosurg.* 2017;103:404–409.
90. Han S, Hyun SJ, Kim KJ, Jahng TA, Lee S, Rhim SC. Rod stiffness as a risk factor of proximal junctional kyphosis after adult spinal deformity surgery: comparative study between cobalt chrome multiple-rod constructs and titanium alloy two-rod constructs. *Spine J.* 2017;17(7):962–968.
91. Kim HJ, Lenke LG, Shaffrey CI, Van Alstyne EM, Skelly AC. Proximal junctional kyphosis as a distinct form of adjacent segment pathology after spinal deformity surgery: A systematic review. *Spine (Phila Pa 1976).* 2012;37(22 Suppl):S144–164.
92. Mendoza-Lattes S. Proximal junctional kyphosis and proximal junctional failure following spinal deformity surgery. *Tech Orthop.* 2021;36(1):1.
93. Wang T, Zhao Y, Liang Y, Zhang H, Wang Z, Wang Y. Risk factor analysis of proximal junctional kyphosis after posterior osteotomy in patients with ankylosing spondylitis. *J Neurosurg Spine.* 2018;29(1):75–80.
94. Kim YJ, Bridwell KH, Lenke LG, Kim J, Cho SK. Proximal junctional kyphosis in adolescent idiopathic scoliosis following segmental posterior spinal instrumentation and fusion: Minimum 5-year follow-up. *Spine (Phila Pa 1976).* 2005;30(18): 2045–2050.
95. Nguyen NLM, Kong CY, Hart RA. Proximal junctional kyphosis and failure—diagnosis, prevention, and treatment. *Curr Rev Musculoskelet Med.* 2016;9(3):299–308.
96. Hart R, McCarthy I, O'brien M, et al. Identification of decision criteria for revision surgery among patients with proximal junctional failure after surgical treatment of spinal deformity. *Spine (Phila Pa 1976).* 2013;38(19):E1223–1227.
97. Miller DJ, Jameel O, Matsumoto H, et al. Factors affecting distal end & global decompensation in coronal/sagittal planes 2 years after fusion. *Stud Health Technol Inform.* 2010;158:141–146.
98. Arlet V, Aebi M. Junctional spinal disorders in operated adult spinal deformities: Present understanding and future perspectives. *Eur Spine J.* 2013;22(Suppl 2):S276–295.
99. Kwon BK, Elgafy H, Keynan O, et al. Progressive junctional kyphosis at the caudal end of lumbar instrumented fusion: Etiology, predictors, and treatment. *Spine (Phila Pa 1976).* 2006; 31(17):1943–1951.
100. Tan JH, Tan K-A, Hey HWD, Wong H-K. Distal junctional failure secondary to L5 vertebral fracture—a report of two rare cases. *J Spine Surg.* 2017;3(1):87–91.
101. Bridwell KH, Edwards CC, Lenke LG. The pros and cons to saving the L5-S1 motion segment in a long scoliosis fusion construct. *Spine (Phila Pa 1976).* 2003;28(20):S234–242.
102. O'Neill KR, Bridwell KH, Lenke LG, et al. Extension of spine fusion to the sacrum following long fusions for deformity correction. *Spine (Phila Pa 1976).* 2014;39(12):953–962.
103. Edwards CC, Bridwell KH, Patel A, et al. Thoracolumbar deformity arthrodesis to L5 in adults: The fate of the L5-S1 disc. *Spine (Phila Pa 1976).* 2003;28(18):2122–2131.
104. Zuckerman SL, Cerpa M, Lenke LG, et al. Patient-reported outcomes after complex adult spinal deformity surgery: 5-year results of the Scoli-Risk-1 study. *Global Spine J.* 2022;12(8): 1736–1744.
105. Ryu WHA, Cheong M, Platt A, et al. Patient satisfaction following minimally invasive and open surgeries for adult spinal deformity. *World Neurosurg.* 2021;155:e301–e314.
106. Kyrölä K, Kautiainen H, Pekkanen L, Mäkelä P, Kiviranta I, Häkkinen A. Long-term clinical and radiographic outcomes and patient satisfaction after adult spinal deformity correction. *Scand J Surg.* 2019;108(4):343–351.
107. Hamilton DK, Kong C, Hiratzka J, et al. Patient satisfaction after adult spinal deformity surgery does not strongly correlate with health-related quality of life scores, radiographic parameters, or occurrence of complications. *Spine (Phila Pa 1976).* 2017;42 (10):764–769.
108. Scheer JK, Lafage R, Schwab FJ, et al. Under correction of sagittal deformities based on age-adjusted alignment thresholds leads to worse health-related quality of life whereas over correction provides no additional benefit. *Spine (Phila Pa 1976).* 2018;43(6):388–393.
109. Samuel AM, Morse KW, Pompeu YA, et al. Preoperative opioids before adult spinal deformity surgery associated with increased reoperations and high rates of chronic postoperative opioid use at 3-year follow-up. *Spine Deform.* 2022;10(3):615–623.

Index

Note: Page numbers followed by "*f*" indicate figures, "*t*" indicate tables, "*b*" indicate boxes.